List of Chapters by Body System

Advanced Health Assessment and Clinical Diagnosis in Primary Care

6TH EDITION

Joyce E. Dains, DrPH, JD, RN, FNP-BC, FNAP, FAANP
Professor and Chair, ad interim, Department of Nursing
Director Advanced Practice Nursing
The University of Texas MD Anderson Cancer Center
Houston, Texas

Linda Ciofu Baumann, PhD, APRN, BC, FAAN
Professor Emerita
University of Wisconsin–Madison
School of Nursing
Madison, Wisconsin

Pamela Scheibel, MSN, RN, PNP
Clinical Professor Emerita
University of Wisconsin–Madison
School of Nursing
Madison, Wisconsin

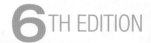

ELSEVIER

ELSEVIER

3251 Riverport Lane
St. Louis, Missouri 63043

ADVANCED HEALTH ASSESSMENT AND CLINICAL DIAGNOSIS
IN PRIMARY CARE, SIXTH EDITION

ISBN: 978-0-323-55496-1

Notices

Practitioners and researchers must always rely on their own experience and knowledge in evaluating and
using any information, methods, compounds or experiments described herein. Because of rapid advances in
the medical sciences, in particular, independent verification of diagnoses and drug dosages should be made.
To the fullest extent of the law, no responsibility is assumed by Elsevier, authors, editors or contributors for
any injury and/or damage to persons or property as a matter of products liability, negligence or otherwise, or
from any use or operation of any methods, products, instructions, or ideas contained in the material herein.

Library of Congress Cataloging-in-Publication Data

Dains, Joyce E., author.
  Advanced health assessment and clinical diagnosis in primary care / Joyce E. Dains, Linda Ciofu Baumann,
Pamela Scheib. -- 6th edition.
    p. ; cm.
  Includes bibliographical references and index.
  ISBN 978-0-323-26625-3 (pbk. : alk. paper)
  I. Baumann, Linda Ciofu, author. II. Scheibel, Pamela, author. III. Title.
  [DNLM: 1. Diagnosis, Differential. 2. Diagnostic Techniques and Procedures. 3. Primary Health Care. WB 141.5]
  RC71.5
  616.07'5--dc23
  2015006322

Executive Content Strategist: Lee Henderson
Director, Content Development: Laurie Gower
Content Development Specialist: Elizabeth Kilgore
Publishing Services Manager: Shereen Jameel
Senior Project Manager: Umarani Natarajan
Design Direction: Brian Salisbury

Printed in China

Last digit is the print number: 9 8 7 6 5 4 3 2

Working together
to grow libraries in
developing countries

www.elsevier.com • www.bookaid.org

Reviewers

Margaret R. Benz, MSN(R), APRN, ANP-BC, FAANP
Assistant Professor of Nursing
Saint Louis University
St. Louis, Missouri

Torry Grantham Cobb, MPH, MHS, DHSc, PA-C
Assistant Professor
St. Francis University
Loretto, Pennsylvania

Amy J. Culbertson, DNP, FNP-BC
Assistant Professor and Certified Family Nurse Practitioner
School of Nursing and Health Studies
Georgetown University
Washington, DC

Tamika Dowling, FNP-C, DNP
Nursing Adjunct Faculty
Aspen University
Denver, Colorado

Dawn Lee Garzon, PhD, CPNP-PC, PMHS, FAANP
Clinical Professor and Associate Director
College of Nursing
Washington State University Vancouver
Vancouver, Washington

Wendy L. Halm, DNP, FNP-BC, APNP
Clinical Assistant Professor of Nursing
University of Wisconsin–Madison
Madison, Wisconsin

Cheryl Jackson, DNP, CRNP
Assistant Professor of Nursing
Bloomsburg University
Bloomsburg, Pennsylvania

Kathleen S. Jordan, DNP, MS, FNP-BC, ENP-BC, ENP-C, SANE-P, FAEN
Clinical Associate Professor, School of Nursing
The University of North Carolina at Charlotte
Nurse Practitioner
Emergency Department
Mid-Atlantic Emergency Medicine Associates
Charlotte, North Carolina

Barbara B. Kelly, MSN, APN, FNP-BC
Assistant Professor of Nursing
Graduate Nursing Program
University of Indianapolis
Indianapolis, Indiana

Yvette Lowery, DNP, MSN/Ed, FNP-C, CCRN, CEN, PCCN
Saint Joseph's College at Maine, Women's Health
Jacksonville, Florida

Donna M. Mannello, DC
Professor of Clinical Science
Logan University
Chesterfield, Missouri

Gina M. Oliver, PhD, APRN, FNP-BC, CNE
Associate Teaching Professor
Sinclair School of Nursing
University of Missouri
Columbia, Missouri

Michael Wayne Rager, PhD, DNP, MSN, FNP-BC, APRN, CNE
Dean of Nursing
Daymar College
Owensboro, Kentucky

Jennifer Ruel, DNP, RN, FNP-BC, ENP-BC
Associate Clinical Professor
McAuley School of Nursing
University of Detroit Mercy
Detroit, Michigan

Julie G. Stewart, DNP, MPH, MSN, FNP-BC, APRN, FAANP
Associate Professor of Nursing, Director of FNP and DNP Programs
Sacred Heart University
Fairfield, Connecticut

Colleen Taylor, PhD, MSN, RN, FNP-C
Assistant Professor of Nursing
University of Toledo
Toledo, Ohio

Daniel Thomas Vetrosky, PA-C, PhD, DFAAPA
Associate Professor (Retired), Urology
University of South Alabama
Pensacola, Florida
Physician Assistant
Cordova Urology
Mobile, Alabama

Lisa M. Young, DNP, APRN
Assistant Professor
College of Nursing and Health Sciences
Ashland University
Mansfield, OH

Acknowledgments

No text is ever written as a solitary effort, and we have many thanks to offer. We have benefited from the extraordinary support and help of friends, family, and colleagues. We would like to acknowledge each one. Our thanks are heartfelt; we honor your place in our lives.

To our colleagues at Elsevier who have continued to believe that this text is necessary and who have contributed their time, talent, and expertise—thank you. The remarkable efforts of each member of the publishing team are evident in the final product.

We would also like to acknowledge the contributors to our first edition. Each is a superb clinician and each shared incredible expertise. This text is richer because of them.

Katharine E. Hohol, MS, APRN, BC, APNP
Sandra K. Roof, MSN, APRN, BC, APNP
Robert W. Vogler, PhD, RN, CS, FNP
Pam Willson, PhD, RN, CS, FNP

Finally, we want to express our profound appreciation for those faculty, students, and clinicians who have discovered and used this book, for those who have shared their enthusiasm with us, and for those who have offered helpful suggestions and comments that have enhanced the content of this text. Thank you.

Joyce E. Dains
Linda C. Baumann
Pamela Scheibel

Introduction

This text is designed for beginning clinicians and for students who will be using history and physical examination skills in the clinical setting. Its purpose is to take the student to the "next step" of health assessment, that is, beyond basic history and physical examination to using a diagnostic reasoning process. The book is intended to fill the gap between basic physical examination texts and the medical texts that are aimed primarily at disease management. It is not intended as a substitute for a clinical management text, nor does it address management of disorders or diseases. Rather, it is designed specifically to focus on the clinical evaluation of common problems that present in primary care settings using the tools of history and physical examination to engage in the process of clinical diagnosis.

The sixth edition of this text has several changes to further assist the transition to that "next step" of health assessment. A new chapter has been added on care of transgender patients (Chapter 42). Consistent with the rest of the text, the chapter provides health history questions and physical examination considerations that are specific to transgender patients in the primary care setting. New to this edition, one list of selected references for each chapter appears at the end of the book. These references support the information provided in each chapter and are suggested for further in-depth learning about the problem. We continue to include *Evidence-Based Practice* boxes in each chapter. The focus of *Advanced Health Assessment* is primary care patients. Both adults and children are included, with divergence in questions, examination, or interpretation of findings noted when pertinent. This text does not attempt to address all possible patient concerns, but rather seeks to focus on the most common concerns as exemplars of the diagnostic reasoning process.

HOW TO USE THIS BOOK

Each chapter is structured in the context of a commonly occurring chief concern rather than a specific diagnosis or disease entity. Patients generally seek care for relief of symptoms and undiagnosed conditions. The initial challenge for primary care providers is to begin the process of differential diagnosis to determine the cause of a problem based on history and physical examination and laboratory and other diagnostic tests. However, the steps of the diagnostic reasoning process are seldom articulated in a sequence that reflects the clinician's thought process. Novice clinicians are often left to their own devices to figure out, for example, which history questions are the most important, which should be asked first, and which can be left for later or to determine which parts of the physical examination must be done as opposed to which will yield little information for a given concern. This text tries to articulate the reasoning process, order the history questions in a meaningful way, and focus the physical examination for a specific chief concern.

The diagnostic or clinical reasoning process is woven into each presenting problem. Each symptom begins with a brief introduction, providing an overview of causative mechanisms and processes. The clinical problem-solving process begins with *Focused History,* which walks through the thinking process involved in obtaining a pertinent, relevant, problem-specific history that will assist with differential diagnosis. The section is designed around questions that experienced clinicians ask themselves to order and organize the questions to be asked of the patient. These "self-questions" are structured according to what information the clinician needs first or most immediately about the presenting complaint followed by self-questions that help sort through the possible differential diagnoses. The content and order of the self-questions vary, depending on the presenting problem. Sometimes the self-questions are based on what the condition is most likely to be; sometimes they are based on what is too important to miss.

For each of the self-questions there is a list of *Key Questions* to ask of the patient or about the patient if a family member is giving the history. The *Key Questions* are followed by an interpretation or explanation of what the patient responses might signify. For ease of format, the *Key Questions* are written as though the clinician were addressing the patient. Certainly with young children and sometimes with adults, the clinician will be asking questions of another person about the patient. The intent is to convey what questions to ask rather than to provide every possible format for each question.

Following these two sections is the *Focused Physical Examination* section. It instructs you in what focused physical examination to perform to assist the diagnostic process. The section is not intended to teach basic physical examination; it assumes you know how, using the techniques of inspection, auscultation, percussion, and palpation. This section, rather, provides focus for the examination, explains how to do more advanced maneuvers, and offers an interpretation of the findings.

Following is the section titled *Laboratory and Diagnostic Studies*. This section provides a brief outline of what kinds of laboratory or diagnostic studies would be appropriate for the chief concern or suspected diagnosis. Because the goal of the text is clinical diagnosis, the laboratory and diagnostic studies included are those that would be a logical starting point, although perhaps not an ending point.

The final section of each presenting concern is the *Differential Diagnosis*. It contains the most common differential diagnoses for the chief concern and summarizes, in a narrative format, the history and physical examination findings, along with the laboratory and diagnostic studies indicated. The section finishes with one or more *Differential Diagnosis* tables, mirroring the narrative summary, which can be used as a quick reference. An index to the *Differential Diagnosis* tables is provided in the text inside the back cover.

Perfecting advanced health assessment skills is a lifelong endeavor. It is our hope that this edition continues to assist you in expanding the diagnostic reasoning process.

Joyce E. Dains
Linda C. Baumann
Pamela Scheibel

CHAPTER

1

Clinical Reasoning, Evidence-Based Practice, and Symptom Analysis

Basic health assessment involves the application of the practitioner's knowledge and skills to identify and distinguish normal from abnormal findings. Basic assessment often moves from a general survey of a body system to specific observations or tests of function. Such an approach to assessment and clinical decision making uses a deductive process of reasoning. For example, a specialist examining a patient with known hyperthyroidism would conduct a physical examination to test for deep tendon reflexes. Brisk or hyperreflexic reflexes would lead the practitioner to conclude that a hyperthyroid state is a likely cause of these findings. This would greatly narrow the choices of diagnostic tests and treatment decisions.

Advanced assessment builds on basic health assessment yet is performed more often using an inductive or inferential process, that is, moving from a specific physical finding or patient concern to a more general diagnosis or possible diagnoses based on history, physical findings, and the results of laboratory and diagnostic tests. The practitioner gathers further evidence and analyzes this evidence to arrive at a hypothesis that will lead to a further narrowing of possibilities. This is known as the process of diagnostic reasoning.

DIAGNOSTIC REASONING

Diagnostic reasoning is a scientific process in which the practitioner suspects the cause of a patient's symptoms and signs based on previous knowledge. The practitioner gathers relevant information, selects necessary tests, makes an accurate diagnosis, and recommends therapy. The difference between an average and an excellent practitioner is the speed and focus used to arrive at the correct conclusion and initiate the best course of evidence-based treatment with minimum harm, cost, inconvenience, and delay. This expertise of the practitioner is acquired through knowledge and a skill set developed through experience in clinical practice. Repeated practice with real cases helps to develop memory schemes for relating clinical problems and store them in long-term memory.

By using diagnostic reasoning, the practitioner is able to accomplish the following:
- Determines and focuses on what needs to be asked, what data need to be obtained, and what needs to be examined
- Performs examinations and diagnostic tests accurately
- Clusters all pertinent findings
- Analyzes and interprets the findings
- Develops a list of likely or differential diagnoses

THE DIAGNOSTIC PROCESS

The Primary Care Context

The process of assessment in the primary care setting begins with the patient or caregiver stating a reason for the visit or a chief concern. Most visits to primary care providers involve concerns or symptoms presented by the patient, such as an earache, vomiting, or fatigue. The initial evidence is collected through a patient history. Demographic information, such as gender, age, occupation, and place of residence, is obtained to place the patient in a risk category that may rule out certain diagnoses immediately. In most primary care settings, routine vital signs are obtained, which can include height and weight, temperature, pulse, respiratory rate, blood pressure, last menstrual period, and smoking status. While obtaining the history, the practitioner also makes observations of the patient's appearance, interaction with family members, orientation, and mental and physical condition. The practitioner notes any unusual presentations that could help focus the assessment process.

Symptom Analysis

Presenting symptoms need to be explored with further questions. One useful mnemonic for gathering this information is COLDSPA.

Character: How does it feel, look, smell, sound?

Onset: When did it start?

Location: Be specific. Where is it? Does it radiate?

Duration: How long does it last? Does it recur?

Severity: How do you rate your pain on a scale from 0 (no pain) to 10 (worst pain I've ever had)?

Pattern: What makes it better? What makes it worse? What have you done and did it help?

Associated factors: What other symptoms do you have? How much does it interfere with your usual activities?

Another mnemonic is OLDCARTS: **o**nset, **l**ocation, **d**uration, **c**haracter, **a**ggravating or associated factors, **r**elieving factors, **t**emporal factors, and **s**everity.

Information can also be gleaned from the review of systems. A final step is to ask about the patient's or caregiver's perception of the meaning of the symptom(s). The practitioner then clusters the information into logical groups based on prior knowledge of symptom clusters associated with specific diagnoses or body systems. At the conclusion, the history of the presenting concerns should give the practitioner a good idea of the most likely differential diagnoses. These hypotheses may be further strengthened during the physical examination.

Performing a Physical Examination

This section may be performed as a complete physical examination or as a focused or localized examination that emphasizes the body or organ systems most likely affected by the patient's presenting symptoms.

Formulating and Testing a Hypothesis

The practitioner then formulates a hypothesis based on expertise and knowledge of possible pathological, physiological, or psychological processes. Further interpretation of evidence refines the hypothesis to a working or probable diagnosis. Hypothesis generation begins during the assessment of the patient's age, gender, race, appearance, and presenting problem. Age is often the most significant variable in narrowing the probabilities of a problem. Hypothesis generation forms the context in which further data are collected. This context includes the setting in which care is delivered, such as in a hospital, in an outpatient setting, or in another community-based setting where more than a single individual could be affected. Clinical decision making can be filled with uncertainty and ambiguity. Because available evidence is almost never complete, hypothesis formation involves some element of subjective judgment.

The hypothesis must then be tested and assessed for the following characteristics.

- *Coherence:* Are the physiological links, predisposing factors, and complications for this disease present in the patient?
- *Adequacy:* Does the suspected disease encompass all of the patient's normal and abnormal findings?
- *Parsimony:* Is it the simplest explanation of the patient's findings? The surest way to make this determination is to ask the patient or the caregiver the reason for seeking care and the current understanding of the problem and possible treatment options. This is a crucial step because patients must find the treatment recommendation acceptable.
- *Diagnostic probability:* Is the diagnosis confirmed by radiographic or laboratory tests? A rational diagnostic hypothesis is one that, if confirmed by the select tests, limits the need for additional confirmation.
- *Eliminate a competing hypothesis:* What other diseases could explain the patient's symptoms?

To confirm the hypothesis, the practitioner establishes a "most likely" diagnosis as a basis for a treatment plan and evaluates the outcome. The goal of a clinical decision is to choose an action that is most likely to result in the health outcomes the patient desires. This step of the decision-making process involves personal preference as to whether the benefits outweigh the harms involved, whether the cost is reasonable, and whether the most desired outcomes are short or long term.

Practitioners make extensive use of heuristics, or rules of thumb, to guide the inductive or inferential process of diagnostic reasoning. Heuristics are generally accurate and useful rules to make the task of information gathering more manageable and efficient—rules such as familiarity, salience, and resemblance to a patient who has a known disease. On occasion, however, heuristics can be faulty, particularly if the presentation is atypical or the condition is rare. The practitioner must always be open to a low probability of a serious diagnosis. Heuristics can have negative effects when stereotypes or biases influence judgment. For example, assuming that a patient is heterosexual can lead to errors in clinical reasoning and differential diagnosis when evaluating the symptom of rectal pain.

EXPERT VERSUS NOVICE PRACTITIONERS

Students of advanced assessment have a variety of backgrounds, with many coming from specialized areas of clinical practice. Such students could have difficulty broadening the scope of their observations and clinical possibilities. In any case, nonexperts tend to be nonselective in data gathering and in the clinical reasoning strategies they use. Experts, however, are able to focus on a problem, recognize patterns, and gather only relevant data, with a high probability of a correct diagnosis. The goal for a novice practitioner is to aim for competence and expertise.

A competent practitioner will execute the following steps:

1. *Identify the most important cues.* These cues are obtained largely through thorough symptom analysis (e.g., COLSDPA or OLDCARTS), functional assessment, and history to assess the patient's beliefs and understanding or explanatory model of the illness. Research evidence shows that a person's beliefs or explanatory models of an illness or a symptom include a cause, an opinion about the timeline (acute or chronic), consequences of the condition (minor or life threatening), and some type of verbal label used to identify the cluster of symptoms or sensations (e.g., "the flu," "the blues"). Practitioners need to distinguish between the presence of disease, which has a biological basis, and illness, which is the human experience of being sick that could have little correlation with the objective evidence available.

2. *Understand and perform advanced examination techniques.* These techniques can include special maneuvers and closer observation of fine details during the physical examination, more in-depth interviews using valid and reliable instruments to assess the patient's risk for a specific diagnosis, and "gold standard" diagnostic tests for the identification of a specific disorder.

3. *Test differential or competing diagnoses.* A differential diagnosis results from a synthesis of subjective and objective findings, including laboratory and diagnostic tests, with knowledge of known and recognized patterns of signs and symptoms. When using the "rule-out" strategy, the practitioner looks for the absence of findings that are frequently seen with a specific condition; the absence of a sensitive finding is strong evidence against the condition being present. When using the "rule-in" strategy, the practitioner looks for the presence of a finding with high specificity (low false-positive and high true-negative values); the presence of this finding is strong evidence that the condition is present.

4. *See a pattern in the information gathered.* A pattern or cluster of findings can emerge from the subjective and objective data. This pattern could be evident during one patient encounter, or it could depend on a pattern of signs and symptoms that develops over time. Often an expert practitioner can eliminate competing diagnoses only after the initial treatment prescribed is ineffective or after the symptoms either disappear sooner than expected or persist longer than expected.

DEVELOPING CLINICAL REASONING

Clinical reasoning is a situational, practice-based form of reasoning that acknowledges the many variables that are present in an actual clinical situation, such as environmental and social factors involving the patient, family, community, and a team of health care providers. Clinical reasoning involves developing a brief summary in which patient-specific details are translated into appropriate diagnostic terminology. This process requires a background of scientific and evidence-based knowledge about general cases and a practical ability to evaluate the relevance of the evidence behind general scientific and technical knowledge and how it applies to a particular patient. In doing so, the clinician considers the patient's particular clinical trajectory; her or his concerns, values and preferences; and her or his particular vulnerabilities (e.g., having multiple comorbidities) and sensitivities to care interventions (e.g., known drug allergies and past responses to therapies) when formulating clinical decisions or conclusions.

NEGOTIATING GOALS AND EXPECTATIONS OF A PATIENT ENCOUNTER

It is important, especially in an ambulatory care setting, to identify the patient's goals, expectations, and resources to determine what needs to be achieved during an encounter. A patient who seeks care because of a bothersome symptom could be more interested in having the symptom relieved by a particular date than in knowing the cause or diagnostic explanation for the symptom. Other patients might want reassurance that a symptom or sign is not a serious condition and yet do not expect treatment to alleviate the sensations they are experiencing. An explicit discussion between the practitioner and patient is necessary to establish what the goals and focus of an encounter will be. Goals can be mutually negotiated to assure clinicians that serious conditions can be "ruled out" and to assure patients that their needs and desires are acknowledged.

EVIDENCE-BASED PRACTICE

Evidence-based practice (EBP) is the integration of clinical expertise with the most current, relevant, and sound research evidence to guide clinical practice decisions. Using evidence-based guidelines in practice, informed through research evidence, improves patient outcomes. EBP integrates the best research evidence with clinical expertise and the patient's values and preferences and involves the use of simple rules of logic to apply evidence from research to an individual patient. Some of these rules include evaluating the validity, reliability, and generalizability of the evidence. The levels of evidence range from the "gold standard" of the randomized clinical trial to case studies, correlational studies, and expert opinion. Practitioners and patients increasingly gather evidence from web-based sources, such as the Cochrane Library, which includes databases of systematic reviews of a clinical topic, abstracts of reviews of effectiveness, a controlled trial registry, and review methodology. These databases have gathered the "best evidence" related to clinical problems (Evidence-Based Practice box). Access to web-based data requires that the practitioner develop skills in health informatics—the application of computer technology to health care delivery—to develop skills in searching for and appraising evidence in the literature to guide care for a specific patient in a specific clinical context.

Evidence-Based Practice Boxes

A feature of the fifth edition of this text is to include Evidence-Based Practice boxes in each chapter. The studies cited represent evidence from epidemiologic studies, meta-analyses, systematic reviews, and randomized clinical trials that informs and guides primary care practitioners in delivering clinical services.

SUMMARY

In the context of primary care practice, the orientation to the patient should be holistic and general and toward the most prevalent or common conditions in a particular population group. This orientation requires that the expert practitioner develop skills in inductive

EVIDENCE-BASED PRACTICE *Web Sources*

National Guideline Clearinghouse	www.guideline.gov	Evidence-based practice guidelines and best practices
The Cochrane Collaboration	www.cochrane.org	Cochrane Library of systematic literature reviews about treatments and interventions
Cumulative Index to Nursing and Allied Health Literature	www.cinahl.com	CINAHL database on all aspects of nursing, allied health, alternative health, and community medicine
Medscape (from WebMD)	www.medscape.com	MEDLINE database maintained by the National Library of Medicine for biomedical content for dentistry, veterinary medicine, and nursing
Agency for Healthcare Research and Quality	www.ahrq.gov	A resource for information related to improving quality, safety, efficiency, and effectiveness of care
U.S. Preventive Services Task Force	www.ahrq.gov/clinic/uspstfix.htm	Evidence-based guidelines for screening children and adults in primary care settings
Clinical Evidence	www.clinicalevidence.org	A compendium of resources for informing treatment and patient care decisions
UpToDate	www.uptodate.com	Evidence-based clinical decision support database useful at the point of care
ConsultGeri	www.consultgeri.org	A clinical website developed by The Hartford Institute for Geriatric Nursing

reasoning to arrive at a diagnosis and to develop a treatment plan that is acceptable to the patient. An ongoing relationship with the patient over time greatly enhances the database from which the practitioner works to arrive at the best clinical judgments. Treatment plans in primary care settings rely on low-level technology and stress prevention and encourage self-care behaviors as well as open and effective patient–provider communication.

Practitioners need to be able to search for and evaluate the best evidence to guide assessment, treatment, and evaluation of diagnostic efficacy on health outcomes. A practitioner can progress from novice to expert and become more efficient in exercising clinical judgment by asking the right questions, seeking pertinent and high-quality information from available scientific evidence, and using clinical reasoning to apply the best evidence to clinical practice.

Evidence-Based Clinical Practice Guidelines

Although most primary care visits are related to acute symptoms, the focus of this chapter is health screening conducted in primary care settings on asymptomatic adults and children and the process of developing evidence-based clinical practice guidelines for prevention, counseling, and screening interventions. The National Academy of Medicine, formerly the Institute of Medicine, defines clinical practice guidelines as "recommendations intended to optimize patient care, informed by a systematic review of evidence and an assessment of the benefits and harms of alternative care options." The benefits of delivering evidence-based services include improving the quality of care, achieving desired health outcomes, and reducing health care costs. The ability to analyze and evaluate evidence requires a knowledge base and critical thinking skills.

STEPS IN EVIDENCE-BASED PRACTICE

First, begin with a clinical problem. To examine the suitability of exploring a topic to develop practice guidelines, assess its public health importance. Criteria used include the burden of having a disorder poses to a population and the anticipated effectiveness of a preventive service or intervention to reduce that burden.

Second, pose a clinical question that focuses on a patient problem and potential preventive service. A useful format that incorporates key components of a well-constructed question is PICO: *p*roblem, *i*ntervention or exposure, *c*omparison, and *o*utcome.

An analytic framework can be useful in illustrating the chain of evidence that needs to be evaluated in moving from a screening or preventive intervention to health outcomes, such as improved quality and quantity of life (Fig. 2.1). Following the overarching question of "Does screening for X reduce morbidity and/or mortality?" (key question 1) is a series of questions to establish the clinical logic to support the implementation of a preventive service in a primary care setting:

1. Can a group at high risk for X be identified by clinical characteristics?
2. Are there accurate (i.e., sensitive and specific) screening tests available?
3. Are treatments available that make a difference in intermediate outcomes when the disease is caught early or detected by screening?
4. Are treatments available that make a difference in morbidity or mortality when the condition is caught early or detected by screening?
5. How strong is the association between the intermediate outcomes and patient health outcomes?
6. What are the harms of the screening test?
7. What are the harms of the treatment?

When evaluating the chain of evidence, both certainty and magnitude of evidence for each key question is assessed to address the multiple opportunities for bias.

Third, select appropriate resources and conduct a literature search of each of the key questions that discuss comparisons of interventions and strategies used to examine outcomes of interest. Appraise the evidence for its validity and applicability. To begin a search, large databases such as PubMed or the Cochrane Library will access primary sources. Secondary sources such as the American College of Physicians (ACP) Journal Club, Essential Evidence Plus, and Clinical Evidence provide assessments of the original study

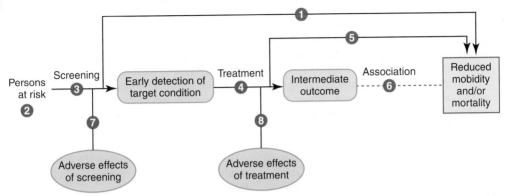

FIGURE 2.1 Template of an analytic framework. See text discussion for the key questions that correspond to the numbers in the template. (From U.S. Preventative Services Task Force. Methods and processes: procedure manual, Figure 3, n.d. Retrieved from https://www.uspreventiveservicestaskforce.org/Page/Name/section-3-topic-work-plan-development.)

(see Chapter 1). In analyzing the results, consider the following terms:

- *Relative risk (RR)* is the ratio of risk in the experimental group compared with the risk in the control group.
- *Clinical versus statistical significance* can be a matter of judgment and often depends on the magnitude of the effect being studied. "Is the difference between groups large enough to be worth achieving?"
- *Odds ratio (OR)* is the odds of previous exposure in a case divided by the odds of exposure in a control patient. For example, an OR of 3.0 means that the control cases were three times more likely to have been exposed than were treatment patients.
- *Confidence intervals (CIs)* are a measure of the precision of results. Wider CIs indicate lower precision. For example, "36 (CI, 27–51)" indicates that if the trial was repeated 100 times, 95% of the time the values would fall between 27 and 51.

Finally, apply this knowledge to patients and their preferences. It is important to assess whether the population from which the evidence is gathered matches that of a patient. For example, population-based mammography screening guidelines would not be applied to a person with a history of breast cancer.

SOURCES OF EVIDENCE

A hierarchy of evidence refers to study designs that allow for less bias or systematic error and may lead to a wrong conclusion. Randomized controlled clinical trials (RCTs) can provide sound evidence of cause and effect and can control for bias. Some limitations of RCTs are threats to the representativeness of the study population and consistency of implementation of the intervention. Meta-analysis examines a number of valid studies on a topic and mathematically combines the results to report them as if they were one large study. Expert opinion is evidence based on clinical experience, collective experience, and knowledge of professional organizations, such as the American Heart Association or the American College of Obstetrics and Gynecology. Case reports, cohort studies, and qualitative research provide less robust evidence of cause and effect and have less reliability and validity than higher levels of evidence.

LEVELS OF PREVENTION

The three levels of prevention are primary, secondary, and tertiary. Primary prevention involves activities directed at improving general well-being while also providing specific protection for selected diseases. Interventions can include screening, counseling, or preventive medicines, such as immunizations or dental sealants. Counseling about behavioral risks, such as using seat belts or bicycle helmets, can reduce injury and death. A common model used to guide behavioral counseling is the 5 *A*s model: **a**sk about the behavior, **a**dvise about health risks and benefits of change, **a**gree to set a goal, **a**ssist with identifying and overcoming barriers, and **a**rrange for follow up.

The goal of secondary prevention is to identify and detect disease in its earliest stages before symptoms appear. Screening interventions can identify elevated blood pressure or risk of diabetes with a hemoglobin A1C measurement. With early detection and diagnosis, it may be possible to cure a disease, slow its progression, prevent or minimize complications, and limit disability.

Tertiary prevention programs aim to improve the quality of life for people with various conditions by limiting complications and disabilities, reducing the severity and progression of disease, and providing rehabilitation therapy to maximize functionality and self-sufficiency. Tertiary prevention can occur over a long period of time, such as optimizing treatment for chronic conditions such as asthma, physical or cognitive disability, and diabetes.

POPULATION VERSUS TARGETED SCREENING

Population screening includes all members of a particular population; for example, all newborns are screened for congenital hypothyroidism at birth. Targeted screening is more selective and focuses on a population at risk. An example is sexually transmitted infection (STI) screening done in sexually active adolescents and young adults in a specific age group (e.g., those 24 years and younger have the highest rates of infection) and who have increased risk factors for STI such as new or multiple sexual partners, inconsistent condom use, and sex work.

ETHICAL GUIDELINES FOR SCREENING

Not all diseases or conditions are appropriate for screening. The purposes of screening must be ethically acceptable, information must be

used for appropriate purposes, tests must be of high quality, individuals should know what is taking place and be informed of their results, counseling must be available to interpret results, and results must be kept confidential. Additionally, genomic medicine has created a new urgency in recognition and application of screening guidelines to assess the value of population screening for genetic susceptibility to diseases and conditions.

Guidelines for determining if a disease or condition warrants screening include the following:

Is the condition significant in the community?

The condition must have a significant impact on the quality or quantity of life, must be measured using morbidity and mortality data, and must be measured by the quality of life. The incidence, or the number of new or undiagnosed cases, of the condition must be sufficient to justify the cost of screening.

Can the condition be screened?

Tests that are acceptable to patients must be available at a reasonable cost to detect the condition in its asymptomatic period. Measures used to determine acceptability of tests include sensitivity (ability to provide a true positive) and specificity (ability to provide a true negative), as well as measures of reliability (reproducibility) and validity (does it measure what you think it measures?). Other considerations include potential harms of screening, such as labeling and stigma, or morbidity associated with the screening test, as well as patient preference.

Should the condition be screened?

Before screening can be recommended, acceptable treatments must be available. Contextual variables, such as ethnicity and cultural beliefs and practices, socioeconomic conditions, and geographic location, need to be considered. The disease or condition must have an asymptomatic period and a period in which detection and treatment significantly improve health outcomes compared with a diagnosis obtained based on symptoms. Hypertension is

| Table 2.1 | **Matrix for Arriving at a Grade Recommendation** |

| | | MAGNITUDE OF NET BENEFIT | | |
CERTAINTY OF NET BENEFIT	SUBSTANTIAL	MODERATE	SMALL	ZERO/NEGATIVE
High	A	B	C	D
Moderate	B	B	C	D
Low	Insufficient			

From U.S. Preventive Services Task Force: Procedure manual, n.d. Retrieved from https://www.uspreventiveservicestaskforce.org/

an asymptomatic condition that affects a large number of adults, blood pressure can be measured accurately with minimal harm, and evidence-based risk reducing behavioral counseling and medications can improve health outcomes.

United States Preventive Services Task Force

The United States Preventive Services Task Force (USPSTF) was established in 1984 as an independent group of experts in prevention and evidence-based medicine. The work of the task force is to make recommendations about clinical preventive services such as screenings, counseling, and preventive medications.

The Task Force works with Evidence-Based Practice Centers (EPCs) that conduct in-depth systematic reviews of the available evidence and develop an analytic framework or research plan that includes a set of key questions and outcomes of interest that the review must answer (see Fig. 2.1). After deliberation with input and comments from the public and other experts, a recommendation is reached by calculating the balance between the certainty and magnitude of the net benefit (Table 2.1) and is then assigned a grade (Table 2.2). Box 2.1

| Table 2.2 | **What the USPSTF Grades Mean and Suggestions for Practice** |

GRADE	GRADE DEFINITIONS	SUGGESTIONS FOR PRACTICE
A	The USPSTF recommends the service. There is high certainty that the net benefit is substantial.	Offer or provide this service.
B	The USPSTF recommends the service. There is high certainty that the net benefit is moderate or there is moderate certainty that the net benefit is moderate to substantial.	Offer or provide this service.
C	The USPSTF recommends selectively offering (or providing) this service to individual patients based on professional judgment and patient preferences. There is at least moderate certainty that the net benefit is small.	Offer or provide this service for selected patients depending on individual circumstances.
D	The USPSTF recommends against the service. There is moderate or high certainty that the service has no net benefit or that the harms outweigh the benefits.	Discourage the use of this service.
I Statement	The USPSTF concludes that the current evidence is insufficient to assess the balance of benefits and harms of the service. Evidence is lacking, of poor quality or conflicting, and the balance of benefits and harms cannot be determined.	Read "Clinical Considerations" section of USPSTF Recommendation Statement. If offered, patients should understand the uncertainty about the balance of benefits and harms.

USPSTF, U.S. Preventative Services Task Force.
Grade Definitions. U.S. Preventive Services Task Force, Rockville, MD. (Current as of November 2017). https://www.uspreventiveservicestaskforce.org/Page/Name/grade-definitions

Box 2.1	**Questions to Consider When Evaluating Evidence**

1. Do the studies have the appropriate research design to answer the key question(s)?
2. To what extent are the existing studies of high quality?
3. To what extent are the results of the studies generalizable to the general US primary care population and situation?
4. How many studies have been conducted that address the key question(s)?
5. How consistent are the results of the studies?
6. Are there additional factors that assist with drawing conclusions?

contains the six questions posed when evaluating evidence. The Task Force recommendations are considered the gold standard for clinical preventive services.

Electronic Preventive Services Selector (ePSS) is a resource that practitioners can use to electronically access Task Force recommendations. It is designed to assist primary care practitioners in determining appropriate clinical preventative services for their patients (see http://epss.ahrq.gov/PDA/index.jsp).

The National Guideline Clearinghouse (www.guideline.gov) is a public resource maintained by the Agency for Health Care Research and Quality that provides summaries of guidelines from major medical and specialty organizations. To be included in the Clearinghouse, guidelines must meet criteria of incorporating a systematic review and including an assessment of the harms and benefits.

SUMMARY

Evidence alone was never meant to replace experience and intuition. There are always the human concerns to account for in clinical decision making. However, primary care practitioners will increasingly be engaged in delivering both preventive and acute care services. Practitioners need to be aware of evidence-based practice guidelines and make clinical decisions based on good-quality scientific evidence as well as clinical judgment considerations with individual patients and families.

CHAPTER

3   Abdominal Pain

Abdominal pain is a subjective feeling of discomfort in the abdomen that can be caused by a variety of problems. The goal of initial clinical assessment is to distinguish acute life-threatening conditions from chronic/recurrent or acute mild, self-limiting conditions. Assessment is complicated by the dynamic rather than static nature of acute abdominal pain, which can produce a changing clinical picture, often over a short period of time. In addition, both children and older adults tend to deviate from the usual and anticipated clinical pattern of abdominal pain. The following three processes can produce abdominal pain: (1) tension in the gastrointestinal (GI) tract wall from muscle contraction or distention, (2) ischemia, and (3) inflammation of the peritoneum. Pain can also be referred from within or outside the abdomen.

Colic is a type of tension pain. It is associated with forceful peristaltic contractions and is the most characteristic type of pain arising from the viscera. Colicky pain can be produced by an irritant substance, from infection with a virus or bacteria, or by the body's attempt to force its luminal contents through an obstruction. Another type of tension pain is caused by acute stretching of the capsule of an organ, such as the liver, spleen, or kidney. The patient with this visceral pain is restless, moves about, and has difficulty getting comfortable.

Ischemia produces an intense, continuous pain. The most common cause of intestinal ischemic pain is strangulation of the bowel from obstruction.

Inflammation of the peritoneum usually begins at the serosa covering the affected and inflamed organ, causing visceral peritonitis. The pain is a poorly localized aching. As the inflammatory process spreads to the adjacent parietal peritoneum, it produces localized parietal peritonitis. The pain of parietal peritonitis is more severe and is perceived in the area of the abdomen corresponding to the inflammation. A patient with parietal pain usually lies still and does not want to move.

Pain can be referred from within the abdomen or from other parts of the body (Box 3.1).

Referral of pain occurs because tissues supplied by the same or adjacent neural segments have the same common pathways inside the central nervous system. Thus, stimulation of these neural segments produces the sensation of pain. For example, nerves that supply the appendix are derived from the same source as those that supply the small intestine, resulting in the onset of appendicitis pain in the epigastric area.

Abdominal pain in adults can be classified as acute, chronic, or recurrent. The term "acute abdomen" refers to any acute condition within the abdomen that requires immediate attention because surgical intervention may be required. Acute abdominal pain refers to a relatively sudden onset of pain that is severe or increasing in severity and has been present for a short duration. Chronic pain is characterized by its persistent duration or recurrence. Recurrent episodes of pain can be either acute or chronic in nature.

In adults, acute pain requiring immediate surgical intervention is commonly caused by appendicitis, perforated peptic ulcer, intestinal obstruction, peritonitis, perforated diverticulitis, ectopic pregnancy, or dissection of aortic aneurysm. Other common causes of acute pain include cholelithiasis, gastroenteritis, peptic gastroduodenal syndrome, pancreatitis, pelvic inflammatory disease (PID), or urinary tract infection (UTI). Chronic or recurrent pain can be caused by GI disorders, such as Crohn disease, irritable bowel syndrome (IBS), diverticulitis, or esophagitis; pelvic disorders, such

| Box 3.1 | **Some Causes of Pain Perceived in Anatomical Regions** |

RIGHT UPPER QUADRANT
- Duodenal ulcer
- Hepatitis
- Hepatomegaly
- Pneumonia
- Cholecystitis

RIGHT LOWER QUADRANT
- Appendicitis
- Salpingitis
- Ovarian cyst
- Ruptured ectopic pregnancy
- Renal or ureteral stone
- Strangulated hernia
- Meckel diverticulitis
- Regional ileitis
- Perforated cecum

PERIUMBILICAL
- Intestinal obstruction
- Acute pancreatitis
- Early appendicitis

- Mesenteric thrombosis
- Aortic aneurysm
- Diverticulitis

LEFT UPPER QUADRANT
- Ruptured spleen
- Gastric ulcer
- Aortic aneurysm
- Perforated colon
- Pneumonia

LEFT LOWER QUADRANT
- Sigmoid diverticulitis
- Salpingitis
- Ovarian cyst
- Ruptured ectopic pregnancy
- Renal or ureteral stone
- Strangulated hernia
- Perforated colon
- Regional ileitis
- Ulcerative colitis

Modified from Judge R, Zuidema G, Fitzgerald F: *Clinical diagnosis,* ed. 5, Boston, 1988, Little Brown.

as dysmenorrhea or uterine fibroids; genitourinary disorders, such as recurrent UTI or chronic prostatitis; or conditions outside the abdomen, such as costochondritis, hip disease, or hernia.

In children, abdominal pain can be classified as acute or recurrent. Common causes of acute pain include appendicitis, food poisoning, UTI, viral gastroenteritis, and bacterial enterocolitis. Recurrent abdominal pain (RAP) is defined as more than three episodes of pain in 3 months in children older than 3 years. It affects 10% to 15% of children between the ages of 3 and 14 years; of these children, 90% will not have an organic etiology.

DIAGNOSTIC REASONING: FOCUSED HISTORY

Is this an acute condition?

Key Questions
- How long ago did your pain start?
- Was the onset sudden or gradual?
- How severe is the pain (on a scale of 1–10)?

- If a child: What is the child's level of activity?
- Does the pain wake you up from sleep?
- What has been the course of the pain since it started? Is it getting worse or better?
- When was your last bowel movement?
- Have you ever had this pain before? What was diagnosed? How was it treated?

Onset and Duration

Acute onset of pain that is getting progressively worse could signal a surgical emergency. In general, patients who present with severe pain 6 to 24 hours from the onset probably have an acute surgical condition. Acute abdominal pain can signal a few potentially life-threatening conditions that must be considered first. The following are possible surgical emergencies that require immediate evaluation and intervention:

- *Perforation or ruptured appendix:* look for signs and symptoms of peritonitis (Box 3.2)
- *Ectopic pregnancy:* suspect in any woman of childbearing age

Box 3.2	**Features of Peritonitis**
P	Pain: front, back, sides, shoulders
E	Electrolytes fall; shock ensues
R	Rigidity or rebound of anterior abdominal wall
I	Immobile abdomen and patient
T	Tenderness with involuntary guarding
O	Obstruction
N	Nausea and vomiting
I	Increasing pulse rate, decreasing blood pressure
T	Temperature falls and then rises; tachypnea
I	Increasing girth of abdomen
S	Silent abdomen (no bowel sounds)

Modified from Shipman JJ: *Mnemonics and tactics in surgery and medicine*, ed. 2, Chicago, 1984, Mosby.

- *Obstruction:* sudden onset of crampy pain usually in umbilical area
- *Ruptured abdominal aortic aneurysm:* when back pain is present
- *Intussusception:* in infants
- *Malrotation:* in infants usually younger than 1 month old

Pain of sudden onset is more likely associated with colic, perforation, or acute ischemia (torsion, volvulus). Slower onset of pain generally is associated with inflammatory conditions, such as appendicitis, pancreatitis, and cholecystitis.

Acute pain that comes and goes can be related to intestinal peristalsis. The onset of pain in relation to food ingestion provides diagnostic clues: pain occurring several hours after a meal suggests a duodenal ulcer (pain with stomach empty), but pain immediately after eating occurs with esophagitis.

In children, RAP occurs in attacks usually lasting less than 1 hour and rarely longer than 3 hours and frequently interferes with daily routines. Between episodes, the pain resolves completely. When interviewing a child, remember that the child might not be old enough to have a clear sense of time.

Severity and Progression

Severity is the most difficult symptom to evaluate because of its subjective quality. It is helpful to use a scale of 1 to 10 in adults.

Children often respond to the use of the FACES pain scale or the Oucher pain scale (Fig. 3.1).

Determine whether the pain is an acute episode or a chronic or recurrent episode. Acute abdominal pain requires immediate attention because it can signal an acute surgical condition in the abdomen. Chronic or recurrent episodes of pain can be handled in a more temperate manner.

Pain that is steady, severe, and progressive is worrisome. Pain that causes one to awake from sleep is serious. A sudden pain severe enough to cause fainting suggests perforated ulcer, ruptured aneurysm, or ectopic pregnancy. A severe knifelike pain usually indicates an emergency. Tearing pain is characteristic of an aortic aneurysm. Appendicitis is often described as an initial ache that gets progressively worse. Colicky pain that becomes steady can indicate appendicitis or strangulating intestinal obstruction.

Children are poor historians regarding the severity of pain. The caregiver should indicate how severe the child's pain is by a description of the activity level of the child. In general, avoidance of favorite activities or motion indicates an organic problem. Organic disease awakens the child from sleep.

Last Bowel Movement

Obstipation (the absence of stools) occurs with complete obstruction, but diarrhea can be present with partial obstruction. Lack of a bowel movement for 3 days could signal constipation. Children have a poor sense of stool patterns and may not know what it means to be constipated. Parents often do not recognize abnormal stooling patterns in the child. The onset of constipation can cause severe abdominal pain.

Previous Pain

Chronic pain could result when a potential surgical event is partially controlled but is not totally resolved. Chronic pain that has been present for longer than 1 year generally is not caused by a neoplasm; consider instead IBS or colorectal, endometrial, or inflammatory causes.

Recurrent attacks of acute pain could be caused by inflammation and exacerbation of a

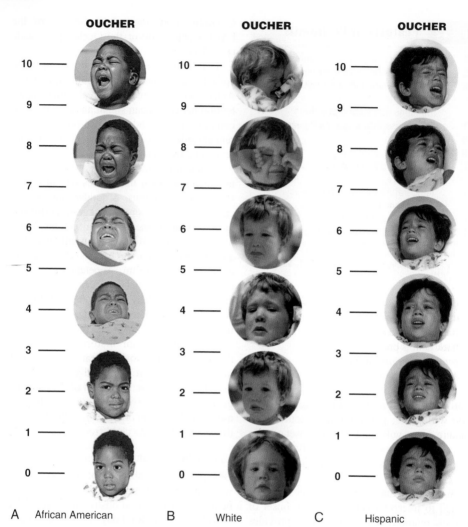

A   African American   B   White   C   Hispanic

FIGURE 3.1 The Oucher Pain Scale illustrated with African American (**A**), white (**B**), and Hispanic (**C**) children to best fit the child's cultural identity. The African American child version of the Oucher was developed and copyrighted in 1990 by Mary J. Denyes, PhD, RN, FAAN (Wayne State University) and Antonia Villarruel, PhD, RN, FAAN (University of Michigan) at the Children's Hospital of Michigan. Cornelia P. Porter, PhD, RN and Charlotta Marshall, MSN, RN contributed to the development of this scale. The white child version of the Oucher was developed and copyrighted in 1983 by Judith E. Beyer, PhD, RN, currently at Graceland University School of Nursing in Independence, Missouri. Photographs were taken by Lynn Juliano, RN, BSN at Martha Jefferson Hospital in Charlottesville, Va. The Hispanic child version of the Oucher was developed and copyrighted in 1990 by Antonia M. Villarruel, PhD, RN (University of Michigan) and Mary J. Denyes, PhD, RN (Wayne State University). Photographs were taken at Children's Hospital of Michigan in Detroit.

chronic condition, such as functional colonic pain, IBS, cholecystitis, chronic pancreatitis, diverticulitis, or ulcer disease. Other causes of acute attacks of pain are recurrent infection, such as pyelonephritis or cystitis, and urinary tract stones.

Will the location of pain give me any clues?

Key Questions
- Where is the pain? Can you point to it?
- Does it travel (radiate) anywhere?

Location of the Pain

The viscera are innervated bilaterally so that pain is perceived in the midline. It is often described as a deep, dull, diffuse pain. Visceral pain originates from epigastric, periumbilical, and hypogastric causes; from intraabdominal, extraperitoneal organs (pancreas, kidneys, ureters, great vessels, pelvic organs); or from a referred source.

Parietal (also known as peritoneal or somatic) pain is more localized and is described as a sharp pain. Parietal pain originates from intraabdominal and intraperitoneal organs.

Inflammation (e.g., with appendicitis) can produce either visceral or parietal peritonitis. Initially, the inflammation is limited to the serosa covering an inflamed organ. The pain is visceral and is felt diffusely. As the inflammation progresses to the adjacent parietal peritoneum, it produces a more severe localized pain that is perceived in the corresponding area of the abdomen. Children generally have a poor ability to localize pain and are not helpful in the majority of cases.

The Apley rule states that the further the localization of pain from the umbilicus, the more likely it is that there is an underlying organic disorder.

When blood, pus, or gastric fluid suddenly floods the peritoneal cavity, the pain is frequently reported as "all over the abdomen" at first. However, the maximum intensity of pain at the onset is likely to be in the upper abdomen with gastric problems and in the lower abdomen with tubal and appendix rupture. Irritating fluid from a perforated duodenal ulcer produces pain in the right hypochondrium, lumbar, and iliac regions.

Pain arising from the small intestine is felt in the epigastric and umbilical areas of the abdomen. The 9th and 11th thoracic nerves supply the small intestine via the common mesentery nerve. Appendicular nerves are derived from the same source as those that supply the small intestine, resulting in the onset of pain in the epigastric area with appendicitis.

Table 3.1 describes the structures involved in specific pain locations.

Radiation of Pain

Radiation of pain can help in diagnosis. Pain that radiates will do so to the area of distribution of the nerves coming from that segment of the spinal cord that supplies the affected area. Whereas biliary colic or gallbladder pain is frequently referred to the region just under

Table 3.1	**Pain Location and Involved Structures**
PAIN LOCATION	**INVOLVED STRUCTURES**
Epigastric	Esophagus, stomach, duodenum, liver, gallbladder, pancreas, spleen
Upper abdominal	Esophagus, stomach, duodenum, pancreas, liver, gallbladder, or thorax
Right upper quadrant	Usually esophagus, stomach, duodenum, pancreas, liver, gallbladder, or thorax; often indicates acute cholecystitis
Left upper quadrant	Spleen
Periumbilical	Jejunum, midgut, ileum, appendix, ascending colon; pain caused by inflammation, ischemic spasm, or abnormal distention
Lower abdominal	Colon, sigmoid colon, rectum, and genitourinary structures—bladder, uterus, prostate
Right lower quadrant	Appendix, fallopian tube, ovary
Left lower quadrant	Sigmoid colon, fallopian tube, ovary
Flanks	Kidney(s)
Localized	Occurs from local inflammation of skin or peritoneum, as with appendicitis; lateralized pain occurs in paired organs—kidneys, ureters, fallopian tubes, gonads
Generalized	Produced by diffuse inflammation of gastrointestinal tract, peritoneum, or abdomen wall

the right scapula (eighth dorsal segment), renal colic in males is frequently felt in the testicle of the same side. Pain from a ruptured spleen is often referred to the top of the left shoulder.

What do the pain characteristics tell me?

Key Questions
- Can you describe the pain (e.g., burning, sharp, achy, crampy)?
- What makes it worse or better?

Character of Pain

Colicky or cramping pain occurs with obstruction of a hollow viscus that produces distention. Generally, there are pain-free intervals when the pain is much less intense but still present, although it is subtle. During the painful episodes, the patient is exceedingly agitated and restless and often pale and diaphoretic. The pain from obstruction of the small intestine is rhythmic, peristaltic pain with intermittent cramping. When the obstruction site is in the proximal small intestine rather than in the more distal portion, the paroxysms of cramping occur with greater frequency.

Steady pain is associated with perforation, ischemia, inflammation, and blood in the peritoneal cavity. Burning pain is characteristic of esophagitis. Pain from a duodenal ulcer has been described as burning or "gnawing." Pain of pancreatic origin is steady, epigastric, and prostrating. Pricking, itching, or burning pain comes from superficial causes such as herpes zoster. Dull, aching pain indicates deeper pain. In children, abdominal pain is generally characterized as colicky or inflammatory.

Remember, however, that despite descriptions of characteristic or typical abdominal pain, presentation in children and older adults is often atypical and might not fit any pattern.

Precipitating or Aggravating Factors

Lying down or bending forward often produces pain from esophagitis. Alcohol can aggravate gastritis or an ulcer. Eating before sleeping can aggravate gastroesophageal reflux.

Pain that is made worse by deep inspiration and is stopped or diminished by a respiratory pause indicates a pleuritic origin. If the cause is peritonitis, intraperitoneal abscess, or abdominal distention from intestinal obstruction, pain will increase on deep inspiration. Biliary colic is made worse by forced inspiration. The pain from biliary colic often causes inhibition of movement of the diaphragm.

A patient with visceral pain is restless, moves about, and has difficulty getting comfortable. A patient with parietal pain usually lies still and does not want to move. Children with inflammatory pain secondary to peritoneal irritation usually appear quiet and motionless because movement exacerbates the pain.

Relieving Factors

Food or antacids can relieve pain caused by an ulcer or gastritis. Antacids often relieve pain from gastroesophageal reflux disease (GERD). Both colicky pain and inflammatory pain are alleviated significantly with analgesics. However, the pain of a vascular accident will not respond to analgesics.

Are there any precipitating events that will help narrow my diagnosis?

Key Questions
- Is the pain related to any other activity (e.g., eating, lying down)?
- Can you identify any trigger?

Relation to Other Events

Pain that is relieved by defecation, flatus, laxatives, or diet changes implicates the intestine. Pain associated with meals implicates the GI tract.

Pain with sexual activity (dyspareunia) suggests a pelvic origin. Pain that occurs with position changes can be referred from the spine, hips, sacroiliac joint, pelvic bones, or abdominal musculature. Exertional pain can be of cardiac origin.

What does the presence of vomiting or diarrhea tell me?

Key Questions
- Are you vomiting? Did the vomiting start before or after the pain?

- What does the vomitus look like?
- What do your stools look like?
- How frequent are your stools?

Vomiting

Vomiting that precedes the onset of abdominal pain is unlikely to signal a problem requiring surgery. Vomiting suggests that the pain is visceral in origin. Anorexia is a nonspecific symptom, but its absence makes serious disease less likely.

Vomiting associated with an acute condition of the abdomen may be from one of the following three causes:

- Severe irritation of the nerves of the peritoneum or mesentery. Sudden stimulation of many sympathetic nerves causes vomiting to occur early and to be persistent.
- Obstruction of an involuntary muscular tube. Obstruction of any of the muscular tubes causes peristaltic contraction and consequent stretching of the muscle wall, which results in vomiting. The area behind the obstruction becomes dilated, and as each peristaltic wave occurs, the tension and stretching of the muscular fibers are temporarily increased; therefore, the pain of colic usually occurs in spasms. Vomiting usually occurs at the height of the pain.
- The action of absorbed toxins on the medullary centers. The chemoreceptor trigger zone is stimulated by drugs such as cardiac glycosides, ergot alkaloids, and morphine or by uremia, diabetic ketoacidosis, or general anesthetics. Impulses to the medullary vomiting center activate the vomiting process.

Pain with vomiting

In sudden and severe stimulation of the peritoneum or mesentery, vomiting comes soon after the pain. In acute obstruction of the urethra or bile duct, vomiting is early, sudden, and intense. In intestinal obstruction, the timing of the vomiting indicates the location of the obstruction. If the duodenum is obstructed, vomiting occurs with the onset of pain. Obstruction of the large bowel causes very late or infrequent vomiting.

Vomiting is not usually seen in ectopic pregnancy, gastric or duodenal perforation, or intussusception. Vomiting occurring before pain indicates gastroenteritis. With appendicitis, pain almost always precedes the vomiting.

Appearance of vomitus

Clear vomitus suggests gastric fluid; bile-colored vomitus is from upper GI contents. Feculent vomitus occurs with distal intestinal obstruction. Coffee grounds or black color indicates GI bleeding. Patients with gastric outlet obstruction vomit fluid that contains food particles if the patient has eaten recently, but later the vomitus becomes clear. Infants with duodenal atresia and small bowel volvulus will vomit bilious fluid, but in pyloric stenosis, no bile is seen.

Diarrhea

Diarrhea (see Chapter 12) is associated with inflammatory bowel disease (IBD), IBS, diverticulitis, early obstruction, or infection. The presence of blood in the stool suggests that the pain originates in the intestinal tract. Blood can indicate neoplasm, intussusception, inflammatory lesions, or an invasive organism.

Diarrhea can precede perforation of the appendix as a result of irritation of the sigmoid colon by an inflammatory mass. Some patients will report gas stoppage symptoms: the sensation of fullness that suggests the need for a bowel movement. With appendicitis, the patient often attempts to defecate but without relief.

In children, mild diarrhea associated with the onset of pain suggests acute gastroenteritis but can also occur with early appendicitis. A low-lying appendix, close to the sigmoid colon and rectum, can induce an inflammatory process of the muscle wall of the sigmoid colon. Any distention of the sigmoid by fluid or gas, signals the child to pass gas and small amounts of stool. The cycle repeats a few minutes later. In gastroenteritis, typically the child will have large liquid stools. Children can also have abdominal pain from chronic constipation. Constipation that precedes pain suggests disease of the colon or rectum.

Are there any clues to implicate a particular organ system?

If the patient gives a positive response to the following history questions, refer to the topic or chapter indicated for additional discussion. Pain that is not abdominal in origin could be referred to or perceived to be in the abdomen. Accompanying symptoms of headache, sore throat, and general aches and pains suggest a viral, flulike cause.

Key Questions

Cardiovascular system (see Chapter 8):

- Does the pain occur with exertion or at rest?
- Do you have any chest pain, palpitations, fast heartbeat, or pain that goes to the arm or jaw?

Referred pain from the chest is common. Pain on exertion signals coronary artery disease (CAD) and angina. Right upper quadrant (RUQ) pain can be caused by congestive heart failure. Myocardial infarction (MI) and pericarditis can also cause abdominal pain.

Key Questions

Gastrointestinal system (see Chapters 10 and 12):

- Do you have any GI symptoms (e.g., gas, diarrhea, constipation, vomiting, heartburn)?
- Have you had any changes in your bowel habits, stools, or eating pattern?
- Is the pain relieved by defecation or burping?

Gas, bloating, diarrhea, constipation, and rectal bleeding can occur with pain that is intestinal in origin. Heartburn and dysphagia are characteristic of esophagitis and GERD. Changes in bowel habits can signal obstruction or neoplasm. Constipation alternating with diarrhea is characteristic of IBS. The patient often also reports distention, bloating, belching, gas, and mucus in the stools.

Pain relieved by defecation or the passage of gas suggests IBS or gas entrapment in the large intestine. Pain relieved by burping suggests distention of the stomach by gas.

Key Questions

Genitourinary system (see Chapters 5, 18, 27, and 35 to 37):

- When was your last menstrual period (LMP)? Was it normal for you? Could you be pregnant?
- Do you have any vaginal symptoms or problems, such as unusual discharge, unusual bleeding, or pain with sexual intercourse?
- Do you have any menstrual irregularity or unusual bleeding? (Sexual history could provide information relevant to the possibility of sexually transmitted infections [STIs], PID, and pregnancy.)
- Do you have any urinary symptoms (e.g., frequency, urgency, dysuria, blood in urine, change in urine color)?
- Do you have pain in the back (flank)? Can you point to it?

Menstrual irregularities, vaginal discharge, unusual bleeding, or dyspareunia indicates a pelvic origin of the pain. Sexually active adolescent girls are at the highest risk for contracting PID. Patients with PID may complain of both vaginal discharge and abnormal vaginal bleeding, although pain is often the only presenting symptom. The pain is usually severe and progressive. Pain just before the onset of menses indicates endometriosis. Pain related to ovulation (mittelschmerz) occurs midcycle. In women of childbearing age, always consider ectopic pregnancy. Regard women of childbearing age as pregnant until pregnancy is ruled out.

Urinary symptoms (dysuria, hematuria, hesitancy, or frequency) point to a urinary tract cause of the pain. In young children abdominal pain and vomiting may be signs of a UTI. Flank pain is usually associated with renal calculi or pyelonephritis. Upper abdominal pain that radiates to the groin signals ureterolithiasis.

Key Questions

Musculoskeletal system (see Chapters 22 to 24):

- Does the pain occur with change in position or movement?
- Do you have any joint pain, heat, swelling, noises, or limitation in range of motion?
- Do you have any difficulty walking?

Pain produced by musculoskeletal problems and referred to the abdomen can be provoked by position changes or walking. Costochondritis can produce pain with respiration. Symptoms of joint involvement point to either a local cause with referred pain, or a systemic cause, such as rheumatoid arthritis.

Key Questions

Respiratory system (see Chapters 11 and 14):
- Do you have a cough or difficulty breathing?
- Do you have any shortness of breath?
- Does the child complain of a sore throat?

Pneumonia, especially of a lower lobe, is a common cause of pain perceived in the abdomen, especially in children. Pleurisy can produce pain on deep inspiration. Persistent coughing can produce musculoskeletal soreness that may be referred to the abdomen. Children with strep throat may present with abdominal pain.

Is the pain psychogenic, organic, or functional?

Key Questions

- Do you feel unhappy, sad, depressed?
- Are you able to eat, sleep, or engage in usual activities?
- Have you had recent problems with diarrhea or constipation?
- How is your energy level?
- Have you ever been diagnosed with or treated for a mental health or psychiatric problem?

Abdominal pain can be functional or psychogenic in origin and presents somewhat differently from organic pain (Table 3.2). In children, functional abdominal pain is caused by one of four or a combination of more than one of the following: functional dyspepsia, functional abdominal pain syndrome, IBS, or abdominal migraine.

The presence of vegetative symptoms suggests depression (see Chapter 4).

What else do I need to consider?

Key Questions

- What medications (prescribed and over the counter) are you taking? Why are you taking them?
- Have you had any operations? What were they?
- Have you recently had an involuntary weight loss?
- Have you been camping?
- If a child: Is the child in a day care setting?

Medications

Gastrointestinal distress is a common adverse reaction to many medications. Erythromycin and tetracycline are commonly associated with abdominal pain. Aspirin and nonsteroidal antiinflammatory drugs (NSAIDs) can cause pain associated with gastritis and ulcer formation.

Surgery

Prior surgery can produce adhesions that cause intestinal obstruction. Adhesion of organs to

Table 3.2	**Organic versus Functional Pain**	
HISTORY	**ORGANIC PAIN**	**FUNCTIONAL PAIN**
Pain character	Acute, persistent pain increasing in intensity	Less likely to change or get more severe
Pain localization	Sharply localized	Various locations
Pain in relation to sleep	Awakens at night	Does not affect sleep
Pain in relation to umbilicus	Farther away	At umbilicus
Associated symptoms	Fever, anorexia, vomiting, weight loss, anemia, elevated ESR	Headache, dizziness, and multiple system complaints
Psychological stress	None reported	Present

the abdominal wall can also produce pain. Prior appendectomy does not preclude appendicitis; the stump can become inflamed.

Involuntary Weight Loss

Involuntary weight loss raises the index of suspicion for colon cancer. Identify other factors that would lead you to suspect neoplasms, such as a recent change in bowel habits in a middle-aged patient, family history of colorectal or gynecologic cancer, and the presence of blood in the stool.

Camping or Day Care

Ingestion of untreated water can result in intestinal parasites. Transmission of intestinal parasites is also common in day care settings. Children with intestinal parasites may present with abdominal pain as the only symptom; therefore, stools should be evaluated for ova and parasites.

DIAGNOSTIC REASONING: FOCUSED PHYSICAL EXAMINATION

Note General Appearance

Patients with visceral pain are restless, move about, and have difficulty getting comfortable. These are patients with colicky type pain, often indicative of biliary obstruction, ureterolithiasis, obstruction, gastroenteritis, or early peritonitis.

Patients with parietal pain usually lie still and do not want to move. These are patients with localized peritonitis indicative of appendicitis, rupture, or perforation.

In children, note whether the child looks sick (see Chapter 17). Children can react to pain differently than adults. With peritoneal irritation, they are typically quiet and motionless with their knees flexed and drawn up. Children who are septic or have serious diseases, such as perforation or intussusception, generally lie still and look lethargic, withdrawn, and apprehensive. A child with colicky pain frequently writhes in discomfort, occasionally rocking in a rhythmic fashion.

Assess Vital Signs

In patients who are tachycardic and tachypneic, suspect a serious thoracic, intraabdominal, or pelvic disorder that is producing an acute condition in the abdomen. Shallow respirations could indicate pneumonia or pleurisy with referred pain. Orthostatic hypotension, an unusually low blood pressure, or a normal blood pressure in someone who is usually hypertensive can indicate an acute abdominal condition.

The presence of a fever suggests an acute inflammatory condition. A temperature of greater than 39.4°C (102.9°F) is associated more with pulmonary and renal infection than with an abdominal problem and can indicate pneumonia or pyelonephritis.

In adults, look for documented recent involuntary weight loss, which indicates a neoplasm. Weigh a child to determine weight loss and dehydration status.

Examine the Throat

Note exudate, erythema, and anterior cervical adenopathy suggesting group A β hemolytic streptococcal pharyngitis.

Observe Abdominal Musculature

Whereas a rigid abdomen characterizes peritoneal irritation, a soft abdomen suggests otherwise. A rigid abdomen can signal an acute condition of the abdomen that requires surgical intervention.

Note Coloring of Abdominal Skin

Ecchymosis around the umbilicus (Cullen sign) is associated with hemoperitoneum caused by either pancreatitis or ruptured ectopic pregnancy. Ecchymosis of the flanks (Grey Turner sign) is associated with hemoperitoneum and pancreatitis. Look for skin rashes of viral exanthema.

In children, a rash (palpable purpura) located on the lower extremities, buttocks, and arms indicates Henoch-Schönlein purpura (a syndrome of purpura with urticaria, erythema, arthritis, and GI symptoms).

Note Abdominal Distention

Generalized symmetrical distention can occur as the result of obesity, enlarged organs, fluid, or gas. Distention from the umbilicus to the symphysis can be caused by an ovarian tumor, pregnancy, uterine fibroids, carcinoma, pancreatic cyst, or gastric dilation. Asymmetrical distention or protrusion may indicate hernia, tumor, cysts, bowel obstruction, or enlargement of abdominal organs. Remember the *F* s of distention: fat, fluid, feces, fetus, flatus, fibroid, full bladder, false pregnancy, and fatal tumor.

To determine distention in children, stoop down by the child's side and view across the abdomen. If the skin is tense and taut with a distended abdomen, and if the umbilicus is everted, ascites is often present. Superficial abdominal veins are often distended in children with peritonitis. The healthy child will usually have a flat abdominal profile. A flat abdomen is a straight line from the xiphoid to pelvis with no scaphoiding (abdomen has a concave, sunken appearance). A scaphoid abdomen can occur with marked dehydration or high intestinal obstruction.

Auscultate Bowel Sounds

If bowel sounds are absent, suspect peritonitis or ileus. Hyperactive bowel sounds suggest gastroenteritis, early pyloric or intestinal obstruction, or GI bleeding. High-pitched tinkling bowel sounds can indicate obstruction.

In children, use of the stethoscope can be helpful in palpation to determine abdominal pain. Begin listening to the chest; the child accepts this as painless. Then gently move the stethoscope down to the belly, slightly increasing the pressure, watching the child's face and feeling the resistance when painful.

Percuss for Tones and Guarding

In percussion, look for unexpected dullness. Guarding with percussion suggests peritoneal irritation. Tenderness can be elicited with gentle tapping. Tenderness is usually local and only rarely referred.

Palpate the Abdomen

Start with gentle palpation and palpate the area of pain last. Testing for rebound tenderness should be performed gently. Tenderness, guarding, and rebound tenderness suggest peritoneal irritation. The most reliable clinical indicator of parietal peritonitis is involuntary guarding, which must be distinguished from voluntary guarding because of pain or fear of worsening pain as a result of the examination. Guarding is determined with gentle palpation of the abdomen, not by deep palpation of the underlying organs.

You can induce guarding by having the patient place the chin on the chest or cross the arms on the chest and sit up. Palpate the painful area again. Note that intraperitoneal pain is made less severe by induced guarding. If the severity of pain is not decreased by induced guarding, consider other causes such as functional pain or abdominal wall pain.

Palpate for the liver, gallbladder, spleen, kidneys, aorta, and bladder to detect organ tenderness or involvement. Abrupt cessation of inspiration on palpation of the gallbladder (Murphy sign) indicates acute cholecystitis.

Palpate for Masses

Palpation of a mass can indicate neoplasm, obstruction, hernia, or the presence of feces in the colon. Anatomical structures can be mistaken for an abdominal mass. A mass in the upper abdomen that pulsates laterally suggests an abdominal aortic aneurysm.

A sausage-shaped mass can be felt in the upper mid-abdomen in 85% to 95% of infants with intussusception. An olive-shaped mass may be palpable in the RUQ with pyloric stenosis.

Palpate the Groin

The groin must be examined in everyone who has abdominal pain to exclude an incarcerated hernia or ovary or torsion of the ovary or testicle (see Chapter 18).

Palpate for Hernias

Palpate for inguinal, incisional, femoral, and umbilical hernias. Uncomplicated hernias will reduce; strangulated ones will not. Bowel sounds will be present in uncomplicated hernias.

Percuss for Flank Tenderness

The use of direct or indirect percussion over the costovertebral angle (CVA) can elicit tenderness if the kidney is involved. Flank pain, especially with the occurrence of hematuria, can indicate a kidney stone.

Test for Peritoneal Irritation

Several maneuvers can be used to test for peritoneal irritation.
- *Obturator muscle test.* Perform this test when you suspect a ruptured appendix or

pelvic abscess because these conditions can cause irritation of the obturator muscle. Pain in the hypogastric region is a positive sign, indicating obturator muscle irritation. With the patient supine, flex the right leg at the hip and knee to 90 degrees. Hold the leg just above the knee, grasp the ankle, and rotate the leg laterally and medially.

- *Iliopsoas muscle test.* Perform this test when you suspect appendicitis because an inflamed appendix can cause irritation of the lateral iliopsoas muscle. Pain in the lower quadrant is a positive test result. With the patient supine, place your hand over the lower thigh and have the patient raise the leg, flexing at the hip while you push downward against the leg.
- *Markle (heel drop) test.* Perform this test if you suspect appendicitis. The patient stands with straightened knees and then rises up on the toes. The patient then relaxes and allows the heels to hit the floor, thus jarring the body. The maneuver will cause abdominal pain if positive.
- *Rovsing test.* Perform this test if you suspect appendicitis. Press on the left lower quadrant (LLQ). If pain in the right lower quadrant (RLQ) is intensified, the test result is positive.

Perform a Pelvic Examination in Patients with a Vagina and Uterus

Perform a pelvic examination in women to rule out STI, PID, ovarian pain, ectopic pregnancy, and uterine fibroids. Vaginal discharge may or may not be present with STI or PID. Bleeding can accompany ectopic pregnancy.

Cervical motion tenderness (CMT) is the hallmark of PID. CMT plus adnexal pain (often bilateral) in the presence of abdominal pain and lower abdominal tenderness are criteria for a presumptive diagnosis of PID.

Adnexal tenderness in the region of pain can signal ectopic pregnancy. An adnexal mass may or may not be palpable, and its presence is not diagnostic. Vague adnexal tenderness can be present with STI. Bilateral, inflammatory ovarian pain and tenderness are usually related to PID, appendicitis, or peritonitis. A functional cyst can produce unilateral tenderness. Uterine

fibroids may be palpable as masses in the uterus, or the entire uterus may be enlarged.

Perform Genital and Prostate Examinations in Patients with a Penis and Prostate

Perform genital and prostate examinations in men to rule out STIs and prostatitis. Look for penile discharge as an indicator of STI and perhaps prostatitis. A tender prostate signals prostatitis. In acute prostatitis, make sure the examination is gentle; vigorous examination or massage of the prostate can cause bacterial release and produce septicemia (see Chapter 18).

Perform Digital Rectal Examination

Look for frank blood and test for occult blood. The presence of blood can indicate an acute process or carcinoma. Palpate for masses, polyps, and lesions. Occasionally, patients with a rectocecal appendix and appendicitis can have a tender, localized mass on rectal examination, even though the abdominal examination is normal.

Check Peripheral Pulses

Diminished femoral pulses in the presence of a pulsatile abdominal mass suggest ruptured abdominal aortic aneurysm.

Perform a Generalized Examination as Indicated

Because abdominal pain can be referred from other areas, examine the lungs, cardiovascular system, head and neck structures, and musculoskeletal system. Palpate for regional lymphadenopathy.

LABORATORY AND DIAGNOSTIC STUDIES

Complete Blood Count with Differential

An elevated white blood cell (WBC) count indicates an inflammatory or infectious condition.

Pregnancy Test

Urine or serum testing for the beta subunit of the human chorionic gonadotropin (β-hCG) is used to identify or rule out pregnancy. Use serial quantitative serum testing if you are concerned about ectopic pregnancy.

Erythrocyte Sedimentation Rate

Inflammation or tissue injury causes an increased erythrocyte sedimentation rate (ESR). However, the test is nonspecific and does not indicate the source. The ESR is often elevated as a result of PID, infectious states, or AIDS.

Cardiac Enzymes

Cardiac troponin (T or I; cTnT or cTnI) and creatinine kinase MB isoenzyme (CK-MB) are used in diagnosing MI (see Chapter 8).

Urinalysis

Urinalysis (U/A) is used to evaluate for kidney infection, presence of a kidney stone, renal failure, or a systemic disease. Microscopic hematuria suggests UTI or stone. Glycosuria and ketonuria suggest metabolic disturbances. A positive nitrite test on a U/A dipstick indicates the presence of bacteria, which can be seen on microscopic examination. The finding of 20 or more bacteria per high-powered field (HPF) indicates a UTI. The presence of greater than 0 to 1 RBCs/HPF or greater than 0 to 4 WBCs/HPF on microscopic examination also suggests UTI. RBCs can also be present as a contaminant with vaginal bleeding. The presence of red cell casts suggests kidney disease or renal infarction. White cell casts indicate pyelonephritis.

Urine for Culture and Sensitivity

If you suspect UTI, consider a urine test for culture and sensitivity (C&S). Uncomplicated UTIs may be treated empirically.

Molecular Testing for Sexually Transmitted Infection

DNA probes or nucleic acid amplification tests (NAAT) test for infectious organisms of *Chlamydia trachomatis, Neisseria gonorrhoeae, Trichomonas vaginalis, Gardnerella vaginalis,* and *Candida* spp. Obtain a sample of vaginal or penile discharge with a sterile swab and place it in the medium provided. Urine can also be tested for chlamydia and gonorrhea. The results are rapid and have high sensitivity and specificity. DNA probe testing has largely replaced Gram staining and culture.

Potassium Hydroxide Test

The potassium hydroxide (KOH) test involves direct microscopic examination of material to determine whether fungus is present. View under the microscope for the presence of mycelial fragments, hyphae, and budding yeast cells (see Chapter 37). The presence of fishy odor (the "whiff test") suggests bacterial vaginosis.

Saline Wet Prep

In a female with vaginal discharge, this test can demonstrate the presence of *Trichomonas vaginalis* or *Gardnerella* organisms by microscopic examination. The presence of trichomonads indicates *T. vaginalis.* The presence of bacteria-filled epithelial cells (clue cells) indicates bacterial vaginosis *(Gardnerella)* (see Chapter 37).

Fecal Occult Blood Test

Perform the fecal occult blood test (FOBT) to rule out GI bleeding. The test result is positive if a stool smear on a prepared card turns color (usually blue or green) when a solution is applied. A three-sample series provides more reliable results.

Fecal Immunochemical Test

Also called immunochemical FOBT (iFOBT), the fecal immunochemical test (FIT) uses antibodies to hemoglobin to detect a specific portion of a human blood protein. This test is done essentially the same way as conventional FOBT but is more specific and reduces the number of false positive results. Vitamins or foods do not affect the fecal immunochemical test, and some forms require only one or two stool specimens.

Stool Testing

Stool testing for ova and parasites and giardia can be useful in patients with abdominal pain accompanied by diarrhea and who have traveled recently. Fresh stool is required to preserve the trophozoites of some parasites. Giardia antigen test is a solid phase immunoassay used for the detection of Giardia-specific antigen 65. Only one stool specimen is required, and the test result is available within 1 day.

Rapid Strep Screen

The throat and tonsils are swabbed, and a rapid antigen test is ordered. The test can determine if strep is present. A negative strep result often indicates no group A streptococcus is present.

Electrocardiogram

An electrocardiogram (ECG) can add objective data to the diagnostic process if you suspect the pain is of cardiac origin. ST segment elevation or depression indicates the presence of injured myocardium. T-wave inversion will demonstrate the presence of ischemia. The appearance of both strongly supports ischemia but is not diagnostic of coronary artery disease. Arterial spasm, pericarditis, and electrolyte imbalance can also cause these variations from normal (see Chapter 8).

Helicobacter Pylori Testing

Helicobacter pylori (H. pylori) testing may be useful in high prevalence areas or in patients with epigastric pain when *H. pylori* infection is suspected. Laboratory methods for testing include antibody or antigen testing with serology, urine or stool, or urea breath test.

Radiography

Abdominal radiographs are of limited value in evaluating abdominal pain. An anteroposterior radiograph of the abdomen shows the kidneys, ureters, and bladder (KUB) and adjacent structures. It can be used to exclude free air (perforation) and obstruction (e.g., renal calculi) or to confirm intestinal obstruction. A chest radiograph can reveal the presence of pneumonia or air under the diaphragm (see Chapters 40 and 41).

Abdominal and Pelvic Ultrasound

Abdominal ultrasound is useful if you are considering ectopic pregnancy, abdominal aortic aneurysm, acute cholecystitis, acute pancreatitis, incarcerated hernia, hernia, or diverticular disease.

Computed Tomography and Magnetic Resonance Imaging

Computed tomography (CT) scanning and magnetic resonance imaging (MRI) are appropriate if you suspect retroperitoneal bleeding, pelvic abscess, pancreatitis, obstruction, hernia, incarcerated hernia, or diverticular disease. CT scanning is the preferred imaging study for diagnosing suspected appendicitis and in patients in whom appendiceal perforation is suspected. Noncontrast-enhanced helical CT is used to definitively diagnose urolithiasis. Helical CT scanning with rectal contrast is accurate and efficient in evaluating adults with equivocal presentations for appendicitis.

Colonoscopy or Sigmoidoscopy

If you suspect GI origin of pain, both colonoscopy and sigmoidoscopy are useful in directly visualizing the colon.

Anorectal Manometry

Anorectal manometry is used to evaluate constipation or fecal incontinence. The test measures the pressures of the anal sphincter muscles, the sensation in the rectum, and the neural reflexes that are needed for normal bowel movements.

 EVIDENCE-BASED PRACTICE *Use of Computed Tomography in Diagnosing Appendicitis in Children*

This study evaluated the impact of a clinical algorithm on computed tomography (CT) use and diagnostic accuracy of appendicitis in children. The study included 331 patients with 41% in the preimplementation period and 59% in the postimplementation period. CT use decreased from 39% to 18% ($P < .001$) after implementation of the algorithm. The negative appendectomy rate increased from 9% to 11% ($P = .59$). Use of CT did not have an impact on the risk of negative appendectomy ($P = .64$). The authors concluded that use of CT was significantly reduced after implementing a diagnostic algorithm for appendicitis without having an impact on diagnostic accuracy. Given the concern for increased risk of cancer after CT, these results support use of an algorithm in children with suspected appendicitis.

Reference: Polites et al, 2014.

DIFFERENTIAL DIAGNOSIS

When there is no worrisome history or there are no physical findings, use the specific history questions to point you in the right direction. Then determine whether the clinical findings are consistent. Review the history to see evolution over time, especially of an acute condition.

Identify physical findings that are worrisome as well, such as lower abdominal pain beginning at older age, involuntary weight loss, abnormal bleeding in a perimenopausal or postmenopausal woman, palpable abdominal or pelvic mass, or stool that is positive for occult blood.

Initially, look for surgical problems. Serial abdominal examinations are the best indicator of progression of an abdominal problem. Try to identify what organ seems to be involved and remember that extraabdominal systems can cause abdominal pain (e.g., pneumonia). Try to determine if the pain is organic or functional in origin. Remember that common causes of acute pain differ from common causes of chronic pain. Box 3.3 lists indicators of abdominal emergencies.

Acute Conditions That Cause Abdominal Pain

Appendicitis

The incidence of appendicitis peaks at age 10 to 20 years, although it can occur at any age. The patient reports sudden onset of colicky pain that progresses to a constant pain. The pain can begin in the epigastrium or periumbilicus and later localize to the RLQ. The pain worsens with movement or coughing. Vomiting after the onset of pain sometimes occurs. On physical examination, the patient will be lying still and demonstrate involuntary guarding. Classically, tenderness occurs in the RLQ. The results of other tests for peritoneal irritation will be positive. Rebound tenderness may be present. Variation in presentation is common, particularly with infants, children, and older adults. Diagnostic testing includes complete blood count (CBC) with differential to confirm or rule

Box 3.3	Indicators of Abdominal Emergencies

SUBJECTIVE FINDINGS	OBJECTIVE FINDINGS
• Progressive intractable vomiting	• Involuntary guarding
• Lightheadedness on standing	• Progressive abdomen distention
• Acute onset of pain	• Orthostatic hypotension
• Pain that progresses in intensity over hours	• Fever
	• Leukocytosis and granulocytosis
	• Decreased urine output

EVIDENCE-BASED PRACTICE *Clinical Diagnosis of Appendicitis*

In a review of clinical decision rules to assist in diagnosing appendicitis, the authors concluded that decision models that score combinations of findings from the history and clinical examination are more powerful than any single finding. They point to the Alvarado model as one that balances accuracy with ease of use and familiarity to clinicians. It combines the results for eight findings; a score of 7 or more of a potential 10 indicates the need for surgical intervention. The Alvarado model has a sensitivity of 81% and a specificity of 74%.

ALVARADO SCORE FOR EARLY DIAGNOSIS OF ACUTE APPENDICITIS

VARIABLE	SCORE
Migration of pain	1
Anorexia-acetone	1
Nausea or vomiting	1
Tenderness in the RLQ	2
Rebound pain	1
Elevation of temperature	1
Leukocytosis	2
Shift to the left on differential (neutrophils >75%)	1
Maximum total score	10
Positive score	**≥7[a]**

[a]A score of 7 or more indicates the need for surgical intervention.
References: Wagner and Shojania, 2009; Alvarado, 1986.
RLQ, Right lower quadrant.

out infection and the use of either ultrasonography, CT scan, or MRI. Ultrasonography is the preferred modality, with MRI and CT used if diagnosis remains unclear.

Ectopic pregnancy

Ectopic pregnancy can occur in any sexually active woman of childbearing age, especially those with a history of irregular menses. The patient experiences a sudden onset of spotting and persistent cramping in the lower quadrant that begins shortly after a missed period. On examination, the patient shows signs of hemorrhage, shock, and lower abdominal peritoneal irritation that can be lateralized. On pelvic examination, the uterus is enlarged but smaller than anticipated from dates provided. The cervix is tender to motion, and a tender adnexal mass can be palpable. Diagnosis is confirmed by positive hCG test results and ultrasound. Serial quantitative serum hCG levels can be useful. A ruptured ectopic pregnancy is a surgical emergency.

Peptic ulcer perforation

The patient reports sudden onset of severe, intense, steady epigastric pain that radiates to the sides, back, or right shoulder. The patient can give a history of burning, gnawing pain that worsens with an empty stomach. The patient lies as still as possible. Epigastric tenderness will be present with palpation or percussion. Rebound tenderness is intense. The abdominal muscles are rigid, and bowel sounds can be absent. The diagnosis is confirmed by upright or lateral decubitus radiographs, showing air under the diaphragm or in the peritoneal cavity. Perforation is a surgical emergency.

Dissection of aortic aneurysm

This condition occurs most frequently in men and persons older than 50 years, especially those with a history of uncontrolled hypertension. The patient experiences the sudden onset of excruciating pain that can be felt in the chest or abdomen and may radiate to the legs and back. Vital signs will reflect impending shock, and there can be a deficit or difference in femoral pulses. The diagnosis can be made by CT or MRI. Additional tests include ECG and cardiac enzymes. This is a surgical emergency with a high death rate.

Myocardial infarction

In patients older than 50 years, acute MI can present with abdominal pain and GI symptoms rather than the classic chest pain. If there is no other explanation for the pain, consider a cardiac origin.

Peritonitis

The most common cause of peritonitis is perforation of the GI tract. It occurs more often in older adults. The patient experiences the sudden onset of severe pain that is diffuse and worsens with movement or coughing. On examination, the patient will be guarding and have rebound tenderness. Bowel sounds will be decreased or absent. Diagnostic tools include CBC with differential and abdominal radiographs.

Acute pancreatitis

Acute pancreatitis is more common in patients with cholelithiasis or a history of alcohol abuse. The pain is steady and boring in quality and is unrelieved by change of position. It is located in the left upper quadrant (LUQ) and radiates to the back. The patient can also experience nausea, vomiting, and diaphoresis and will appear acutely ill. Abdominal distention, decreased bowel sounds, and diffuse rebound tenderness will be present on physical examination. The upper abdomen can show muscle rigidity. Examination of the lungs can reveal limited diaphragmatic excursion. Diagnostic testing includes CBC with differential, ultrasonography, radiography, and serum amylase and lipase levels.

Mesenteric adenitis

Adenovirus-induced (commonly *Yersinia* spp.) adenopathy of the mesenteric lymph nodes can result in fever and RLQ abdominal pain that mimics appendicitis. This condition is difficult to diagnose, but the WBC count is elevated and an abdominal radiograph will show abnormalities of the terminal ileus.

Cholecystitis or lithiasis

Cholecystitis or lithiasis occurs more often in adults than in children and more often in females than in males. The pain is colicky in nature and progresses to a constant pain. The patient reports pain in the RUQ, which can radiate to the right scapular area. The typical pain of cholelithiasis is constant, progressively rising to a plateau and falling gradually. The patient can also experience nausea and vomiting and give a history of dark urine or light stools. On physical examination, the patient will be tender to palpation or percussion in the RUQ. The gallbladder is palpable in about half of cases of cholecystitis. Painful splinting of respiration during deep inspiration (Murphy sign) is frequently present with cholecystitis. Diagnostic testing includes CBC with differential, ultrasonography, radiography, and serum amylase and lipase levels.

Ureterolithiasis

The patient reports the sudden onset of excruciating intermittent colicky pain that can progress to a constant pain. The pain is in the lower abdomen and flank and radiates to the groin. The patient can also experience nausea, vomiting, abdominal distention, chills, and fever. There is CVA tenderness on examination along with increased sensitivity in the lumbar and groin areas. Hematuria and increased frequency of urination can be present. U/A should be performed. Urine pH and the presence of crystals can help identify stone composition. Definitive diagnostic testing is via noncontrast-enhanced helical CT.

Urinary tract infection and pyelonephritis

Abdominal pain associated with UTI or pyelonephritis is common in children and could be the only presenting complaint. U/A and C&S are done to confirm the diagnosis.

Pelvic inflammatory disease and salpingitis

Pelvic inflammatory disease occurs most commonly in women younger than 35 years of age who are sexually active and have more than one sexual partner. Infection results from organisms transmitted via intercourse, through childbirth, or with abortion. PID is most often caused by *Chlamydia trachomatis* and *Neisseria gonorrhoeae*. Infection begins intravaginally in most cases and then spreads upward, causing salpingitis. The tubal infection produces an exudate, and as it spreads, peritonitis can result. The onset is usually shortly after menses. Patients have lower abdominal pain that becomes progressively more severe. On examination, abdominal tenderness, CMT, and adnexal tenderness (usually bilateral) are present. With peritonitis, patients can also have guarding and rebound tenderness. Patients can also have a fever, irregular bleeding, vaginal discharge, or vomiting. WBC count and ESR are usually elevated. DNA probes, cultures, and Gram staining can assist with diagnosis.

Obstruction

Obstruction occurs most often in newborns, older adults, and those with recent GI surgery. The patient presents with a sudden onset of

---

EVIDENCE-BASED PRACTICE *Clinical Diagnosis of Acute Cholecystitis*

In both the original and updated systematic reviews, the authors concluded that no single clinical finding, or known combination of clinical history and physical examination findings, efficiently establishes a diagnosis of acute cholecystitis. Individual findings with the highest diagnostic value are a Murphy sign and right upper quadrant tenderness. The authors concluded the clinician's gestalt is the most important piece of evidence from the clinical evaluation and that bedside ultrasonography by a trained clinician may be useful in diagnosis.

Reference: Trowbridge et al, 2009.

crampy pain, usually in the umbilical area of the epigastrium. Vomiting occurs early with small intestinal obstruction and late with large bowel obstruction. Obstipation occurs with complete obstruction, but diarrhea can be present with partial obstruction. Hyperactive, high-pitched bowel sounds can be present in small bowel obstruction. A mass can be palpable in lower obstruction. Abdominal distention can be present. The rectum will be empty on digital examination. Diagnosis is confirmed with abdominal radiographs (supine and sitting), MRI, or CT.

Ileus

Ileus is associated with intraperitoneal or retroperitoneal infection, metabolic disturbances, and intraabdominal surgery. The patient experiences abdominal distention, vomiting, obstipation, and cramps. On auscultation, there is minimal or absent peristalsis. Abdominal radiographs show gaseous distention of isolated segments of both the small and large intestines.

Intussusception

Bowel obstruction in children ages 2 months to 2 years usually occurs in the ileocecal region and classically presents with vomiting, colicky abdominal pain with drawing up of the legs, and eventual currant jelly stools. The onset is dramatic. The child is asleep or awake when suddenly he or she cries out with severe pain. The child twists and squirms; nothing gives any relief until, almost suddenly, there is a lull with absence of pain followed by a similar painful episode. The abdomen has a sausage-shaped mass that can be felt in the RUQ. The stool tests positive for blood.

Malrotation and volvulus

Improper rotation and fixation of the duodenum and colon can cause an artery to obstruct, and the patient experiences ischemic necrosis. This disorder of the embryonic gut is usually seen in the first month of life. The infant presents with bilious emesis followed

by abdominal distention and GI bleeding. Shock occurs from progression of the ischemia.

Henoch-Schönlein purpura

In Henoch-Schönlein purpura, crampy, acute abdominal pain and bleeding are secondary to edema and hemorrhage of the intestinal wall. This disease is an immunoglobulin A (IgA)–mediated vasculitis that affects very small vessels. An urticarial rash occurring on the buttocks and lower extremities progresses to papular purpuric lesions. The laboratory findings show an elevated WBC count but a normal platelet count. A mild increase in ESR, an increase in IgA concentration, and negative antinuclear antibodies (ANA test) are also found.

Incarcerated hernia

Incarcerated hernia occurs most commonly in older adults. The patient reports a constant severe pain in the RLQ or LLQ that worsens with coughing or straining. Physical examination reveals a hernia or mass that is nonreducible. Diagnosis is confirmed by MRI or CT. Surgical intervention is indicated.

Pneumonia

Pneumonia is a frequently overlooked cause of abdominal pain in children. The pain is referred from right lower lobe pneumonia because of associated phrenic nerve irritation, which can cause muscular spasm, ileus, and pain referred to the RLQ. The WBC count in pneumonia is typically higher than that in early appendicitis.

CHRONIC CONDITIONS THAT CAUSE LOWER ABDOMINAL PAIN

Irritable bowel syndrome

Irritable bowel syndrome begins in adolescent and young adult years. It produces crampy hypogastric pain that is of variable, infrequent duration. The pain is associated with bowel function, gas, bloating, and distention. Relief is often obtained with the passage of flatus or feces. The patient has a normal abdominal examination and the stool is negative for blood. Consider a proctosigmoidoscopy or barium enema (BE) if onset is at middle age or older, if the stool is positive for blood, if there is a family history of colorectal cancer or polyps, or if the patient fails to improve after 6 to 8 weeks of therapy.

Crohn disease

Crohn disease is an inflammatory bowel disease that presents with abdominal pain or cramping, abdominal tenderness, and diarrhea (see Chapter 12). Rectal bleeding may accompany the diarrhea.

Lactose intolerance

Lactose intolerance produces crampy pain and diarrhea after the consumption of milk or milk product foods (see Chapter 12). It is caused by a deficiency in lactase, an enzyme that decreases in activity with increasing age. It is more common in Asians, Native Americans, and African Americans. A trial elimination of offending foods can aid in diagnosis. The use of the Hydrogen Breath Test for diagnoses is popular but lacks sensitivity and specificity.

Diverticular disease

Diverticular disease causes localized abdominal pain and tenderness. The patient will have a fever, elevated ESR, and leukocytosis. Perform a barium enema or proctoscopy or colonoscopy if there is rectal bleeding.

Simple constipation

In adults, constipation is associated with infrequency, or difficulty passing dry, hard stools and abdominal bloating.

Children with constipation frequently report abdominal pain. The pain is usually colicky in nature but can be dull and steady. The pain varies and is not persistent or progressively worsening. Mild, poorly localized periumbilical tenderness, and perhaps guarding are reported. A fecal mass may be palpable.

Habitual constipation

With habitual constipation, the patient presents with a lifelong history of constipation with onset as a young adult, has a normal physical examination, and does not have occult blood in the stool. Diet, activity, and bowel habits are often causal factors. Consider sigmoidoscopy, anorectal manometry, or colonoscopy if you suspect a metabolic or systemic cause, if the stool is heme positive, or if the patient is middle-aged or older or fails to respond to treatment.

Dysmenorrhea

Dysmenorrhea, a typically lower abdominal pain or cramping, occurs with menstruation. Dysmenorrhea can be classified as primary (no organic cause) or secondary (pathological cause). In primary dysmenorrhea, the onset is usually soon after menarche and gradually diminishes with age. The woman will have a normal pelvic examination. Secondary dysmenorrhea is associated with specific conditions and disorders such as endometriosis, PID, cervical stenosis, and uterine fibroids. Obtain a gynecologic (GYN) consult or pelvic ultrasound for secondary dysmenorrhea, dysmenorrhea with increasing severity, or abnormal findings on pelvic examination.

Uterine fibroids

Fibroids produce pain related to the menstrual cycle and intercourse. The patient can experience dysfunctional uterine bleeding. On examination, palpable myomas are often present. Suspect this cause when there is no suspicion of other pelvic disorder. Order a pelvic ultrasound if ovarian or uterine neoplasm cannot be excluded. Obtain a GYN consult for abnormal bleeding or severe symptoms.

Hernia

A hernia is a loop of intestine that has prolapsed through the inguinal wall or canal or through the abdominal musculature. The patient reports intermittent localized pain that can be exacerbated with exertion or lifting. A physical examination will document the hernia, especially when the patient is instructed in maneuvers or positions to increase intraabdominal pressure. Consider CT or MRI if you suspect strangulation or bowel obstruction.

Ovarian cysts

Ovarian cysts occur most commonly in young women and produce adnexal pain. The cysts may be palpable, late cycle (corpus luteum) cysts. A pelvic ultrasound is indicated. Ovarian cysts can become quite large before producing symptoms.

Abdominal wall disorder

With abdominal wall disorder, the patient can present with a history of trauma. Ecchymosis or swelling may be visible. The patient may report pain with rectus muscle stress. GI and genitourinary symptoms are absent. A hernia may be palpable. Obtain a CT scan if internal disease cannot be excluded.

CHRONIC CONDITIONS THAT CAUSE UPPER ABDOMINAL PAIN

Esophagitis and gastroesophageal reflux disease

With GERD (see Chapter 20), the patient reports a burning, gnawing pain in the mid-epigastrium (heartburn) that worsens with recumbency. Regurgitation of gastric contents (water brash or pyrosis) that occurs with hypersalivation secondary to acid stimulation of the lower esophagus is commonly reported. The pain typically occurs after eating or when lying down and may be relieved with antacids. The physical examination results are negative. Consider endoscopy if symptoms are severe or the patient does not respond to therapy.

Peptic ulcer

The patient reports a burning or gnawing pain that occurs most often with an empty stomach, stress, and alcohol intake. The pain is relieved by food intake. Some patients describe the pain as a soreness, empty feeling, or hunger. Typical pain is steady, mild, or severe and located in the epigastrium. Complaints can be atypical in children and minimal in older adults. There can be epigastric tenderness on palpation. Endoscopy and *H. pylori* testing can aid in diagnosis.

Gastritis

Gastritis pain is a constant burning pain in the epigastric area that can be accompanied by nausea, vomiting, diarrhea, or fever. Alcohol, NSAIDs, and salicylates make the pain worse. The physical examination results are negative. No diagnostic testing is necessary if the patient responds to therapy.

Gastroenteritis

Gastroenteritis can occur at any age and produces a diffuse, crampy pain that is accompanied by nausea, vomiting, diarrhea, and fever. Hyperactive bowel sounds will be heard on auscultation. The condition usually resolves on its own, and no diagnostic testing is needed. If the patient has traveled recently, consider stool testing for ova and parasites and giardia

Abdominal migraine

This condition is most common in female children ages 7 to 10 years old. Patients experience episodic periumbilical pain lasting more than 1 hour that is accompanied by nausea, photophobia, headache, and vomiting. In between episodes, patients are healthy and symptom free. There is frequently a family history of migraines.

Functional dyspepsia

Functional dyspepsia refers to GI symptoms in which a pathological condition is not present or does not entirely explain the clinical presentation, although altered physiological activity can be present. The patient has vague reports of indigestion, heartburn, gaseousness, or fullness. The patient also reports belching, abdominal distention, and occasionally nausea. The physical examination results are negative. Perform a CBC and fecal testing for occult blood. Test for presence of *H. pylori* infection. Consider endoscopy if there is no response to empiric treatment. Consider an upper and lower GI series if the patient also has dysphagia, weight loss, vomiting, or a change in the pattern of the symptoms (see Chapter 20).

Recurrent abdominal pain

Recurrent abdominal pain (RAP) usually presents in children 5 to 10 years of age—rarely after 14 years of age. The patient reports dull, colicky, periumbilical pain that is intermittent, occurs daily, and lasts from 1 to 3 hours with complete recovery between episodes. The pain does not awaken the child from sleep but can interfere with the ability to fall asleep. The child can have a low-grade fever, pallor, headache, and constipation. A history of stress associated with school social activities, parental conflicts, or with loss is frequently elicited. Physical examination results are essentially negative. Initial laboratory tests are CBC, ESR, U/A, fecal blood testing, and stool for ova and parasites (O&P).

> ## DIFFERENTIAL DIAGNOSIS OF *Common Causes of Acute Abdominal Pain*

CONDITION	HISTORY	PHYSICAL FINDINGS	DIAGNOSTIC STUDIES
Appendicitis	Age 10–20 yr, although it can occur at any age; patient reports sudden onset of colicky pain that progresses to constant pain; pain can begin in epigastrium or periumbilicus and then later localizes in RLQ; pain worsens with movement or coughing; vomiting after onset of pain is sometimes present	Patient lying still; involuntary guarding; tenderness in RLQ; other tests for peritoneal irritation positive; rebound tenderness; variation in presentation common, particularly with infants, children, and older adults	CBC with differential, ultrasonography (preferred), CT, MRI
Ectopic pregnancy	Women of childbearing age; sudden onset of spotting and persistent cramping in lower quadrant that begins shortly after missed period	Signs of hemorrhage, shock, and lower abdominal peritoneal irritation that can be lateralized; enlarged uterus; CMT; tender adnexal mass	Positive hCG, ultrasound; ruptured ectopic pregnancy is surgical emergency
Peptic ulcer perforation	Sudden onset of severe intense, steady epigastric pain that radiates to sides, back, or right shoulder; history of burning, gnawing pain that worsens with empty stomach	Patient lying still; epigastric tenderness; rebound tenderness; abdominal muscles rigid; bowel sounds can be absent	Diagnosis confirmed by upright or lateral decubitus radiograph showing air under diaphragm or in peritoneal cavity; perforation is surgical emergency

Continued

> **DIFFERENTIAL DIAGNOSIS OF** *Common Causes of Acute Abdominal Pain—cont'd*

CONDITION	HISTORY	PHYSICAL FINDINGS	DIAGNOSTIC STUDIES
Dissection of aortic aneurysm	Most frequent in older adults, especially if hypertensive; sudden onset of excruciating pain that can be felt in chest or abdomen and can radiate to legs and back	Patient appears shocky, vital signs reflect impending shock; deficit or difference in femoral pulses	CT or MRI; additional tests include ECG and cardiac enzymes; surgical emergency
Myocardial infarction	Upper or diffuse abdominal pain; can be accompanied by nausea, vomiting, dyspepsia	Hypertension or hypotension, cardiac arrhythmia, paradoxical S_2	Serial ECG, serial cardiac enzymes
Peritonitis	Occurs more often in older adults; sudden onset of severe pain that is diffuse and worsens with movement or coughing	Guarding; rebound tenderness; bowel sounds decreased or absent	CBC with differential, abdominal radiographs
Acute pancreatitis	History of cholelithiasis or excessive alcohol use; pain is steady and boring in quality and is unrelieved by change of position; located in LUQ and radiates to back; nausea, vomiting, and diaphoresis	Patient appears acutely ill; abdominal distention, decreased bowel sounds, diffuse rebound tenderness; upper abdomen can show muscle rigidity; can have limited diaphragmatic excursion of lungs	CBC with differential, serum amylase and lipase levels, triglyceride level, calcium level, and liver chemistries; ultrasonography; CT
Mesenteric adenitis	Fever, pain in RLQ, other symptoms suggestive of appendicitis	Pain on palpation in RLQ; there can be pharyngitis, cervical adenopathy	CBC with differential; adenovirus found in tissue of surgical specimen
Cholecystitis or lithiasis	Appears in adults more than in children, females more than males; colicky pain with progression to constant pain; pain in RUQ that can radiate to right scapular area; pain of cholelithiasis is constant, progressively rising to plateau and falling gradually; nausea, vomiting, history of dark urine or light stools; may be aggravated by certain foods	Tender to palpation or percussion in RUQ; gallbladder palpable in about half cases of cholecystitis; positive Murphy sign	CBC with differential, ultrasonography, radiographs, serum amylase and lipase levels

> **DIFFERENTIAL DIAGNOSIS OF** *Common Causes of Acute Abdominal Pain—cont'd*

CONDITION	HISTORY	PHYSICAL FINDINGS	DIAGNOSTIC STUDIES
Ureterolithiasis	Sudden onset, excruciating intermittent colicky pain that can progress to constant pain; pain in lower abdomen and flank and radiates to groin; nausea, vomiting, abdominal distention, chills, and fever; increased frequency of urination	CVA tenderness; increased sensitivity in lumbar and groin areas; hematuria	U/A, noncontrast-enhanced helical CT
Urinary tract infection (UTI) or pyelonephritis	Urinary symptoms with UTI, back pain with pyelonephritis; infants present with fever, failure to thrive, irritability; toddlers report pain in abdomen; may not report dysuria or frequency	Altered voiding pattern, malodorous urine, fever	U/A and culture
Pelvic inflammatory disease (PID)	Lower abdominal pain that becomes progressively more severe; can have irregular bleeding, vaginal discharge, and vomiting; most common in sexually active women	Abdominal tenderness, CMT and adnexal tenderness (usually bilateral); with peritonitis can also have guarding and rebound tenderness; fever and vaginal discharge common	WBC count and ESR usually elevated; DNA testing, cultures and Gram staining for STIs
Obstruction	Sudden onset of crampy pain usually in umbilical area of epigastrium; vomiting occurs early with small intestinal obstruction and late with large bowel obstruction; obstipation or diarrhea	Hyperactive, high-pitched bowel sounds; fecal mass can be palpated; abdominal distention; empty rectum on digital examination	Diagnosis confirmed with CT, abdominal radiographs
Ileus	Abdominal distention, vomiting, obstipation, and cramps	Minimal or absent peristalsis on auscultation	Gaseous distention of isolated segments of both small and large intestines shown on radiographs
Intussusception	Sudden-onset pain in infant; occurs with sudden relief, then pain again	Fever, vomiting, currant jelly stools	Abdominal films, ultrasound
Malrotation or volvulus	Seen in infants up to 1 mo old; irritability, pain	Bilious emesis, abdominal distention	Abdominal films

Continued

▶ DIFFERENTIAL DIAGNOSIS OF *Common Causes of Acute Abdominal Pain—cont'd*

CONDITION	HISTORY	PHYSICAL FINDINGS	DIAGNOSTIC STUDIES
Henoch-Schönlein purpura	Seen in children age 2–8 yr	Rash on lower extremities or buttocks; arthralgias; hematuria	CBC, ESR, serum IgA
Incarcerated hernia	More common in older adults; constant severe pain in RLQ or LLQ that worsens with coughing or straining	Hernia or mass that is nonreducible	MRI, CT, ultrasound
Pneumonia	Children age 2–5 yr can present with only abdominal pain and fever	Tachypnea, retractions, pallor, nasal flaring, crackles	CBC, chest radiograph demonstrating infiltrations
Irritable bowel syndrome (IBS)	Begins in adolescence or as young adult; hypogastric pain; crampy, variable infrequent duration; associated with bowel function; associated with gas, bloating, distention; relief with passage of flatus, feces	Normal examination; heme-negative stool	Proctosigmoidoscopy, colonoscopy if onset at middle age or older, stool positive for blood, family history of colorectal cancer or polyps, failure to improve after 6–8 wk of therapy
Crohn disease	Abdominal pain with chronic bloody diarrhea	Abdominal tenderness; weight loss	Colonoscopy or biopsy
Lactose intolerance	Crampy pain after eating milk or milk products	Negative physical examination results	Trial elimination of offending foods Hydrogen Breath Test may be useful
Diverticular disease	Localized pain, usually LLQ; older patient	Abdominal tenderness; fever	CT, contrast enema, cystography, ultrasound, colonoscopy sometimes useful but not used during acute attack
Simple constipation	Colicky or dull and steady pain that does not progress and worsen	Fecal mass palpable, stool in rectum	None
Habitual constipation	Lifelong history; younger patient	Normal examination; heme-negative stool	Sigmoidoscopy, anorectal manometry, colonoscopy if symptoms are alarming
Dysmenorrhea	Typical premenstrual pain onset soon after menarche, gradually diminishing with age	Normal pelvic examination	Gynecology consult; pelvic ultrasound if secondary dysmenorrhea, increasing disability, or abnormal pelvic examination

> **DIFFERENTIAL DIAGNOSIS OF** *Common Causes of Acute Abdominal Pain—cont'd*

CONDITION	HISTORY	PHYSICAL FINDINGS	DIAGNOSTIC STUDIES
Uterine fibroids	Pain related to menses, intercourse	Palpable myomas; no suspicion of other pelvic disorder	Pelvic ultrasound if ovarian or uterine neoplasm cannot be excluded; gynecology consult if abnormal bleeding or severe symptoms
Hernia	Localized pain that increases with exertion or lifting	Physical examination documents hernia	MRI, CT, ultrasound, BE if suspect strangulation or bowel obstruction
Ovarian cyst(s)	Young woman	Adnexal pain and palpable ovarian cysts, especially in late cycle (corpus luteum)	Pelvic ultrasound
Abdominal wall disorder	History of trauma	Visible ecchymosis or swelling; palpable hernia pain with rectus muscle stress; no GI or GU symptoms	CT if internal disease cannot be excluded
Esophagitis or GERD (see Chapter 20)	Burning, gnawing pain in midepigastrium that worsens with recumbency; water brash; pain occurs after eating and can be relieved with antacids; in infant: failure to thrive, irritability, postprandial spitting and vomiting	Physical examination negative; in infants: weight loss, in some cases aspiration pneumonia	Endoscopy if symptoms are severe or do not respond to therapy; manometry, pH monitoring
Peptic ulcer	Burning or gnawing pain; soreness, empty feeling, or hunger; occurs most often with empty stomach, stress, and alcohol, and relieved by food intake; pain steady, mild, or severe and located in epigastrium; can be atypical in children and minimal in older adults	Can be epigastric tenderness on palpation	*Helicobacter pylori* testing; endoscopy if no response to therapy
Gastritis	Constant burning pain in epigastric area that can be accompanied by nausea, vomiting, diarrhea, or fever; alcohol, NSAIDs, and salicylates make pain worse	Physical examination negative	No diagnostic testing necessary if patient responds to therapy

Continued

DIFFERENTIAL DIAGNOSIS OF *Common Causes of Acute Abdominal Pain—cont'd*

CONDITION	HISTORY	PHYSICAL FINDINGS	DIAGNOSTIC STUDIES
Gastroenteritis	Occurs at any age and produces diffuse crampy pain accompanied by nausea, vomiting, diarrhea, and fever; can have history of recent travel, family members ill	Hyperactive bowel sounds will be heard on auscultation; dehydration if severe	No diagnostic testing needed; if recent travel test for O&P, giardia
Functional dyspepsia	Vague reports of indigestion, heartburn, gassiness, or fullness; belching, abdominal distention, and occasionally nausea	Physical examination negative	*H. pylori* testing; consider endoscopy if no response to empiric treatment; CBC, FOBT, or FIT
Abdominal migraine	Girls age 7–10 yr; episodic periumbilical pain lasting more than 1 hr accompanied by nausea, photophobia, headache, and vomiting; family history of migraines	Physical examination negative	Rule out other causes of episodic pain
Recurrent abdominal pain (RAP)	Children age 5–10 yr; history of environmental or psychological stress	Physical examination negative	CBC, U/A, ESR, FOBT, or FIT, stool for O&P

BE, barium enema; *CBC,* complete blood count; *CMT,* cervical motion tenderness; *CT,* computed tomography; *CVA,* costovertebral angle; *ECG,* electrocardiography; *ESR,* erythrocyte sedimentation rate; *FIT,* fecal immunochemical test; *FOBT,* fecal occult blood test; *GERD,* gastroesophageal reflux disease; *GI,* gastrointestinal; *GU,* genitourinary; *GYN,* gynecological; *hCG,* human chorionic gonadotropin test; *LLQ,* left lower quadrant; *LUQ,* left upper quadrant; *MRI,* magnetic resonance imaging; *NSAID,* nonsteroidal antiinflammatory drug; *O&P,* ova and parasites; *RLQ,* right lower quadrant; *RUQ,* right upper quadrant; *WBC,* white blood cell.

4 Affective Changes

A large percentage of primary care visits have psychological or psychosocial origins. A practitioner must first rule out organic causes for symptoms, mood changes, and behavior changes. Some patients are able to express that their symptoms could be related to situational stress or a psychosocial cause. Others can identify that psychological or emotional difficulties are causing worrisome symptoms or symptoms that interfere with their ability to function. Often the practitioner suspects an underlying psychological or psychosocial disturbance that the patient is not able to articulate. In some cases, a parent has concerns about a child's or adolescent's behavior. This chapter focuses on commonly encountered psychological conditions and psychosocial concerns and provides an approach to elicit more information, determine suicide risk, and evaluate for a diagnosable psychological disorder (Fig. 4.1).

Do not assume that an emotional symptom has a psychosocial cause until physical causes have been fully explored. Anxiety and depression are prevalent in the primary care setting. Although they are distinct diagnoses, they often co-occur. Substance use is either a primary condition that is the cause of psychological concern or a comorbid condition that is a consequence of a psychological or psychosocial condition.

DIAGNOSTIC REASONING: FOCUSED HISTORY

Is this a psychosocial problem?

Key Questions (to self)
- Does the presenting concern provide any clues?
- Are behavioral cues present?

Presenting Concern

Fatigue, lack of energy, sleep disturbance, and an inability to concentrate are symptoms that can bring a patient to the primary care setting. These symptoms are common in patients experiencing situational stress, depression, anxiety, or substance use problems. Prolonged somatic symptoms that have not been diagnosed, such as headache, chest pain, abdominal pain, low back pain, or dizziness, can suggest a psychosocial or psychological cause. It is imperative that you consider these clues as you rule out an organic cause. Also see specific chapters that address these symptoms.

A parent may relate that a child's behavior is different from that of other children. On developmental screening, the very young child may have deficits in social skills and in preverbal language.

Behavioral Cues

A history of frequent primary care or emergency department visits for unexplained symptoms can point to a psychosocial cause. Sometimes the patient's behaviors and general appearance do not match the presenting concern. An emotional response that is not consistent with the severity of the presenting problem or situation can point to a psychosocial problem.

Agitation and restlessness are common manifestations of depression, anxiety, or substance abuse. Changes in personality or in relationships may be associated with substance abuse, depression, and anxiety.

Language and social skills that seem out of sync with general development are important cues that might indicate a more serious condition.

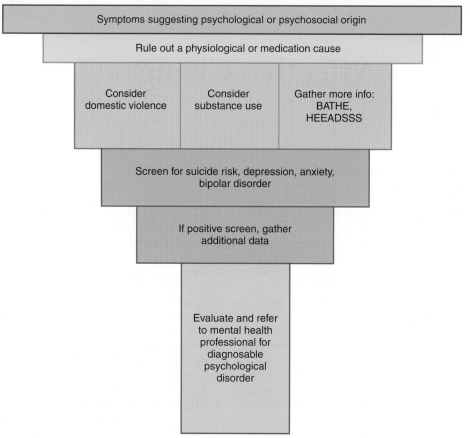

FIGURE 4.1 A suggested approach to the visit. There are areas of overlap. *BATHE,* Background, affect, trouble, handling, and empathy; *HEEADSSS,* home, education and employment, eating, peer-group activities, drugs, sexuality, suicide or depression, and safety.

Could this be a result of a physiological problem?

Key Questions

- Can you describe the symptoms you are having?
- Have you had a major illness recently?
- How long have you had these symptoms?

Symptoms

Physiological problems often present in the patient as abdominal pain (see Chapter 3), chest pain (see Chapter 8), confusion (especially in an older adult; see Chapter 9), dizziness (see Chapter 13), fatigue (see Chapter 16), headache (see Chapter 19), and sleep

disturbances (see Chapter 31). Refer to the specific chapters that discuss the evaluation of the presenting concern and symptom(s).

Major Illness or Chronic Conditions

Mood disorders can occur secondary to a physiological condition. Patients who have had a major health event, such as a myocardial infarction, stroke, or trauma, or who have chronic symptoms, such as pain, are at risk for the development of depression.

The mnemonic THINC MED is useful when evaluating for underlying organic causes of changes in mood or behavior. Box 4.1 identifies conditions that are commonly associated with anxiety and depression.

Box 4.1   THINC MED

Major categories of medical conditions that mimic psychological conditions are as follows:

T	Tumors
H	Hormones (e.g., thyroid, adrenal, gonads, insulin)
I	Infections and immune diseases (e.g., AIDS, lupus, syphilis, Lyme disease)
N	Nutrition
C	Central nervous system (e.g., head trauma, seizures, multiple sclerosis, Parkinson disease, dementia)
M	Miscellaneous (e.g., sleep apnea, anemia, congestive heart failure)
E	Electrolyte abnormalities and toxins (e.g., hypercalcemia, hypo- or hyperphosphatemia, hypo- or hypernatremia)
D	Drugs (including nicotine, caffeine, prescribed medications, illicit drugs, and alcohol)

Box 4.2   Medications Associated with Changes in Mood

MEDICATIONS THAT CAN CAUSE SYMPTOMS OF DEPRESSION
- Accutane
- Antabuse
- Anticonvulsants
- Antiparkinsonian medications
- Antivirals
- Barbiturates
- Benzodiazepines
- Beta-adrenergic blockers
- Calcium channel blockers
- Estrogens
- Fluoroquinolone antibiotics
- Interferon alfa
- Narcotics
- Statins

MEDICATIONS THAT CAN CAUSE SYMPTOMS OF ANXIETY
- Albuterol
- Theophylline
- Thyroid hormones

MEDICATIONS THAT CAN CAUSE SYMPTOMS OF MANIA
- Antabuse
- Anticholinergics
- Antiparkinsonian medications
- Capoten
- Cogentin
- Corticosteroids
- Cyclosporine
- Monoamine oxidase inhibitors
- Opioids
- Tagamet
- Thyroid hormones

Could this be caused by medication?

Key Questions
- What prescribed medications are you currently taking?
- What over-the-counter (OTC) or herbal medicines do you take?
- What dietary supplements are you taking?

Medication History

Many medications can cause psychiatric symptoms and mood changes. Box 4.2 lists medications that can produce symptoms of depression, anxiety, and mania. The Beers criteria identifies potentially inappropriate medications for older adults (available at http://onlinelibrary.wiley.com/doi/10.1111/jgs.13702/full).

OTC medications, herbal medicines, and dietary supplements

Some OTC medications, herbal preparations, dietary supplements, and energy drinks or substances that contain high levels of caffeine can contribute to psychiatric symptoms. A complete list of all preparations that the patient is taking is a starting point for evaluating side effects and interactions.

Is this a situation of domestic or partner violence?

Key Questions
- Have you been hit, kicked, punched, or otherwise hurt by someone within the past year?
- Do you feel safe in your current relationship?

- Is there a partner from a previous relationship who is making you feel unsafe now?

A positive response to any one of these three questions constitutes a positive screen for partner violence (Feldhaus et al, 1997). The first question, which addresses physical violence, has been validated in studies as an accurate measure of 1-year prevalence rates. The latter two questions evaluate the perception of safety and provide estimates of the short-term risk of further violence and the need for counseling, but reliability and validity evaluations have not yet been established. A positive screen result requires further assessment and clinical follow up, including ascertaining patient safety.

Is this a situation of elder abuse?

Key Questions
- Do you feel safe at home?
- Does anyone in your home hurt you?
- Has someone not helped you when you needed help?
- Are you prevented from seeing friends or family members whom you wish to see?
- Has money or property been taken from you without your consent?
- Have your credit or ATM cards been used without your consent?

Older and vulnerable adults who exhibit depression, anxiety, or other psychological symptoms may be experiencing abuse at home or by those providing care. The United States Preventive Services Task Force (USPSTF) has found no valid, reliable screening tools to identify abuse of older or vulnerable adults in the primary care setting (USPSTF, 2013). The above questions are directed at physical, psychological, and financial abuse (Lachs & Pillemer, 2017). A positive response requires further assessment and clinical follow up.

Could this be situational stress or normal grief?

The BATHE model provides a framework for understanding the patient in the context of his or her total life situation (Lieberman, 1997) and serves as a rough screening test for anxiety,

depression, or situational stress disorders; and takes minimal time. BATHE is a mnemonic for **b**ackground, **a**ffect, **t**rouble, **h**andling, and empathy.

Key Questions
Background: ascertains the context of the visit
- What is going on in your life?
- What is going on right now?
- Has anything changed recently?

Affect: elicits the emotional response and allows the patient to label the feeling
- How do you feel about that?
- What is your mood?

Trouble: determines the symbolic meaning of the situation for the patient
- What about the situation troubles you most?
- What worries or concerns you?

Handling: helps to assess patient resources and responses to the situation
- How are you handling that?
- How are you coping?

Empathy: reflects an understanding that the patient's response is reasonable under the circumstances
- That must be very difficult for you.
- I can understand that you would feel that way.

Could this be a result of substance abuse?

Key Questions
- In the past year, have you used alcohol or drugs more than you meant to?
- Have you wanted or needed to reduce your drinking or drug use in the past year?

A positive response to one question indicates a substance use concern and the need for further investigation. When the screen is positive, the CAGE questions can be used to detect alcoholism. Other substances can be substituted for alcohol in the CAGE questionnaire (Box 4.3). Other questionnaires, T-ACE and CRAFFT, for alcohol use are also available (Boxes 4.4 and 4.5).

How can I narrow my diagnosis?

Begin with broad screening questions. If the patient's response to the screening question(s)

CAGE Questionnaire

The CAGE questionnaire developed in 1984 includes four interview questions designed to help diagnose alcoholism. Answering yes to one or more of the four questions raises a high index of suspicion for alcohol abuse and dependence. The acronym CAGE helps practitioners quickly recall the main concepts of the four questions (cutting down, annoyance by criticism, guilty feeling, and eye openers).

The CAGE questionnaire has been used and tested extensively in many populations. It is considered to be a reliable method of screening for alcohol abuse in adults. It has reported sensitivities of 43% to 94% and specificities ranging from 70% to 97%.

The complete questionnaire can be found at http://addictionsandrecovery.org/addiction-self-test.htm.

Reference: Ewing, 1984.

T-ACE Questionnaire

This questionnaire provides a brief screening for prenatal detection of risk-drinking. The acronym stands for tolerance, annoyed, cut down, and eye opener. A positive answer to T alone, or to two of A, C, or E can signal a problem with a high degree of probability, and positive answers to all four indicates great certainty of a problem. The complete questionnaire can be found at https://www.mirecc.va.gov/visn22/T-ACE_alcohol_screen.pdf.

Reference: Sokol et al, 1989.

is positive, proceed to elicit more specific symptoms. Although a negative response to a given screening question decreases the likelihood of a disorder, the sensitivity of such screening is not perfect, and answers should be interpreted within the context of the patient's entire history and physical examination.

Key Questions
- Is there a personal or family history of mental illness?
- Is there a family history of autism?
- Over the past 2 weeks, have you felt down, depressed, or hopeless?

The CRAFFT Questionnaire

The CRAFFT questionnaire was developed as a screening tool for alcohol and substance abuse in adolescents. The CRAFFT acronym helps practitioners remember the main concepts of the six questions: car, relax, alone, forget, friends, and trouble. It is considered a valid screening test among all demographic subgroups of adolescents with reported sensitivities of 76% to 92% and specificities of 80% to 94%

The complete questionnaire can be found at http://archpedi.jamanetwork.com/article.aspx?articleid=203511.

Reference: Knight et al, 2002.

- Over the past 2 weeks, have you had little interest or pleasure in your daily activities?
- Do you tend to be an anxious or nervous person?
- Have you had periods of feeling so happy or energetic that your friends told you were talking too fast or that you were too "hyper"?

Prior Mental Illness, Family History

A personal or family history of prior mental illness increases the likelihood of a current mental illness. Studies support the influence of both behavioral and biological factors in the development of mental health conditions.

Family history of another child with autism increases the risk of autism in a sibling.

Down, Depressed, Hopeless, Loss of Interest or Pleasure

These are cardinal symptoms for depression, and the presence of at least one of these symptoms is required to diagnose clinically significant depression. Research suggests that asking the following two questions is as effective as longer inventories (Whooley et al, 1997):
- Over the past 2 weeks, have you felt down, depressed, or hopeless?
- Over the past 2 weeks, have you felt little interest or pleasure in your daily activities?

The two questions mirror those in the two-item Patient Health Questionnaire

(PHQ-2), which has been validated as a sensitive screening instrument depression (Maurer, 2012) If the screening result is positive, confirm with a more thorough assessment of neurovegetative signs (Box 4.6) and further investigation. In older adults, the Geriatric Depression Scale (see Chapter 9, Fig. 9-2) is positive for depression if the score is above 5.

Anxious or Nervous

Asking patients whether they feel anxious or nervous is useful as a general screen. Clinical experts suggest that unexplained somatic symptoms along with reports of agitation and difficulty maintaining concentration suggest anxiety rather than depression.

A positive response to a question about anxiety or nervousness can prompt further screening:
- Do you have anxiety or panic attacks?
- Have you had to limit your activities because of your anxiety?

The first question helps to differentiate anxiety from panic attacks. The second question points toward panic with agoraphobia. If the patient is not certain what you mean by the term "panic attacks," you can provide a simple description to clarify: "A panic attack is a sudden rush of fear and nervousness that makes your heart pound and makes you afraid you're going to die or go crazy" (Carlat, 1998).

Happy, Energetic, or Hyper

In the presence of depressive symptoms, a positive response to the last key question is helpful in screening for bipolar disorder. If the screen result is positive, the mnemonic DIG FAST can be used to confirm the cardinal symptoms of mania (Box 4.7).

What about special considerations for adolescents?

For adolescents, a psychosocial review of systems can serve as a screen for areas that could be of concern or that have the potential to create problems. The HEEADSSS method of interviewing provides structure and a framework for focusing assessment. The acronym stands for **h**ome, **e**ducation or employment, **e**ating, peer-group **a**ctivities, **d**rugs, **s**exuality, **s**uicide or depression, and **s**afety.

Box 4.6	**SIG E CAPS**

Neurovegetative Signs in Depression

S	Sleep disorder (either increased or decreased sleep)
I	Interest deficit (anhedonia)
G	Guilt (worthlessness, hopelessness, regret)
E	Energy deficit
C	Concentration deficit
A	Appetite disorder (either decreased or increased)
P	Psychomotor retardation or agitation
S	Suicidality

Reference: Carlat, 1988.

 EVIDENCE-BASED PRACTICE *Screening for Depression*

The United States Preventive Services Task Force recommends screening adults for depression in clinical practices that have systems in place to assure accurate diagnosis, effective treatment, and follow up. In primary care settings, the point prevalence of major depression ranges from 5% to 9% among adults, and up to 50% of depressed patients are not recognized as being depressed. Several depression screening instruments are available, and most instruments have relatively good sensitivity (80%–90%) but only fair specificity (70%–85%). Most instruments are easy to use and can be administered in less than 5 minutes. The evidence demonstrates that shorter screening tests, including simply asking questions about depressed mood and anhedonia, appear to detect a majority of depressed patients, with results comparable to longer depression questionnaires. Ultrashort questionnaires such as the PHQ-2 can be administered easily in writing or verbally. There are no brief validated depression screening questionnaires for children in primary care settings.

PHQ-2, Two-item Patient Health Questionnaire.
References: Maurer, 2012; Siu, 2016; Williams & Steffens, 2009.

Box 4.7	**DIG FAST**

Cardinal Symptoms of Bipolar Disorder

D	Distractibility
I	Indiscretion (excessive involvement in pleasurable activities)
G	Grandiosity
F	Flight of ideas
A	Activity increase
S	Sleep deficit (decreased need for sleep)
T	Talkativeness (pressured speech)

Reference: Carlat, 1988.

Key Questions

The HEEADSSS interview progresses from less intimidating questions about home, family members, and the past to more personal and private issues. The essential questions should be asked of all adolescents. The next in importance are these questions that should be asked of most adolescents if time permits. Finally, the in-depth questions can be asked when time allows or the situation demands it. Table 4.1 provides sample items.

Table 4.1	**The HEEADSSS Psychosocial Interview for Adolescents**

ESSENTIAL QUESTIONS	AS TIME PERMITS	FOR MORE IN-DEPTH INFORMATION
HOME		
What are relationships like at home?	Have you ever run away? (Why?)	—
EDUCATION AND EMPLOYMENT		
What are your favorite subjects at school?	Tell me about your friends at school.	Do you feel connected to your school?
EATING		
What do you like and not like about your body?	Do you worry about your weight? How often?	What would it be like if you gained (lost) 10 lb?
ACTIVITIES		
What do you and your friends do for fun? (With whom)	Do you have any hobbies?	—
DRUGS		
Do any of your friends use tobacco? Alcohol? Other drugs?	Do you ever drink or use drugs when you are alone?	—
SEXUALITY		
Have you ever been in a romantic relationship?	Are you interested in boys? Girls? Both?	—
SUICIDE AND DEPRESSION		
Do you feel sad or down more than usual?	Does it seem that you've lost interest in things that you used to really enjoy?	—
SAFETY (SAVAGERY)		
Have you ever been seriously injured? (How?)	Have you ever been in a car or motorcycle accident? (What happened?)	—

Goldenring J; Rosen D: *Getting into adolescent heads: an essential update*, Contemp Pediatr 21:64, 2004

Key Questions

- Have you been feeling that life is not worth living or that you are better off dead?
- Sometimes when a person feels down or depressed, he or she might think about dying. Have you been having thoughts like that?

If the patient answers yes to the preceding questions, then ask the following:

- Do you have a plan?
- What is the plan?
- Do you have the means to carry it out?
- What would cause you to carry out your plan or keep you from carrying it out?
- Have you ever attempted suicide in the past?

Initial Questions

The first set of questions helps determine whether the patient is at risk. Patients rarely volunteer thoughts of suicide, so it is important to ask directly. There is no evidence to suggest that asking about suicide precipitates suicidal thinking or acts.

Follow-Up Questions

The second set of questions helps you evaluate how imminent the risk is. Patients at high risk for suicide should be referred for psychiatric evaluation; those at imminent risk should be admitted for evaluation and treatment. Major risk factors for suicide include hopelessness, substance abuse, and prior suicide attempts.

All positive screening test results for mental health disorders require a full diagnostic follow-up interview using standard diagnostic criteria, such as those from the *Diagnostic and Statistical Manual of Mental Disorders,* ed 5 *(DSM-5),* to determine the presence or absence of specific disorders. The *DSM-5* describes specific symptom criteria for mental disorders and psychosocial problems. Although primary care providers often diagnose and treat patients with symptoms of depression and anxiety, serious impairment of mental or emotional functioning, psychoses, bipolar disorder, and substance abuse disorders require evaluation, diagnosis, and treatment by qualified mental health specialists. Primary care is not a substitute for psychiatric care. When a patient has been screened and is suspected to be at high risk for a condition, the primary care practitioner has a responsibility to refer the patient to an appropriate resource. See the differential diagnosis table at the end of this chapter for the diagnostic criteria for some common psychological disorders.

DIAGNOSTIC REASONING: FOCUSED PHYSICAL EXAMINATION

Physical examination can yield little additional data that are of diagnostic value. No physical finding is specific for any psychological disorder. The physical examination should be directed at identifying organic-based conditions that mimic psychological disorders. Perform a comprehensive and thorough physical examination if the patient has not had one since the onset of symptoms. This chapter presumes that you have performed the physical evaluation for specific presenting symptoms as part of your process to rule out a physiological cause.

Assess Vital Signs

When substance abuse is suspected, vital signs can quickly confirm the presence of an organic condition related to substance intoxication or withdrawal. Abnormal values for body temperature, blood pressure, heart rate, or respiratory rate indicate a need for a thorough evaluation.

Observe General Appearance

Look for signs of depression or substance abuse, such as an unkempt personal appearance, unusual dress, and general state of poor nutrition (skin condition and appearance of hair and nails). Observe the patient's demeanor and appearance for signs of neglect or abuse or a facial expression that might indicate depression. Observe for such behaviors as finger tapping and pacing that indicate anxiety. Methamphetamine users often have self-induced facial lesions secondary to scratching.

Adolescents who are abusing substances sometimes wear clothing or jewelry that displays drug-oriented graffiti.

Observe the infant or child's engagement. Children with autism may make few, if any, attempts, to contact socially with others; prefer to be alone; and ignore attempts to seek attention, affection, or a connection with their surroundings.

Observe Mental Status

Perform a mental status examination. Assess general behavior. Irritability can occur in patients with anxiety. Note body posture, movement, and facial expressions. Assess for suicidal or delusional thought content, which can occur with substance abuse or psychotic disorders. Determine affect for emotional range (broad or restricted), intensity (blunted, flat, or normal), stability, and congruence with the patient's stated mood. Evaluate the patient's cognitive abilities, including attention, concentration, and memory. A number of assessment instruments are available, including the Montreal Cognitive Assessment (MoCA) and the Mini-Cog see Chapter 9, Fig. 9-1 for the MoCA).

Note Speech and Thought Process

Speech tone, quality, and rate reflect mental status. In depression, the speech can be soft and monotonous with little spontaneity. In mania, the speech can be rapid, pressured, and loud, and the speech content consists of a flight of ideas.

Language delay that is not consistent with development should be noted. In some children with autism, language begins to regress instead of increase in skill level.

Examine the Eyes

Substance abusers can have eyes that are injected, jaundiced, puffy, or glassy. The pupils may be dilated or constricted. The patient may have droopy eyelids and a sleepy appearance or a fixed stare. The patient may have difficulty controlling eye movements.

Examine the Ears, Nose, and Mouth

The ears should be examined. If language delay is suspected, hearing loss or deafness should be ruled out.

Substance abusers may have chronic rhinorrhea, frequent nosebleeds, lesions in the nose or around the nostrils, or a perforated nasal septum. The patient may have dry lips, halitosis, or an odor of alcohol, marijuana, or tobacco.

Examine the Skin

Look for skin lesions that reflect depression or anxiety, such as neurogenic scratching, nail biting, and hair pulling. Look for evidence of attempted self-injury or suicide. Adolescents may show evidence of cutting scars or superficial cuts on areas of the body. Although typically not suicide attempts, cutting serves as a coping mechanism for unrelieved feelings.

In substance abusers, the skin may be cold and clammy, itching and burning, tight, swollen, or puffy. The person may perspire excessively, have discolored fingers, or have injection marks along the veins. Tattoos or burn marks, possibly done while under the influence of drugs or alcohol, can disguise injection marks. The patient may have injuries or bruises from falling or fighting.

In older or vulnerable patients, signs of injury particularly to the head, neck, and upper arms may, in the context of other factors and findings, indicate physical abuse. Multiple injuries in various stages of healing should raise the suspicion of abuse. However, the color of bruises does not reliably indicate their age (Wiglesworth, 2009), and older adults can bruise spontaneously. Decubitus ulcers, dehydration, and poor hygiene may indicate neglect.

Assess Balance and Gait

A patient who has a substance abuse problem may have a slow gait or poor balance.

LABORATORY AND DIAGNOSTIC STUDIES

There are no laboratory tests to assist in the diagnosis of most psychological conditions.

Base the laboratory and diagnostic studies on the presenting reports (see specific chapters).

Commonly performed tests to help identify underlying conditions include the following:

Complete Blood Count with Indices and Differential

The complete blood count (CBC) will provide information about the presence of infection or anemia.

Serum Electrolytes

Symptoms of depression can be exacerbated by hyponatremia, hypernatremia, hypercalcemia, and hyperphosphatemia.

Thyroid Function Tests

An elevated level of thyroid-stimulating hormone is related to chronic symptoms of depression. A hyperthyroid state can be associated with anxiety.

Toxicology Screen and Blood Alcohol Level

Urine and blood screening tests can be used to determine alcohol or drug intoxication as a cause of psychological symptoms.

Serum B_{12} and Folate

Deficiencies of vitamin B_{12} and folate are reversible causes of dementia in older adults.

DIFFERENTIAL DIAGNOSIS

Normal Stress

Stress is the nonspecific response of the body to any demand. The perception of a demand as stressful depends on the individual's experience of how much demand for adaptation an event or situation requires. Stressors can be acute or chronic. External stressors include adverse physical conditions (e.g., pain) or stressful psychological environments (e.g., poor working conditions, abusive relationships, or major life events). Internal stressors can be physical (e.g., infections or inflammation), or psychological (e.g., worry). Daily hassles or situational factors influence the stress load because minor annoyances that happen daily can accumulate. Situational factors can exacerbate a depressive disorder in

significant ways. Symptoms of stress include mental, physical, and behavioral symptoms. Common physical symptoms include responses of the autonomic nervous system and musculoskeletal system.

Normal Grief

Grief is a subjective feeling precipitated by the loss of someone or something important to the individual. Normal grief is a process of emotional upheaval, distress, and eventual resolution. Individuals who are grieving often experience both physical and psychological symptoms and can have difficulty functioning. Grief and depression share many of the same characteristics, and normal grief can become clinical depression. An individual with a history of depression is at risk of becoming depressed in times of significant loss. The mood disturbance in depression is typically pervasive and unrelenting. In normal grief, fluctuations in mood are common. Although the pain of grief is intense, the individual is able to experience moments of less intensity or even happiness.

Domestic or Partner Violence

Domestic or partner violence is a pattern of assaultive and coercive behaviors that include physical, sexual, psychological, and economic attacks by adults or adolescents against their intimate partners. Individuals who have experienced abuse could present with an injury that is not consistent with the description of how the injury occurred. The individual may be seen frequently for undiagnosed psychosomatic concerns. This patient can appear depressed or show evidence of suicide attempts.

Elder Abuse

The psychological effects of elder abuse include depression, anxiety, and delirium. Elder abuse encompasses five types of abuse: physical (acts intended to cause physical pain or injury), verbal or psychological (acts intended to cause emotional pain), sexual (nonconsensual contact of any kind), financial (misappropriation of the elder's money or property), and neglect (failure of a designated caregiver to meet the needs of a dependent elder). The overall prevalence of elder abuse in the community is estimated at 10% (Lachs & Pillemer, 2017). There are no standardized instruments or guidelines for assessment of abuse in older adults.

Substance Use Disorders

Substance use disorders are divided into two groups: substance abuse and substance dependence. The categories of substances included are alcohol, amphetamines, cannabis, cocaine, hallucinogens, inhalants, opioids, phencyclidines, sedatives, and hypnotics. Substance abuse occurs when repeated use of alcohol or other drugs leads to significant impairment in functioning and relationships but does not include compulsive use, addiction, or withdrawal symptoms when stopping the substance. Substance dependence includes a history of substance abuse plus continued use despite related problems, an increase in substance tolerance, and withdrawal symptoms if the substance use is stopped.

Autism Spectrum Disorder

Autism spectrum disorder is a difficult disorder to diagnose because there are no laboratory tests and the clinical signs can be subtle. Infants younger than the age of 18 months are very difficult to diagnose. Noting a lack of social interaction can be the first sign. At 18 months of age, the Modified Checklist for Autism in Toddlers (M-CHAT-R/F) has been shown to be useful in screening for autism spectrum disorders. Revision of the original work includes changes to both the screening instrument and the scoring. The revised instrument has been validated in primary care settings for low-risk toddlers (Robins et. al, 2014). Box 4.8 describes the checklist. After age 3 years, the Autism Diagnostic Observation Schedule is more useful. Generally, children with autism spectrum disorder exhibit mild to severe deficits in social interaction and verbal and nonverbal communication and have repetitive behaviors or interests. Box 4.9 describes a screening checklist for toddlers.

Adjustment Disorders

There are several adjustment disorder diagnoses. All of the disorders in this category relate

---

Box 4.8 Modified Checklist of Autism in Toddlers, Revised, With Follow-Up (M-CHAT-R/F)

The M-CHAT-R/F is validated for screening toddlers between 16 and 30 months of age to assess risk for autism spectrum disorders. The 20-item instrument can be scored in less than 2 minutes. Designed to maximize sensitivity, the false positive rate is high, so a structured follow-up interview is available. Children who score in the moderate risk range (3 to 7 at-risk responses) need to be administered the relevant follow-up items. Children whose follow-up score is 2 or more or whose initial M-CHAT-R score is 8 or more should be referred for diagnostic evaluation and early intervention. The instrument and scoring instructions are available for download from http://www.mchatscreen.com.

Reference: Robins et al, 2014.

---

to a significantly more difficult adjustment to a life situation than would normally be expected, considering the circumstances. The condition is acute if the disturbance lasts less than 6 months and chronic if it lasts for 6 months or longer in response to a chronic stressor or one that has enduring consequences.

The disorders in this category can present themselves quite differently. The key to diagnosis is to examine the issue that is causing the adjustment disorder and to determine the primary symptoms associated with the disorder (e.g., anxiety or depression).

Anxiety Disorders

There are several types of anxiety disorders and multiple diagnoses. An anxiety disorder should not be confused with everyday stress and worry. Anxiety disorders are persistent conditions that require careful diagnosis. Anxiety is a group of disorders characterized by a number of both mental and physical symptoms, with no apparent explanation. The primary feature is abnormal or inappropriate anxiety. Apprehension, fear of losing control, fear of going "crazy," fear of

Box 4.9 **The Five Key Items on the CHAT Screen**

ASK THE PARENT

1. Does your child ever pretend (e.g., to make a cup of tea using a toy cup and teapot) or pretend with other things?
2. Does your child ever use an index finger to point, to indicate interest in something?

HEALTH PRACTITIONER OBSERVATION

1. Gain the child's attention and then point across the room at an interesting object and say, "Oh look! There's a (name of toy)!" Watch the child's face. Does the child look across to see what you are pointing at?
2. Gain the child's attention and then give the child a toy cup and teapot and ask, "Can you make me a cup of tea?" Does the child pretend to pour out tea, drink it, and so on?
3. Ask the child, "Where's the light?" or "Show me the light." Does the child point with an index finger at the light? To record "yes" on this item, the child must have looked up at your face around the time of pointing.

CHAT, Checklist for Autism in Toddlers.
Reprinted with permission from Baird G, Charman T, Cox A, et al. Current topic: screening and surveillance for autism and pervasive and developmental disorders. *Arch Dis* 84:471, 2001.

impending danger or death, and uneasiness are among the most common psychological symptoms. Common physical symptoms include dizziness, lightheadedness, chest or abdominal pain, nausea, increased heart rate, and diarrhea.

Generalized anxiety disorder

Chronic anxiety, also referred to as generalized anxiety disorder, manifests as persistent worries, fears, and negative thoughts lasting a minimum of 6 months. Excessive worry over daily activities and a tendency toward headache and nausea are seen. Typically, generalized anxiety disorder (GAD) develops over a period of time and is not noticed until it is significant enough to cause problems with functioning. Anxiety is persistent and pervasive and occurs in many different settings.

Panic disorder

Panic disorder is manifested by sudden attacks of fear accompanied by symptoms that resemble a heart attack (e.g., palpitations, chest pain, dizziness). Often the symptoms develop rapidly and without an identifiable stressor. The individual could have had periods of high anxiety in the past or could have been involved in a recent stressful situation; however, the underlying cause is typically subtle. Panic attacks subside as abruptly as they begin, typically lasting a few minutes, although they can last several hours. The patient could have thoughts of impending disaster, which can lead to repeated emergency medical presentations. The frequency of these attacks can vary from several times a day to only once or twice a year.

Social phobia (social anxiety disorder)

Symptoms include extreme anxiety and fear associated with social or performance situations in which the patient is exposed to unfamiliar people or to scrutiny. The patient recognizes that the fear is excessive or unreasonable but avoids the social or performance situations or endures them with intense distress or anxiety.

Mood Disorders

Mood disorders contain several categories, including dysthymia, depression, and bipolar disorder.

The disorders in this category include those in which the primary symptom is a disturbance in mood with inappropriate, exaggerated, or a limited range of affect. The feelings are extreme, pervasive, and unrelenting.

Dysthymia

The patient experiences feelings that are less intense than major depression but that still disrupt everyday life. The patient experiences a depressed mood for most of the day, for more days than not, for a minimum of 2 years. During this time, there must be two or more of the following symptoms: undereating or overeating, sleep difficulties, fatigue, low self-esteem, difficulty with concentration or decision making, and feelings of hopelessness.

Major depressive disorder

The hallmark symptom of depression is either a depressed mood or a loss of interest or pleasure in usual activities. Major depression can significantly impair a person's ability to function in family, work, and social situations. Patients with depression experience deep, unshakeable sadness and diminished interest in nearly all activities. Crying and feeling depressed or suicidal occur frequently.

Bipolar disorder

Bipolar disorder has two types. Bipolar I disorder requires the occurrence of at least one manic episode even though other episodes, such as major depressive, hypomanic, or mixed, could have occurred. Bipolar II disorder requires at least one hypomanic episode.

Mania is sometimes referred to as the other extreme of depression. The patient experiences an elevated, expansive, or irritable mood with behaviors and symptoms that reflect a "high." The symptoms are sufficient to interfere with usual social activities and relationships with others.

In bipolar II disorder, periods of highs, as described previously, often followed by periods of depression. The high episodes are hypomanic rather than manic. The symptoms are similar but are not severe enough to cause marked impairment in social or occupational functioning and typically do not require hospitalization to ensure the safety of the person.

▶ **DIFFERENTIAL DIAGNOSIS OF** *Common Causes of Psychological Disorders*

CONDITION	HISTORY	PHYSICAL FINDINGS	DIAGNOSTIC STUDIES
Normal stress	Perceived stress related to external or internal stressors, such as daily life events or situations, psychological environments, relationships Can be acute or chronic Can feel unable to cope or adapt Can have mental, physical, and behavioral symptoms	Could appear unkempt, with unusual dress Could have depressed demeanor Facial expression (e.g., dejected, sad, downcast) Tearing, crying Adolescents could show evidence of cutting	None
Normal grief	Loss of someone or something of importance Can have physical and psychological symptoms Mood fluctuations; feels depressed Can have difficulty functioning	May appear unkempt, with unusual dress, general state of poor nutrition Depressed demeanor Facial expression (e.g., dejected, sad, downcast) Tearing, crying Speech could be soft and monotonous with little spontaneity Adolescents can show evidence of cutting	None

Continued

DIFFERENTIAL DIAGNOSIS OF *Common Causes of Psychological Disorders—cont'd*

CONDITION	HISTORY	PHYSICAL FINDINGS	DIAGNOSTIC STUDIES
Domestic or partner violence	Reports physical, sexual, psychological, emotional, or economic attacks from family or partners Could seek care frequently for undiagnosed psychosomatic concerns Could report suicide attempts	Can have injuries inconsistent with history Adolescents can show evidence of cutting	None
Elder abuse	Reports physical, verbal, psychological, sexual abuse, financial exploitation or neglect from family or caregiver	Can have injuries inconsistent with history Multiple injuries in various stages of healing Nonadherence to medication or treatment regimen	None As indicated for physical findings
Substance use disorders[a]	Reports recurrent substance use that results in failure to fulfill major obligations at work, school, or home and substance-related legal problems Use in situations that are physically hazardous (e.g., driving while intoxicated) Continued use despite significant social or interpersonal problems caused or exacerbated by effects of the substance Report increased tolerance of and need for increased amounts of substance Report withdrawal symptoms Report unsuccessful efforts to cut down or control substance use	Skin can be cold and clammy, itching and burning, tight, swollen, or puffy Excess perspiration Discolored fingers or injection marks along the veins Tattoos or burn marks, injuries or bruises Methamphetamine users can have self-induced facial lesions secondary to scratching Eyes can be injected, jaundiced, puffy, or glassy Pupils can be dilated or constricted Eyelids can be droopy with sleepy appearance or fixed stare Can have difficulty controlling eye movements Can have chronic rhinorrhea, lesions in the nose or around the nostrils, perforated nasal septum Can have dry lips, halitosis, or an odor of alcohol, marijuana, or tobacco	Toxicology screen Blood alcohol level

> **DIFFERENTIAL DIAGNOSIS OF** *Common Causes of Psychological Disorders—cont'd*

CONDITION	HISTORY	PHYSICAL FINDINGS	DIAGNOSTIC STUDIES
Autism spectrum disorder[a]	Lack of language developmental milestones; could lose language skills; social interaction lacking	Lack of eye contact, might not smile, does not respond to name with hearing intact	M-CHAT-R/F screening at age 18 mo CHAT screening for toddlers Refer for developmental and cognitive evaluation
Adjustment disorder[a]	The development of emotional or behavioral symptoms in response to an identifiable stressor(s) occurring within 3 mo of the onset of the stressor(s) Distress that is in excess of what would be expected from exposure to the stressor Significant impairment in social or occupational (academic) functioning	None	Refer for psychological evaluation
ANXIETY DISORDERS			
Generalized anxiety disorder[a]	Excessive anxiety and worry for most days of past 6 mo about a number of events or activities (e.g., work or school performance) Difficult to control the worry Associated physical symptoms, such as restlessness, edginess, fatigue, difficulty concentrating, irritability, sleep disturbance, social, occupational, or other areas of functioning	Behaviors such as finger tapping and pacing that indicate anxiety Restlessness, edginess, difficulty concentrating Adolescents could show evidence of cutting	Refer for psychological evaluation

Continued

DIFFERENTIAL DIAGNOSIS OF *Common Causes of Psychological Disorders—cont'd*

CONDITION	HISTORY	PHYSICAL FINDINGS	DIAGNOSTIC STUDIES
Panic disorder[a]	Recurrent unexpected panic attacks: discrete period of intense fear or discomfort with physical symptoms, such as palpitations, pounding heart, or accelerated heart rate, sweating, trembling or shaking, sensations of shortness of breath or smothering, feeling of choking, chest pain or discomfort, nausea or abdominal distress, feeling dizzy, unsteady, lightheaded, or faint, paresthesias, chills or hot flushes Report fear of losing control or going crazy, fear of dying Persistent concern about having additional attacks	None except during attack	Refer for psychological evaluation
Social phobia (social anxiety disorder)[a]	Marked and persistent fear of one or more social or performance situations Anxious about acting in a way that will be humiliating or embarrassing Report panic attack related to exposure to the situation Avoids the situation Avoidance, anxiety, and distress interferes significantly with the person's normal routine, occupational (academic) functioning, or social activities or relationships	None	Refer for psychological evaluation
MOOD DISORDERS			
Dysthymic disorder[a]	Depressed mood for most of the day, for more days than not, for at least 2 yr Reports symptoms of depression such as appetite and sleep disturbance, low energy or fatigue, low self-esteem, poor concentration or difficulty making decisions, feelings of hopelessness	Can appear unkempt, with unusual dress; general state of poor nutrition Depressed demeanor Facial expression (e.g., dejected, sad, downcast) Tearing, crying Speech can be soft and monotonous with little spontaneity Adolescents could show evidence of cutting	Refer for psychological evaluation

> ## DIFFERENTIAL DIAGNOSIS OF *Common Causes of Psychological Disorders—cont'd*

CONDITION	HISTORY	PHYSICAL FINDINGS	DIAGNOSTIC STUDIES
Major depressive disorder[a]	Reports acute symptoms of depressed mood most of the day, nearly every day, or loss of interest or pleasure in all or almost all activities of the day, nearly every day Experiences other symptoms most every day such as appetite disturbance, sleep disturbance, psychomotor agitation or retardation, fatigue or loss of energy, feelings of worthlessness or excessive or inappropriate guilt, diminished ability to think or concentrate, recurrent thoughts of death or suicide	Can appear unkempt, with unusual dress; general state of poor nutrition Depressed demeanor Facial expression (e.g., dejected, sad, downcast) Tearing, crying Speech can be soft and monotonous with little spontaneity Adolescents could show evidence of cutting	Serum electrolytes CBC Thyroid function tests Refer for psychological evaluation
Bipolar disorder[a]	History of at least one manic episode or hypomanic episode A distinct period of abnormally and persistently elevated, expansive, or irritable mood, lasting at least 1 wk Accompanying symptoms of inflated self-esteem or grandiosity, decreased need for sleep, more talkative than usual or pressure to keep talking, insomnia or hypersomnia nearly every day, psychomotor agitation or retardation, flight of ideas or racing thoughts, easy distractibility, increase in goal-directed activity, excessive involvement in pleasurable activities that have a high potential for painful consequences Report history of one or more major depressive episodes (see above)	In mania, the speech can be rapid, pressured, and loud, and the speech content consists of a flight of ideas	Refer for psychological evaluation

[a]For specific diagnostic criteria, see *Diagnostic and statistical manual of mental disorders,* ed. 5, Arlington, VA, 2013, American Psychiatric Association.
M-CHAT, Modified Checklist for Autism in Toddlers.

Table 5.1	**Correlation of Ovarian and Endometrial Cycles (Ideal 28-Day Cycle)**						
MENSTRUAL (1–3 TO 5 DAYS)	**EARLY FOLLICULAR (4 TO 6–8 DAYS)**	**ADVANCED FOLLICULAR (9 TO 12–16 DAYS)**	**OVULATION (12–16 DAYS)**	**EARLY LUTEAL (15–19 DAYS)**	**ADVANCED LUTEAL (20– 25 DAYS)**	**PREMENSTRUAL (26–32 DAYS)**
OVARY						
Involution of corpus luteum	Growth and matura- tion of graafian follicle		Ovulation	Active corpus luteum		Involution of corpus luteum
ESTROGEN						
Diminution	Progressive increase	High concen- tration		Secondary rise		Decreasing
PROGESTERONE						
Absent	Absent	Absent	Appearing	Rising	Rising	Decreasing
ENDOMETRIUM						
Menstrual desqua- mation and involution	Reorgani- zation and pro- liferation	Further growth and watery secretion	—	Active secre- tion and glandular dilation	Accumula- tion of secre- tion and edema	Regressive
PITUITARY SECRETION						
FSH fairly constant until just before ovulation	Moderate increase just before	Rapid decrease in previous levels				
LH fairly constant until just before ovulation	Marked increase just before	Rapid decrease in previous levels				

FSH, Follicle-stimulating hormone; *LH,* luteinizing hormone.
Modified from Thompson JM, McFarland GK, Hirsch JE, Tucker SM: *Mosby's clinical nursing,* ed. 4, St. Louis, 1997, Mosby.

and sexual abuse, with consequent unintended pregnancy. Ask direct questions in private about being hit, pushed, or slapped or about having nonconsensual sex.

Contraceptive Use

The type and use patterns of contraceptives are important in the search for the cause of amenorrhea. Contraceptive failures can account for an unintended pregnancy. Amenorrhea can occur after discontinuation of oral contraceptives. Measurement of serum gonadotropins is affected by long-acting contraceptives, such as medroxyprogesterone acetate (DMPA) (Depo-Provera), implants, or intrauterine devices (IUDs) containing progestogens; these must be discontinued before testing.

Seeking Pregnancy

Knowing that the patient is seeking pregnancy, or if the patient is pregnant, whether it is intended or unintended, allows the interview to be structured appropriately. It also aids in proper counseling and referral. Amenorrheic patients seeking pregnancy, who do not bleed after androgen challenge tests, are most successfully treated by an infertility specialist. Patients seeking pregnancy who are younger than 35 years of age and have been unsuccessful after a year of unprotected sex, and those older than 35 years of age for 6 months should be referred to an infertility specialist.

Is this primary or secondary amenorrhea?

Key Questions
- Have you ever had a menstrual cycle?
- Have you started pubertal development? Can you show me how your breasts and pubic hair look compared with these pictures? Use Tanner stages of development (Figs. 5.2 and 5.3).

M₁—Tanner 1 (preadolescent). Only the nipple is raised above the level of the breast, as in the child.

M₂—Tanner 2. Budding stage; bud-shaped elevation of the areola; areola increased in diameter and surrounding area slightly elevated.

M₃—Tanner 3. Breast and areola enlarged. No contour separation.

M₄—Tanner 4. Increasing fat deposits. The areola forms a secondary elevation above that of the breast. This secondary mound occurs in approximately half of all girls and in some cases persists in adulthood.

M₅—Tanner 5 (adult stage). The areola is (usually) part of general breast contour and is strongly pigmented. Nipple projects.

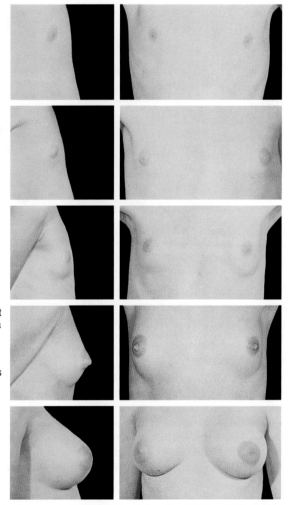

FIGURE 5.2 Five stages of breast development in females. (From Growth diagrams 1965 Netherlands: Second national survey on 0- to 24-year-olds, by J. C. Van Wieringen, F. Wafelbakker, H. P. Verbrugge, J. H. DeHaas. Groningen: Noordhoff Uitgevers BV, The Netherlands.)

P$_1$—Tanner 1 (preadolescent). No growth of pubic hair.

P$_2$—Tanner 2. Initial, scarcely pigmented straight hair, especially along medial border of the labia.

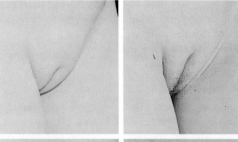

P$_3$—Tanner 3. Sparse, dark, visibly pigmented, curly pubic hair on labia.

P$_4$—Tanner 4. Hair coarse and curly, abundant but less than adult.

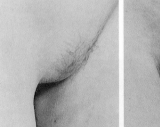

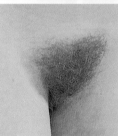

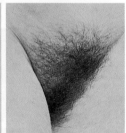

P$_5$—Tanner 5. Lateral spreading; type and triangle spread of adult hair to medial surface of thighs.

P$_6$—Tanner 6. Further extension laterally, upward, or dispersed (occurs in only 10% of women).

FIGURE 5.3 Six stages of pubic hair development in females. (From Growth diagrams 1965 Netherlands: Second national survey on 0- to 24-year-olds, by J. C. Van Wieringen, F. Wafelbakker, H. P. Verbrugge, J. H. DeHaas. Groningen: Noordhoff Uitgevers BV, The Netherlands.)

- At what age did you start your periods?
- When was your last normal menstrual period?
- What is the nature of your periods (e.g., frequency, duration, amount of flow)?

Onset of Menstruation

The age range for menarche in the United States is 9 to 17 years. If the patient has had established menses at intervals of every 21 to 38 days, then the classification of secondary amenorrhea would apply. Established menses indicate that there is no outlet flow problem and that the HPO axis and endometrium are functioning.

Pubertal Development

Female pubertal development begins with a growth spurt 1 year before the development of

breast buds (thelarche) at around age 11 years. Growth continues for 1 year until the peak height velocity is achieved. Pubic hair appears (pubarche) followed by axillary hair and the beginning of menarche. In the United States, the average age of menarche is 12 years, 4 months. The length of time from thelarche to menarche is 2 to 3 years.

A thorough review of pediatric growth charts is helpful in determining the young patient's norm of growth and development and the centimeters attained by the latest growth spurt. Most adolescent girls have a mean height gain of 29 cm (11.4 inches), and the growth spurt lasts approximately 4 years. Adolescents who are overweight for height may be hypothyroid; adolescents who are underweight may have deficiencies in caloric intake or systemic illnesses. Asking adolescents to self-identify their Tanner stages, for breast and pubic development maturity, provides very accurate staging (see Figs. 5.2 and 5.3). Additionally, it gives the opportunity for insight into their feelings about their body and self-esteem.

Age of Menarche

The lack of menstrual periods and secondary sex characteristics by age 14 years or the lack of menses by age 16 years in the presence of secondary sex characteristics is considered primary amenorrhea. Fifty-six percent of all adolescents start menses when pubic hair development is at pubic hair stage 4 and 19% at pubic hair stage 3 (see Fig. 5.3). If the adolescent is pubic hair stage 4 but has not had a menses, then primary amenorrhea should be diagnosed. However, if the adolescent does not meet the age and maturation criteria, then delayed puberty should be suspected, especially if there is a family history of delayed menarche. Almost 80% of amenorrheic adolescents with intact female genitalia and developed breasts have an inappropriate LH feedback, anovulatory cycles, or high levels of androgenic hormones. They will bleed after a PCT and should be monitored for continued menses to avoid endometrial hyperplasia.

Menstrual History

Absence of a menstrual period for the past 3 months in patients with established normal menstruation, or 9 months in patients with previous oligomenorrhea (menstrual periods occurring at intervals of greater than 35 days, with only four to nine periods in a year), is considered secondary amenorrhea. Whereas sudden cessation of menstruation is more likely to indicate pregnancy or stress as a cause, a gradual cessation suggests polycystic ovarian syndrome (PCOS), or ovarian failure. Ovarian failure is considered premature in women younger than 40 years of age. Premature ovarian failure is also called primary ovarian insufficiency, and women may have occasional periods. Women older than age 40 younger who have not had a period within the past 3 to 11 months may be considered perimenopausal.

Are there any constitutional delays causing the amenorrhea?

Key Questions

- Has there been a change in weight, percentage of body fat, or athletic training intensity?
- Are you under unusual stress at school, home, or work?
- Do you or anyone in your family have any congenital disorders or chronic diseases?

Change in Weight, Percentage Body Fat, and Athletic Training Intensity

Underweight people typically have a low body fat–to–lean muscle ratio. Body fat can be assessed using the body mass index (BMI [weight in kilograms/height in meters^2]). The severe stress of anorexia nervosa can produce prolonged amenorrhea. Exercise from various sports—jogging, middle- and long-distance running, ballet dancing, gymnastics, and track and field events—can lower body fat sufficiently to cause menstrual aberrations. Long-distance runners and ballerinas are more apt to be amenorrheic than are swimmers; however, even moderate exercise can cause one or two missed periods a year. The mechanism of action on the HPO axis is unknown but is expressed by delayed puberty, shortened luteal phase, anovulation, and amenorrhea. Obesity can be the cause of amenorrhea or be a sign of PCOS. PCOS causes ovarian dysfunction—elevated androgens, hirsutism, low sex steroid–binding globulin (SSBG), and an elevated LH:FSH ratio.

Emotional State

The stress of athletic competition, family situations, school performance, peer relations, and work can disrupt normal cyclic menses. The HPO axis of a teenager is more sensitive to physical and psychological stress than that of an adult.

Congenital or Chronic Diseases

Turner syndrome features (see the discussion on performing a head and neck examination later in this chapter) or similar physical findings suggest the probability of an abnormality of one or all components (CNS, structural anomalies, or HPO axis) necessary for menstruation. Most structural anomalies that would prevent outflow of the menstrual blood are detectable on physical examination. Chronic diseases, such as anorexia nervosa, diabetes mellitus, Crohn disease, systemic lupus erythematosus, glomerulonephritis, cystic fibrosis, pituitary adenoma, adrenal diseases, and thyroid dysfunction, can cause amenorrhea.

> *Could this be thyroid dysfunction?*

Key Questions
- Have you noticed changes in the texture of your hair or skin?
- Are you bothered by hot or cold temperatures?
- Have you had any changes in your energy level?
- Have you had any changes in your bowel function?

Hair and Skin Changes and Temperature Intolerance

Hypothyroidism and hyperthyroidism are expressed by changes in hair and skin texture. Women with hypothyroidism may report dry hair along with thinning of hair. Hyperthyroidism often makes women intolerant of the heat, and this is sometimes confused with menopausal syndrome symptoms. Cold intolerance is frequently exhibited by people with a low-functioning thyroid.

Energy and Bowel Changes

Whereas increased functioning of the thyroid causes restlessness and diarrhea, decreased functioning results in constipation and fatigue. Even mild thyroid dysfunction can cause menstrual irregularities; therefore, a thyroid function test is needed to assess the thyroid status.

> *Could this be caused by hyperprolactinemia?*

Key Questions
- Are you able to express a discharge or liquid from your nipples?
- Is there increased stimulation to your nipples?

- Have you had any surgery or disease of the breasts or chest wall?

Galactorrhea

A patient may notice breast nipple discharge that is not associated with breastfeeding or medications. Causative medications are listed in Box 5.1 and include primarily the dopamine antagonist agents and estrogens.

Nipple Stimulation and Chest Wall Stimulation

Nipple stimulation from clothing irritation during jogging, from nipple manipulation, or from stimulation during sexual activity may cause galactorrhea. Surgical interventions such as lymph node dissection or disease processes such as herpes zoster can also lead to galactorrhea, triggered by peripheral neural stimulation.

> *Could the amenorrhea be caused by medications?*

Key Questions
- What prescription medicines are you taking?
- Have you used any street drugs? What kind of drugs have you used?
- Do you use oral contraceptives?

Box 5.1 Drugs That May Cause Amenorrhea

PROLACTIN INCREASE
- *Antipsychotics:* phenothiazines, haloperidol, pimozide, clozapine
- *Antidepressants:* tricyclic antidepressants, monoamine oxidase inhibitors
- *Antihypertensives:* calcium channel blockers, methyldopa, reserpine

ESTROGENIC EFFECT
- Digitalis, marijuana, flavonoids, oral contraceptives

OVARIAN TOXICITY
- Busulfan, chlorambucil, cisplatin, cyclophosphamide, fluorouracil

Modified from Kiningham RB, Apgar BS, Schwenk TL: Evaluation of amenorrhea, *Am Fam Physician* 53:1186, 1996.

Medication History

Some medications, such as phenothiazines or oral contraceptives, can cause amenorrhea. These drugs increase prolactin levels, induce an estrogenic effect, or are toxic to the ovaries (see Box 5.1). Use of illicit drugs, such as heroin and methadone, also leads to menstrual abnormalities

Is a pituitary tumor causing the amenorrhea?

Key Questions
- Have you experienced any visual changes?
- Are you having an increased number of headaches?

Visual Changes and Headaches

A pituitary tumor could be responsible for hyperprolactinemia. Enlarging pituitary tumors cause headaches. As the tumor grows out of the sella turcica, it compresses the optic chiasm and nerves. The common visual defect is bitemporal hemianopia, although other defects can occur. Changes in visual fields are often self-diagnosed when the patient recognizes vision problems while reading or driving an automobile. Clinical changes in vision warrant a referral to an ophthalmologist and magnetic resonance imaging (MRI) workup for a tumor of the sella turcica. A high prolactin level indicates a pituitary adenoma that presents with or without galactorrhea.

Is this a problem of the hypothalamic–pituitary–ovarian axis?

Key Questions
- Have you experienced any problems with infertility?
- Do you have excess hair on your face or chest?

- Are you having any menopausal symptoms (e.g., hot flashes, vaginal dryness)?
- Did you hemorrhage during childbirth?

Infertility

Many cases of infertility are caused by failure of ovulation. PCOS affects women between the ages of 15 and 30 years. Basal body temperature charts and endometrial biopsies can reveal anovulatory cycles. Vaginal ultrasound shows enlarged ovaries with multiple small, fluid-filled cysts. Infertility can be caused by low or high estrogen levels. Measurement of gonadotropins, vaginal maturation index (MI), and progesterone levels, provide insight into the functioning of the HPO axis.

Androgen Excess

About 50% of women diagnosed with PCOS are hirsute and obese and have difficulty conceiving. Few other signs of masculinization are present. LH is elevated with PCOS. Truncal obesity, acne, and male pattern baldness can signify androgen excess.

Estrogen Deficiency

Amenorrhea can indicate a menopausal state. During perimenopause, ovulation and menses occur irregularly because of fluctuations in the hormones of the HPO axis. Hot flashes or flushes, changes in mood, and difficulty sleeping are common menopausal symptoms that women with low estradiol levels can experience. A dry vagina is often accompanied by dyspareunia and sometimes dysuria. The dysuria can be secondary to the hypoestrogenic state of the urethra and not be the result of a urinary tract infection. Prolonged hypoestrogenic status leads to osteopenia, regardless of age.

> **EVIDENCE-BASED PRACTICE** *Predictors of Menopause*
>
> Brambilla and colleagues (1994) found that 3 to 11 months of amenorrhea or irregular periods among women age 45 to 55 years were most predictive of menopause within the following 3 years (sensitivity, 72%; specificity, 76%). A systematic review by Bastian and colleagues (2003) showed that besides menstrual history, the strongest indicators of perimenopause were hot flashes, night sweats, and vaginal dryness.

References: Brambilla DJ et al, 1994; Bastian et al,, 2003.

Hemorrhage at Childbirth

Amenorrhea can occur subsequent to a pregnancy and delivery if there was severe hemorrhage at the time of delivery. Obstetric hemorrhage causes pituitary ischemia and infarction and results in pituitary insufficiency. This pathological process is known as Sheehan syndrome. In this instance, refer the patient to an endocrinologist.

> *Is this a problem of the uterus?*

Key Question

- Have you had a miscarriage or abortion, uterine infection, or any surgery or procedure involving your uterus?

Gynecologic Problem

Endometritis, incomplete abortion, or aggressive curettage of the uterus can lead to denuding of the endometrial layer, scarring, and Asherman syndrome. A patient with Asherman syndrome will not bleed after the PCT, nor will she bleed after the uterus is primed with estrogen and challenged with DMPA. The diagnosis can be made by performing weekly serum progesterone tests to determine if any value is within the ovulatory range (>3 ng/mL), yet there are no periods. The diagnosis can also be made by the gynecologist via hysteroscopy, hysterosalpingography, or measuring endometrial thickness by ultrasonography.

> *What symptoms support a structural outflow problem?*

Key Questions

- Do you have cyclic abdominal bloating or cramping?
- Have you been amenorrheic since you had a cervical procedure?

Presence of Premenstrual Symptoms or Dysmenorrhea

Cyclic symptomatology of dysmenorrhea, in the absence of menses, can be caused by an incomplete outflow tract. Physical examination validates a vaginal opening, imperforate hymen, intact uterus, or congenital imperforate cervical os. If there is no indication of a uterus by examination or lower abdominal ultrasound, a karyotype is needed to determine the congenital disorder. A referral to an endocrinologist or gynecologic surgeon could be indicated for removal of any abdominal male gonads, which would be a risk for cancerous degeneration.

Amenorrhea After Cervical Procedure

Stenosis of the cervical os can occur after gynecological office surgeries, such as cervical biopsies and cryotherapy. However, it is more common after cone biopsies of the cervix, such as the loop electrosurgical excision procedure or carbon dioxide laser treatment.

DIAGNOSTIC REASONING: FOCUSED PHYSICAL EXAMINATION

Note General Appearance

The body morphology of the patient can provide clues to the cause of amenorrhea; often disorders can be diagnosed secondary to short stature, underweight, or overweight. A height less than 5 feet (short stature) in a girl who is 14 years old or older could indicate a congenital chromosomal problem. Assess the patient's general state of health to determine if there are signs of systemic, chronic, or congenital disease.

Assess Nutritional Status and Plot Measurements on the Growth Chart in Adolescents

Assess nutritional status, looking for signs of undernutrition or overnutrition. Measure the height, weight, and arm span of the adolescent. Plot on a growth chart if delayed puberty is a consideration. Anorexia nervosa is often found while evaluating an adolescent who has short stature and is underweight.

Assess Sexual Maturity

Use the Tanner stages to assess and rate the stage of breast and pubic hair development. A sexual maturity rating (SMR) can be calculated by averaging the girl's stages of pubic hair and breast development. The stage of breast and pubic hair development in an adolescent girl is related to her chronological age,

age at menarche, and evidence of growth spurt. The breasts often develop at different rates, so some asymmetry is common. Menarche generally occurs at SMR 4 or breast stage 3 to 4. Plot these physiological events on the growth curve.

Screen for Eating Disorders

If you suspect anorexia nervosa or bulimia, administer a screening instrument to help determine the diagnosis. Refer to the *Diagnostic and Statistical Manual of Mental Disorders, ed 5 (DSM-5)* for diagnostic criteria. About half of those with eating disorders will have short stature.

Calculate the Body Mass Index

Seventeen percent body fat is needed for menarche, and about 22% body fat is necessary for ovulation. Calculate the BMI (Box 5.2). A BMI of 19 kg/m^2 usually indicates about 17% body fat, which can cause amenorrhea.

Obesity causes amenorrhea secondary to ovarian dysfunction. A BMI of greater than 27 kg/m^2 corresponds to being more than 20% overweight. Adipose cell stroma convert androstenedione to estrogen (estrone) as the body fat increases. Obesity also increases SSBG, thereby increasing free steroid levels. Both processes can cause an imbalance in the HPO axis and lead to amenorrhea.

Box 5.2 **Body Mass Index**

Body mass index (BMI) is helpful in assessing the nutritional status and total body fat of the patient. You can use the BMI chart in Appendix C to determine the BMI. You can also calculate the BMI by using the following formula.

Multiply the patient's weight in pounds by 704. Take that number (product) and divide by the patient's height in inches. Once again, divide by the height in inches.

Example: Weight = 75 lb; height = 4 feet 2 inches or 50 inches

75 × 704	=	52,800
52,800 ÷ 50	=	1056
1056 ÷ 50	=	21.12
BMI	=	21

Examine the Skin and Hair

Observe for signs of thyroid dysfunction or adrenal excess. Features of hypothyroidism include dry, coarse, flaky skin; coarse hair that tends to break; and thick, brittle nails. Hyperthyroidism is characterized by fine, warm skin that is hyperpigmented at pressure points. Nails often separate from the nail plate (onycholysis), and hair is fine, thin, and limp. Cushingoid features include truncal obesity, striae, and "moon face." Observe for other signs of androgen excess, which include hirsutism, acne, and male pattern baldness.

Perform a Head and Neck Examination

During the head and neck examination, note any visual changes, including visual field defects that might indicate a pituitary tumor. Anosmia might denote a congenital absence of GnRH, resulting in no secretion of LH or FSH from the pituitary. Without LH or FSH production, there is no ovulation; anovulatory cycles are amenorrheic. Also look for Turner syndrome features—a webbed neck and low-set ears. (Other signs are a shield-like chest and short fourth metacarpal.)

Palpate the Thyroid Gland and Lymph Nodes

Palpate the thyroid gland for diffuse enlargement, asymmetry, and nodules. Auscultate for thyroid bruits and count the pulse rate. Assess for supraclavicular and infraclavicular lymphadenopathy or carcinogenic masses of the sternal notch and abdomen, which could arise from a tumor of germ cell, adrenal, or pituitary origin.

Perform Clinical Breast Examination

Physical examination verifies sexual maturation level. The growth spurt occurs before breast development (thelarche), which is followed by the appearance of axillary hair. Perform a breast examination and assess breast maturity level using Tanner stages. More than 95% of adolescents are menarchal 1 year after they reach a breast stage of 4. Check for galactorrhea (see Chapter 6).

Perform a Pelvic Examination

Observe for maturation of the female genitalia and secondary sex characteristics. Assign a

Tanner stage for pubic hair development. A congenital problem might manifest as vaginal or uterine agenesis and is identified by the absence of a vagina, cervix, or uterus. There could be a small invagination of the perineum below the urinary meatus. It can be explored using a cotton-tipped applicator and otoscope with a large ear speculum or nasal speculum to determine the dimensions of the vault and presence of a cervix. A clitoris larger than 1 cm is suggestive of androgen excess.

Assess for other outlet problems, including an imperforate hymen (painful, bluish bulging of the perineum), stenotic cervix (bulging os, or inability to pass a cotton-tipped applicator through the os), or a transverse vaginal septum. The development of hematocolpos, hematometra, or hematoperitoneum from menses behind an obstructed outflow tract needs immediate intervention to prevent inflammatory changes and endometriosis. Needle aspiration is not recommended because it might potentiate infection. Refer to a reconstructive gynecologic surgeon for MRI, and often, extensive surgery.

If the introitus is small, use a pediatric or other appropriately sized speculum or a Huffman vaginoscope. Vaginal walls that are pale and dry, have few rugae, and are friable are estrogen deficient. Low estrogen levels cause scant cervical mucus. Vaginal cytology reports for women exhibiting such symptoms show an MI lacking or low in estrogen.

The bimanual examination can be performed with only an index finger in the vagina if the vaginal vestibule is small. If the hymen is rigid, a rectal bimanual examination can be completed instead of the usual vaginal bimanual examination. On pelvic bimanual examination, enlarged ovaries are palpated about half the time in patients with PCOS. Assess for position, size, shape, and consistency of the cervix, uterus, and ovaries.

LABORATORY AND DIAGNOSTIC STUDIES

Pregnancy Test

Urine or serum testing for the beta subunit of the human chorionic gonadotropin (β-hCG) is used to identify or rule out pregnancy and is an essential test on all patients presenting with amenorrhea.

Thyroid-Stimulating Hormone

A serum thyroid-stimulating hormone test identifies hypothyroidism. When hormonal supplementation is provided, menses usually resume for these patients. If the amenorrhea is associated with galactorrhea and hyperprolactinemia, the prolactin level must be measured again after the thyroid function levels become normal.

Prolactin Levels

About one-third of women with no obvious cause of amenorrhea will have an elevated prolactin level. When the patient's fasting prolactin level is within reference range (< 50 ng/mL), a PCT is indicated. If the fasting prolactin level is high(>50 ng/mL) or if the patient has galactorrhea, an MRI of the hypothalamic–pituitary area is done to rule out a pituitary adenoma. A level greater than 200 ng/mL is highly suggestive of a prolactinoma. A prolactin elevation less than 100 ng/mL but higher than normal is most frequently caused by prescribed or illicit drugs. The hyperprolactinemia usually subsides a few weeks after stopping the offending drug. Prolactin levels are normal in PCOS. Microscopic examination of breast discharge will reveal fat globules and no red blood cells (see Chapter 6).

Serum Follicle-Stimulating Hormone Levels

Ovarian failure, which causes a low estradiol secretion, will raise the FSH level higher than 40 mU/mL. If both the FSH and LH levels are greater than 50 mU/mL, then primary ovarian failure is established. If the patient is older than 30 years, menopause is diagnosed; if she is younger than 30 years, a karyotype should be done. An FSH measurement of less than 40 mU/mL denotes a hypothalamic–pituitary dysfunction and secondary ovarian failure.

Serum Luteinizing Hormone Levels

A serum LH level greater than 35 mU/mL is frequently seen in patients with PCOS. An

LH:FSH ratio higher than 2:1 is suggestive of PCOS, and a ratio higher than 3:1 is considered diagnostic of PCOS.

Dehydroepiandrosterone Sulfate

Mildly elevated levels of dehydroepiandrosterone sulfate (DHEA-S) are seen in women with PCOS. A significantly elevated level of DHEA-S (>700 mg/dL) indicates congenital adrenal hyperplasia.

Central Nervous System Imaging

If both FSH and LH levels are low or the prolactin level is greater than 100 ng/mL, indicating a problem of the pituitary, imaging of the CNS is warranted. MRI of the hypothalamic–pituitary area can determine whether there is an abnormality.

Pelvic Ultrasound and Vaginal Ultrasound

Pelvic and vaginal ultrasound studies are used to determine the presence of a uterus, the anatomical size and endometrial thickness of a uterus, and whether fibroids or other tumors exist. Ultrasound is used to measure ovarian size, to identify cysts, and to evaluate follicular development. In primary amenorrhea, ultrasound is helpful in assessing müllerian agenesis and gonadal dysgenesis because there could be internal organs and no conduit to the perineum. One-third of these patients also have urinary tract abnormalities; therefore, an abdominal ultrasound can be obtained at the same time to evaluate that system.

Progesterone Challenge Test

Also called the progesterone withdrawal test, the PCT consists of the administration of oral DMPA 10 mg/day for 7 to 10 days or parenteral progesterone in oil 200 mg intramuscularly. The patient should respond to the medication within 2 to 7 days. If there is a positive PCT response, the patient bleeds. This demonstrates that there are sufficient endogenous estrogens to prepare the endometrium and confirms that there is a functioning outflow tract. It substantiates an intact HPO axis. Other forms of progesterone can be used: micronized progesterone 400 mg/day orally for 7 to 10 days or norethindrone 5 mg/day orally for 7 to 10 days.

Estrogen/Progesterone Challenge Test

The estrogen/progesterone challenge test (E/PCT) consists of the administration of conjugated estrogens 1.25 mg/day or estradiol 2 mg/day for 21 days followed by progesterone as given in the PCT. If there is no menstrual flow, administer the regimen a second time. If there is no flow after both courses of therapy, the cause is either the outflow tract or the uterine endometrium. The E/PCT result is positive if there is menstrual flow within 2 to 7 days. A positive test result denotes that there is inadequate estrogen production either from inadequate functional ovarian follicles or from inadequate pituitary gonadotropic stimulation.

Chromosome Analysis (Karyotyping)

Karyotyping is done to delineate probable chromosomal abnormalities. Mullerian agenesis and androgen insensitivity are causes of primary amenorrhea. Turner syndrome is a cause of secondary amenorrhea. Karyotyping is used in the workup for ambiguous genitalia, primary amenorrhea, oligomenorrhea, delayed puberty, or abnormal development at puberty.

Endometrial Biopsy

Endometrial biopsy can be used to show the hormonal response of the uterine endometrium.

Basal Body Temperature Charting

Taking and recording the awakening body temperature each day can determine if ovulation is occurring. This test is based on the fact that progesterone increases the body temperature by 0.5° to 0.8°F for 11 days during the luteal phase. If this increase in temperature occurs, ovulation has occurred and a positive estrogen component is inferred.

Maturation Index

The MI indicates the degree of maturation of the vaginal epithelium and provides an objective assessment of vaginal hormone response as well as overall hormonal environment. The sample is collected by scraping the vaginal wall near the cervix. The index is read from left to right and refers to the percentage of parabasal, intermediate, and superficial squamous cells appearing on a smear, with the total of all three values equaling 100%. For example, an MI of 0/40/60 represents 0% parabasal cells, 40% intermediate cells, and 60% superficial cells. Lack of estrogen effect is demonstrated by the predominance of parabasal cells. Low estrogen effect is demonstrated by the predominance of intermediate cells. Increased estrogen effect is demonstrated by the predominance of superficial cells. Both increased and decreased estrogen effects can be reflective of a hormonal imbalance of the HPO axis.

Progesterone Levels

Serum progesterone levels collected at weekly intervals can establish whether ovulation has occurred. A value greater than 3 ng/mL is found with ovulation.

DIFFERENTIAL DIAGNOSIS

Pregnancy

Pregnancy is the most common reason for amenorrhea in women of childbearing age. Determining the pregnancy status of the patient is the first step in the amenorrhea workup.

Constitutional Problems

Delayed puberty

A pituitary adenoma must be ruled out for all patients with delayed puberty. Yearly prolactin levels should be performed for those with delayed puberty because of the possibility of occult pituitary adenomas.

Anorexia nervosa and bulimia

Anorexia nervosa and bulimia are disorders that are psychiatric in origin. Affected patients have such a fear of being fat that they do not eat or they purge after eating. Often these patients are overachievers and have low self-esteem. The majority are adolescents, with a mean age of 13 to 14 years. Amenorrhea is caused by extreme weight loss or a cachectic state.

Exercise-induced amenorrhea

This amenorrhea is common in competitive athletes, but exercise can also cause skipped menses in the casual trainer. Gymnasts, ballerinas, and long distance runners are at high risk, especially if they started their training at a very early age. Body fat of 17% is needed for menarche, and 22% body fat is necessary for ovulation. The BMI estimates the level of body fat.

Congenital or Chronic Disorders

Turner syndrome

Turner syndrome causes primary amenorrhea because of ovarian agenesis. The typical features are short stature, a webbed neck, a shield-like chest, and delayed secondary sex characteristics.

Cushing syndrome

Cushing syndrome is caused by an excess secretion of adrenocorticotropic hormone (ACTH) from a pituitary or adrenal adenoma. Classically, patients present with a moon face, acne, hirsutism, kyphosis, purplish striae of the abdomen, and hypertension. Diagnostic imaging can reveal pituitary or adrenal adenoma.

Thyroid dysfunction

Amenorrhea from thyroid dysfunction subsides as soon as serum thyroid levels return to normal. Hypothyroidism frequently causes amenorrhea and is characterized by fatigue, constipation, cold intolerance, and dry skin.

Polycystic ovarian syndrome

In PCOS, the patient typically is obese, is hirsute, has oligomenorrhea, and has large cystic ovaries. However, women with chronic anovulatory cycles and hyperandrogenemia meet the criteria for PCOS even if they are slim and without hirsutism. The LH:FSH ratio is greater than 3:1. The level of DHEA-S is elevated.

Uterine and Outflow Tract Problems

Imperforate hymen

The patient with an imperforate hymen could present with a painful, bulging perineum. There is lack of an intact outflow tract, which causes the primary amenorrhea.

Cervical os stenosis

Stenosis of the cervical os can be the cause of either primary or secondary amenorrhea. Stenosis is often caused by therapeutic procedures of the cervix such as cryotherapy or cone biopsies. These procedures cause scarring and stenosis of the os, obstructing the outflow tract.

Asherman syndrome

Asherman syndrome occurs when the uterine endometrial lining is denuded or scarred, usually by infection or curettage. The patient does not respond to either a PCT or an E/PCT.

Hypothalamic–Pituitary–Ovarian Axis Problem

Ovarian failure

Menopause occurs when the ovaries fail, secondary to depletion of ova. The average age of menopause in the United States is 51 years. It is a state of hypoestrogenemia. The gonadotropin levels rise (FSH >40 mU/mL), and the estradiol levels fall (<15 pg/mL). Clinical symptoms are hot flashes, night sweats, insomnia, mood changes, and amenorrhea for 12 months. If this occurs before age 40 years, it is considered premature. Common causes of premature ovarian failure include genetic and enzyme disorders, immune disturbances, and chemotherapy.

Sheehan syndrome

Sheehan syndrome is activated by severe obstetrical hemorrhage, which causes pituitary ischemia and infarction. The pituitary gland becomes dysfunctional.

Medications

Prescription and illicit drugs can increase prolactin levels, which in turn promote galactorrhea. Offending drugs are primarily dopamine antagonist agents, estrogens, and marijuana.

Chest wall or nipple stimulation

Prolactin inhibits the pulsatile secretion of GnRH, unbalancing the HPO axis and possibly causing amenorrhea. The higher the prolactin level, the greater the likelihood that the patient will be amenorrheic.

Pituitary adenoma

Pituitary macroadenomas and microadenomas should be suspected if the prolactin level is greater than 100 ng/mL or if there are any abnormalities of the MRI of the hypothalamic–pituitary area. Patients with pituitary adenomas should be referred to an endocrinologist. Patients with prolactin levels exceeding 1000 ng/mL probably have an invasive tumor.

▶ DIFFERENTIAL DIAGNOSIS OF *Common Causes of Amenorrhea*

CONDITION	HISTORY	PHYSICAL FINDINGS	DIAGNOSTIC STUDIES
PREGNANCY			
Pregnancy	Breast tenderness, morning sickness, urinary frequency	Globular, enlarged uterus; soft, bluish color cervix	β-hCG pregnancy test result positive; ultrasonography positive

Continued

▶ **DIFFERENTIAL DIAGNOSIS OF** *Common Causes of Amenorrhea—cont'd*

CONDITION	HISTORY	PHYSICAL FINDINGS	DIAGNOSTIC STUDIES
CONSTITUTIONAL PROBLEMS			
Delayed puberty	No menstruation beyond age 16 yr; more than 5 yr between initiation of breast growth and menarche	Breast stage 1 persists beyond age 13.4 yr; pubic hair stage 1 persists beyond age 14.1	Prolactin normal; TSH, T_4 normal; CBC, U/A normal; chemistry profile normal; bone age normal; skull radiograph normal
Anorexia nervosa or bulimia	Mean age, 13–14 yr; fear of being fat; low self-esteem; depression; isolation; overachiever; food is parental battleground; preoccupation; hair loss; abdominal bloating, pain, constipation	Amenorrhea before or after weight loss; cachexia; low body fat; short stature; yellow, dry, cold skin; acrocyanosis: increased lanugo hair; hypotension, systolic murmurs, often mitral valve prolapse	TSH normal; prolactin normal; FSH and LH usually low; glucose normal; ECG: bradycardia, low-voltage changes, T wave inversions, and occasional ST-segment depression
Exercise-induced amenorrhea	Began athletic training at young age; more common with long-distance runners, ballerinas, gymnasts	BMI <17% body fat	TSH normal; prolactin normal
CONGENITAL OR CHRONIC DISORDERS			
Turner syndrome	Congenital; short stature; infantile sexual development	Characteristics: webbed neck, low-set ears, shield-like chest, short fourth metacarpal	Karyotype (45,X)
Cushing syndrome	Weight gain; weakness; back pain	Moon face, acne, hirsutism, purple striae of abdomen	Cortisol increased; 17-ketosteroids increased; CT adenoma
Thyroid dysfunction	Hypothyroid: delayed growth, weight gain, fatigue, constipation, cold intolerance; hyperthyroid: weight loss, nervousness, heat intolerance	Hypothyroid: dry skin, fine hair, galactorrhea; hyperthyroid: moist skin, hyperpigmentation over bones, thin hair, goiter	Hypothyroid: TSH high; hyperthyroid: TSH low; T_3 high; T_4 high
Polycystic ovary syndrome	Infertility	Hirsutism; obesity; enlarged ovaries	LH:FSH ratio higher than 3:1; DHEA-S may be elevated
UTERINE AND OUTFLOW TRACT PROBLEMS			
Imperforate hymen or stenotic cervical os	Monthly bloating, cramping, and pelvic pressure; no menses; cryotherapy or other procedure to cervix	Fibrotic hymen without patent opening; stenotic cervical os	Clinical diagnosis by history and findings
Asherman syndrome	History of uterine infection; tuberculosis, schistosomiasis; uterine iatrogenic scarring; curettage, irradiation	Pelvic examination normal	PCT negative; E/PCT negative; hysteroscopy adhesions

> **DIFFERENTIAL DIAGNOSIS OF** *Common Causes of Amenorrhea—cont'd*

CONDITION	HISTORY	PHYSICAL FINDINGS	DIAGNOSTIC STUDIES
HYPOTHALAMIC–PITUITARY–OVARIAN AXIS PROBLEM			
Ovarian failure	Hot flashes, night sweats, insomnia, mood changes	Pale, dry vaginal mucosa; few rugae	FSH and LH high; estradiol low
Sheehan syndrome	Recent history of postpartum hemorrhage and shock during delivery	Hair loss; depigmentation of skin; mammary and genital atrophy	Pituitary and end-organ hormones low; hemoglobin low
Medications or chest wall or nipple stimulation	Breast nipple discharge; history of dopamine antagonists, estrogens, or illicit drugs; stimulation of nipples: exercise or sexual; history of chest wall surgery or herpes zoster	Nipple discharge: bilateral; multiduct; milky, clear, or yellowish discharge	Wet mount or hemoccult of nipple discharge: negative for RBCs; prolactin high; MRI of hypothalamic–pituitary areas
Pituitary adenoma	Delayed puberty; history of visual changes, increasing headaches	Visual field defects; galactorrhea	Prolactin high; MRI of hypothalamic–pituitary area

β-hCG, Beta human chorionic gonadotropin; *BMI*, body mass index; *CBC*, complete blood cell count; *CT*, computed tomography; *DHEA-S*, dehydroepiandrosterone sulfate; *ECG*, electrocardiogram; *E/PCT*, estrogen/progesterone challenge test; *FSH*, follicle-stimulating hormone; *LH*, luteinizing hormone; *MRI*, magnetic resonance imaging; *PCT*, progesterone challenge test; *RBCs*, red blood cells; *T₃*, triiodothyronine; *T₄*, thyroxine; *TSH*, thyroid-stimulating hormone; *U/A*, urinalysis.

Breast Lumps and Nipple Discharge

Up to 90% of all breast lumps are found by the patient or partner before detection by clinical breast examination (CBE) or mammography. The three most common breast lumps are fibroadenomas, fibrocystic breast changes, and breast carcinoma. Fibroadenomas are benign solid tumors most frequently seen before age 30 years. Fibrocystic breast changes are a heterogeneous group of nonproliferative changes of stromal or glandular (or both stromal and glandular) elements of the breast tissue that include benign cysts, diffuse and localized nodularity, nipple discharge, and breast tenderness. Fibrocystic symptoms are seen with great frequency in patients ages 30 to 50 years but less often in those who are menopausal.

Breast carcinoma is the most common cancer in women and the second leading cause of cancer-related death. The risk of breast cancer in patients with female breasts rises steadily with age and accelerates rapidly after the age of 50 years. Although benign conditions that affect the breast are more common, the presence of a lump raises legitimate fears. The goal of the assessment process is to reach a diagnosis that addresses the possibility of breast cancer.

Nipple discharge is a common complaint among postmenarchal patients. It is often related to pregnancy, recent breastfeeding, or estrogenic medications. In patients who are not lactating, nipple discharge is most frequently caused by intraductal papilloma, duct ectasia, or cancer. Nipple discharge is more commonly caused by benign lesions than by cancerous ones. Physiological stimulation (e.g., sucking, pregnancy, mechanical stimulation) of the breasts can produce discharge, as can breast trauma and inflammation (e.g., herpes zoster, mammoplasty), pituitary disorders (e.g., pituitary adenoma), or tranquilizing drugs (e.g., phenothiazines, methyldopa).

DIAGNOSTIC REASONING: FOCUSED HISTORY FOR BREAST LUMPS

Is this lump likely to be malignant?

- How long has the lump been present?
- Is the lump changing (e.g., getting bigger, worse, or more painful)?
- Is the lump in one breast only, or are there lumps in both breasts?
- When was your last menstrual period?
- Is there any discharge from the nipple? If so, describe it.
- Have you recently been treated for a breast infection?

Duration and Growth

The primary presenting complaint of a malignant lesion is that of a single, hard, painless lump in the breast that is unchanged by the cyclic hormonal milieu. A change from the patient's normal physical findings is the most persuasive criterion for considering a diagnosis of breast cancer.

Malignant lumps are more likely to be new lumps that show progressive increase in size. The lump grows until there is an alteration in the contour of the breast tissue. An unchanged lump of long duration (years) is almost always benign. Half of all newly appearing benign cysts resolve within two or three menstrual cycles.

Unilateral versus Bilateral

Breast lumps found bilaterally in identical quadrants of the breast are more likely to be benign. A solitary unilateral lump, although usually a cyst, fibroadenoma, or lipoma (rare), raises more suspicion for malignancy.

Postmenopausal

Cyclic cysts of the breast are less common after menopause and necessitate diagnostic investigation. A postmenopausal patient with unilateral mastalgia (breast pain) has a greater risk for breast cancer. Perimenopausal and postmenopausal patients are also at greater statistical risk for breast cancer because of the higher incidence of breast cancer as they age. A new breast lump in a postmenopausal patient warrants a high degree of suspicion for cancer.

Nipple Discharge with a Lump

The occurrence of nipple discharge, with the presence of a lump, is worrisome because it can represent a ductal cancer. This condition demands further investigation such as mammogram, ultrasonography, ductogram, and biopsy.

Infection

Any residual masses in the breast after antibiotic therapy are suspicious for malignancy and require biopsy.

Does the person have additional risk factors for breast cancer?

Key Questions
- Have you ever had breast cancer or ductal cancer in situ?
- Have you ever had a breast biopsy that showed atypical cells?
- Do you have a family history of breast cancer (i.e., first-degree relative)?
- Have you ever had ovarian, endometrial, colon, or thyroid cancer?
- Do you have a family history of ovarian, endometrial, colon, or prostate cancer?
- Have you ever received radiation to the chest or had a malignancy in childhood?

Risk Factors

The presence of risk factors in a patient who has a lump raises the index of suspicion for malignancy. It is important to remember that the absence of such risk factors is not cancer protective. About 70% to 80% of all breast cancers occur in patients who have no risk factors for malignancy. Patients with a personal history of breast cancer, ductal carcinoma in situ (DCIS), atypical ductal hyperplasia (ADH) or atypical lobular hyperplasia (ALH), or lobular carcinoma in situ (LCIS) are usually evaluated every 6 months because of their increased risk for malignancy. Malignant breast tumors in adolescents are more likely to be a metastasis such as Hodgkin lymphoma, rhabdomyosarcoma, or neuroblastoma rather than a primary tumor. A history of chest wall irradiation is a risk factor. See Box 6.1 for a

---

Box 6.1   Primary Risk Factors for Breast Cancer

FEMALE BREASTS

AGE
75% of all cases occur after age 50 years; there is no plateau effect with age.

PERSONAL HISTORY OF BREAST CANCER OR CANCER IN SITU
DCIS is a precursor of cancer and increases the risk for invasive breast cancer, usually in the same breast.

PREVIOUS HISTORY OF BREAST BIOPSIES FOR NONMALIGNANT BREAST DISEASE
Biopsy-proved proliferative changes or atypical epithelial hyperplasia; fibrocystic histological findings that indicate increased risk of breast cancer are moderate or severe hyperplasia (1.5 to 2 times the risk), atypical hyperplasia (5 times the risk), and LCIS (8 to 10 times the risk); LCIS is a marker for cancer rather than a precursor; the cancer may occur in either breast.

LABORATORY EVIDENCE OF SPECIFIC GENETIC MUTATION
Presence of breast cancer mutation genes *BRCA1* or *BRCA2*

PERSONAL HISTORY OF CANCER
Ovarian, endometrial, colon, or thyroid cancers

FAMILY HISTORY OF BREAST CANCER
In first-degree relatives (mother, sister, or daughter) or in two or more close relatives

DCIS, Ductal carcinoma in situ; *LCIS*, lobular carcinoma in situ.

summary of characteristics that could increase the risk for breast cancer.

Is this condition more likely to be benign?

Key Questions
- How old are you?
- Do you have a history of cystic breast changes or lumpy breasts?
- Does this lump feel like other lumps you have had?
- Do the lumps change with your periods?
- Have you ever had a mammogram or ultrasound? Why was it done? What were the results?
- Have you ever had a lump drained or biopsied? What was the diagnosis?
- Do you have breast implants?

Age

Fibrocystic breast changes occur predominantly between the ages of 20 and 30 years. Fibroadenomas are more frequent between the ages of 15 to 39 years. Whereas intraductal papilloma and ductal ectasia occur in the age range of 35 to 55 years, breast carcinoma is most prevalent in ages 40 to 70 years. Any patient older than 25 years who has a breast lump should be evaluated by CBE, diagnostic mammography with tomosynthesis, or ultrasonography. Magnetic resonance imaging (MRI) sometimes can be used in addition to mammography and ultrasonography. Additional evaluation with tissue biopsy may be required.

Timing, Consistency, and Duration

The most frequent breast complaint is that of a painful, mobile lump that increases in size and tenderness as the menstrual cycle approaches. The lump commonly has discrete borders that allow for measurement of the length, width, and depth of the lesion by the patient (e.g., size of a pea). The lump remains prominent on breast self-examination, is almost always painful to palpate, and frequently causes pain with changes in position of the arm on the affected side. Fibrocystic breast changes exist on a continuum that corresponds with the menstrual cycle. Tenderness and size variations occur throughout the month.

Previous Mammograms or Biopsies

History or documentation of cyclic changes in lumps or the presence of glandular breast tissue on a mammogram or ultrasound supports a clinical diagnosis of benign disease. More convincing evidence of benign disease occurs when there is a clear fluid aspirate from the cyst, with no residual or recurring breast lump, with the caveat that benign disease and malignant disease can occur simultaneously.

Breast Implants

With a ruptured implant, augmented breast tissue is pushed away from the chest wall by the implant.

Could this lump be mastitis related to lactation?

Key Questions
- Have you recently given birth?
- Are you currently breastfeeding or breast suckling?
- Are your nipples sore or cracked?
- Have you had pierced nipples?
- Is your breast painful or hot? Are there any areas of redness?
- Have you had a fever?

Childbirth

Engorgement or congestive mastitis begins on day 2 or 3 after delivery and affects both breasts. A breast mass in a lactating patient is usually associated with mastitis, an inflammation of breast tissue, and a blocked duct. It occurs most often in primiparous nursing mothers and is usually caused by coagulase-positive *Staphylococcus aureus*. It can also occur during periods of weaning, when the flow of milk is disrupted. Inflammatory breast cancer in lactating patients is rare but must be considered.

Sore, Cracked, or Pierced Nipples

Cracked or pierced nipples can be a site for the introduction of infection.

Painful or Hot Breast

Mastitis is characterized by a breast that is painful, hot, and red. In lactating patients, the most frequent symptom is a painful, erythematous lobule in an outer quadrant of the breast. Although mastitis is most common in lactating patients, it can also occur in nonlactating patients, usually as the result of a generalized dermatitis occurring from insect bites, sunburn, or allergic reactions. However, the most common cause of an inflamed breast in nonlactating women is inflammatory breast cancer. In inflammatory breast cancer, the entire breast is swollen, heavy, and edematous.

Fever

Fever is a sign of infectious mastitis and occurs most often in association with lactation and breastfeeding. High fever does not occur because of simple breast engorgement in the postpartum period. Fever does not usually occur in inflammatory breast cancer and is rare in dermatitis reactions.

DIAGNOSTIC REASONING: FOCUSED HISTORY FOR NIPPLE DISCHARGE

A focused history can help sort out the causes of the most frequently presenting cases of nipple discharge. Questioning should address normal lactation, high circulating levels of prolactin, and malignancy.

Is this normal lactation?

Key Questions

- When was your last normal menstrual period? How frequent are your cycles?
- Is it possible that you are pregnant? What are you using for birth control?
- When was your last delivery or miscarriage? How long were you pregnant?
- Did you breastfeed? For how long? When did you stop?
- Is the nipple discharge clear or milky?
- How long have you had the nipple discharge?

Menstrual Cycle

Frequently, fibrocystic breast changes are most marked just before menses and manifest as a spontaneous multiple duct discharge that can be either unilateral or bilateral.

Pregnancy and Lactation

Pregnancy is the most common cause of breast tenderness and clear or milky nipple discharge (galactorrhea). A bloody nipple discharge during pregnancy is usually the result of vascular engorgement and clears within weeks. Recent pregnancy or breastfeeding (within 8 weeks) can account for a prolonged, clear, or milky discharge that is successfully suppressed by decreased breast stimulation or by the administration of dopamine agonist therapy (bromocriptine or pergolide). If the patient has had prolonged lactation, there can be milk formation even though prolactin levels are normal.

Color of Discharge

Normal lactation produces a discharge that is milky and nonpurulent. Mastitis associated with breastfeeding can produce purulent discharge. A subareolar abscess can also produce a purulent discharge. Mastitis and abscesses that produce purulent nipple discharge must be distinguished from inflammatory breast cancer by biopsy or by evoking remission with antibiotic therapy.

Oral contraceptives can cause a clear, serous, or milky discharge from single or multiple ducts. Ductal ectasia and papillomatosis can produce a greenish or brownish nipple discharge. A serous or serosanguineous discharge from a single duct is usually indicative of an intraductal papilloma but can be from an intraductal cancer. A bloody nipple discharge can occur with benign or cancerous conditions.

Duration of Discharge

Patients who breastfeed sometimes experience a milky discharge long after the termination of nursing. New-onset discharge in a patient who is not pregnant or lactating requires further investigation.

Is the discharge related to high prolactin levels?

Key Questions

- What medications are you taking?
- Do you jog or run? If yes: Do you wear a sports bra? Do your nipples rub on your clothing?

- Are your breasts fondled, squeezed, or suckled during sexual activity?
- Do you have a thyroid condition?
- What medical conditions or health problems do you have?
- If a newborn: Has the discharge been present since birth?

Medicines

Patients taking multiple tranquilizing medications are often found to have nipple discharge. Discontinuation of the medication(s) usually eliminates most clear, or milky, bilateral nipple discharge. However, the condition might not warrant a drug cessation trial. See Box 6.2 for medications that can produce nipple discharge.

Behavioral Activities

Nipple stimulation (sexual or during jogging) increases prolactin levels, as does the use of marijuana. Only about 13% of men with hyperprolactinemia will develop gynecomastia and galactorrhea. Patients with increased prolactin levels commonly experience both galactorrhea and amenorrhea.

Box 6.2	**Drugs That Can Produce Nipple Discharge**

ESTROGENS OR DRUGS THAT INCREASE ESTROGEN
- Digitalis
- Marijuana
- Heroin

DOPAMINE RECEPTOR BLOCKERS
- Phenothiazines
- Haloperidol
- Metoclopramide
- Isoniazid

CNS DOPAMINE DEPLETERS
- Tricyclic antidepressants
- Reserpine
- Methyldopa
- Cimetidine
- Benzodiazepines

CNS, central nervous system.

Other Causes of Galactorrhea

Certain genetic disorders, medical conditions, and central nervous system (CNS) lesions can be responsible for galactorrhea.

- *Genetic disorders:* Chiari-Frommel syndrome, Argonz-del Castillo (Forbes-Albright) syndrome
- *Medical conditions:* chronic renal failure, sarcoidosis, Schüller-Christian disease, Cushing disease, hepatic cirrhosis, hypothyroidism
- *CNS lesions:* pituitary adenoma, empty sella, hypothalamic tumor, head trauma

Newborns

The breasts of a newborn can be abnormally enlarged secondary to the effects of maternal estrogens. A discharge that is usually white can be present, and is commonly referred to as *witch's milk.*

Can the nipple discharge be a sign of malignancy?

Key Questions

- Is the nipple discharge spontaneous, or must it be expressed?
- Does it come from one or both nipples?
- Does it come from one or multiple nipple ducts?
- Do you also have a breast lump?
- Are you postmenopausal?

Spontaneous versus Expressed Discharge

Spontaneous discharge is more concerning than expressed discharge. Bilateral spontaneous discharge is likely related to lactation or systemic causes (e.g., hyperprolactinemia). Unilateral spontaneous discharge is associated with intraductal papilloma or cancer.

Unilateral versus Bilateral Discharge

Unilateral discharge is usually associated with an intraductal papilloma or cancer. Bilateral breast findings seldom represent cancer.

Single-Duct versus Multiple-Duct Discharge

Single-duct involvement is more suspicious for intraductal papilloma or cancer. Multiple-duct discharges usually are caused by hyperprolactinemia or duct ectasia.

Associated Mass

An associated mass could be benign or malignant. Further evaluation is mandatory. Ultrasonography is helpful in differentiating solid from cystic lesions and is often the first step in the evaluation of a cyst or a mass in a patient with firm, dense breast tissue.

Postmenopausal

Postmenopausal patients have a higher incidence of breast cancer. Other risky signs for a cancerous cause of nipple discharge are the presence of a mass or lump, unilateral nipple discharge, abnormal cytology, and an abnormal mammogram.

Nipple discharge that is spontaneous, unilateral, and from a single duct is suspicious for a cancerous etiology.

DIAGNOSTIC REASONING: FOCUSED PHYSICAL EXAMINATION

Perform a multiposition physical examination of the breasts and nipples. See the Evidence-Based Practice box on the effectiveness of CBE.

Inspect the Breasts and Nipples

Inspect the breasts while the patient is sitting with her arms at her sides, arms pushing down on hips (to contract the pectoralis muscles), arms elevated above the head, and while the patient is bending forward from the waist (gravity pulling on breast tissue). Look for changes in breast shape or contour, a lump, or dimpling. Contraction of underlying muscles in the different arm positions will accentuate skin findings caused by a fixed adherent lesion characteristic of cancer. Look for breasts that are notably asymmetrical. The skin over the lesion could then flatten or dimple inward, or the nipple could be directed differently than the nipple of the opposite breast. Normal nipples are everted and point in like directions. Lifelong inversion, either unilateral or bilateral, is also normal, but a new inversion is suspicious. Engorgement (congestive mastitis) involves both breasts, which are enlarged and tense. Infectious mastitis usually involves one lobe or a quadrant of one breast.

Observe Skin of Breasts and Nipples

Observe the patient's skin color for erythema and unilateral prominent blood vessels, which may be a presentation of breast cancer. Prominent vessels, plus a tender cordlike vein, suggest thrombophlebitis of the superficial veins of the breast. Both conditions require a CBE and a mammogram to look for a mass. Paget disease begins as a scaling eczematoid area on the nipple and progresses to a deep lump behind the nipple well. Paget disease can produce darkly pigmented lesions that are suspicious for malignant melanoma. An excisional or punch biopsy is recommended to distinguish Paget disease from malignant melanoma

EVIDENCE-BASED PRACTICE *Effectiveness of Clinical Breast Examination in Detecting Breast Cancer*

In this systematic review of randomized clinical trials, the authors estimated clinical breast examination (CBE) sensitivity at 54% and specificity at 94%. The ability of CBE to detect breast cancers missed on screening mammograms ranged from 3% to 45%. The lack of standardized examination techniques contributed to differences in findings among clinicians. A longer time spent in performing CBE and use of specific techniques were associated with greater accuracy. The authors concluded that CBE should be performed as part of screening for breast cancer. The authors' bottom line for the CBE procedure: position the patient properly; use a vertical-strip pattern covering all breast tissue; make circular motions with the pads of the fingers, depressing tissue with light, medium, and deep pressure; and spend at least 3 minutes examining each breast.

Reference: Barton et al, 1999.

or other ulcerative lesions such as Bowen disease, eczema, or papillomatosis. Observe the condition of the skin of the nipples for cracks or dried exudate or the presence of nipple flattening or retraction.

Palpate the Breasts with the Patient Sitting

Stand in front of the patient and place the palm of your right hand at the patient's right clavicle at the sternum. Sweep downward from the clavicle to the nipple, feeling for superficial lumps. Repeat the sweep until you have covered the entire right chest wall. Repeat the procedure using your left hand for the left chest wall.

Perform bimanual digital palpation. Place one hand, palmar surface facing up, under the patient's right breast. Position your hand so that it acts as a flat surface against which to compress the breast tissue. With the fingers of the other hand, walk across the breast mound, feeling for lumps as you compress the tissue between your fingers and your flat hand. Repeat the procedure for the other breast.

If the patient has augmentation of breast tissue, small masses, including those from ruptured implants, can best be felt with the patient in the sitting position.

Palpate Lymph Nodes

Palpate the supraclavicular, infraclavicular, and axillary lymph nodes (Fig. 6.1). The supraclavicular lymph nodes can be accessed by having the patient shrug her shoulders; then feel deep in the supraclavicular hollow. Feel for lymph nodes, noting their size, shape, consistency, and mobility. The presence of a small (<1 cm), single, rubbery, and mobile lymph node can be a sign of inflammation; rarely is it a sign of early malignancy. However, finding one or more lymph nodes in the same region that are larger than 1 cm, firm, fixed to the chest wall, or of a matted consistency is highly suggestive of metastatic disease.

Palpate the Breasts and Nipples with the Patient Supine

With the patient supine, ask her to position one arm above her head. Place a small towel

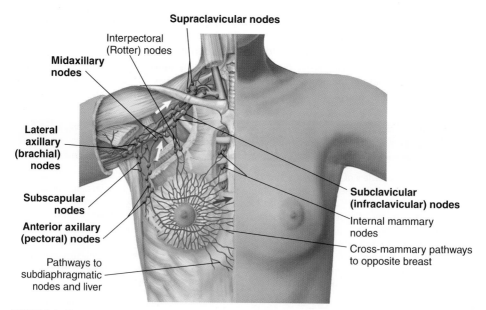

FIGURE 6.1 Six groups of lymph nodes accessible to palpation. (From Ball JW, Dains JE, Flynn JA, et al: *Seidel's guide to physical examination,* ed. 9, St. Louis, 2018, Elsevier.)

behind the scapula to aid in flattening the breast tissue. Palpate all areas of breast tissue, feeling for lumps or nodules. Remember that the breast tissue extends from the second or third rib to the sixth or seventh rib and from the sternal margin to the midaxillary line. It is essential to include the tail of Spence in palpation. Recall that the greatest amount of glandular tissue lies in the upper outer quadrant of the breast, with tissue extending from this quadrant into the axilla, to form the tail of Spence.

Palpate using your finger pads because they are more sensitive than your fingertips. Palpate systematically, pushing gently but firmly toward the chest, with your fingers rotating in a clockwise or counterclockwise pattern. At each point, press inward using three depths of palpation: light, then medium, and finally deep palpation. Strip, concentric circle, or wedge methods are commonly used for ensuring palpation of the entire breast. The vertical strip method has evidence of greater accuracy. Be sure that every part of the breast is palpated. Regardless of the method, glide your fingers from one point to the next. Avoid lifting your fingers off the breast tissue because doing so makes it easy to miss tissue.

Assess the Nipple Well

At the completion of the examination, return to the nipple, and with two fingers, gently depress the tissue inward into the well behind the areola. Your fingers and tissue should move easily inward. A normal nipple well is a smooth concave structure. Most lumps in this area are found at the areola border. Repeat with the other breast.

Examine the Nipple for Discharge

Palpate for discharge only if the patient presents with a report of nipple discharge. Place the thumb and first finger 1 to 2 cm outside the border of the areolar complex and gently compress, sliding the fingers toward the nipple in a milking fashion. Repeat this maneuver twice, cephalocaudally and laterally. Determine if the discharge is unilateral or bilateral. Look closely to determine if the discharge is from a single duct or multiple ducts. Palpation of a single site on the areola border may reproduce the discharge and reveal the responsible duct. Specimen collection is often easier and of a larger quantity when the patient is sitting.

Inflammatory symptoms and a purulent nipple discharge are suggestive of a breast abscess.

Transilluminate Breast Masses

Transillumination of a breast mass (best performed in a darkened room) sometimes provides diagnostic clues. A fluid-filled cyst will transilluminate, but a solid mass will not. A solid lump is more frequently a malignant mass, and a cystic, fluid-filled lump is more commonly benign.

Characterize Lumps

Accurately measure any lumps by marking the edges with a pen and measure the width and length with a centimeter ruler. Estimate the depth of the lesion, contour, shape, fluctuation, firmness, and mobility.

Fluctuation can be determined by holding the edges of the mass against the chest wall and pressing the center with finger pads. Fluctuation ("bouncy" consistency) occurs with cysts, lipomas, and abscesses. Cysts are frequently tender, especially premenstrually. Reexamination in 1 or 2 weeks will usually demonstrate cyclic hormonal changes of the tissue, and lump size and tenderness will have changed. In a postmenopausal patient, hormone replacement therapy can stimulate similar symptoms of breast lumps and pain (mastodynia). A single, firm, asymmetrical, immobile mass in a postmenopausal patient will, when biopsied, prove to be cancerous 75% of the time.

LABORATORY AND DIAGNOSTIC STUDIES

The diagnostic accuracy of ultrasonography, mammography, and aspiration biopsy ranges from about 70% to 80% and varies with the training and skills of the clinician or technician. Therefore, a high degree of suspicion for cancer and excellent patient follow-up should be sustained for a breast lump or nipple discharge.

Ultrasonography

Ultrasonography is helpful in differentiating solid from cystic lesions. In women younger than age 30 years, ultrasonography is often the first step in the evaluation of a cyst or a mass. The ultrasound finding of a cystic lesion can be followed by aspiration of the cyst, eliminating it to make sure it is not concealing another abnormal breast finding. The ultrasound identification of a solid mass can be followed by tissue biopsy.

Mammography: Diagnostic

In the presence of a palpable mass or nipple discharge, a diagnostic mammogram is necessary to identify palpable lumps or further evaluate abnormal screening mammograms. It consists of additional views to the features and location of palpable masses. Additional views could include spot clarify compression, magnification, exaggerated craniocaudal (CC) to the medial or lateral side, tangential, and 90-degree lateral views. Mammography is of less diagnostic value in patients younger than age 30 because of the density of the breast tissue. Mammogram with tomosynthesis creates a three-dimensional image that minimizes tissue overlap and improves detection of masses.

Magnetic Resonance Imaging

Magnetic resonance imaging is used primarily to evaluate abnormal areas that are seen on a mammogram, and to assess breast implants for leaks or ruptures. MRI is sometimes useful in viewing breast abnormalities that can be felt but are not visible with mammography or ultrasound. It also can be used to image dense breast tissue, which is often found in younger patients. Contrast is used to enhance the vascularity of malignant lesions. Although MRI is highly sensitive (85%–100%), it lacks specificity. MRI is inferior to mammography in detecting in situ cancers and cancers smaller than 3 mm. The role of MRI in the evaluation of nipple discharge is evolving.

Fine-Needle Aspiration and Cytologic Examination

Fine-needle aspiration (FNA) biopsy uses a small-gauge needle to obtain fluid and cellular material. FNA is a routinely performed office procedure that is both diagnostic and therapeutic. It immediately determines if the lump is a cyst or a solid tumor. The aspirate is sent for cytologic evaluation to determine the presence or absence of malignant cells. If cytology findings of the aspirate are negative, the mass completely goes away and is not present on follow-up examinations, no further treatment is necessary.

Stereotactic or Needle Localization Biopsy

Fine-needle aspiration can also be used with ultrasonography or stereotactic imaging to further assess and obtain adequate sampling in poorly defined palpable masses. The lesion is located, marked, and verified by imaging to assist in the identification of the tissue to be sampled.

Core Needle Biopsy

Core needle biopsy uses a large-gauge needle to obtain several cores of tissue. It produces a larger tissue sample than FNA. It can be used in conjunction with ultrasonography or stereotactic imaging for small or difficult-to-palpate lesions. Local anesthesia is required.

Excisional Biopsy

Excisional biopsy is the gold standard for evaluating breast masses. It is performed in an operating room using local or general anesthetic, and the entire lesion is removed. Excisional biopsy is indicated if there is a large breast mass or for lesions in which more conservative biopsy has produced equivocal results. The surgical specimen is evaluated histologically.

Microscopy

Microscopy of nipple discharge can reveal fat cells of galactorrhea, leukocytes of infection, or red blood cells. Care must be taken to prevent the slide from drying out. Place a coverslip on the slide immediately after obtaining the specimen and review the slide shortly after it is prepared.

Cytologic Smear

A cytologic specimen of discharge is placed directly from the nipple onto the slide, or if there is only a small amount of discharge, it can easily be collected with a saline-saturated cotton-tipped applicator and spread onto the slide. The slide is then fixed in the same manner as a cervical specimen. This technique can expose cancerous cells. However, a smear with negative findings is not conclusive, and additional workup is mandated.

Ductography (Ductogram)

A ductogram is useful in evaluating the cause of nipple discharge. Contrast medium is injected into the discharging duct followed by a mammogram. The mammogram may show a filling defect (commonly an intraductal papilloma), a dilated or cystic appearance (duct ectasia or fibrocystic disease), or an abrupt obstruction (malignancy).

Serum Prolactin Level

Elevated serum prolactin levels can produce nipple discharge. Hyperprolactinemia should be suspected when the prolactin level exceeds 20 to 25 ng/mL. Prolactin elevation secondary to medications is generally less than 100 ng/mL. Prolactinomas are found when the prolactin level exceeds 150 ng/mL.

Thyroid Function Testing

Thyroid-stimulating hormone (TSH) is high in hypothyroidism. About 20% of patients with hyperprolactinemia have hypothyroidism. TSH testing is done to rule out primary hypothyroidism as a cause of the hyperprolactinemia and associated nipple discharge.

DIFFERENTIAL DIAGNOSIS

Single Breast Mass

Cancer

Breast cancer can occur at any time after puberty, but it occurs more frequently with increasing age. Classically, breast cancer is a single lump that is hard, nontender, and immobile and with borders that are not clearly delineated from the rest of the breast tissue. It occurs most commonly in the upper, outer quadrant of the breast. Malignant tumors eventually affix to the skin, ligaments, or chest wall and cause retractions. Cancers infrequently cause pain or tenderness on palpation, but some do. The tumors continually increase

in size (although at varying rates) and do not come and go. Other suspicious signs of cancer include nipple inversion, dimpling of the breast, bloody nipple discharge, and axillary lymphadenopathy. Occasionally, breast cancer presents as diffuse swelling, pain, or breast erythema. Unilateral breast pain in a postmenopausal patient is suggestive of cancer. A mammographic finding of a nonpalpable mass or preinvasive lesion associated with macrocalcifications could be the only evidence of a malignant breast mass. Benign lumps are usually smooth, round, and freely movable. However, colloid, medullary, and expansive intraductal cancers can feel like benign tumors.

Fifteen percent of patients younger than 40 years who have breast cancer are diagnosed during pregnancy or the postpartum period. Pregnant and postpartum women with breast cancer make up about 2% of total number of patients with breast cancer. The normal physiological changes of the breast tissue during these times necessitate a thorough history and physical examination. A breast lump during pregnancy or lactation is more difficult to sample for a biopsy because of the increased vascularity of the breasts. Additionally, a lactating breast can act as an ideal medium for bacterial infection and is slower to heal.

Cysts

Benign cysts occur with higher frequency than any other type of breast lump. They are typically round or elliptical, soft or fluctuant, and mobile. Cysts are not attached to the surrounding breast, nipple, or chest wall, so there is no dimpling of breast tissue or nipple retraction. There are often multiple cysts, frequently in the upper outer quadrants of each breast. Cysts vary in size throughout the menstrual cycle and are usually at their smallest and least tender stage at the end of menses (end of the secretory phase). Transillumination of a cyst allows light to pass through the lump and supports the clinical diagnosis.

Fibroadenoma

Fibroadenoma usually occurs as a single, nontender, rubbery, firm, ovoid, or lobulated mass that measures 1 to 5 cm in diameter. The lump is freely mobile; thus, there is no dimpling or retractions. Fibroadenomas do not vary in size with the menstrual cycle. Fibroadenomas are multiple or bilateral about 25% of the time. They are the most commonly occurring breast mass in adolescence. Only biopsy can distinguish them from dysplasia, cancer, or cystosarcoma phyllodes.

Cystosarcoma phyllodes is a type of fibroadenoma in which the tumor grows rapidly and reaches a large size. Surgical removal of the tumor, with a margin of normal breast tissue, or simple mastectomy is sometimes necessary to prevent recurrence. The tumor is rarely malignant.

Abscess

A peripheral abscess is found more than 1 cm away from the areola and is usually caused by *S. aureus* or streptococcal organisms. A subareolar abscess is located in the nipple complex and can be associated with duct ectasia. Anaerobic organisms are the likely cause of subareolar abscesses. A chronic abscess can be encapsulated by fibrous tissue, causing the mass to be an irregularly shaped, firm mass that is nontender. An abscess should be incised, drained, and cultured.

Fat necrosis

Fat necrosis occurs as the result of thickened and retracted scar tissue from an injury and subsequent hematoma. A biopsy alone can differentiate this single, fixed, and often irregular tumor from carcinoma.

Lipoma

A lipoma is a fatty tumor of the breast, with borders that are smooth and well defined. The mass has a fluctuant consistency and is usually nontender and mobile.

Tuberculosis

Tuberculosis is an uncommon breast finding but should be considered, especially in immunocompromised patients. In early stages, tuberculosis can appear as a solitary, firm, irregular, nontender mass.

Ruptured implant

With a ruptured implant, augmented breast tissue is pushed away from the chest wall by the implant. Masses found in these patients often are best palpated with the patient in the sitting position. The definitive diagnosis is made by mammogram, ultrasound, or MRI.

Inflammatory Breast Mass

Mastitis and acute abscess

An acute abscess typically follows lactational mastitis. It is exquisitely tender on palpation and is very warm to the touch. The breast is erythematous and swollen, and the abscess usually involves only one-fourth of the breast. The mass has a fluctuant consistency. Chills and fever can be present. Axillary lymphadenopathy suggests an abscess, but inflammatory breast cancer must be considered.

Inflammatory breast cancer

Inflammatory breast cancer presents similarly to acute mastitis but differs from mastitis in that almost all or the entire breast is swollen, and fever is rarely present. Axillary lymphadenopathy can be present. Inflammatory breast cancer is a rapidly progressing disease; therefore, close follow up and prompt referral are necessary.

Multiple or Bilateral Breast Lumps

Fibrocystic breast changes

Fibrocystic breast changes usually present as multiple, bilateral painful masses, which frequently intensify premenstrually during the luteal phase of the menstrual cycle. The masses often rapidly fluctuate in size, are transient in appearance, and cause cyclic mastodynia (see Chapter 7). They occur most often between the ages of 30 to 50 years and are rare in the postmenopausal years. Some are require biopsy. On biopsy, nonproliferative lesions have no increased risk for breast cancer. Proliferative findings that indicate increased risk of breast cancer are atypical hyperplasia (5 times the risk) and lobular carcinoma in situ (8 to 10 times the risk).

Nipple Discharge

Intraductal papilloma

Intraductal papillomas are the most common benign lesions to cause a bloody nipple discharge. They usually are unilateral, subareolar lesions occurring during the perimenopausal years. Solitary papillomas do not increase breast cancer risk.

Duct ectasia

Mammary duct ectasia occurs most frequently after menopause. The subareolar ducts become blocked with desquamating secretory epithelium, necrotic debris, and chronic inflammatory cells. This condition is frequently bilateral and is characterized by pain, tenderness, periods of inflammation, and a nipple discharge that is spontaneous, sticky, multicolored, and from multiple ducts. Nipple retraction can occur. There is no known association with malignancy.

Neonatal discharge (witch's milk)

Newborns of either sex can have breast enlargement and a white nipple discharge secondary to maternal estrogens. This condition disappears within 1 to 2 weeks after birth.

Hyperprolactinemia

Hyperprolactinemia can cause nipple discharge in both male and female breasts. The nipple discharge is usually bilateral, milky, and from multiple ducts. Additional symptoms include amenorrhea, decreased libido, or gynecomastia. Most patients who present with galactorrhea and amenorrhea have hyperprolactinemia. A prolactin-secreting tumor can produce additional symptoms such as headaches and visual disturbances. Normal serum-fasting prolactin levels are generally less than 30 ng/mL. A prolactinoma is likely if the prolactin level is greater than 250 ng/mL and less likely if the level is less than 100 ng/mL.

Male Breast Disease

Acute mastitis

Acute mastitis in males occurs from trauma (e.g., nipple chafing from jogging) and presents as previously discussed in the section on mastitis.

Cancer

Breast cancer in male breasts is extremely rare and represents about 1% of all breast cancers. It begins as a painless induration, retraction of the nipple, and an attached mass. It progresses to include lymphadenopathy, and skin and chest wall lesions.

▶ **DIFFERENTIAL DIAGNOSIS OF** *Common Causes of Breast Lumps and Nipple Discharge*

CONDITION	HISTORY	PHYSICAL FINDINGS	DIAGNOSTIC STUDIES
SINGLE BREAST MASS			
Cancer	Usually older than age 35 yr; unilateral new lump	Hard, nontender, fixed lump; borders irregular or not discrete; can be erythema dimpling, increased vessel patterns; can have nipple discharge	Diagnostic mammogram; ultrasound; tissue biopsy
Cysts	Younger age, often younger than age 35 yr; may be single or multiple	Round or elliptical; soft or fluctuant; mobile	Clinical examination; FNA: clear aspirate; mammogram; ultrasound: cyst(s)

Continued

> **DIFFERENTIAL DIAGNOSIS OF *Common Causes of Breast Lumps and Nipple Discharge—cont'd***

CONDITION	HISTORY	PHYSICAL FINDINGS	DIAGNOSTIC STUDIES
Fibroade-noma	Common in adolescence	Single, sharply circumscribed, mobile lump	Diagnostic mammogram; ultrasound; biopsy
Abscess	History of mastitis	Single mass; irregular shape; chronic abscess can be nontender	Incision and drainage with culture
Fat necrosis	Can have history of injury at site	Single, fixed, and often irregular tumor	Biopsy
Lipoma	Can have others on arms, trunk, buttocks, or back; usually nontender	Single tumors; smooth, well-defined; fluctuant consistency	Biopsy
Tuberculosis	History of tuberculosis, positive PPD, or chest radiography; immunocompromised patient status	Single; irregular shape; nontender	Biopsy
Ruptured implant	History of augmentation; change in size or shape of breast	Nodule palpated best when patient is sitting	Diagnostic mammogram; ultrasound; MRI
INFLAMMATORY BREAST MASS			
Mastitis and acute abscess	Primigravidas more often than multigravidas; >1 wk after delivery; breastfeeding; tender nipples	Red, warm, tender; usually unilateral, one fourth of breast, or one lobule; breast engorgement; fever; nipple discharge: pus	Culture positive for *Staphylococcus aureus, Escherichia coli,* streptococci; elevated WBC count
Inflammatory breast cancer	History of mastitis or inflammatory process of breast	Entire breast swollen; fever rarely present; axillary lymphadenopathy	Biopsy
MULTIPLE OR BILATERAL BREAST LUMPS			
Fibrocystic breast changes	Multiple breast lumps of both breasts; cyclic changes that worsen at time of menses	Bilateral nodularity, dominant lumps; tender, mobile	FNA; ultrasound; mammogram
NIPPLE DISCHARGE			
Intraductal papilloma	Bloody nipple discharge; usual age is 40–50 yr	Unilateral, subareolar	Diagnostic mammogram; ultrasound; ductogram; maybe MRI

> ## DIFFERENTIAL DIAGNOSIS OF *Common Causes of Breast Lumps and Nipple Discharge—cont'd*

CONDITION	HISTORY	PHYSICAL FINDINGS	DIAGNOSTIC STUDIES
Fibrocystic breast changes	Milky nipple discharge; cyclic changes that worsen at time of menses	Spontaneous, clear or milky, bilateral, multiduct nipple discharge; multiple breast lumps of both breasts	Diagnostic mammogram; ultrasound; ductogram; maybe MRI
Duct ectasia	Green nipple discharge	Greenish or brownish nipple discharge	Diagnostic mammogram; ductogram; maybe MRI
Neonatal discharge (witch's milk)	Milky discharge 1–2 wk after birth	Enlarged breast tissue, milky discharge lasting 1–2 wk after birth	None
Hyperprolactinemia	Milky or clear nipple discharge; amenorrhea; history of medications: estrogenic, dopamine blockers, or dopamine depleters; hypothyroidism; pregnancy; postabortion; nipple stimulators; visual changes	Spontaneous, unilateral or bilateral, multiduct; clear or milky nipple discharge	Serum prolactin levels; TSH; MRI if indicated
MALE BREAST DISEASE			
Acute mastitis	History of clothing rubbing nipple (e.g., jogging); swelling or lump of chest wall; tenderness of site	Red, warm, tender; usually unilateral, one fourth of breast, or one lobule; breast engorgement; fever; nipple discharge or pus	Culture positive for *S. aureus, E. coli*, streptococci; elevated WBC count
Cancer	Family history of male breast cancer; painless lump of chest wall	Induration, retraction of nipple or mass in nipple well; fixed, nontender; lymphadenopathy	Mammogram; FNA; tissue biopsy

FNA, fine-needle aspiration; *MRI*, magnetic resonance imaging; *PPD*, purified protein derivative (tuberculin); *TSH*, thyroid-stimulating hormone; *WBC*, white blood cell count.

7 Breast Pain

Breast pain (mastalgia) is a frequent presenting health concern in primary care. A common problem in menstruating patients, breast pain is less common in postmenopausal patients. The pain can be mildly annoying or severe, and it can be periodic or nearly constant. Breast pain can occur in one or both breasts or in the axillary region of the body. It can be diffuse or localized.

Because of awareness about breast cancer, many patients worry that breast pain indicates malignancy. The cause of breast pain is not known. Its relationship to the menstrual cycle and its occurrence in premenopausal patients suggest a hormonal etiology. Breast pain alone is rarely associated with breast cancer and is usually related to fibrocystic changes. Breast pain associated with gynecomastia is seen in some young males. An abnormal ratio of estrogen to androgen causes the breast tissue to grow and become tender. It is also seen with Klinefelter syndrome, a sex chromosomal disorder (XXY) that occurs in males.

DIAGNOSTIC REASONING: FOCUSED HISTORY

Could this be inflammatory breast cancer?

Key Questions
- Is your breast hot, red, or swollen?
- Are you breastfeeding?

Hot, Red, or Swollen Breast
The most common cause of an inflamed breast in nonlactating patients is inflammatory breast cancer. In inflammatory breast cancer, the entire breast can be painful or tender, swollen, heavy, and red. Mastitis is characterized by a painful breast with localized heat and redness. In lactating patients, the most frequent symptom is a painful erythematous lobule in an outer quadrant of the breast. Although mastitis is most common in lactating patients, it can also occur in nonlactating patients, usually as the result of generalized dermatitis occurring from insect bites, sunburn, or allergic reactions.

Could age help explain the cause?

Key Questions
- How old are you?

Breast tissue changes with age. Female breasts in patients younger than age 25 years have more stromal and lobular breast characteristics, and fibroadenomas are more frequently seen in this kind of tissue. Between the ages of 25 to 40 years, breasts are more likely to be nodular, and breast pain is more likely to be cyclic. mastalgia and nodularity. After age 40 years, female breasts begin to involute and are more likely to develop duct ectasia. Patients with female breasts who are older than age 50 years have an increased risk of breast cancer.

In adolescents, an abnormal ratio of estrogen to androgens can occur, causing breast tissue to grow and become tender.

Is this cyclic or noncyclic mastalgia?

Key Questions
- Are you still menstruating?
- What is the relationship of the pain to your menstrual cycle?

Premenopausal or Postmenopausal
Cyclic mastalgia occurs premenopausally and is associated with the menstrual cycle. Postmenopausal pain is not cyclic.

Relationship to Menstrual Cycle

Cyclic mastalgia occurs in relation to the menstrual cycle. Typically, it is most severe before the menses and goes away spontaneously with or after the menses. Premenstrual water retention in the breasts has also been proposed as a cause of breast pain.

What other characteristics of the pain will help me with a diagnosis?

Key Questions
- Can you describe the pain?
- Is the pain diffuse or localized?
- Where in the breast(s) is it?
- Does the pain radiate?

Pain Description

Cyclic mastalgia is usually described as a heaviness, most likely caused by hormonal changes that affect the breast tissue, resulting in edema and increased nodularity. Noncyclic mastalgia is described as sharp and burning.

Localization and Radiation

Cyclic mastalgia is usually bilateral and diffuse. Patients often describe it as radiating to the axillae and arms. Noncyclic mastalgia is often unilateral and well localized. Diffuse breast pain without redness is less worrisome than localized pain.

Is the pain associated with a lump or discharge?

Key Questions
- Have you felt a lump?
- Do you have a history of cystic breast changes or lumpy breasts?
- Do the lumps come and go or change with your periods?
- Have you ever had a mammogram or ultrasound? Why was it done? What were the results?
- Have you ever had a lump drained or biopsied? What was the diagnosis?
- Do you have any nipple discharge?

Lumps

Noncyclic mastalgia is occasionally secondary to the presence of a fibroadenoma or cyst.

Cysts that increase in size and tenderness as the menstrual cycle approaches can contribute to breast pain. Cyclic cysts of the breast are less common after menopause and necessitate diagnostic investigation. A postmenopausal patient with unilateral breast pain with a lump has a greater risk of a diagnosis of breast cancer.

Previous Mammograms or Biopsies

History or documentation of cyclic changes in lumps or the presence of cystic or glandular breast tissue on a mammogram or ultrasound supports a clinical diagnosis of benign disease.

Nipple Discharge

Pregnancy is the most common cause of breast tenderness and clear or milky nipple discharge (galactorrhea). Mastitis associated with breastfeeding can produce purulent discharge. A subareolar abscess can also produce a purulent discharge. For evaluation of nipple discharge, see Chapter 6.

What else could be causing the pain?

Key Questions
- When was your last period?
- Have you missed any periods?
- Could you be pregnant?
- Does the pain get worse with deep inspiration?
- What medications are you taking?
- Have you been hit or injured in your chest area?
- Are you a runner or jogger?
- Have you had chicken pox or shingles?

Missed Periods and Pregnancy

Pregnancy is the most common cause of breast tenderness.

Pain with Deep Inspiration

Pain with deep inspiration suggests a musculoskeletal etiology. Costochondritis especially affects the second and third ribs.

Medications

In postmenopausal patients, hormone therapy can stimulate symptoms of breast lumps and pain. Many herbal products, such as soybean, ginseng, and dong quai, can also cause some patients to experience an onset of breast pain. Patients on liquid diet supplements that have a soy base can experience breast changes and discomfort.

Gynecomastia can occur as a result of such medications as corticosteroids, hormonal medications, diazepam, and illicit drugs (particularly marijuana).

Trauma to the Chest

Chest trauma can cause breast pain. In adolescents, breast pain has been linked to sexual abuse.

Runner or Jogger

Patients who run or jog frequently report breast pain that is either induced or aggravated by running.

Chicken Pox or Shingles

People who have had varicella infection are susceptible to reactivation of latent varicella-zoster virus (VZV) infection in dorsal root ganglia or cranial nerve ganglia. Herpes zoster eruption can occur in the chest area, producing breast pain, before or concurrent with and months or years after the skin eruption.

Could the pain be related to another system?

Key Questions

• Have you ever had chest pain or shortness of breath?
• Have you had abdominal pain with this breast pain?

Chest Pain or Shortness of Breath

See Chapter 8 for a discussion of chest pain. It is important to rule out cardiac disease when assessing any type of chest pain, including breast pain. The most common cause of death in North American women is heart disease with atypical presenting symptoms.

Abdominal Pain

See Chapter 3 for a discussion of abdominal pain. Gallbladder disease and hiatal hernia can also refer pain to the breast region. These conditions must be ruled out when evaluating breast pain.

DIAGNOSTIC REASONING: FOCUSED PHYSICAL EXAMINATION

Perform a Breast Examination

Perform a multiposition examination of the breasts, nipples, and regional lymph nodes, as described in Chapter 6. In the vast majority of patients with breast pain, the clinical breast examination findings are normal. A red and swollen breast may indicate mastitis or inflammatory breast cancer. In mastitis, tenderness, redness, and swelling are usually localized. In inflammatory breast cancer, the findings are more diffuse and involve at least a third of the breast. Skin that has a *peau d'orange* (orange peel) appearance points to cancer. In children, assess for breast development using the Tanner stages of breast development (see Chapter 5).

Characterize Lumps

If you find a mass on physical examination, determine its size, depth, contour, shape, fluctuation, firmness, and mobility. Fluctuation can be determined by holding the edges of the mass against the chest wall and pressing the center with finger pads. Fluctuation ("bouncy" consistency) occurs with cysts, lipomas, and abscesses. Cysts are frequently tender, especially premenstrually. Reexamination in 1 or 2 weeks usually demonstrates cyclic, hormonal changes of the tissue, and change in lump size and tenderness. See Chapter 6 for evaluation of a breast lump.

Examine the Chest Wall

Palpate the intercostal spaces for costochondral margin tenderness and swelling. Palpation that reproduces the pain, especially affecting the second and third ribs, suggests costochondritis.

Skin

Look for the vesicular eruption along a single dermatome. Unilateral pain precedes the eruption of herpes zoster by 3 to 5 days (see Chapter 28).

Examine the Genital Area in the Male

In some adolescent boys, the first sign of Klinefelter syndrome is breast pain and gynecomastia. Boys with Klinefelter syndrome have sparse or absent pubic hair and small testes and penis. Testicular palpation

should be performed to estimate the size of the testicles. Sexual maturation should be assessed by using the Tanner stages for genital (testes and penis and scrotum) development (Fig. 7.1) and pubic hair development (Fig. 7.2). Sexual maturation rating for boys is calculated by averaging the boy's stages of genital and pubic hair development.

G_1—Tanner 1. Testes, scrotum, and penis are the same size and shape as in a young child.

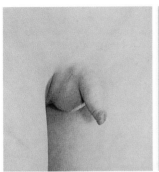

G_2—Tanner 2. Enlargement of scrotum and testes. The skin of the scrotum becomes redder, thinner, and wrinkled. Penis no larger or scarcely so.

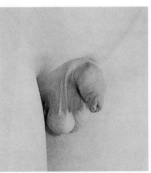

G_3—Tanner 3. Enlargement of the penis, especially in length; further enlargement of testes; descent of scrotum.

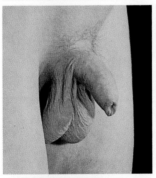

G_4—Tanner 4. Continued enlargement of the penis and sculpturing of the glans; increased pigmentation of scrotum. This stage is sometimes best described as "not quite adult."

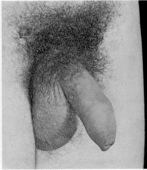

G_5—Tanner 5 (adult stage). Scrotum ample, penis reaching nearly to bottom of scrotum.

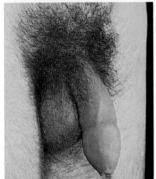

FIGURE 7.1 Five stages of genital (penis, testes, and scrotal) development in boys. (Growth diagrams 1965 Netherlands: Second national survey on 0- to 24-year-olds, by J. C. Van Wieringen, F. Wafelbakker, H. P. Verbrugge, J. H. DeHaas. Groningen: Noordhoff Uitgevers BV, The Netherlands.)

P₁—Tanner 1 (preadolescent). No growth of pubic hair; that is, hair in pubic area no different from that on the rest of the abdomen.

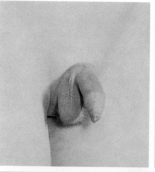

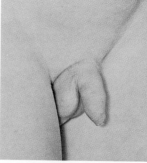

P₂—Tanner 2. Slightly pigmented, longer, straight hair, often still downy; usually at base of penis, sometimes on scrotum. Stage is difficult to photograph.

P₃—Tanner 3. Dark, definitely pigmented, curly pubic hair around base of penis. Stage 3 can be photographed.

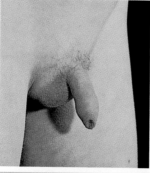

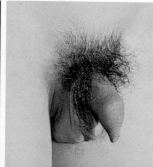

P₄—Tanner 4. Pubic hair definitely adult in type but not in extent (no further than inguinal fold).

P₅—Tanner 5 (adult distribution). Hair spread to medial surface of thighs but not upward.

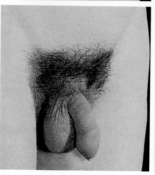

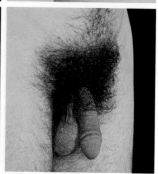

P₆—Hair spread along linea alba (occurs in 80% of men).

FIGURE 7.2 Six stages of pubic hair development in boys. (Growth diagrams 1965 Netherlands: Second national survey on 0- to 24-year-olds, by J. C. Van Wieringen, F. Wafelbakker, H. P. Verbrugge, J. H. DeHaas. Groningen: Noordhoff Uitgevers BV, The Netherlands.)

LABORATORY AND DIAGNOSTIC STUDIES

Pregnancy Testing

Test urine or blood for human chorionic gonadotropin (β-hCG) to rule out pregnancy.

Mammography

Diagnostic mammography is indicated in patients 30 years of age and older to assess clinical findings that include a palpable lump, persistent focal area of pain or tenderness, nipple discharge, erythema, and *peau d'orange* appearance of the skin.

Ultrasound

If a mass is found on mammography, ultrasound is helpful in differentiating solid from cystic lesions. Ultrasound, rather than mammogram, is indicated in women younger than age 30 years with breast symptoms or findings.

> **EVIDENCE-BASED PRACTICE** *Breast Imaging in Patients with Breast Pain*
>
> Although the role of mammogram and ultrasound is well established in the evaluation of a palpable breast lump, imaging guidelines for evaluation of breast pain are less well established. In clinical practice, mammogram is typically ordered first in patients older than 40 years followed by ultrasound only if the mammogram detects a finding. In a recent clinical study of 257 patients with focal breast pain without an associated palpable abnormality, the efficacy of mammogram alone, ultrasound alone, and in combination to detect breast cancer was evaluated. All modalities had a sensitivity of 100% and a negative predictive value (NPV) of 100% in detecting breast cancer. Specificities ranged from 83.7% to 92.5%. The authors concluded that mammogram alone showed a high sensitivity and negative predictive value for detection of breast cancer in patients presenting with localized breast pain. However, in 36 (25%) of 142 women with negative mammogram findings, an underlying lesion, including a solid mass in 6 cases, was found on ultrasound. Therefore, the NPV of mammography alone for detecting underlying mass lesions (benign or malignant) was only 75%, which suggests an important role for ultrasound. However, the costs of adding ultrasound include additional testing and surveillance. In this study, the addition of ultrasound to a mammogram in 206 patients resulted in 8 additional biopsies and 14 additional 6-month follow-up examinations without detecting any additional cancer.
>
> Reference: Leddy et al, 2013.

Karyotyping

Chromosomal testing determines the presence of the XXY chromosomal disorder or related chromosomal variants.

DIFFERENTIAL DIAGNOSIS

Cyclic Mastalgia

Cyclic mastalgia—pain that corresponds to changes in the menstrual cycle—is the most common type of breast pain and accounts for as much as two-thirds of the occurrence of breast pain. Cyclic mastalgia is usually bilateral; is often greatest in the upper outer breast quadrant; and is described as dull, heavy, and aching, often radiating to the axilla and arm. The pain has a variable duration and is often relieved after menses. Typically, for several days preceding the menstrual flow, the breasts enlarge, become lumpy and tender to touch, and produce a generalized aching. The nipples can become extremely sensitive and very uncomfortable. Cyclic mastalgia is usually bilateral, diffuse, and poorly localized. Compared with noncyclic mastalgia, cyclic mastalgia occurs more often at a younger age.

Cyclic mastalgia is attributed to the fluctuations of hormones during the menstrual cycle. Because the breasts prepare for pregnancy each month, by increasing the number of milk-producing cells, as much as 15 to 30 mL of fluid can be stored in each breast. This fluid can cause breast enlargement and the possibility of tenderness and pain. Additional factors that contribute to cyclic mastalgia include caffeine intake, high-sodium diets, and high-fat diets. Thyroid conditions have also been shown to cause cyclic mastalgia.

Noncyclic Mastalgia

Noncyclic mastalgia is most common in between the ages of 40 to 50 years. It accounts for about one-fourth of breast pain cases. The duration of symptoms tends to be shorter than that of cyclic mastalgia, and noncyclic mastalgia resolves spontaneously in 50% of cases. The pain is localized to a specific area in the breast and is described as sharp, stabbing, burning, and throbbing. Noncyclic mastalgia is occasionally secondary to the presence of a fibroadenoma or cyst, and the pain can be relieved by treatment of the underlying breast lesion.

Noncyclic mastalgia has no relationship to the menstrual cycle. It can be constant or intermittent, with irregular exacerbations, and increased nodularity is often noted on physical examination. Cysts, fibroadenomas, duct ectasia, mastitis, breast injury, and breast abscesses have been associated with noncyclic mastalgia. Additional causes include referred pain from infected teeth, medication-induced pain, and musculoskeletal pain.

Mastitis or Abscess

Mastitis is inflammation and infection of the breast tissue characterized by a sudden onset of localized swelling, tenderness, erythema, and heat, which is usually accompanied by chills, fever, and an increased pulse rate. Most infections are staphylococcal, often *Staphylococcus aureus*. Mastitis is most common in lactating patients after milk is established, usually the second to third week after delivery; however, it can occur at any time. Mastitis is not an indication to discontinue breastfeeding unless an abscess forms. An abscess presents as a large, hardened mass with a discharge of pus (suppuration) and an area of fluctuation, erythema, and heat. The underlying pus-filled abscess can impart a bluish tinge to the skin.

Inflammatory Breast Cancer

A rare and aggressive cancer, inflammatory breast cancer can be mistaken for mastitis. The patient reports sensations of heaviness, burning, or tenderness in the breast; a rapid increase in breast size; or a nipple that is inverted. On clinical breast examination, look for erythema that involves at least a third of the breast. *Peau d'orange* may be present. Symptoms are a result of lymphedema caused by cancer cells blocking lymph drainage. Sometimes an underlying mass may be felt but often not. Diagnostic mammogram, ultrasound, and ultimately tissue biopsy are required for diagnosis.

Mammary Duct Ectasia

Mammary duct ectasia occurs most frequently after menopause. The subareolar ducts become blocked with desquamating secretory epithelium, necrotic debris, and chronic inflammatory cells. This condition is frequently bilateral and is characterized by pain, tenderness, periods of inflammation, and nipple discharge. Nipple retraction can occur. There is no known association with malignancy. Mammogram and ultrasound can show ectasia.

Pregnancy

Pregnancy is the most common cause of breast tenderness. Test the urine or serum for β-hCG to rule out pregnancy.

Costochondritis

A common musculoskeletal cause of breast pain is Tietze syndrome or costochondritis, which is inflammation of the cartilage of the ribs. This pain, which originates in the area of the sternum and the ribs, is localized close to the sternum and causes tenderness on palpation when moving the rib cage or when taking a deep breath.

Herpes Zoster (Shingles)

Herpes zoster is caused by reactivation of the VZV from a dorsal root ganglion to a cutaneous nerve and the adjacent skin. Herpes zoster eruption can occur in the chest area, producing breast pain. An area of erythema and pain can precede the development of grouped vesicles or may occur years or months later.

Klinefelter Syndrome

This sex chromosomal disorder (XXY) occurs in males and is characterized by gynecomastia and prepubertal testes. In some adolescent boys, the first signs of Klinefelter syndrome are breast pain and gynecomastia. Patients may lack secondary sexual characteristics because of a decrease in androgen production. This results in sparse facial, body, pubic, and axillary hair; a high-pitched voice; a female type of fat distribution; and small testes and penis. By late puberty, 30% to 50% of boys with Klinefelter syndrome manifest gynecomastia, which is secondary to elevated estradiol levels, and an increased estradiol-to-testosterone ratio. The risk of developing breast carcinoma is at least 20 times higher than that of males without Klinefelter syndrome.

Breast Lumps or Nipple Discharge Associated with Breast Pain

See Chapter 6 for a discussion of breast lumps and nipple discharge.

> **DIFFERENTIAL DIAGNOSIS OF** *Common Causes of Breast Pain*

CONDITION	HISTORY	PHYSICAL FINDINGS	DIAGNOSTIC STUDIES
Cyclic mastalgia	Corresponds to changes in menstrual cycle Bilateral; pain often greatest in upper, outer breast quadrant Dull, heavy, and aching pain; radiates to axilla and arm; varying duration	Often no physical findings; breasts can be tender	None; history and clinical examination
Noncyclic mastalgia	Age 40–50 yr No relationship to menses Pain localized to specific area in breast; described as sharp, stabbing, burning, throbbing	Often no physical findings; breast can be more nodular; lump can be present	Mammogram; ultrasound
Mastitis or abscess	Sudden onset of swelling, tenderness, erythema, and heat, which is usually accompanied by chills, fever, and increased pulse rate Lactating patients after milk is established, usually second to third week after delivery	Swelling, redness, tenderness Possible abscess formation with hardened mass, area of fluctuation, erythema, and heat Underlying pus-filled abscess can impart bluish tinge to skin	None; clinical examination
Inflammatory breast cancer	Sensations of heaviness, burning, or tenderness in the breast; rapid increase in breast size; or a nipple that is inverted (facing inward)	Swelling, redness that covers more than one-third of the breast, tenderness; *peau d'orange*	Mammogram; ultrasound; biopsy
Mammary duct ectasia	Menopausal Bilateral or unilateral pain, tenderness; periods of inflammation; nipple discharge	Often no physical findings Nipple retraction can occur; lump may be present	Mammogram; ultrasound
Pregnancy	Missed period; contraceptive use failure	Breast tenderness and swelling	Urine or serum for β-hCG
Costochondritis	Pain in area of sternum and ribs; pain with deep inspiration	Tenderness on palpation, when moving rib cage, or when taking a deep breath	None; trial of NSAIDs
Herpes zoster	Pain; history of chicken pox or shingles	Vesicular eruption along a cutaneous dermatome	None history and clinical examination
Klinefelter syndrome	Adolescent boy with breast tenderness and enlargement	Testes prepubertal, gynecomastia, decreased body hair	Karyotyping
Breast lumps associated with breast pain	See Chapter 6 for discussion on breast lumps and nipple discharge.		

β-hCG, Human chorionic gonadotropin; *NSAID*, nonsteroidal antiinflammatory drug.

CHAPTER

8 Chest Pain

The first step in the evaluation of a patient with chest pain is to determine whether the pain is a life-threatening condition. Acute coronary syndrome includes myocardial ischemia and myocardial infarction (MI), aortic dissection, pulmonary embolism (PE), or pneumothorax. These are life-threatening causes of chest pain and must be assessed rapidly so emergent treatment can be initiated. A quick diagnosis of acute MI greatly increases the patient's chances of survival. Aortic dissection is a rare but catastrophic cause of chest pain. PE is accompanied by the sudden onset of dyspnea.

If acute ischemic heart disease is an unlikely cause, other causes of acute chest pain should be considered, such as pulmonary, gastrointestinal (GI), psychological, musculoskeletal, or other conditions (e.g., pericarditis). A significant proportion of patients whose presenting symptoms include acute chest pain have esophageal spasm or gastroesophageal reflux disease (GERD); however, harmless conditions can mimic more serious disease. Pericarditis and valvular diseases, such as aortic stenosis and mitral valve prolapse (MVP), are less emergent causes of cardiac pain.

Pain in any organ or system can be the result of inflammation, obstruction or restriction, or distention or dilation. All pain arising from the GI, musculoskeletal, respiratory, cardiac, and pulmonary systems transmits to the same spinal cord segments—T1 through T5—and makes identification of the specific origin of discomfort difficult. Many causes of noncardiac chest pain relate to chest anatomy, specifically skin, muscles, ribs, cartilage, pleura, lungs, esophagus, mediastinum, and thoracic vertebrae.

In an infant, sweat on the forehead can indicate congenital heart disease (CHD).

A decrease in cardiac output causes a compensatory sympathetic overactivity, resulting in a cold sweat on the forehead.

In children, chest pain is rarely associated with serious organic disease. The most common causes of chest pain in children are costochondritis, trauma, muscle strain to the chest wall, and respiratory conditions associated with cough. Chest pain from rheumatic heart disease or other cardiac disease is relatively rare in children. However, patients and families often associate chest pain with heart disease and can be anxious about the condition because of reports of sudden death in young athletes.

DIAGNOSTIC REASONING: FOCUSED HISTORY

The identification of potentially acute, life-threatening situations must be made immediately. After you have determined that there is no immediate risk of severe oxygen deprivation to vital organs (e.g., MI, aortic dissection, and PE), proceed with a focused history.

First, is this a life-threatening condition?

Key Questions
- Can you describe the pain? What does it feel like? (Dull, sore, stabbing, burning, squeezing?)
- Does the pain radiate?
- When did it start?
- What were you doing when it started?
- How long have you had the pain?
- What other symptoms have you noticed?

Characteristics of Pain

Typical anginal pain is described as substernal heaviness, pressure, or a squeezing sensation that is provoked by exertion and relieved with rest or nitroglycerin. The substernal pain or discomfort radiates to the left shoulder and down the left arm and can extend to the neck and lower jaw. An abrupt tearing pain, located in the anterior or posterior chest, characterizes aortic dissection. This pain can migrate to the arms, abdomen, back, or legs. Patients with Marfan syndrome are at risk for aortic dissection.

Pneumonia, PE, and pneumothorax present with chest pain. The patient with PE is able to point to the area of pain over the affected lung and usually describes a gripping, stabbing pain that is moderate to severe in intensity. The pain can radiate to the neck or shoulders. Patients experiencing a pneumothorax most frequently report mild to severe chest pain of sudden onset, located in the lateral thorax, and radiating to the ipsilateral shoulder. The quality of pain is described as sharp or tearing. Chest pain of pneumonia is located over the area of infiltration and does not radiate. It frequently has a burning or stabbing quality and is associated with cough (see Chapter 11).

Remember that chest pain is subjective and that prior experience, personal attitudes, and cultural values form the patient's perception of pain. Assessment of the intensity of the pain is done using a 0 to 10 analog scale, with 0 being no pain and 10 being the worst pain ever experienced.

Onset of Pain

Determine if the onset of pain was sudden or gradual and what the patient's activity was at the time of onset. The typical onset of angina occurs during exercise, exertion, or emotional stress and is relieved by rest or nitroglycerin. Chest pain of MI can occur at any time and is relieved by rest in 2 to 5 minutes. A sudden onset of chest pain and dyspnea is common with PE. In a pneumothorax, the patient usually reports a sudden onset of severe coughing, exertion, or straining that precipitated the chest pain. Chest pain caused by pneumonia occurs gradually over several hours or days. Chest pain in adolescents that occurs after activity can indicate organic cardiac disease.

Most MIs occur in the morning hours, with a peak on Mondays. Patients might also report acute chest pain hours after heavy exertion, such as snow shoveling, sexual intercourse, or other physical activity.

In children, ask about recent choking episodes or swallowing a foreign body if the pain increases with attempts to swallow. Pain that usually occurs when lying down after eating is associated with GERD. Trauma to the chest wall from a fall or strenuous activity can cause rib fractures or chest contusions.

Duration

The most life-threatening conditions produce an acute onset of chest pain. The more chronic the pain, the less likely it is that a specific cause will be found. Intermittent chest pain that occurs frequently probably indicates a more serious problem, such as angina, than one episode of brief, mild pain. Unstable angina is a persistent chest pain, lasting about 30 minutes, not related to activity, compared with stable angina pain, which lasts 2 to 5 minutes and is relieved with rest.

Associated Symptoms

A person experiencing an acute MI frequently reports nausea, vomiting, diaphoresis, shortness of breath, and syncope. PE is often associated with shortness of breath, apprehension, hemoptysis, and chest pain that increases with deep breathing. Fever, cough, and thick sputum production usually accompany chest pain caused by pneumonia.

Does the patient have risk factors for coronary artery disease?

Key Questions
- How old are you?
- Do you smoke?
- Do you have high blood pressure, diabetes, or heart disease?
- Do you have a history of MI?
- Has anyone in your family had a heart attack, or stroke before the age of 60 years?

Risk Factors

According to the report of the US Preventive Services Task Force, clinically significant coronary artery disease (CAD) is uncommon in men younger than 40 years of age and premenopausal women, but risk increases with advancing age. The presence of risk factors such as smoking, hypertension, diabetes, high cholesterol level, obesity, and family history of heart disease increase the risk of CAD. The National Cholesterol Education Program identifies the following major risk factors for CAD: cigarette smoking, hypertension, low high-density lipoprotein cholesterol level (<40 mg/dL), a family history of premature coronary heart disease, age (men 45 years and older; women 55 years and older), and diabetes. In addition, a fasting lipoprotein panel should be obtained that includes low-density lipoprotein (<100 mg/dL is optimal), and total cholesterol values (< mg/dL is desirable).

> *If this is not a life-threatening condition, what does a description of the pain tell me?*

Key Questions
- Is the pain acute or chronic?
- What were you doing when the pain first occurred?
- Point to where the pain is located. Does it spread to any other part of your body?
- What seems to trigger the pain?
- Does the pain awaken you from sleep?

Acute or Chronic

After life-threatening causes of acute chest pain are ruled out, sudden-onset pain can be associated with trauma, musculoskeletal injury, or inflammation. Chronic, gradual-onset chest pain is rarely an emergent situation. Chest pain can be the sequel to an upper respiratory tract infection. Pain from GERD often occurs at night or after a large meal.

Location and Character of Pain

Pain arising from the thoracic skin and other superficial tissues, such as that associated with furuncles, contusions, and abrasions, is sharply localized.

Irritation of the intercostal nerves can result in a neuritis that produces sudden onset of a stabbing, burning pain and tenderness. The pain is easy to locate at the intercostal spaces and along inflamed nerves with three maximal pain points: adjacent to the vertebrae, in the axillary lines, and along the parasternal lines. Pain can be severe when the patient breathes deeply, coughs, or moves suddenly.

Dorsal root irritation associated with herpes zoster can present with intense burning or knifelike pain along the spine to the lateral thoracic wall and the anterior midline. This pain can restrict movement of the trunk and respirations. Generally, this pain is continuous and increases in severity.

Nerve root pain is caused by mechanical irritation or edema of the nerve root. This pain can be felt at the point of irritation but is frequently referred to points along the peripheral course of the nerve. Thoracic spinal segment root pain is often referred to the lateral and anterior chest wall and is seen with spinal diseases and thoracic deformities.

Costal cartilage that loosens from the fibrous attachment most often causes localized, dulling, aching pain and tenderness over the eighth, ninth, and tenth ribs on either side; however, the pain can be acute, paroxysmal, or stabbing.

Musculoskeletal pain is produced by irritation of tissues and transmitted through the sensory nerves. The stimulus travels through the nerve to the dorsal ganglion and up the spinal afferent pathway to the central nervous system.

Bone pain results from irritation of sensory nerve endings in the periosteum, is intense, and is well localized. Chronic diseases affecting the bone marrow can cause a poorly localized pain of varying severity. Ribs are common sites for metastatic malignant deposits, probably because of their rich vascularity. Metastasis to the rib and the periosteum results in pain. Referred pain from a dermatome is described as intense, aching, and boring.

When tumors involve the mediastinum, chronic aching or dull substernal chest pain is produced by pressure of the tumor against the spine or ribs.

Bronchial pain is caused by the involvement of adjacent structures. The trachea and large bronchus are innervated by the vagus nerve (cranial nerve X). The finer bronchi and lung parenchyma are free of pain innervation; therefore, extensive disease can occur in the periphery of the lungs without pain until the process extends to the parietal pleura. Pleural pain, or pleuritis, results from the loss of normal lubricating function and irritation of the serous membranes of the pleural surfaces. The pain waxes and wanes with respirations, movement, and cough. Diaphragmatic pleural pain can be referred to the base of the neck or abdomen. Children often report chest pain from tachyarrhythmia because they are unable to differentiate between true pain and the discomfort of the arrhythmia. Cardiac causes of chest pain in children are usually associated with congenital anomalies or acquired diseases of the coronary artery, such as Kawasaki disease.

Sleep

Distinguish between awakening with pain and awakening from pain. Awakening because of pain signals a more serious problem of organic origin, such as cardiac ischemia. Psychogenic chest pain in adolescents commonly accompanies sleep disturbances.

What do associated symptoms tell me?

Key Questions
- Do you have a cough or a change in your usual cough?
- Do you bring up sputum? If so, how much and what color?
- Do you have a fever?
- Are you lightheaded or dizzy?
- Do you feel like your heart is racing?

Cough and Sputum Production

Chest pain associated with cough and colored sputum production is usually caused by an acute infection, such as pneumonia. Pain results from a pleural effusion, or the collection of fluid in the pleural space. Sputum associated with pneumonia can be dark green, rust color, or red. Frequent lower respiratory tract infections can be caused by CHD, with large left-to-right shunts, and an increase in pulmonary blood flow. Children and older adults with persistent cough can experience chest pain related to the musculoskeletal strain associated with coughing. A person with asthma can develop chest pain from straining of the chest wall muscles caused by tachypnea, coughing, or retraction.

Fever

Fever can indicate pneumonia, myocarditis, pericarditis, or PE. It is possible that older and immunosuppressed people will not have fever, even with bacterial infections.

Lightheadedness, Dizziness, or Fainting

Arrhythmias caused by hypoxia, trauma, or electrical shock can cause insufficient coronary blood flow and chest pain. Paroxysmal atrial tachycardia (PAT) can cause lightheadedness. Diastole is shortened in PAT, and thus cardiac output is decreased. Most cases of syncope in adults are caused by cardiac problems such as structural heart disease, arrhythmias, and coronary insufficiency. Most cases of syncope in children are benign and are the result of breath holding, orthostatic syncope, hyperventilation, or vasovagal syncopal episodes. Syncope during exercise could signal a nonbenign cause (see Chapter 33).

Palpitations

Caffeine, stress, and hormonal changes can cause the sensation of a rapid or forceful heartbeat. MVP can present with a history of palpitations.

Theophylline, levothyroxine, and β-adrenergic agents can cause arrhythmias such as supraventricular tachycardia, which can be perceived as palpitations.

Is the pattern of pain related to activity and position change?

Key Questions
- Can you describe your recent physical activities?
- Have you had any injury to the chest?
- Does chest movement or position make the pain better or worse?

Recent Activities

Recent strenuous exercise (especially weight lifting) or horseplay can strain the pectoral, trapezius, latissimus dorsi, serratus anterior, and shoulder muscles. Rib fractures, musculoskeletal strains, and contusions can cause significant chest pain, especially with movement. Musculoskeletal disorders are the most common cause of chest pain in children and younger adults.

Decreased exercise tolerance can result from significant heart disease such as shunts, arrhythmias, or CAD. In children, congenital coronary anomalies can arise abnormally (as from the pulmonary artery), take an abnormal course, or have fistula connections to other structures, resulting in exertional chest pain. Any episode of moderate to severe chest pain during or after exercise should be investigated as cardiac in origin.

History of Chest Trauma

A careful history of preceding activities should be obtained to detect any recent muscle strain. Posttraumatic pericardial effusion can develop 1 to 3 months after chest trauma. Blunt injury can cause hemothorax, pneumothorax, soft tissue injury, and rib fracture. A ruptured spleen can cause irritation of the phrenic nerve, producing shoulder pain.

Pain with Movement

Pain of cardiac origin, except for pericarditis, is not affected by respiration. Pain on inspiration suggests pleural etiology. A sharp, pleuritic pain, relieved by sitting upright and leaning forward, suggests pericarditis. Pain that is aggravated by chest wall movement, especially along the sternal border, is most frequently costochondritis; both adults and children can experience this inflammatory condition of the costal cartilage. Lying flat, consuming alcohol, taking aspirin, eating spicy meals, and wearing tight clothing often precipitate the pain of esophagitis. Frequently, patients report that this pain occurs after lying down following eating a meal.

Is there a gastrointestinal origin for the patient's chest pain?

Key Questions
• Does the pain get better or worse from eating?
• Do you have blood in your stools?
• Have you vomited any blood?

Food Association

Differentiating between esophageal and cardiac origin of chest pain can present a challenge because the character and location of the pain can be very similar. Nitroglycerin can relieve both the pain of angina and the pain of esophagitis. In these instances, an electrocardiogram (ECG) is indicated.

Esophagitis, usually as a result of GERD, is the most frequent GI cause of chest pain. Patients describe this pain as "heartburn," or a dull, burning sensation in the epigastric and retrosternal area. The esophagus is more pain sensitive in its proximal portion. Therefore, chest pain that is temporally related to eating meals or particular foods should suggest esophagitis.

Sometimes associated symptoms of a sour taste in the mouth and mild nausea are associated with esophagitis. An esophageal tear or spasm causes more acute, severe chest pain, described as a "tearing" or "crushing" sensation. Frequently, the patient experiencing pain of GI origin reports mild to moderate chest pain occurring intermittently over days to months.

Peptic ulcer and cholecystitis can cause chest pain. Hematemesis (blood in the emesis) or hematochezia (blood in the stool) frequently accompanies peptic ulceration. Cholecystitis is frequently reported as right anterior chest pain that radiates to the shoulder or upper back.

Acute pancreatitis should be considered if the chest pain is severe and constant and is reported in the epigastric area of the abdomen, radiating to the chest, shoulder, and arm. Pancreatitis is often accompanied by hypotension. Physical examination and diagnostic tests are necessary to differentiate it from chest pain of cardiovascular origin.

Could this pain be from a systemic cause?

Key Questions
• Do you have any skin problems?
• Do you have any chronic health problems?

Skin Symptoms

If the patient reports persistent unilateral chest pain of pruritic, burning, or stabbing quality, consider herpes zoster. This pain will follow the distribution of a cervical or thoracic nerve root. A vesicular rash in the area of pain is characteristic; this rash occurs several days after the occurrence of chest pain.

Systemic Conditions

Chest muscle pain can be caused by localized inflammation of the muscles in collagen diseases, such as polymyositis, fibromyalgia, or systemic lupus erythematosus. Arthritic inflammatory changes of the cervical and thoracic spine and shoulders can produce upper chest pain. This pain is aggravated by range of motion of the affected joints.

Sickle cell disease (SCD) can cause chest pain. In sickle cell anemia, the erythrocytes become rigid and "sickle," leading to capillary occlusion and sickle cell crisis. The heart increases the stroke volume to compensate for the anemia. The heart gradually dilates and heart failure ensues. Chest pain in a patient with SCD can also originate from acute coronary syndrome. In this condition, chest pain, fever, dyspnea, and cough are caused by infarction of lung tissue or an infectious agent.

Marfan syndrome is a hereditary connective tissue disease. Cardiovascular involvement occurs in more than 50% of people by age 21 years. Mitral valve involvement is common, with auscultatory findings of mitral regurgitation and MVP. Marfan syndrome is associated with an increased risk of aortic dissection.

Kawasaki disease often has a long-term complication of CAD, coronary occlusion, or MI.

What does the family history tell me?

Key Questions
- Has anyone in your family had heart disease, chest pain, or sudden death from cardiac arrest?
- Was anyone in your family born with heart problems?
- Does anyone in your family have high cholesterol?

Family History

A history of CHD in close relatives increases the chances of its occurrence in a child. When one child has the condition, the risk of siblings having the condition increases by one-third. Essential hypertension and CAD show a strong family pattern. Hypertrophic cardiomyopathy has a positive family history, with autosomal dominant transmission in one-third of patients.

Children who have a homogenous family history of hypercholesterolemia can present with CAD before the age of 20 years.

What is the emotional state of the patient?

Key Questions
- In the past 6 months, have you had a spell or an attack in which you suddenly felt frightened, anxious, or very uneasy?
- In the past 6 months, have you had a spell or an attack in which for no apparent reason your heart suddenly began to race, you felt faint, or you could not catch your breath?

Panic Disorder

A response of "yes" to the above key questions can be a highly sensitive screen for a psychogenic component of pain and is a positive screen for panic disorder. Patients with anxiety or depression often describe feelings of chest heaviness or tightness that can last for days and dyspnea unrelated to exertion or rest. Patients can also report difficulty taking a deep breath.

DIAGNOSTIC REASONING: FOCUSED PHYSICAL EXAMINATION

A focused physical examination of the patient experiencing chest pain will provide objective data for the assessment. A thorough examination of the cardiovascular, pulmonary, upper GI, dermatologic, and upper body musculoskeletal systems is essential. The ECG greatly improves the accuracy of the diagnosis of acute chest pain and should be obtained early in the assessment if cardiac causes are suspected.

Observe the General Appearance

Initial observation of the patient will provide clues to the severity of the problem. Observe for grimacing, diaphoresis, pallor, cyanosis, tachypnea, use of accessory muscles for breathing, splinting of chest wall, and unequal chest wall excursion. People experiencing an MI can be diaphoretic, pale, and anxious. Patients manifesting PE appear diaphoretic and anxious, respirations are rapid, splinting of the chest is common, and peripheral cyanosis can be present. People with fractured ribs or significant chest wall contusions splint their chest wall and take shallow breaths to avoid aggravating pain with respiratory expansion.

Observe the height and weight of a child. Abnormal findings for age can indicate chronic disease.

Measure the Vital Signs and Note Respiratory Patterns

Vital signs for people experiencing angina can be within normal ranges. Frequently, however, with acute MI, blood pressure is elevated, and cardiac arrhythmias are present. Hypotension can indicate cardiogenic shock.

The patient with aortic dissection can be hypotensive with unequal peripheral pulses. Pericarditis can be accompanied by fever, rapid and shallow respirations, and hypertension. Myocarditis can present with fever, respiratory distress, and paradoxical pulse.

In heart failure, decreased stroke volume reduces the systolic blood pressure, and compensatory vasoconstriction maintains a constant diastolic pressure. This can result in a decreased pulse pressure.

Pneumothorax is manifested by tachypnea and unequal chest wall excursion. The patient with pneumonia can also be tachypneic, with signs of infection that include fever and a productive cough.

In children, chest pain with tachycardia and hypotension is generally caused by hypovolemia, secondary to a hemothorax, hemopneumothorax, or vascular injury. Pain can also be caused by rhythm disturbance.

The rate, rhythm, and depth of respirations in patients experiencing costochondritis, GI disease, or herpes zoster are not usually altered.

Hyperventilation can cause chest pain as a result of hypercapnic alkalosis or coronary artery vasoconstriction. Most hyperventilation is associated with a stressful event or emotional upset; however, aspirin overdose, severe pain, and diabetic ketoacidosis can be organic causes.

Inspect the Skin

Cool, pale, moist skin can accompany an acute MI, PE, or aortic dissection. Observe the skin overlying the area of chest pain for signs of the vesicular rash of herpes zoster. Petechial rash on the face and shoulders can be a sign of protracted coughing as a result of pneumonia, asthma, or upper respiratory tract infection. Bruises can indicate trauma or abuse.

Palpate Trachea and Chest

Tracheal shift can occur with pneumothorax and in children with atelectasis, involving a significant portion of one lung. To assess the trachea for lateral displacement, position your index finger first on the right side of the suprasternal notch and then the left. If the trachea has shifted to the side, you will feel the wall on one side but only soft tissue on the other. In a pneumothorax, the trachea is deviated to the opposite side during exhalation and toward the side of the pneumothorax during inspiration. The trachea is displaced toward a lung that is atelectatic, with the displacement exaggerated during inspiration.

Palpate the entire chest wall for tenderness, depressions, or bulges. Fractured ribs and contusions result in tenderness to palpation and possible deformity. Palpate each costochondral and chondrosternal junction. Costochondritis is manifested by pain with palpation over the cartilage between the sternum and the ribs. Palpation and range of joint motion can elicit arthritic pain in the shoulder or cervical spine. Musculoskeletal chest pain is usually reproduced with palpation or by moving the arms and chest through a variety of positions. Subcutaneous emphysema may be palpable at the neck or upper chest wall. Rib pain on palpation in children without a reported history of trauma can indicate child abuse.

To check the chest wall for symmetry, first test for diaphragmatic expansion of both the anterior and the posterior thorax between the eighth and tenth ribs. As the patient takes a deep breath, the practitioner places each hand over the chest with thumbs inward. Each thumb should move the same distance from the spine or costal margins. Pneumothorax, pneumonia, and fractured ribs can alter this finding.

Percuss the Chest

Percussion in the area of pneumothorax will result in a hyperresonant sound of an air-filled cavity. Areas of infiltration, as in pneumonia, will produce a dull or flat sound.

Auscultate Breath Sounds

Instruct the patient to breathe through the mouth slowly and deeply. Auscultate systematically from the lung apexes to the lower lobes anteriorly, posteriorly, and laterally (Table 8.1).

Auscultation of bronchial or bronchovesicular breath sounds over the peripheral lungs can indicate consolidation. If breath sounds are diminished over all lung fields, suspect chronic obstructive pulmonary disease (COPD). Obese patients can have breath sounds that are difficult to auscultate. Breath sounds will be inaudible in areas of pneumothorax.

Auscultate for Adventitious Sounds

Adventitious lung sounds are superimposed on normal sounds and can be auscultated over any area of the lung field during inspiration or expiration. Documentation of abnormal lung sounds should include the type of sound heard, location, and changes during both inspiration and expiration phases of respiration.

Crackles or rales are discontinuous popping sounds heard most often during inspiration. Any disease process that increases peripheral airway resistance, obstructs the peripheral airway, or causes a loss of elastic recoil will produce crackles. These indicate the presence of fluid, mucus, or pus in the smaller airways. Fine crackles are soft and high pitched.

Medium crackles are louder and lower pitched. Crackles might be heard over the site of a PE.

Wheezing is frequently described as a whistling sound and can be heard during inspiration, expiration, or both. The sound is high pitched and musical. Wheezing indicates that there is fluid in the large airways, such as in severe heart failure; more often it is associated with bronchospasm, as seen in asthma. Wheezing occurs on exhalation because that is when small airways collapse. During inhalation, the negative pressure in the chest tends to hold open the airways. However, during exhalation, positive pressure in the alveoli is conducted from the outside of the small airways and tends to collapse them. The sound is usually polyphonic; this means that multiple, slightly different, high-pitched sounds are heard at the same time. Most of the causes of wheezing affect many small airways at the same time; each one collapses at a slightly different time, creating a slightly different tone. The presence of a single-tone wheeze suggests a single area of blockage, such as with a foreign body. A prolonged expiratory phase of respiration is produced by intrathoracic airway obstruction associated with lower respiratory tract involvement.

Rhonchi are continuous, deep-pitched, coarse breath sounds usually heard during expiration. They are generated by turbulent air passing through secretions in large airways. Rhonchi can be present when the patient has pneumonia.

Pleural friction rub is a grating or squeaking sound heard in the lateral lung fields during inspiration and expiration. It indicates that

Table 8.1	**Normal Breath Sounds**		
BREATH SOUND	**LOCATION**	**QUALITY**	**INSPIRATION-TO-EXPIRATION RATIO**
Bronchial	Heard on chest over sternum and on back between scapulae	Loud, high pitched	Expiration longer than inspiration
Bronchovesicular	Heard over bronchi at first and second intercostal spaces anteriorly and between scapulae posteriorly	Loud, medium pitched	Equal inspiratory and expiratory phases
Vesicular	Heard over most of peripheral lung fields	Soft, low pitched	Inspiration longer than expiration

inflamed parietal and visceral pleural linings are rubbing together.

If abnormal lung sounds are detected, additional auscultation for bronchophony, egophony, and whispered pectoriloquy are indicated (see Chapter 14).

Auscultate Heart Sounds

Auscultate for normal heart sounds in all positions, identifying S_1, S_2, rate, and rhythm. Identification of myocardial ischemia cannot be reliably performed by physical examination alone. An ECG must be obtained to assess electrical conduction and the condition of myocardial function. Abnormal sounds, such as paradoxical S_2 during pain, are a sign of coronary ischemia. A transient, paradoxical S_2 could indicate a transient left ventricular dysfunction, congestive heart failure, or left bundle branch block. A transient S_3 (ventricular gallop) or mitral regurgitation murmur at the apex can occur occasionally with myocardial ischemia or congestive heart failure. An S_4 (atrial gallop) typically indicates a stressed heart, which can be the result of hypertension, MI, or CAD causing heart failure. A summation gallop is the result of an S_3, S_4, and rapid rate; this can also occur with heart failure. Abnormal rhythms and heart rates are often heard during MI. ECGs are necessary to identify the specific rhythm.

Also note any murmurs and their location, grade, and radiation. Incompetent heart valves produce murmurs and can be the cause of heart failure. In children, a loud murmur, best audible at the upper right sternal border, or upper left sternal border with a thrill, can indicate a congenital heart defect.

Aortic diastolic murmur can be present with a dissecting aorta. In aortic valve stenosis, a harsh ejection systolic murmur, with radiation to the neck, is heard on auscultation.

Midsystolic click or late systolic murmur (honk) is heard with MVP. The patient must be examined in both the supine and upright positions to elicit the characteristic sounds.

Observe the Spine for Evidence of Scoliosis

People with scoliosis are at increased risk for pulmonary problems because of structural variations that can cause compression of intrathoracic contents.

Examine the Abdomen

Auscultate for bowel sounds. Palpate the abdomen for tenderness and masses. Epigastric pain with palpation can occur with pancreatitis, esophagitis, or peptic ulcer disease. Cholelithiasis or cholecystitis can be manifested by pain on palpation in the right upper quadrant. Pancreatitis can produce epigastric pain radiating to the back.

Examine the Extremities

Clubbing of the fingers can be an indication of chronic hypoxia resulting from CHD in children or COPD in adults. Peripheral cyanosis indicates hypoxia if accompanied by central cyanosis. Consider exposure to a cold environment or anxiety if peripheral cyanosis is observed. Lower extremity edema is a sign of heart failure or venous stasis. Note the progression of the edema or whether there is pitting edema up the leg.

Absent peripheral pulse(s) can be a sign of atherosclerotic vessel disease or dissecting aortic aneurysm. Compare the quality of the pulses bilaterally.

LABORATORY AND DIAGNOSTIC STUDIES

Diagnostic tests are indicated when cardiovascular, pulmonary, or GI pathology is the suspected cause of chest pain. Musculoskeletal and neurological causes of pain usually do not require diagnostic tests.

Electrocardiogram

An ECG can add objective data to the diagnostic process in evaluating chest pain. ECGs are most valuable when there is a previous ECG with which to compare the findings or when serial ECGs are obtained. ST-segment elevation or depression indicates the presence of injured myocardium. T-wave inversion demonstrates the presence of ischemia. The appearance of both strongly supports ischemia but is not diagnostic of CAD. Arterial spasm, pericarditis, and electrolyte imbalance can also cause these variations from normal.

Q waves are indicative of myocardial muscle loss but are not diagnostic of CAD.

Evidence of ischemia is not always obvious on an ECG even when the patient is reporting anginal pain. This is crucial to keep in mind as you are evaluating a patient with chest pain; a normal ECG rules out ischemia in the setting of ongoing chest pain.

Stress Testing

Patients who experience intermittent chest pain, have a normal ECG, and are not taking digoxin should have an exercise stress ECG for diagnostic and prognostic purposes. Treadmill exercise testing uses a standardized protocol of increasing workload with continuous ECG recording. Stress tests provide information on myocardial function determined by blood flow. An important objective of stress testing is to identify patients who have a high risk of severe (left main or three-vessel) CAD. The sensitivity of the test ranges from 65% to 70%.

Exercise Myocardial Perfusion Imaging

This imaging has greater accuracy than the standard treadmill test when the resting ECG result is abnormal, the patient has diabetes, or the patient has a history of known CAD. Because of its higher sensitivity, the test is able to localize and characterize the extent of myocardial ischemia and to provide direct measurement of left ventricular function. This test is costlier than a treadmill test.

Echocardiography

An echocardiogram is a noninvasive cardiac ultrasound examining the heart that provides information about the cardiac muscle function, left ventricular ejection fraction, position, size, and movements of the valves and chambers, as well as the velocity of blood flow by means of reflected ultrasound. This test is used to determine biologic and prosthetic valve dysfunction and pericardial effusion, to evaluate velocity and direction of blood flow, to furnish direction for further diagnostic study, and to monitor patients with cardiac disease over an extended period.

Computed Tomography Scanning

Computed tomography (CT) scans produce cross-sectional images of anatomical structures without superimposing tissues on each other. Aortic dissections and tumors of the lung and pancreas can be detected with CT scans. Spiral CT uses a cone-shaped x-ray beam in a helical trajectory to focus on a width of tissue with high image resolution, revealing more detail than a traditional CT.

Ventilation–Perfusion Lung Scan

Ventilation–perfusion (V/Q) scanning was the first-line diagnostic tool for diagnosing PE before spiral CT and is still an acceptable alternative in select settings. With PE, the blood supply distal to the embolus is restricted. V/Q scanning uses a radioactive substance to show how well oxygen and blood are flowing to the lungs. Perfusion imaging will show poor or no visualization of the affected area. The ventilation scan demonstrates movement or lack of movement of air in the lungs. The perfusion scan demonstrates blood supply to the affected area of the lungs. The V/Q scan is reported as one of three categories: normal, high probability, and nondiagnostic.

Pulmonary Angiography

A pulmonary angiogram (arteriogram) is necessary if an embolectomy is considered. Radiographic contrast medium is injected into the pulmonary arteries, and the vasculature is visualized. This test can detect emboli as small as 3 mm in diameter. The test sensitivity is 98%, and the specificity is 96%. This test is the gold standard for diagnosing PE, but it is expensive and carries a small risk of cardiac arrhythmias, anaphylaxis, and death.

Radiography

Pneumothorax and pneumonia can be identified by chest radiography. Whereas pneumothorax reveals evidence of pleural air, pneumonia is seen on radiographs as a parenchymal infiltrate. Chest radiography, with suspected PE, is usually nonspecific; the findings can be normal, an elevated hemidiaphragm can be seen, or pulmonary infiltrate can be present. Rib radiographs will confirm rib fracture.

Cervical and thoracic spine and shoulder radiographs can show degenerative joint changes.

Magnetic Resonance Imaging

Magnetic resonance imaging is a noninvasive technique that produces cross-sectional images of the body through exposure to magnetic energy sources. It does not involve radiation and is used to differentiate healthy and diseased body tissues. It is useful in detecting tumors, infection sites, cardiac muscle perfusion and function, and diseased vessels.

Abdominal Ultrasound

Abdominal ultrasound is a noninvasive procedure to visualize solid organs. It is useful in detecting abdominal aortic aneurysm and dissection, masses, fluid collections, and infection. Pancreatitis and gallbladder disease can be detected with ultrasound.

Bronchoscopy

Bronchoscopy permits visualization of the trachea, bronchi, and select bronchioles. It is useful to diagnose tumors, hemorrhage, and trauma; to obtain brushings for cytologic examinations; and to remove foreign bodies from the lower respiratory tract.

Endoscopy

Upper endoscopy, with biopsy, is necessary to document the type and extent of tissue damage in GERD. A normal endoscopy, however, does not rule out mild gastric reflux disease.

Esophageal pH

When GERD is suspected, 24-hour esophageal pH monitoring is performed to document pathological acid reflux.

Cardiac Enzymes

Patients presenting with chest discomfort, consistent with an acute cardiac event, should have biomarkers of myocardial injury measured. Current clinical practice is to measure creatine kinase (CK, or CK-MB) and cardiac troponin (T or I; cTnT or cTnI) and cardiac enzymes when an MI is suspected. CK is released into the bloodstream 4 to 6 hours after heart cell damage occurs, and peak blood levels of CK are seen after 24 hours. A patient who has had an MI will have a CK-MB result that is five or more times the normal value.

Elevated CK levels usually indicate heart muscle damage; however, CK levels can be increased with damage to other kinds of cells as well.

Troponin is released into the bloodstream 2 to 6 hours after heart cell damage, and blood levels peak in 12 to 26 hours. Elevated levels of troponin are regarded as a more reliable indicator of heart muscle damage than elevated CK levels. Because troponin is an "earlier" marker of cardiac cell damage than CK, it is the preferred marker today for diagnosing MI. Troponin levels remain elevated for 7 to 10 days after the cardiac event.

D-Dimer Assay

The D-dimer assay is a blood test performed in patients with suspected thrombotic disorders. D-dimers are not normally present in human blood plasma except when the coagulation system has been activated. An abnormal result rules out thrombosis; however, a normal result can indicate thrombosis but does not rule out other potential causes. Its main use is to exclude thromboembolic disease where the probability is low.

Arterial Blood Gases

Arterial blood gases (ABGs) are obtained to detect respiratory alkalosis resulting from hyperventilation, decreased carbon dioxide pressure (PCO_2), and sometimes decreased oxygen pressure (PO_2) (hypoxemia). Hypoxemia often correlates with the extent of the lung area occluded in a PE. ABGs decrease with heart failure resulting in pulmonary edema.

Activated Partial Thromboplastin Time and Prothrombin Time

Activated partial thromboplastin time (aPTT) is a clotting test that screens for coagulation disorders and is used to monitor the effectiveness of heparin therapy. Prothrombin time (PT) measures a potential defect in stage II of the clotting mechanism through analysis of the clotting ability of five plasma coagulation factors. PTs are commonly ordered to measure the effects of oral anticoagulant therapies. Ineffective anticoagulation therapy places the patient at risk for PE.

These tests can also be ordered to search for the cause of PE.

Serum Amylase and Lipase

Amylase is an enzyme that helps convert starch to sugar; it is produced in the pancreas, liver, salivary glands, and fallopian tubes. If there is inflammation of the pancreas or salivary glands, increased levels of amylase enter the bloodstream. Lipase is the enzyme responsible for the breakdown of fats to fatty acids and glycerol. The pancreas is the main source of lipase. Pancreatic damage results in elevated serum lipase levels. Therefore, determining the levels of serum amylase and lipase is useful in the diagnosis of pancreatitis. Amylase levels return to normal before lipase levels.

Complete Blood Count

A complete blood count (CBC) is obtained to detect an elevated white blood cell count that occurs with infection. Hemoglobin and hematocrit levels are useful if anemia is suspected as an underlying cause of chest pain.

Erythrocyte Sedimentation Rate

The erythrocyte sedimentation rate (ESR) value is elevated with inflammation, such as in arthritis and pericarditis. The test is not specific for a particular disease.

DIFFERENTIAL DIAGNOSIS OF COMMON CAUSES OF EMERGENT CHEST PAIN

Acute Myocardial Infarction

Assessment of the patient experiencing acute chest pain must first focus on the potential diagnosis of MI to facilitate prompt initiation of treatment to limit infarct size and cardiac damage. The patient with an acute MI generally describes a sudden onset of pain at rest. It is a persistent, often severe, deep, central chest pain and can radiate, as does angina, to the throat or neck, across both sides of the chest to the shoulder, or down the medial aspect of either or both arms but more often to the left. Rest or nitroglycerin does not relieve the pain. The chest pain is often associated with shortness of breath, nausea, vomiting, and diaphoresis.

The quality of the pain or discomfort is generally more intense than any previously experienced anginal symptoms. Patients can also express a sense of impending doom. Quick review for positive risk factors (men 45 years and older; women 55 years and older; cigarette smoker; hyperlipidemia; hypertension; diabetes; obesity; history of CAD; family history of CAD) is useful. Objective evidence of an MI can include skin pallor, cool diaphoretic skin, and transient paradoxical S_2. The patient can be hypertensive or hypotensive.

A patient with severe chest pain or a suspected MI should be placed on a cardiac monitor as soon as possible. Observe for premature ventricular contractions and classic electrocardiographic changes that indicate MI, including ST segment elevations, T-wave inversions, and Q waves. Performing a 12-lead ECG and determining levels of cardiac isoenzymes will help confirm or rule out an MI.

Aortic Dissection

The patient often is in a great deal of distress, describing unrelenting chest pain as ripping and tearing, and radiating to the interscapular region, jaw, neck, or lower back. Hypertension is a risk factor in 70% of cases, and it most commonly affects men 50 to 70 years of age. Physical examination reveals hypotension or an increased pulse pressure and rapid or weak pulses if the tear produces bleeding into and along the wall of the aorta. However, specific circulatory changes depend on the location of the dissection. Chest radiography demonstrates a wide mediastinum with extension of the aortic wall beyond the calcific border. Diagnosis can be made by aortic angiogram, with CT of the chest and abdomen using a contrast dye injection to visualize the aorta and its branches. A transesophageal ultrasound can also be ordered. Patients with suspect aortic dissection should be immediately referred for emergent care. Studies have demonstrated in-hospital, witnessed aortic dissection carries a mortality rate of more than 96%.

Acute Coronary Insufficiency

Acute coronary insufficiency refers to situations in which chest pain is caused by lack of oxygen to the myocardium but there is no evidence of infarct. The patient reports severe, oppressive, constricting, retrosternal discomfort lasting longer than 30 minutes. The patient may report prior history of MI or angina. The ECG can show intermittent ischemic changes or be normal. Cardiac enzymes are normal.

Pulmonary Embolus

Patients presenting with PE usually report sudden onset of severe sharp, crushing, non-radiating chest pain if there is an embolus impacted in a major artery. Infarction of the pulmonary parenchyma closer to the pleural surface will cause pleuritic chest pain, often accompanied by the sudden onset of dyspnea and hemoptysis. Patients frequently express feelings of impending doom.

A review of risk factors will likely reveal one or more of the following: older age, prior venous thromboembolism, prolonged immobility or paralysis, cancer, heart failure, other chronic disease, pelvic or lower extremity surgery, recent pregnancy or delivery, obesity, oral contraceptive use, or varicose veins. Physical findings include restlessness, tachycardia, tachypnea, fever, diminished breath sounds, crackles or wheezes, and possible pleural friction rub. There can be signs of thrombophlebitis of the extremities. Initial diagnostic tests should include chest radiography and ECG; the results of both can be normal, but if clinical signs still point to PE, referral for consultation and further tests, including ABGs, venous Doppler studies, spiral CT scan, V/Q scan, and pulmonary angiography, is indicated.

Pneumothorax

Pneumothorax can be a life-threatening event, especially if the patient has underlying COPD or asthma. The patient reports sharp or tearing chest pain that can radiate to the ipsilateral shoulder. Sudden onset of shortness of breath is also associated with spontaneous pneumothorax. Objective findings include decreased or absent breath sounds on the affected side, tachycardia, tachypnea, and possible deviated trachea. A chest radiograph is needed to evaluate the possible complete or partial collapse of the lung.

Arrhythmias

Patients report palpitations or forceful heartbeats. These arrhythmias can be the result of myocardial ischemia, cocaine abuse, conditions such as prolapsed mitral valve, or anxiety. Syncope associated with palpitations indicates a more serious cardiac arrhythmia.

Congenital Coronary Anomalies

The coronary arteries can arise abnormally, take an abnormal course, or have fistulous connections to other structures, resulting in exertional chest pain that can lead to sudden death in the young athlete. The child or adolescent can have a history of moderate to severe chest pain during or after exercise. Risk factors include a family history of sudden death at an early age, heart disease, seizures, a history of lightheadedness or loss of consciousness during exercise, and a tall and lanky body type with double jointedness. Referral to a pediatric cardiologist is warranted.

Common Causes of Nonemergent Chest Pain

Stable angina

Stable angina refers to chest pain typically described as substernal chest pressure or

---

 EVIDENCE-BASED PRACTICE *Recognizing Myocardial Infarction*

Although certain signs and symptoms have been identified as being important in recognizing myocardial infarction (MI), data from the Framingham study estimate that 25% of infarctions may go unrecognized because of either lack of chest pain or the presence of atypical symptoms. The main predictive factors of silent MI are age, hypertension, history of cardiovascular disease, and diabetes duration. Silent MI is associated with as poor a prognosis as symptomatic MI.

Reference: Valensi et al, 2011.

heaviness, radiating to the left shoulder and arm, neck, or jaw. The pain onset is usually gradual, brought on and exacerbated by exercise and stress; it is associated with nausea, diaphoresis, and shortness of breath and is alleviated with rest or nitroglycerin. Pain typically lasts 2 to 10 minutes. Physical examination results are usually normal. An S_4 gallop can be transiently present during an episode of pain. Tests for angina include performing an ECG during an episode of pain, which can show ST-segment depression and T-wave inversions, or the findings can be normal. In contrast, unstable angina pain is intense, lasts as long as 30 minutes, and does not subside with rest or nitroglycerin. Unstable angina is an impending emergency.

Myocarditis

Myocarditis is an inflammation of the myocardium and is commonly caused by viruses. The heart is unable to contract properly because the inflammatory process interferes with the contractile function of the myocardial cells and eventually leads to cell death. It is frequently accompanied by pericarditis. The chest pain is caused by ischemia or arrhythmia. Patients have fever and dyspnea and can have evidence of heart failure. Heart murmurs and friction rubs can be heard. Chest radiographs show cardiomegaly. ECG will detect signs of irritation to the heart muscle and arrhythmia.

Pericarditis

The pain associated with pericarditis is described as sharp, located in the center of the chest, short-lived, episodic, and radiating to the back in the trapezial area. The pain is worse when the patient is supine and sitting; leaning forward often reduces the intensity of the pain. Shallow breathing can be an associated symptom, in an effort to avoid pain. Dyspnea can be present with compression of the bronchial tree by a large pericardial effusion. Risk factors for pericarditis include recent viral or bacterial infection, recent MI, uremia, myxedema, and history of autoimmune disease. Objective signs include fever before the onset of pain, tachycardia, and pericardial friction rub. The rub is pathognomonic for pericarditis but is found in only 60% to 70% of patients with pericarditis. Diagnostic tests show elevated white blood cells and ESR and ECG showing diffuse ST-segment elevation in the early stages. Chest radiography can be normal or show effusion with an increase in cardiac shadow.

Aortic stenosis

Aortic stenosis can cause exertional chest pain. Associated symptoms include fatigue, palpitations, dyspnea on exertion, dizziness, and syncope. Physical examination reveals a loud, harsh crescendo–decrescendo murmur, best heard at the second right intercostal space, with the patient leaning forward. The murmur can radiate to the neck and is often associated with a thrill. An echocardiogram will provide diagnostic evidence of aortic stenosis.

Mitral regurgitation

Symptoms of mitral regurgitation are similar to those of aortic stenosis: they include exertional substernal chest pain, fatigue, palpitations, dizziness, dyspnea on exertion, and syncope. The murmur associated with mitral regurgitation is holosystolic and blowing and often is heard best at the apex in the left lateral position. The murmur decreases with inspiration and can radiate to the left axilla and occasionally to the back. Again, echocardiography will provide evidence of mitral regurgitation.

Pneumonia

Signs and symptoms of pneumonia include pleuritic chest pain; a productive, moist cough with dark sputum; shortness of breath; and fever and chills. Risk factors include ineffective cough reflex, inability to swallow, advanced age, or very young age. Auscultation of the lungs reveals diminished breath sounds over affected areas, and crackles and wheezes can be heard. Rales and rhonchi are frequently heard on auscultation. Dullness with percussion is heard over areas of consolidation. Vocal fremitus is heard. In addition, physical findings can include tachycardia, tachypnea, bronchophony, and egophony. Chest radiography, sputum culture, and ABGs will further support the diagnosis of pneumonia. Follow-up chest radiographs are indicated after pneumonia because lung tumors can be hidden by pneumonia. Very young and very old patients may be hospitalized for observation and treatment of pneumonia.

Mitral valve prolapse

Patients with chest pain from MVP report a range of signs and symptoms, including arrhythmias, palpitations, fatigue, and anxiety. Patients may have a history of rheumatic fever. Physical examination can be normal or a mid-systolic click can be heard over the apex, while the patient is sitting or squatting. An echocardiogram will provide evidence of MVP.

Pleuritis

Pleuritic chest pain occurs suddenly and is worsened by deep breathing, coughing, and sneezing. Pleuritic chest pain can be a manifestation of pneumonia or can represent pleural inflammation, usually after a viral upper respiratory tract infection. Physical examination of the chest can be normal or a pleural friction rub can be heard over the area of inflammation. The patient's respiration rate is normal but often shallow or guarded. Unless pneumonia is suspected, no diagnostic tests are indicated because the cause of pleuritic chest pain is likely of viral etiology.

Esophagitis

Esophagitis or esophageal spasm symptoms often mimic angina. In fact, sublingual nitroglycerin can also relieve the symptoms, but usually relief takes longer than the 3 to 5 minutes to relieve angina. Patients frequently report that the pain is worse after eating spicy foods or large meals or if they lie down after eating. They sometimes report a sour taste in their mouth. Physical examination is normal, except for possible epigastric tenderness with palpation. The most reliable way to detect reflux as the cause of chest pain is to correlate episodes of chest pain with results of 24-hour esophageal pH monitoring.

Chest trauma

Rib fractures usually follow trauma. Pain is made worse by deep breathing. The patient's respirations are shallow, and pain is exacerbated by palpation in the area of the fracture. Chest or rib radiographs will confirm suspected rib fractures.

Rheumatic diseases

Rheumatic diseases, such as rheumatoid arthritis and ankylosing spondylitis, may cause thoracic pain. In children, lasting joint pain and inflammation are common with rheumatic fever but can also indicate rheumatic heart disease.

Costochondritis and Tietze syndrome

Costochondritis and Tietze syndrome are both identified by severe pain with palpation along the anterior cartilage where the ribs meet the sternum. Deep breathing and movement of the chest wall intensify the pain. In Tietze syndrome, swelling also occurs along this border.

Herpes zoster

Herpes zoster is manifested by unilateral chest pain that follows a dermatome. The pain is usually described as burning, stabbing, or pruritic. Early in the course of the disease, no objective manifestations are present. As the course of herpes zoster progresses, a vesicular rash appears in the area of pain (see Chapter 28).

Peptic ulcer disease

Subjective manifestations of peptic ulcer disease include episodes of pain 1 to 3 hours after eating. The pain can awaken the patient at night and is frequently relieved by antacids or eating. The patient can report hematemesis or melena. A CBC can show iron-deficiency anemia. Personal or family history of ulcer disease can be a risk factor, as well as cigarette smoking and excessive alcohol use. Upper GI radiography and endoscopy are diagnostic tests that can confirm peptic ulcer disease.

Cholecystitis

Cholecystitis is reported as colicky, intermittent epigastric or right-upper-quadrant pain that often follows a high-fat meal. Nausea and vomiting can accompany the pain, which often radiates to the right infrascapular area. Physical examination can show a positive Murphy sign, as indicated by tenderness in the region of the gallbladder. The gallbladder can be distended and palpable. Gallbladder ultrasonography is the most important diagnostic test in the evaluation of this problem.

Acute pancreatitis

Acute pancreatitis occurs as the sudden onset of severe, steady upper epigastric, or left-upper-quadrant abdominal pain, which frequently radiates to the left anterior chest, shoulders, or back. The pain is worse in the supine position. The patient appears restless, and pain can be associated with nausea and severe vomiting, hypotension, and unexplained shock. Left-upper-quadrant abdominal pain with palpation is present. Determination of serum amylase and lipase levels confirms the diagnosis. A rise in amylase level is seen 2 to 12 hours after the onset of symptoms. The lipase level returns to normal slower than the amylase level and thus is more useful in diagnosing pancreatitis later in its course. Pancreas ultrasonography and CT are necessary to show positive evidence of pancreatitis.

Lung and mediastinal tumors

Lung and mediastinal tumors can be manifested by chest pain. Associated symptoms include shortness of breath, cough, and hemoptysis. Pneumonia is often the initial diagnosis, and persistence of symptoms after treatment can lead to further investigation for tumors. Risk factors include a smoking history and family history of cancer. Physical examination can be normal or reveal diminished breath sounds in the area of the tumor. Dull sounds on percussion of the chest can be an objective manifestation of a chest mass. Chest radiography and CT of the chest are diagnostic tools to identify these lesions. Bronchoscopy is performed to obtain a biopsy.

Cocaine and amphetamines

Cocaine and amphetamines increase the metabolic requirement of the heart for oxygen and decrease the supply of oxygen, producing myocardial ischemia and chest pain. Cocaine causes adrenergic stimulation, thus increasing heart rate, blood pressure, and left ventricular contractility. Concomitantly, myocardial oxygen supply declines because of cocaine-induced vasoconstriction of the coronary arteries. ECGs, serial cardiac enzymes, and urine drug screens are useful diagnostic tools.

Psychogenic origin

Adults and adolescents with a history of a recent stressful situation can present with chest pain. Physical examination results are normal.

Pleurodynia

Group B coxsackieviruses can cause pleurodynia. The presentation is usually a sudden, severe onset of stabbing, paroxysmal pleuritic pain over the lower rib cage and substernal area. Deep breathing aggravates the pain. Fever, headache, malaise, and unproductive cough are usually present. The chest examination results are normal except for a pleuritic friction rub in 25% of cases. The condition lasts from 1 to 14 days.

Precordial catch syndrome

Recurrent brief episodes of sudden, sharp pain occurring at rest or during mild exercise can indicate precordial catch syndrome. It is localized near the apex of the heart, and along the left sternal border, or beneath the left breast. It is seen in children and adolescents and is benign in nature.

> **DIFFERENTIAL DIAGNOSIS OF** *Common Causes of Nonemergent Chest Pain*

CONDITION	HISTORY	PHYSICAL FINDINGS	DIAGNOSTIC STUDIES
Stable angina	Substernal chest pressure following exercise or stress and relieved by rest or nitroglycerin; nausea, SOB, diaphoresis, sternal chest pressure	Normal examination; possible transient S_4	ECG during episode of chest pain, treadmill stress testing, myocardial perfusion imaging
Myocarditis	Chest pain; history of fever, dyspnea	Heart murmur, friction rub, fever	ECG, chest radiograph, echocardiogram
Pericarditis	Sharp, stabbing pain referred to left shoulder or trapezius ridge, usually worse during coughing or deep breathing; can be relieved by sitting forward; history of viral or bacterial infection, autoimmune disease	Fever before onset of pain, tachycardia, pericardial friction rub	WBC, ESR, ECG, chest radiograph, echocardiogram
Aortic stenosis	Chest pain on exertion, substernal and anginal in quality; fatigue, palpitations, DOE, dizziness, syncope	Radial pulse diminished; narrow pulse pressure; loud, harsh, crescendo-decrescendo murmur heard best at second right ICS with patient leaning forward; thrill	Echocardiogram, ECG, chest radiograph
Mitral regurgitation	Exertional chest pain, fatigue, palpitations, dizziness, DOE, syncope	Holosystolic, blowing, often loud murmur heard best at apex in left lateral position and decreases with inspiration; murmur can radiate to axilla and possibly back	Chest radiograph, ECG, echocardiogram
Pneumonia	Productive cough of yellow or green or rust sputum, dyspnea, pleuritic pain	Fever; tachycardia, tachypnea; inspiratory crackles; vocal fremitus; percussion dull or flat over area of consolidation; bronchophony; egophony	Chest radiograph, sputum cultures, ABGs
Mitral valve prolapse	Chest pain, varies in location and intensity; palpitations; anxiety; nonexertional pain of short duration; history of Marfan syndrome	Arrhythmias, possible midsystolic click heard over apex; heard best while patient is in sitting or squatting position; thoracoskeletal deformity common in children	ECG, echocardiogram
Pleuritis	Mild, localized chest pain, worse with deep breathing; recent URI	Shallow respirations, local tenderness, pleural friction rub	Chest radiography

DIFFERENTIAL DIAGNOSIS OF *Common Causes of Nonemergent Chest Pain—cont'd*

CONDITION	HISTORY	PHYSICAL FINDINGS	DIAGNOSTIC STUDIES
Esophagitis	Substernal pain worse after eating and lying down; sour taste in mouth	Epigastric pain with palpitation	Esophageal pH
Chest trauma (rib fracture)	History of injury or trauma; pain with deep breaths; splinting of chest wall	Shallow respirations; chest wall pain on palpitation	Chest radiograph
Costochondritis	Pain along sternal border, increases with deep breaths; history of exercise, URI, or physical activity	Pain with palpitation over costochondral joints; normal breath sounds	None
Herpes zoster	Unilateral chest pain; painful rash	Normal breath sounds; vesicular rash along dermatome	None
Peptic ulcer disease	Epigastric pain 1–2 hr after eating, can be relieved by antacids; hematemesis and melena; risk factors include smoking and alcohol overuse	Tenderness to palpitation in epigastric area; signs of hypovolemia	Upper GI radiograph, upper endoscopy, CBC
Cholecystitis	Right-upper-quadrant abdominal pain radiating to right chest, often after eating high-fat meal; nausea and vomiting	Positive Murphy sign; palpable gallbladder	Gallbladder ultrasound
Acute pancreatitis	Severe epigastric or left-upper-quadrant abdominal pain radiating into left chest; pain worse in supine position; nausea, vomiting, fever	Left upper abdominal pain with palpation; hypotension	Amylase, lipase, pancreas ultrasound or CT scan
Lung tumors	Chest pain, SOB, cough, hemoptysis, history of cigarette smoking; history of pneumonia	Normal examination or diminished breath sounds over tumor and dull percussion sound over tumor	Chest radiograph, spiral CT of chest, bronchoscopy
Cocaine and amphetamine use	Chest pain, SOB, diaphoresis, nausea; can relate to substance use	Tachycardia, hypertension	ECG, serial cardiac enzymes, drug screen
Psychogenic origin	Precordial chest pain, history of stressful situations	Normal examination	ECG, chest radiograph, treadmill stress test if cardiac risk factors present
Pleurodynia	Severe, acute onset, stabbing, paroxysmal, pleuritic pain over lower rib cage and substernal edge; headache, malaise, nonproductive cough	Pleural friction rub 25% of time; chest examination normal; fever usually present	Chest radiograph

Continued

> **DIFFERENTIAL DIAGNOSIS OF** *Common Causes of Nonemergent Chest Pain—cont'd*

CONDITION	HISTORY	PHYSICAL FINDINGS	DIAGNOSTIC STUDIES
Precordial catch syndrome	Sudden, sharp, nondistressing pain near apex of heart; seen in adolescents	Normal examination	Chest radiography, ECG

CBC, complete blood cell count; *CT*, computed tomography; *DOE*, dizziness on exertion; *ECG*, electrocardiogram; *ESR*, erythrocyte sedimentation rate; *GI*, gastrointestinal; *ICS*, intercostal space; *SOB*, shortness of breath; *URI*, upper respiratory tract infection; *WBC*, white blood cell count.

Confusion in Older Adults

Confusion is a symptom rather than a disease state. It is the inability to think quickly or coherently. A confused patient is disoriented to time, person, or place and may demonstrate impaired cognitive function. Older adults are far more likely to experience an acute confusional state as a result of hospitalization or surgery, systemic or electrolyte imbalance, organ failure, excessive medication, nutritional deficiency, systemic infection, or cerebral insufficiency (e.g., stroke or transient ischemic attacks [TIAs]). When an older patient presents with confusion, the differential diagnosis includes delirium, dementia, and depression.

Delirium, caused by alterations in brain metabolism, is characterized by an abrupt onset, reduced level of acute consciousness, and sleep–wake cycle disturbance. *Delirium is a medical emergency* and can occur as a result of medications, alcohol use or alcohol withdrawal, narcotic reaction or narcotic withdrawal, Wernicke-Korsakoff syndrome (vitamin B_{12} deficiency), hepatic encephalopathy, acute illness, chronic illness, interacting diseases, or trauma (e.g., head injury).

Dementia, a chronic generalized impairment of brain function, affects thinking but not the level of consciousness (LOC). A common early complaint in dementia is forgetfulness, with loss of concentration and loss of memory. Causes of dementia can be classified as reversible (or partially reversible), modifiable, or irreversible (Box 9.1).

Depression as a cause of confusion, especially in older adults, is considered a reversible cause of dementia. When anxiety symptoms are also present, depression can manifest as mild delirium (see Chapter 4).

DIAGNOSTIC REASONING: FOCUSED HISTORY

Obtaining an appropriate history from a confused patient involves the use of another person as the historian. Preferably that person is someone who has had consistent contact with the patient and can report about usual behavioral patterns and the conditions involved with this episode.

Is this a condition that requires immediate intervention?

Key Questions
- How abruptly did the confusion start?
- Is the patient alert and aware of time, person, and place?
- Has the patient expressed thoughts of suicide (in words or actions)?
- Does the patient use alcohol or other drugs?

Confusion that is acute in onset and persistent can indicate delirium, a cerebrovascular event, cerebral infection, subdural hematoma, or neoplasm. A history of altered LOC along with the current confusion indicates a condition that requires immediate intervention. Acute-onset confusion can produce paranoia and aggression. Suicidal ideation can accompany depression and is an indication for immediate intervention and further evaluation. If the patient has been misusing alcohol or other chemical substances, acute withdrawal can require immediate medical intervention.

If the onset is gradual and the patient is not seriously ill, consider depression or dementia. Unless the patient is suicidal or seriously ill, both depression and dementia can be handled in a more temperate manner.

| Box 9.1 | **Causes of Dementia** |

REVERSIBLE CAUSES OF DEMENTIA
D   Drugs or medications
E   Emotional illness or depression
M   Metabolic or endocrine disorders
E   Eye or ear involvement or environmental
N   Nutritional or neurologic
T   Tumors or trauma
I   Infection
A   Alcoholism, anemia, or atherosclerosis

MODIFIABLE CAUSES OF DEMENTIA
• Normal-pressure hydrocephalus
• Hepatic encephalopathy
• HIV encephalopathy (AIDS dementia complex)

IRREVERSIBLE CAUSES OF DEMENTIA
• Alzheimer disease
• Multi-infarct dementia
• Dementia with Lewy bodies
• Frontotemporal lobar degeneration

What distinguishing characteristics of confusion does this patient exhibit?

Key Questions
• Was the onset of the confusion abrupt (i.e., over a period of minutes or hours) or gradual (i.e., a few days, weeks, or months)?
• Does the confusion change within a 24-hour period (stable or fluctuating)?
• Is there a change in the sleep pattern?
• Is the patient alert and aware?
• Has the patient experienced seeing, hearing, or feeling things that are not there?
• Is there any history of head trauma?

Onset and Duration

Confusion that is abrupt in onset but short-lived can indicate a TIA. Sudden onset, usually over a period of hours, is characteristic of delirium. In delirium, the condition is persistent but has been present for no longer than 1 month. In an acute confusion episode, the symptoms are less severe than with delirium and have a less sudden onset. The onset of confusion in depression is usually gradual, over a period of weeks, and is persistent over time. In dementia, the onset is insidious and gradual; the condition has often been present for many weeks or months.

Fluctuation in Symptoms

With delirium, the symptoms can fluctuate over the course of a day and frequently are worse at night and with fatigue. The course is more stable with both depression and dementia, with little variation over a 24-hour period.

Disturbance in Sleep–Wake Cycle

The sleep–wake cycle in delirium is impaired. Either the patient gets little or no sleep or has night insomnia and is drowsy and tired during the day. Thus, the sleep–wake cycle is usually fragmented, and the patient tends to be restless and agitated and hallucinates while awake during the night.

Level of Consciousness

In both dementia and depression, the individual is likely to be both alert and aware, although the mood can be depressed. With delirium, the patient will have a decreased LOC, be less alert and aware, and can be difficult to arouse. In an acute confusional state, the person will demonstrate impaired concentration and make errors in thinking.

Hallucinations

Visual, tactile, and auditory hallucinations are common with delirium, especially at night when changes in environment or activity occur. Hallucinations are uncommon in both depression and dementia, although hallucinations can occur in late-stage dementia. Visual hallucinations are the symptoms of Lewy body disease and precede cognitive impairment. The occurrence of visual hallucination early in the symptom history is Lewy body disease until proven otherwise

Head Trauma

Head trauma can produce confusion and disorientation. In older adults, common causes of head trauma include motor vehicle crashes, physical abuse, and falls.

Are there any associated symptoms that will point me in the right direction?

Key Questions
• Has the patient shown any tremor, especially at rest?

- Has the patient had any trouble walking?
- Has the patient reported severe headache or nausea?
- Has the patient had a fever?
- Has the patient gained or lost weight?
- Does the patient engage in his or her usual activities?

Tremor and Gait Disturbance

Tremors are associated with parkinsonism, human immunodeficiency virus (HIV), encephalopathy, and liver disease. Gait disorder is associated with parkinsonism, medication reactions, and head trauma.

Headache, Nausea, and Fever

Headache and nausea are associated with head trauma, stroke, and tumor. Fever is usually present with HIV-associated infection, other systemic infections, or acute alcohol withdrawal.

Change in Weight and Usual Activities

Patients with depression can exhibit vegetative symptoms (e.g., cessation of talking, eating, dressing, and toileting; insomnia; weight loss or gain; diminished interest in most activities or former pleasures) and feelings of worthlessness.

What does the pattern of cognitive losses tell me?

Key Questions
- What specific problems with mental abilities or thinking have you noticed?
- What behavioral changes or personality changes have you noticed?

Changes in Mental Abilities and Behaviors

Patients with delirium have global cognitive losses that involve memory, thinking, perception, and judgment. These patients can become disoriented, irritable, and fearful. They can be difficult to arouse or conversely have insomnia. Families sometimes note visual hallucinations.

Patients in an acute confusional state can be disoriented, especially for time, less for place, and almost never for self. They show impaired concentration, experience sensory misperceptions, and make errors in thinking.

Early dementia presents with more selective cognitive losses. Family members report that patients cannot remember recent events; are disoriented, irritable, or depressed; have poor hygiene; show poor judgment; make financial errors; are socially withdrawn; have difficulty finding or saying the right words; are clumsy or fall; have urinary incontinence; have deteriorating interpersonal relationships; and show personality changes. Memory loss is typical of Alzheimer disease. Loss of executive function occurs early with vascular causes of dementia. Language disturbance is typical of frontotemporal lobe dementia, and clumsiness or falling typifies Lewy body disease.

Fewer cognitive losses occur with depression. These individuals can exhibit cognitive losses consistent with confusion—apathy and drowsiness, impaired concentration, and errors in thinking. The most common cognitive symptoms are severe negative thinking, guilt, and remorse.

Is the confusion caused by a concurrent health problem?

Key Questions
- Does the patient have any chronic health conditions?
- Has the patient been hospitalized recently, and if so, for what reason?
- Has the patient been acutely ill recently?
- Is there a history of mental illness or similar thought disturbance?

Current and Past Health Status

Obtain past medical records for a complete health history. Most likely, you will have to use a relative or close friend to determine current and past health status. Many systemic conditions and disorders can produce alteration in mental status, particularly in older patients (Box 9.2). Chronic health problems (e.g., alcoholism, renal failure, liver disease, severe anemia, chronic obstructive pulmonary disease [COPD], severe cardiovascular disease, and HIV) predispose individuals, especially older adults, to the development of

Box 9.2	**Systemic Conditions Associated with Confusional States**

ENDOCRINE
- Hypo- or hyperthyroidism

METABOLIC
- Anemia (severe)
- Hypo- or hypercalcemia
- Hypo- or hypercortisolism
- Hypo- or hyperglycemia
- Hypomagnesemia
- Hypo- or hypernatremia
- Wilson disease (copper disorder)
- Porphyria

INFECTIOUS
- AIDS
- Cerebral amebiasis
- Cerebral cysticercosis
- Cerebral toxoplasmosis
- Cerebral malaria
- Fungal meningitis

- Lyme disease
- Neurosyphilis
- TB meningitis

CARDIOVASCULAR
- Congestive heart failure
- Hyperviscosity

CEREBROVASCULAR
- Cerebral insufficiency (TIA, CVA)
- Postanoxic encephalopathy

PULMONARY
- COPD
- Hypercapnia
- Hypoxemia

RENAL
- Renal failure
- Uremia

NEUROLOGIC
- Hepatic encephalopathy
- Hypertensive encephalopathy
- Limbic encephalitis
- Head trauma

OTHER
- Alcoholism
- Anemia (severe)
- Leukoencephalopathy
- Metastatic cancer to brain
- Sarcoidosis
- Sleep apnea
- Vasculitis (e.g., SLE)
- Vitamin deficiencies (vitamin B_{12}, folate, niacin, thiamine)
- Whipple disease

CVA, Cerebrovascular accident; *SLE,* systemic lupus erythematosus; *TB,* tuberculosis; *TIA,* transient ischemic attack.

confusion. Patients with multiple chronic health problems are particularly at risk.

Could the confusion be caused by medication?

Key Questions
- What medications is the patient taking?
- Is the patient taking the medications correctly?

Medications

Drugs that can produce altered mental status include the following:
- Alcohol
- Antibiotics (e.g., isoniazid, aminoglycosides)
- Anticholinergic agents
- Anticonvulsants
- Antidepressants
- Antihypertensive agents (e.g., reserpine, β-blockers, methyldopa, clonidine, hydralazine)
- Antiparkinsonian agents
- Cardiac drugs (e.g., digitalis, lidocaine, β-blockers, vasodilators, diuretics)
- Chemotherapeutic agents (e.g., methotrexate)
- Gastrointestinal drugs (e.g., H_2 blockers, metoclopramide)
- Illicit drugs (e.g., amphetamines, cocaine, opiates)
- Narcotics
- Over-the-counter cold or allergy preparations
- Sedatives

Taking Medication Correctly

Combinations of these medications increase the probability of medication-induced confusion. People who are confused may be taking medications improperly, which compounds the problem. Older adults may need lower doses or a gradual increase in dosages of medications used to treat both acute and chronic conditions. The exception to the "start low, go slow" rule is antidepressants in older adults because of the high rate of suicide. In that case, start low but be aggressive in titrating up to goal dose. Chronic kidney disease, common in older adults, can affect drug metabolism and elimination, so dosing adjustments and monitoring may be necessary to ensure therapeutic benefit.

What risk factors do I need to consider?

Key Questions

- How old is the patient?
- How many medications is the patient taking?
- Is the patient HIV positive?
- Has the patient experienced recent life losses?

Age

Older adults are at risk for the development of confusion, delirium, dementia, and depression. Factors that place them at risk include the use of multiple medications, the existence of multiple medical conditions, and the physiological changes associated with aging. Dementia occurs in approximately 5% to 10% of adults 65 to 80 years of age, 20% of those older than 80 years, and almost half of those older than 85 years.

Polypharmacy

Older adults who are taking multiple medications are at risk for medication interactions and resulting confusion (see also the preceding list of medications that can produce altered mental status).

Human Immunodeficiency Virus

Patients with HIV infection or those who are immunocompromised are at increased risk for the development of HIV, encephalopathy (AIDS dementia complex), or dementia caused by central nervous system opportunistic infections.

Recent Bereavement

Recent loss and the lack of a social network place an individual at risk for depression. Both cause profound biopsychosocial stress that can easily exceed the person's resources and skills. Extreme mourning or isolation can be physically and emotionally draining.

DIAGNOSTIC REASONING: FOCUSED PHYSICAL EXAMINATION

Take the Vital Signs

The presence of a fever can indicate infection or alcohol withdrawal. In the presence of confusion, a diastolic blood pressure greater than 120 mm Hg suggests hypertensive encephalopathy; a systolic blood pressure less than 90 mm Hg can indicate impaired cerebral perfusion.

Note the Level of Consciousness

In both dementia and depression, the individual is likely to be alert and aware, although the mood can be depressed. With delirium, the patient will have a decreased LOC, be less alert and aware, and can be difficult to arouse. In an acute confusional state, the patient will demonstrate impaired concentration and have difficulty thinking.

Perform a Mental Status Examination

A thorough mental status examination is essential. Mental status assessment is used to determine cognitive function. A number of assessment instruments are available, including the Montreal Cognitive Assessment (available at http://www.mocatest.org) and the Mini-Cog (available at http://mini-cog.com). Patients with delirium may be unable to cooperate or answer questions. Patients with dementia are cooperative and willing to try but make mistakes and give incorrect or "near-miss" answers. Patients with depression are less cooperative and are more likely to give "don't know" answers, refuse to answer questions, or be less willing to try.

Global cognitive loss is consistent with delirium. Losses occur in the following areas: memory, thinking, perception, information acquisition, information retention, information processing, information retrieval, and information use. Dementia, particularly early in the disorder, presents with selective cognitive losses that can occur in one or more of the following areas:

- Apraxia (i.e., cannot draw simple geometric figures)
- Visuospatial problems (e.g., cannot draw intersecting pentagons)
- Cannot perform commands
- Selective cognitive loss
- Loss of abstract reasoning
- Problems with orientation
- Problems with recent memory
- Problems with number retention

Fewer cognitive losses occur with depression than with dementia. Loss of concentration is an important symptom of depression. The individual is aware of losses and can highlight disabilities, especially memory loss. Along with loss of memory, impaired concentration, and errors in judgment are common.

In older adults, the Geriatric Depression Scale (Fig. 9.1) is positive for depression if the score is above 5. The Personal Health Questionnaire (PHQ-9) has also been validated in older adults and is positive for depression if the score is 10 or greater (available at http://www.cqaimh.org/pdf/tool_phq9.pdf).

The Confusion Assessment Method (CAM) can be used to assess delirium. The CAM instrument assesses the presence, severity, and fluctuation of nine delirium features: acute onset, inattention, disorganized thinking, altered LOC, disorientation, memory impairment, perceptual disturbances, psychomotor agitation or retardation, and altered sleep/wake cycle. The CAM diagnostic algorithm is based on four cardinal features of delirium: (1) acute onset and fluctuating course, (2) inattention, (3) disorganized thinking, and (4) altered LOC. Obtain permission to use the CAM and the training manual for it at https://www.hospital elderlifeprogram.org/delirium-instruments/

Geriatric Depression Scale (short form)

Choose the best answer for how you felt over the past week.

1. Are you basically satisfied with your life? — yes/no
2. Have you dropped many of your activities and interests? — yes/no
3. Do you feel that your life is empty? — yes/no
4. Do you often get bored? — yes/no
5. Are you in good spirits most of the time? — yes/no
6. Are you afraid that something bad is going to happen to you? — yes/no
7. Do you feel happy most of the time? — yes/no
8. Do you often feel helpless? — yes/no
9. Do you prefer to stay at home rather than going out and doing new things? — yes/no
10. Do you feel you have more problems with memory than most? — yes/no
11. Do you think it is wonderful to be alive now? — yes/no
12. Do you feel pretty worthless the way you are now? — yes/no
13. Do you feel full of energy? — yes/no
14. Do you feel that your situation is hopeless? — yes/no
15. Do you think that most people are better off than you are? — yes/no

This is the scoring for the scale. One point for each of these answers. Cut-off: normal (0–5); above 5 suggests depression.

1. no	6. yes	11. no
2. yes	7. no	12. yes
3. yes	8. yes	13. no
4. yes	9. yes	14. yes
5. no	10. yes	15. yes

FIGURE 9.1 Geriatric Depression Scale (short form). (From Sheikh JI, Yesavage JA: Geriatric Depression Scale: recent evidence and development of a shorter version, *Clin Gerontol* 5:165, 1986.)

EVIDENCE-BASED PRACTICE *Does the Patient Have Delirium?*

This systematic review compared several bedside instruments to assess their accuracy in diagnosing the presence of delirium in hospitalized adults. The authors concluded that the confusion assessment method (CAM) is quick and easy to use and has the evidence to support its use at the bedside. Of the instruments evaluated, the MMSE (score <24) was the least useful in identifying a patient with delirium. A caveat: none of the studies in the systematic review included patients in the primary care setting.

Reference: Wong CL et al, 2010.
MMSE, Mini-Mental State Examination

Perform a Complete Neurologic Examination

Normal neurologic findings are typical of early dementia and depression. Abnormal findings suggest other organic involvement.

Cranial nerves

Check vision, hearing, and sensory impairment as contributing factors in confusion. Dilated pupils suggest alcohol withdrawal; pinpoint pupils can indicate narcotic excess or use of eye drops. Changes in pupil size can also indicate neurologic changes, such as those that occur with stroke or neoplasm. The sense of smell is often impaired in dementia. Patients with parkinsonism can exhibit a typical facial presentation: masked facial expression, poor blink reflex, and drooling. Speech is slowed, slurred, and monotonous.

Proprioception and cerebellar function

Test coordination through rapid alternating movements (RAMs), accuracy of movement, balance (Romberg test), and gait. Slowed RAMs are characteristic of early HIV encephalopathy. Tremor and restlessness are associated with alcohol intoxication or withdrawal. Tremor (especially resting), rigidity, and bradykinesia indicate parkinsonism. Asterixis, sometimes referred to as liver flap or liver tremor, is an involuntary tremor of the hands, tongue, and feet that is characteristic of hepatic or metabolic encephalopathy. Postural tremor is present with HIV encephalopathy. Writhing movements (chorea) typify Huntington disease.

Gait abnormalities are found with multi-infarct dementia (MID), normal pressure hydrocephalus, and HIV encephalopathy.

Sensation (Primary and cortical)

Agnosia (failure to identify or recognize objects despite intact sensory function) is present with dementia.

Deep tendon reflexes

Test deep tendon reflexes (DTRs) and the superficial plantar reflexes. Hyperreflexia and primitive reflexes are present in late dementia. Hyperreflexia is also present in MID, HIV encephalopathy, and cerebrovascular accident (CVA).

A positive Babinski sign on testing the plantar reflex is present in MID, CVA, and head injury. Cogwheeling (resistance to a passively stretched hypertonic muscle, resulting in a rhythmical jerk similar to a ratchet) suggests parkinsonism.

Motor tone and function

Apraxia (impaired ability to carry out motor activities despite intact motor function) indicates dementia. Motor weakness, especially of the legs; loss of coordination; and impaired handwriting are consistent with early HIV encephalopathy.

Language

Aphasia (language disturbance) is often present in dementia and can occur with CVA and head injury.

Localizing and lateralizing signs in the central nervous system

Focal neurologic signs (i.e., exaggerated DTRs, positive Babinski sign, gait abnormalities, and hemiparesis) are consistent with MID. Focal deficits also occur with cerebrovascular injury.

Patients with late HIV encephalopathy demonstrate weakness that is greater in the legs than in the arms, ataxia, spasticity and hyperreflexia, positive Babinski sign, myoclonus, and bladder and bowel incontinence.

Psychomotor agitation or retardation is consistent with depression. An agitated confusional state without focal signs can occur with head trauma.

Perform a Respiratory Examination

Monitor the rate and effort of respirations. Auscultate the lung fields. Tachypnea suggests hypoxia. Bibasilar crackles indicate congestive heart failure (CHF) with hypoxia. Asymmetrical crackles suggest pneumonia with hypoxia. Patients with dementia or depression, in the absence of concomitant lung disease, will have normal findings.

Evaluate the Cardiovascular System

Perform a careful cardiovascular examination. Tachycardia suggests sepsis, hyperthyroidism, hypoglycemia, agitation, anxiety, or alcohol withdrawal. Be alert for indicators of cardiovascular problems that can produce hypoxia, such as CHF or myocardial infarction (MI).

Examine the Abdomen

Examine the abdomen and percuss for costovertebral angle (CVA) tenderness. Specific findings can indicate a local or systemic cause for the confusion. For example, urinary retention suggests urinary tract infection, CVA tenderness points to pyelonephritis, and an enlarged liver can indicate hepatic encephalopathy.

LABORATORY AND DIAGNOSTIC STUDIES

Diagnostic testing is aimed at detecting or confirming a metabolic or organic cause of the confusion. If dementia seems likely, these same tests can rule in or rule out reversible or modifiable causes of the dementia. Most tests will be normal when the diagnosis is depression.

Complete Blood Count

Leukocytosis suggests infection. Anemia as a cause of confusion in chronic illness can also be detected.

Blood Chemistry

High or low potassium and sodium levels, dehydration, and acidosis can all produce confusion. Elevated or depressed magnesium and calcium levels, hypoglycemia, and hyperglycemia can also cause confusion. Elevated blood urea nitrogen (BUN) and creatinine levels or an elevated BUN-to-creatinine ratio can indicate renal failure. Elevation in liver enzymes suggests liver dysfunction.

Thyroid Function Tests

Abnormal levels of thyroid-stimulating hormone (TSH) can indicate thyroid dysfunction, either thyroid toxicosis or a hypothyroid state. An elevated TSH level is related to chronic symptoms of depression.

Serum B$_{12}$ and Folate

Deficiencies of vitamin B$_{12}$ and folate are reversible causes of dementia.

Serology for Syphilis

Perform if indicated by medical or social history. A positive test result can indicate neurosyphilis as the cause of confusion.

Arterial Blood Gases

Arterial blood gases are used to determine the presence or degree of hypoxia.

Toxicology Screen and Blood Alcohol Level

These tests can be used to determine alcohol or drug intoxication as a cause of confusion.

Urinalysis

Urinalysis is used to detect infection and can point to renal indicators of systemic disease.

Chest Radiograph

A chest radiograph is used to detect infection, CHF, COPD, pneumonia, or other respiratory-associated causes of hypoxia.

Lumbar Puncture

Lumbar puncture (LP) is used to rule out bacterial, fungal, or tumor meningitis (see Chapter 19). LP is used to test cerebrospinal fluid for Alzheimer disease biomarkers and tau-opathies. High-volume LP decompresses a normal-pressure hydrocephalus (NPH), which may or may not reverse the dementia syndrome, depending on how long the NPH has been present and how long it has compressed the brain.

Electrocardiography

Electrocardiography is used to rule out certain cardiovascular causes of hypoxia, such as MI or dysrhythmias.

Electroencephalography

Electroencephalography can be used to identify a seizure disorder as a cause of or a contributing factor to confusion.

Computed Tomography or Magnetic Resonance Imaging

Computed tomography or magnetic resonance imaging is used to diagnose whether cerebrovascular bleeding, injury, abscess, tumor, or whether focal neurologic signs are present. In the diagnosis of dementia, structural imaging yields limited but helpful diagnostic information. Signs may include decreased hippocampal size (Alzheimer disease), microvascular change (vascular dementia), or atrophy in frontotemporal lobes greater than in other areas.

Positron Emission Tomography Scan

Positron emission tomography (PET) is useful in confirming the diagnosis of Alzheimer disease. PET is also useful in differentiating Alzheimer disease from other forms of dementia, such as vascular dementia, and from other memory disorders such as clinical depression.

DIFFERENTIAL DIAGNOSIS

Delirium

The incidence of delirium increases progressively after the fourth decade of life. Because delirium is associated with an increased risk of death, it should be considered first in older patients who exhibit cognitive impairment or behavioral changes.

Delirium is characterized by reduced ability to maintain attention to external stimuli, disorganized thinking, decreased LOC, perceptual disturbances, disturbed sleep–wake cycle, disorientation, and memory impairment. The patient will evidence a decreased LOC and impaired arousal, increased or decreased psychomotor activity, and irritability. The onset is rapid, and the condition can last from hours to weeks. Fluctuations over the course of the day are common, with lucid intervals during the day and worse symptoms at night. The thought process is disorganized, and the patient is usually disoriented, most commonly to time. There is a tendency for the patient to mistake the unfamiliar for familiar places and people. Hallucinations, usually visual, are common. Physical examination findings depend on the underlying cause of the delirium. The patient often exhibits asterixis or tremor. Speech is incoherent, hesitant, slow, or rapid. Table 9.1 shows the distinguishing characteristics of delirium.

Confusion

Confusion is less abrupt and less severe than delirium, with less severe disorientation and more subtle motor signs. The diurnal variation is less severe than in delirium. The person can be apathetic and drowsy and will show disorientation, especially for time, less for place, and almost never for self. Concentration is impaired, and the person lacks direction and selectivity and is easily distracted. Errors in thinking are common. The person may exhibit tremor and difficulty in motor relaxation.

Dementia

Dementia is characterized by acquired persistent and progressive impairment of intellectual function, with compromise in at least two of the following areas:
- Language (aphasia)
- Memory
- Visuospatial skills (apraxia, agnosia)
- Emotional behavior or personality
- Cognition (e.g., calculation, abstraction, judgment)

Table 9.1	**Distinguishing Characteristics of Delirium, Dementia, and Depression**		
CHARACTERISTIC	**DELIRIUM**	**DEMENTIA**	**DEPRESSION**
Onset	Sudden	Insidious, relentless	Sudden or insidious
Duration	Hours, days	Persistent	>2 weeks
Time of day	Increases and decreases during the day	Stable, no change	Throughout the greater part of the day
Consciousness	Altered	Not impaired except in severe cases	Not impaired
Cognition	Impairment of memory, attentiveness, consciousness, numerous errors in assessment tasks	Minimal cognitive impairment initially, progresses to impaired abstract thinking, judgment, memory, thought patterns, calculations, agnosia	Impaired concentration, reduced attention span, indecisiveness, slower thought processes, impaired short- and long-term memory
Activity	Increased or decreased; can fluctuate	Unchanged from usual behavior	Insomnia or excessive sleeping, fatigue, restlessness, anxiety, increased or decreased appetite
Speech or language	Rambling and irrelevant conversation, illogical flow of ideas, incoherent	Disordered, rambling, incoherent; struggles to find words	Slower speech
Mood and affect	Rapid mood swings; fearful, suspicious	Depressed, apathetic, uninterested	Sad, hopeless, feels worthless, loss of interest or pleasure
Delusions or hallucinations	Misperceptions, illusions, hallucinations, and delusions	Misperceptions usually absent, delusions, no hallucinations	No delusions or hallucinations
Reversibility	Potential	No, progressive	Can be treated; can recur
Pathophysiology	Associated with infections, medications, electrolyte and metabolic disorders, major organ failure, brain insults, and acute alcohol withdrawal	Usually related to structural diseases of the brain	Associated with grief, a stressful life event, reaction to medical or neurologic diseases, or a change in lifestyle

Refer to Table 9.1 for the distinguishing characteristics of dementia.

The onset of symptoms is insidious, with the course stable through the day and night. The condition can be present for months or years, with progressive deterioration. Recent and remote memory is impaired. The patient is alert, and attention is relatively unaffected, although orientation is usually impaired. Hallucinations are usually absent until late in the course of the disease. Speech is usually unimpaired, although the person has difficulty finding words. Sleep is often fragmented. On mental status examination, the patient tries hard and provides "near-miss" answers. Physical findings are often absent. The olfactory sense can be impaired. Box 9.3 lists common presentations of dementia, Box 9.4 lists phases of Alzheimer-type dementia, and Box 9.5 describes a staging system for Alzheimer disease.

Alzheimer-type dementia can sometimes be distinguished from vascular or MID by

<table>
<tr><td>

Box 9.3   Common Presentations of Dementia

- Memory loss
- Depression
- Irritability
- Poor hygiene
- Insomnia
- Paranoia
- Weight loss
- Poor work performance
- Financial errors
- Poor judgment
- Delirium
- Language difficulty

- Social withdrawal
- Behavioral change
- Urinary incontinence
- Hallucinations (late)
- Anxiety
- Failure to thrive
- Falls, clumsiness
- Deteriorating interpersonal relationships
- Personality changes

</td></tr>
</table>

obtaining a cardiovascular history, determining the progression of symptoms, and detecting the presence or absence of focal neurologic signs and symptoms (Box 9.6).

Depression

Depression can produce confusion, especially in older adults. The onset of the confusion is often abrupt, with some diurnal variation. Generally, depression is more consistent over time than delirium. The confusion is of short duration compared with dementia. A past history of psychiatric problems, including undiagnosed depressive episodes, is common. During mental status examination, the patient tends to highlight disabilities, especially memory loss.

Box 9.4   Phases of Alzheimer-Type Dementia

Progression of symptoms corresponds with the progression of underlying nerve cell degeneration. Damage typically begins with cells involved in learning and memory and gradually spreads to cells that control thinking, judgment, and behavior. The damage eventually affects cells that control and coordinate movement.

LIMBIC
- 2–3 years after onset
- Olfactory system involved
- Memory loss
- Can perform tasks

PARIETAL
- 3–6 years after onset
- Loss of comprehension of spoken language

- Cannot name common objects
- Apraxia: cannot perform motor skills, although motor system intact
- Agnosia: failure to identify or recognize objects despite intact sensory function
- Misinterprets visual and auditory stimuli
- Delusions

LATE FRONTAL
- 6–8 years after onset
- Motor disturbances: walking, swallowing, moving
- Primitive reflexes
- Seizures
- Sensation remains intact

Box 9.5   Stages of Alzheimer Disease

Staging systems for Alzheimer disease vary. The Alzheimer Association uses seven stages to describe the progression of Alzheimer disease.

STAGE 1
No impairment (normal function)

STAGE 2
Very mild cognitive decline (may be age-related changes or earliest signs of Alzheimer disease)
- Memory lapses, especially in forgetting familiar words or names or the location of everyday objects

- Symptoms not evident during a medical examination or apparent to friends, family, or coworkers

STAGE 3
Mild cognitive decline
- Problems with memory or concentration; may be measurable in clinical testing or apparent during a detailed medical interview
- Friends, family, or coworkers begin to notice deficiencies.
- Common difficulties include:
  - Word- or name-finding problems noticeable to family or close associates

Continued

| Box 9.5 | Stages of Alzheimer Disease—cont'd |

- Decreased ability to remember names when introduced to new people
- Performance issues in social or work settings
- Reading a passage and retaining little material
- Losing or misplacing a valuable object
- Decline in ability to plan or organize

STAGE 4

Moderate cognitive decline (mild or early-stage Alzheimer disease)
- The affected individual may seem subdued and withdrawn, especially in socially or mentally challenging situations.
- Clear-cut deficiencies in the following areas:
  - Decreased knowledge of recent occasions or current events
  - Impaired ability to perform challenging mental arithmetic (e.g., counting backward from 100 in 7s)
  - Decreased capacity to perform complex tasks, such as marketing, planning dinner for guests, or paying bills and managing finances
  - Reduced memory of personal history

STAGE 5

Moderately severe cognitive decline (moderate or midstage Alzheimer disease)
- Major gaps in memory and deficits in cognitive function emerge. Some assistance with day-to-day activities becomes essential.
- Individuals may:
  - Be unable during a medical interview to recall such important details as their current address, their telephone number, or the name of the college or high school from which they graduated.
  - Become confused about where they are or about the date, day of the week, or season.
  - Have trouble with less challenging mental arithmetic (e.g., counting backward from 40 in 4s or from 20 in 2s).
  - Need help choosing proper clothing for the season or the occasion.
  - Usually retain substantial knowledge about themselves and know their own name and the names of their spouse or children.
  - Usually require no assistance with eating or using the toilet.

STAGE 6

Severe cognitive decline (moderately severe or midstage Alzheimer disease)
- Memory difficulties continue to worsen, significant personality changes may emerge, and affected individuals need extensive help with customary daily activities
- Individuals may:
  - Lose most awareness of recent experiences and events as well as of their surroundings.
  - Recollect their personal history imperfectly, although generally able to recall their own name.
  - Occasionally forget the name of their spouses or primary caregivers but generally can distinguish familiar from unfamiliar faces.
  - Need help getting dressed properly; without supervision, may make such errors as putting pajamas over daytime clothes or shoes on wrong feet.
  - Experience disruption of their normal sleep–wake cycle.
  - Need help with handling details of toileting (flushing toilet, wiping, and disposing of tissue properly).
  - Have increasing episodes of urinary or fecal incontinence.
  - Experience significant personality changes and behavioral symptoms, including suspiciousness and delusions; hallucinations; or compulsive, repetitive behaviors.
  - Tend to wander and become lost.

STAGE 7

Very severe cognitive decline (severe or late-stage Alzheimer disease)
- This is the final stage of the disease when individuals lose the ability to respond to their environment, the ability to speak, and, ultimately, the ability to control movement.
  - Lose capacity for recognizable speech, although words or phrases may occasionally be uttered.
  - Need help with eating and toileting and there is general incontinence of urine.
  - Lose the ability to walk without assistance and then the ability to sit without support, the ability to smile, and the ability to hold their head up.
  - Reflexes become abnormal and muscles grow rigid; swallowing is impaired.

From Reisberg B, Ferris SH, de Leon MJ, Crook T: The global deterioration scale for assessment of primary degenerative dementia, *Am J Psychiatry* 139:1136, 1982. Copyright 1983 by Barry Reisberg, MD. Reproduced with permission.

Box 9.6 Multi-Infarct versus Alzheimer-Type Dementia

FACTORS SUGGESTING DEMENTIA	HACHINSKI ISCHEMIA POINT SCORE[a]	FACTORS SUGGESTING DEMENTIA	HACHINSKI ISCHEMIA POINT SCORE[a]
Abrupt onset	2	History of hypertension	1
Stepwise deterioration	1	History of strokes	2
Fluctuating course	2	Evidence of associated arteriosclerosis	1
Emotional lability	1		
Relative preservation of personality	1	Focal neurologic symptoms[b]	2
Depression	1	Focal neurologic signs[b]	2
Somatic complaints	1		

[a]A score of 4 or more is indicative of Alzheimer-type dementia. A score of 7 or more is indicative of multi-infarct dementia.
[b]Focal neurologic signs or symptoms: exaggerated deep tendon reflexes, positive Babinski sign, gait abnormalities, hemiparesis.

The memory loss is equal for recent and remote events. The cognitive losses, however, are fluctuating rather than stable over time. The patient manifests a depressed or anxious mood, including sleep and appetite disturbance. Hallucinations are usually absent, although the patient may have suicidal thoughts. Depression as a cause of confusion can be easy to miss because it is often associated with anger, anxiety, and unclear thinking as well as denial (see Chapter 4). Refer to Table 9.1 for the distinguishing characteristics of depression.

▶ DIFFERENTIAL DIAGNOSIS OF *Common Causes of Delirium, Confusion, Dementia, and Depression*

CONDITION	HISTORY	PHYSICAL FINDINGS	DIAGNOSTIC STUDIES
Delirium	Onset abrupt; fluctuations over course of day common with lucid intervals during day and worst symptoms at night; lasts hours to weeks; unable to maintain attention to external stimuli; disorganized thinking, perceptual disturbances, disturbed sleep–wake cycle; hallucinations, usually visual, common	Decreased LOC, impaired arousal, decreased psychomotor activity; disoriented, most commonly to time; physical examination findings depend on underlying cause of delirium; patient often exhibits asterixis, tremor, and difficulty in motor relaxation; speech incoherent, hesitant, slow, or rapid	CBC, electrolytes, glucose, BUN, creatinine, LFTs, TFTs, serum B$_{12}$, folate, serology for syphilis, ABGs, toxicology screen, blood alcohol level, U/A, ECG, EEG, chest radiograph, lumbar puncture, CT or MRI (when CVA or injury suspected)
Confusion	Less abrupt, less severe than delirium; diurnal variation less severe than delirium; concentration impaired, easily distracted; errors in thinking common	Apathetic, drowsy; disoriented especially for time, but less for place, almost never for self; less severe disorientation, more subtle motor signs than in delirium	CBC, electrolytes, glucose, BUN, creatinine, LFTs, TFTs, serum B$_{12}$, folate, serology for syphilis, ABGs, toxicology screen, blood alcohol level, U/A, ECG, EEG, chest radiograph, lumbar puncture, CT or MRI (when CVA or injury is suspected)

Continued

> **DIFFERENTIAL DIAGNOSIS OF** *Common Causes of Delirium, Confusion, Dementia, and Depression—cont'd*

CONDITION	HISTORY	PHYSICAL FINDINGS	DIAGNOSTIC STUDIES
Dementia	Onset insidious, course stable through day and night; present for months or years, with progressive deterioration; recent and remote memory impaired; hallucinations usually absent until late in course of disease; sleep often fragmented	Alert, attentive; orientation usually impaired; on mental status examination, patient tries hard, provides "near-miss" answers; demonstrates one or more of following cognitive disturbances: aphasia (language disturbance); apraxia (impaired ability to carry out motor activities despite intact motor function); agnosia (failure to identify or recognize objects despite intact sensory function); disturbance in executive functioning (planning, organizing, sequencing, abstracting); physical findings often absent in Alzheimer type; olfactory sense can be impaired; speech usually unimpaired, although difficulty with finding words; findings in MID include focal neurologic signs or symptoms: exaggerated DTRs, positive Babinski sign, gait abnormalities, hemiparesis	Cognitive testing CBC, electrolytes, glucose, BUN, creatinine, LFTs, TFTs, serum B$_{12}$, folate, serology for syphilis, ABGs, toxicology screen, blood alcohol level, U/A, ECG, EEG, chest radiograph, lumbar puncture, to test CSF for Alzheimer disease biomarkers and tauopathies; CT or MRI (when CVA or injury suspected; does not yield useful information for dementia); PET scan
Depression	Onset of confusion often abrupt, with some diurnal variation, generally more consistent over time than delirium; confusion of short duration compared to dementia; past history of psychiatric problems common, including undiagnosed depressive episodes; cognitive losses fluctuating rather than stable over time; sleep/appetite disturbance; hallucinations usually absent although person can have suicidal thoughts	Depressed or anxious mood; tends to highlight disabilities, especially memory loss; memory loss equal for recent and remote events; physical examination often normal	Geriatric Depression Scale; PHQ-9; CBC, electrolytes, glucose, BUN, creatinine, LFTs, TFTs, serum B$_{12}$, folate, serology for syphilis, ABGs, toxicology screen, blood alcohol level, U/A, ECG, EEG, chest radiograph, lumbar puncture, CT or MRI (when CVA or injury suspected)

ABGs, arterial blood gases; *BUN,* blood urea nitrogen; *CBC,* complete blood count; *CT,* computed tomography; *CVA,* costovertebral angle; *DTRs,* deep tendon reflexes; *ECG,* electrocardiography; *EEG,* electroencephalography; *LFTs,* liver function tests; *LOC,* level of consciousness; *MID,* multi-infarct dementia; *MRI,* magnetic resonance imaging; *PET,* positron emission tomography; *TFTs,* thyroid function tests; *U/A,* urinalysis.

Constipation is a common symptom and is a subjective interpretation of a disturbance of bowel function. There is lack of general agreement on the norms for stool frequency, size, or consistency, with considerable uncertainty on how much deviation is required to warrant the label of constipation. Generally, constipation refers to a failure to completely evacuate the lower colon. This is associated with difficulty in defecating, infrequent bowel movements, straining, abdominal pain, and pain on defecating. It can also refer to hardness of stool or a feeling of incomplete evacuation. Obstipation refers to intractable constipation or the regular passage of hard stools at 3- to 5-day intervals.

There are five areas in the defecation process when interference can cause a disturbance in motility and lead to clinical problems: (1) the peristaltic reflex, (2) the spinal arc, (3) relaxation of the anal sphincter, (4) contraction of the voluntary muscle associated with defecation, and (5) the autonomic and cortical control of defecation. Both functional and organic disturbances can cause constipation.

Acute constipation refers to a sudden change for that individual. This suggests an organic cause, such as mechanical obstruction, adynamic ileus, or traumatic interruption of the nervous system from medications or following anesthesia. *Persistent constipation* occurs when the condition lasts for weeks or occurs intermittently with increasing frequency or severity. Partial obstruction or local anorectal conditions could be the cause.

Chronic constipation occurs as the result of disruption of the storage, transport, and evacuation mechanisms of the colon. Functional causes are the most common and include poor bowel habits; inadequate intake of dietary fiber, bulk, and fluids; and anal fissure

pain. Genetic predisposition to constipation seems to exist.

DIAGNOSTIC REASONING: FOCUSED HISTORY

Is this really constipation?

Key Questions
- How many stools do you have per day?
- What is the consistency of the stool?

Frequency of Stool

Stool frequency is the easiest parameter to quantify. In the general adult population, the "normal" frequency of bowel movements ranges from 3 to 12 per week. Having fewer than three bowel movements per week is considered constipation.

Infants and children have decreasing stool frequency with age, from more than 4 stools per day during the first week of life to 1.2 per day at age 4 years. Infants who have a lower number of stools than average are at greater risk of developing constipation.

Alternating episodes of constipation and diarrhea are characteristic of irritable bowel syndrome (IBS). Patients describe their constipation stools as hard, round balls.

Stool Consistency

Dry, hard stools suggest a lack of sufficient dietary fluids or fiber. Stools that are marginally frequent but are soft and moist do not indicate constipation. The same number of stools that are hard and dry would indicate constipation. Liquid stool and fecal incontinence, particularly in children and older adults, can represent stool impaction and overflow.

The Bristol Stool Form Scale is useful in characterizing stool consistency (Fig. 10.1)

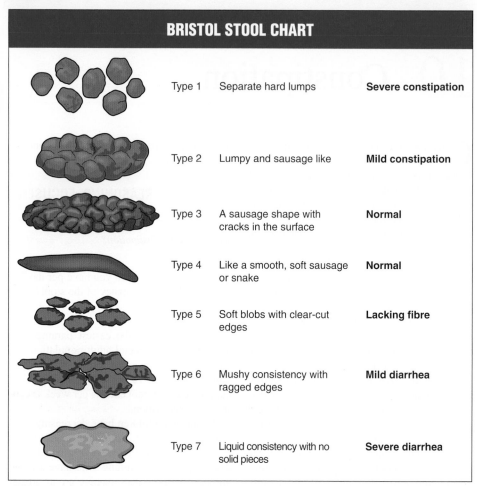

FIGURE 10.1 Bristol Stool Form Scale. By Cabot Health, Bristol Stool Chart (http://cdn.intechopen.com/pdfs-wm/46082.pdf) [CC BY-SA 3.0 (https://creativecommons.org/licenses/by-sa/3.0)], via Wikimedia Commons)

What red flags do I need to consider?

Key Questions

- Is there any rectal bleeding or blood in the stool?
- Have you had an unintentional weight loss of more than 5% of your body weight?
- Have you had inflammatory bowel disease?
- Have you or your family members had colorectal cancer?

Bleeding

Black stools can indicate bleeding from a site in the upper gastrointestinal (GI) tract. Bright red blood indicates bleeding from the lower GI tract and may indicate a mass. Hemorrhoids and anal or rectal fissures can also produce bleeding. Brisk bleeding is uncommon with hemorrhoids and requires immediate investigation.

Unintentional Weight Loss

In an adult, an unintended weight loss of more than 5% of usual body weight over a 6- to 12-month period may signal an underlying cancer (see Chapter 39) or development of frailty syndrome in an older adult.

History of Inflammatory Bowel Disease or Colorectal Cancer

Patients with a history of inflammatory bowel disease (IBD; Crohn disease or ulcerative colitis) or with a personal or family history of colorectal cancer are at increased risk for colorectal cancer. A change in bowel habits can signal an intestinal tumor.

Is the constipation acute or chronic?

Key Questions

- When did the constipation start?
- How long have you been constipated?
- Is this an individual episode or is it chronic?
- At what age did the constipation first begin?

Onset and Duration

Recent onset usually reflects changes in lifestyle or physical health such as dietary changes, activity changes, new medications, partially obstructing lesions, or recent illness. Chronic constipation or constipation of long duration (more than 3 weeks) is usually associated either with functional causes, such as lack of dietary fiber and bulk, or with concurrent systemic disorders such as diabetes or hypothyroidism.

Age of Onset

New-onset constipation in adults older than age 40 years is suspicious for colon lesions. Constipation in the newborn is likely to have an anatomical cause. In infants, the cause is likely inadequate fluid and fiber in the diet. In children, the cause is likely to be diet as well as developmental and psychological factors. In adults, the cause is usually related to dietary and bowel habits.

If the constipation is acute, what conditions should I consider?

Key Questions

- Have you been ill recently?
- Have you had a fever?
- Do you have any chronic health problems?

Recent Illness

Dehydration and fever cause hardening of the stools by diminishing intestinal secretions and increasing water absorption from the colon. A transient period of constipation is common during an acute febrile illness. Reflex ileus is sometimes seen with pneumonia.

Chronic Illness

Hardened stools are found in patients with renal acidosis and diabetes insipidus. Infants and children with hypotonia of the abdominal and intestinal musculature from neurologic conditions are predisposed to constipation.

Neurologic gut dysfunction, myopathies, endocrine disorders, and electrolyte abnormalities can cause constipation. Constipation in infants can be an early symptom of congenital hypothyroidism.

If the constipation is chronic or recurrent, what should I consider?

Key Questions

- What do you usually eat in a day?
- How many glasses of liquid do you drink each day?
- Do you eat breakfast?
- What are your usual bowel habits?
- How active are you?
- What medications are you taking?
- Do you use laxatives? How often do you take laxatives? How long have you used laxatives?

Dietary Pattern

A 3-day dietary history is more accurate than a 24-hour recall, although a 24-hour recall can provide a reasonable picture of the patient's dietary habits. Diets that lack roughage result in lack of fecal bulk, causing an inadequate stimulus for peristaltic movement. Diets high in protein result in complete digestion of the protein, leaving little residue to stimulate movement. Diets high in calcium content lead to the formation of calcium caseinate in the stools, which does not stimulate peristalsis. Teenagers often drink several quarts of milk per day, causing constipation. Inadequate fluid intake (less than six 8-oz glasses per day) contributes to dry, hard, and infrequent stools.

Breakfast

Colonic motility is greatest after breakfast. Skipping this meal decreases the postprandial effect associated with food intake.

Bowel Habits

Postponing a bowel movement because of time constraints or other reasons suppresses the normal gastrocolic reflex and can produce constipation.

Activity Level

Constipation is a common problem in individuals with a sedentary lifestyle. The lack of physical activity reduces the peristaltic reflex. Overactivity can also cause constipation as a result of the lack of adequate fluid replacement.

Medications

Medications that commonly cause or contribute to constipation include narcotics, imipramine, diuretics, calcium channel blockers, anticholinergics, psychotropic agents, antacids, decongestants, anticonvulsants, iron, bismuth, and lead. Opioid-induced constipation (OIC) occurs in almost half the patients on long-term opioids.

Use of Enemas, Laxatives, and Suppositories

Use of stimulants to empty the colon removes the peristalsis stimulus for 2 to 3 days. Diarrhea is usually followed by infrequent stools for several days. Chronic use of stimulants can produce chronic atonic constipation.

How can I further narrow the causes?

Key Questions
- Is the stool size large or small?
- What is the general shape of the stool (e.g., small, round, ribbon-like)?
- Is the stool formed or liquid?
- Have you had any involuntary loss of stool?
- Does the constipation alternate with periods of diarrhea?

Size or Caliber of Stool

Infrequent passage of small, hard stools can indicate congenital aganglionic megacolon. Very large stools can indicate functional constipation, with the size of the stools a function of the size of the colon. Ribbon-like stools suggest a motility disorder, such as IBS. They can also be caused by narrowing of the distal or sigmoid colon from an organic lesion. A progressive decrease in the caliber of stool suggests an organic lesion. Stools with a toothpaste-like caliber suggest fecal impaction.

Consistency of Stool and Fecal Incontinence

Dry, hard stools suggest a lack of sufficient dietary fluids or fiber. Liquid stool and fecal incontinence, particularly in older adults, can represent stool impaction and overflow. Overflow incontinence in children can indicate constipation from a fecal impaction.

Alternating Constipation and Diarrhea

Alternating episodes are characteristic of IBS. Patients often describe the stool during the constipation episodes as hard and pellet-like.

What else do I need to consider?

Key Questions
- Do you have the urge to defecate?
- Do you have any urinary tract symptoms?
- Do you have any nausea or vomiting?
- Is there any pain with defecation?
- Is there any bleeding with defecation? How much?
- What color are your stools? Are the stools very dark colored or black?

Urge to Defecate

Children with Hirschsprung disease (aganglionic megacolon) do not have an urge to defecate because the stool accumulates proximal to the lower portion of the rectum where the proprioceptors for defecation are located. Evidence of stiffening, squeezing, and crying indicates stool is being propelled to the rectum. Adults who overuse laxatives or other stimulants also may not experience the urge to defecate.

Associated Urinary Tract Problems

Voiding problems can indicate an abdominal mass. Day and night enuresis is seen in some children with encopresis (fecal soiling). Typically, a neurologic lesion that produces fecal incontinence also disturbs bladder control.

Vomiting

Bilious vomiting can indicate intestinal obstruction in the newborn. Vomiting associated with pain in adults can indicate obstruction.

Pain

Chronic recurrent abdominal pain is commonly present in constipation. Pain is intermittent and can be localized to the periumbilical region. Crampy lower abdominal pain is usually caused by bowel distention, which can result from IBS, intermittent obstruction, or adhesions. Noncrampy dull pain in the left abdomen is associated with diverticulosis. Pain on defecation can indicate an anal or a rectal lesion such as hemorrhoids or anal fissures.

Bleeding

Bright red blood in the stool indicates hemorrhoid, fissure, or possible rectal mass. Black stools can indicate bleeding from a site in the upper GI tract because blood mixed with gastric acid makes the stools appear black. Brisk bleeding is uncommon with hemorrhoids and requires immediate thorough investigation.

Color

Red stools can be the result of using laxatives of vegetable origin or ingestion of foods such as red beets. A black or very dark brown color can be caused by drugs such as iron and bismuth, both of which contribute to constipation.

> *If this is a child, is there anything else I need to consider?*

Key Questions
- Is there crying with defecation?
- Is there fecal soiling of underpants?
- If an infant: Is there a history of delayed passage of meconium stool?
- Has the child begun to drink milk?
- Has the child recently started toilet training?
- Does the child have urinary frequency?

Crying with Defecation

Small children with constipation will cry with movement when a fissure is present. With large hard stools, the child will not want to defecate because of the pain and will do stool-holding mannerisms such as sitting and standing still.

Fecal Soiling of Underpants

Repeated fecal soiling, from involuntary passage of small amounts of feces into the underpants of children older than age 4 years, is consistent with encopresis. This is generally caused by functional megacolon secondary to chronic constipation. This constipation is usually secondary to painful defecation, with a resultant anal fissure. Coercive bowel training, fear of the toilet, or reactive voluntary withholding of bowel movements can also cause this condition.

History of Delayed Passage of Meconium Stool

Such a history can indicate congenital aganglionic megacolon (Hirschsprung disease).

Change in Diet

Cow's milk is a common cause of constipation in young children who have been on breast milk or formula.

Toilet Training

Some children develop stool withholding when toilet training is initiated.

History of Urinary Frequency

Urinary frequency, enuresis, incontinence (especially in frail older adults), and urinary tract infections (UTIs) can be the result of constipation. Fecal soiling can cause UTI by the introduction of the fecal flora. Furthermore, an enlarged dilated rectum can push on the bladder, causing a frequent need to urinate.

> *Is there a family history or genetic predisposition?*

Key Questions
- Is there a family history of constipation or IBS?

Genetic predisposition to constipation seems to exist. It is common for more than one family member to have a history of chronic constipation or IBS.

DIAGNOSTIC REASONING: FOCUSED PHYSICAL EXAMINATION

Plot Growth Curve in Children

Slow growth can indicate congenital aganglionic megacolon. Incorrect formula mixing, underfeeding, starvation, and anorexia nervosa can first be recognized by a report of constipation.

Perform an Abdominal Examination

Observe abdominal contour, looking for distention. Abdominal distention is frequently not marked in patients with functional constipation but can be present with other causes. Auscultate for bowel sounds. Silent or abnormal bowel sounds can indicate an organic cause such as obstruction. On palpation, stool can be felt as mobile, nontender masses in the left lower quadrant (LLQ). Firm, rubbery masses of stool palpable in the right lower quadrant (RLQ) in newborns can indicate meconium ileus. Palpable abdominal masses or organomegaly points to an organic cause. Note tenderness, which can indicate an organic cause, although a tender bowel can be palpable in IBS. Inspect the sacral region of the back. The presence of dimpling could indicate a spinal deformity contributing to the constipation.

Look for hernias. Large abdominal wall hernias can interfere with the ability to generate the intra-abdominal pressure that is required to initiate defecation.

Perform Digital Rectal Examination

On perianal inspection, look for skin excoriation, skin tags, fissures, strictures, tears, or hemorrhoids, any of which can cause painful defecation. Early fissures have the appearance of superficial erosions. More advanced lesions are linear or elliptical breaks in the skin. Long-standing fissures are deep and indurated. Internal fissures are seen when the anal sphincter relaxes as the examining finger is withdrawn. To examine for a fissure in a child, place the infant or child in the knee–chest position and spread the buttocks to reveal the mucocutaneous junction of the anus.

Table 10.1	**Superficial and Deep Tendon Reflexes and Spinal Level Tested**
REFLEX	**SPINAL LEVEL TESTED**
SUPERFICIAL	
Upper abdominal	T7, T8, T9
Lower abdominal	T10, T11
Cremasteric	T12, L1, L2
DEEP	
Biceps	C5, C6
Brachioradial	C5, C6
Triceps	C6, C7, C8
Patellar	L2, L3, L4
Achilles	S1, S2

Look for rectal prolapse and feel for a rectocele, which might interfere with defecation. A normal anal sphincter with an empty rectal ampulla can indicate Hirschsprung disease. In functional constipation, expect to find a large dilated rectum full of stool. Assess sphincter tone, both at resting and with a squeezing effort. Sphincter tone is increased in functional problems and strictures but is decreased in neurologic diseases. The presence of a mass in the rectum indicates an impaction or obstructive lesion. A pilonidal dimple is seen with spinal bifida occulta.

Perform a Focused Neurologic Examination

Test relevant deep tendon and superficial reflexes. Interruption of the T12 to S3 nerves causes loss of voluntary control of defecation (Table 10.1).

LABORATORY AND DIAGNOSTIC STUDIES

Fecal Occult Blood Test

A positive guaiac-based fecal occult blood test (gFOBT) indicates blood in the stool, which can be the result of ulcerative or malignant lesions. The sensitivity of this test in detecting colorectal cancers and adenomas ranges from 50% to 90%. It is an inexpensive and noninvasive method to screen for bleeding lesions. Three days of serial testing can be

The American Cancer Society, US Multi-Society Task Force on Colorectal Cancer, and the American College of Radiology jointly developed consensus guidelines for colorectal cancer screening in asymptomatic adults 50 years of age and older who are at average risk. The screening tests were grouped into those that primarily detect cancer and those that can detect both cancer and adenomatous polyps, which provides the opportunity for cancer prevention through polypectomy. The panel supports screening primarily for cancer prevention. Specific recommendations may be found at http://www.cancer.org/cancer/colonandrectumcancer/moreinformation/colonandrectumcancerearlydetection/colorectal-cancer-early-detection-acs-recommendations.

The US. Preventive Services Task Force (USPSTF) concludes that there is convincing evidence that colorectal cancer screening substantially reduces deaths from colorectal cancer and does not emphasize specific screening tests.

References: Levin et al, 2008; USPSTF, 2016.

done using stool cards at home, that are returned by mail for analysis. Annual gFOBT, beginning at age 50 years, is one of the recommended screening tests for colon cancer. The Evidence-Based Practice box describes the current recommendations.

Fecal Immunochemical Test

Fecal immunochemical test (FIT), also called immunochemical FOBT (iFOBT), can be used as an alternative to FOBT. FIT uses antibodies to human globin to detect a specific portion of a human blood protein and does not react with nonhuman hemoglobin or peroxidase, so food restrictions before the test are not necessary. Immunochemical FOBTs are also more specific for lower GI tract bleeding because they target the globin portion of hemoglobin, which does not survive passage through the upper GI tract. This test is done essentially the same way as conventional FOBT but is more specific and reduces the number of false-positive results. Vitamins or foods do not affect the FIT and some forms require only one or two stool specimens.

Fecal or Stool DNA

Cells from precancerous polyps and cancerous tumors are shed in the stool and contain recognizable DNA markers. A stool DNA test can identify several of these markers, indicating the presence of precancerous polyps or colon cancer.

Complete Blood Count

Obtain a complete blood count when you suspect bleeding. Hematocrit and hemoglobin levels will be below the expected reference range with a bleeding lesion.

Serum Electrolytes

Severely ill patients can develop hypokalemia and hypercalcemia, which are causes of constipation. Patients on thiazide diuretics can develop hypokalemia and subsequent constipation.

Serum Thyroid-Stimulating Hormone

An elevated thyroid-stimulating hormone (TSH) level may be suggestive of hypothyroidism, which can be a cause of constipation. Screen for elevated TSH levels in people with other symptoms suggestive of hypothyroidism such as sparse, coarse, dry hair; hirsutism; dry skin; or hoarse speech.

Urinalysis

A urinalysis and culture should be done if a child has an associated rectosigmoid impaction because of encopresis.

Anoscopy

Anoscopy is indicated if digital rectal examination detects hemorrhoids, fissures, strictures, or masses in the anus or rectum. It enables a view of the immediate internal anal canal that is not possible on manual digital rectal examination. A handheld anoscope is warmed, lubricated, and slowly eased into the anus while the patient bears down to relax the external sphincter muscle. A light source is necessary; a head lamp is preferable. Anoscopy may not be possible initially with a fissure or abscess because of the pain. However, it should be performed on a follow-up visit to detect IBD or rectal cancer.

Flexible Sigmoidoscopy and Colonoscopy

These tests are indicated for patients in whom conservative treatment fails, for people older than age 50 years or with new-onset constipation, and for those with anemia or fecal occult blood. Colonoscopy is indicated for the patient with rectal bleeding.

Barium Enema

This contrast technique can be used to detect diverticula, polyps, and masses. It is also used to determine the extent of dilated bowel in megacolon. The barium enema in children is reserved to rule out Hirschsprung disease. A barium enema is contraindicated if enterocolitis is suspected.

Colon Transit Studies

Colon transit studies are useful for patients with severe chronic constipation that responds poorly to treatment.

Anorectal Manometry

This test measures the pressure of the anal sphincter muscles, the sensation in the rectum, and the neural reflexes that are needed for normal bowel movements. The manometry probe, a thin tube of soft plastic or rigid metal, is inserted into the rectum about 4 inches and then slowly withdrawn halfway. As the probe is withdrawn, the transducer continuously records the pressure at different points. Alternatively, the pressure can be measured with a balloon manometry system, a hollow metal cylinder to which three balloons are attached to measure pressure during anal contraction. A balloon at the tip of the probe is inflated to determine whether the patient feels a sensation of rectal fullness and an urge to defecate.

DIFFERENTIAL DIAGNOSIS

Despite the high prevalence of constipation, only a small number of adults or children with constipation have a significant abnormality. In otherwise healthy individuals, first consider functional causes, particularly dietary, fluid, bowel, and laxative habits. In adults, depression can be associated with constipation.

Simple Constipation

Typically, individuals with simple constipation report a diet low in fiber and bulk or inadequate fluid intake. A sedentary lifestyle is common. They also often report pain before and with bowel movements because of the hard, dry nature of the stools. Patients can also report loss of appetite. The results of the physical examination of the abdomen and rectum are normal. It may be possible to feel fecal masses in the colon and rectum. No diagnostic workup is needed unless the patient does not respond to therapy.

Functional Constipation

Functional causes of constipation include poor bowel habits; inadequate intake of dietary fiber, bulk, and fluids; and chronic use of laxatives. Patients may report straining during defecation, hard or lumpy stools, and sensations of incomplete evacuation or anorectal obstruction. The abdomen may or may not be distended. The external sphincter is intact.

Functional constipation is seen in children who have large, hard stools that become difficult or painful to pass. The resulting fecal retention sets up a cycle in which the sensitivity of the defecation reflex and the effectiveness of peristalsis lessen. Watery stool from the proximal colon soils the underwear. On physical examination, stool is present in the LLQ, and the rectum is dilated and filled with packed stool. The external sphincter is intact.

Irritable Bowel Syndrome

Irritable bowel syndrome is common in adults, with onset usually in young adulthood. The presenting symptoms can be either predominantly diarrhea (IBS-D), constipation (IBS-C), or mixed (IBS-M), using the Bristol Stool Form to classify abnormal stool consistency—IBS-C is defined as having hard stools more than 25% of the time and loose stools less than 25% of the time. IBS-M is defined as having both hard and soft stools more than 25% of the time. Abdominal pain related to defecation often occurs, usually in the LLQ, and the bowel may be tender to palpation (see Chapter 12).

Fecal Impaction

Fecal impaction is common in older adults and in those who are confined to bed. The passage of hard stools at 3- to 5-day intervals can occur. Some people with impaction have continuous diarrhea-like passage of stools and can experience incontinence. Stools can be of small caliber, sometimes described as tooth-paste-like. On rectal examination, large quantities of hard feces are palpable in the rectal ampulla. On abdominal examination, feces-filled bowel may be palpable.

Idiopathic Slow Transit

This condition is most common in older people, especially those who are less active and have inadequate dietary fiber and fluid intake. These patients experience decreased stool frequency; stools are typically dry and hard.

Hirschsprung Disease (Congenital Aganglionic Megacolon)

Hirschsprung disease is present from birth and is usually detected in young children. Delayed passage of meconium stool can indicate Hirschsprung disease in infants. Children with Hirschsprung disease do not have an urge to defecate because the stools accumulate proximal to the lower portion of the rectum where the proprioceptors for defecation are located. Evidence of stiffening, squeezing, and crying indicates stool is being propelled to the rectum. On examination, the rectal ampulla is empty.

Secondary Constipation from Anorectal Lesion

Because defecation is painful with an ano-rectal lesion, the patient suppresses it. With the eventual passage of hard stools, the patient can report blood on the surface of the stool, on the toilet paper, or in the toilet. On digital rectal examination, look for hemorrhoids (rare in children), fissures, tears, or abrasions.

Drug-Induced Constipation

Drug-induced constipation is consistent with a history of chronic laxative use or taking medications that can produce constipation. It occurs most often in older adults. Abdominal and rectal examinations are usually normal. OIC is defined as a change from baseline bowel habits upon initiation of opioids that is characterized by any of the following symptoms: reduced bowel movement frequency, development or worsening of straining to pass stool, a sense of incomplete rectal evacuation, and harder stool consistency.

Tumors

Tumors are uncommon in children, but the frequency increases in the population over the age of 40 years. Colicky abdominal pain and distention can occur in people with bowel tumors. People with rectosigmoid tumors may report rectal discomfort, stool leakage, urgency, and tenesmus. The patient may report rectal bleeding or blood in the stool. Stool may test positive for occult blood. An abdominal mass may be palpable. Older adult patients who present with constipation, anemia, anorexia, and weight loss are at high suspicion for colorectal cancer. Constipation occurs in less than one-third of people with colon cancer; diarrhea is more common. The onset is recent, and there can be progressive narrowing of stool caliber.

▶ DIFFERENTIAL DIAGNOSIS OF *Common Causes of Constipation*

CONDITION	HISTORY	PHYSICAL FINDINGS	DIAGNOSTIC STUDIES
Simple constipation	Low dietary fiber and bulk; inadequate fluid intake; physical inactivity; pain before and with bowel movements; anorexia	Normal abdominal and rectal examination; can feel fecal masses in colon and rectum	None if resolved; consider colonoscopy or sigmoidoscopy, anorectal manometry, colon transit studies if not resolved

Continued

▶ DIFFERENTIAL DIAGNOSIS OF *Common Causes of Constipation—cont'd*

CONDITION	HISTORY	PHYSICAL FINDINGS	DIAGNOSTIC STUDIES
Functional constipation	Adults: bowel habits; chronic use of laxatives; straining during defecation, hard or lumpy stools, a sensation of incomplete evacuation or anorectal obstruction Preschool and school-age children: history of abdominal pain and stool soiling	Abdomen may or may not be distended. The external sphincter is intact. Palpable stool in LLQ; large dilated rectum with packed stool; external sphincter intact	Abdominal radiography, unprepped barium radiography
Irritable bowel syndrome (IBS)	Onset in young adulthood IBS-C: hard stools >25% of the time and loose stools <25% of the time IBS-M: both hard and soft stools >25% of the time	Can have tender, palpable colon	Colonoscopy or sigmoidoscopy if indicated
Obstipation or impaction	Passage of hard stool at 3- to 5-day intervals; diarrhea, small caliber stools; common in those confined to bed	Hard feces in rectal ampulla; may have palpable feces-filled bowel	Colonoscopy or sigmoidoscopy if indicated
Slow transit	Common in older adults; physical inactivity; decreased stool frequency; stool dry and hard	Normal abdominal and rectal examination	Colonoscopy, FOBT, or FIT to rule out tumors; consider anorectal manometry, colon transit studies
Hirschsprung disease	Delayed passage of meconium at birth; no urge to defecate	Empty rectal ampulla on examination	Colonoscopy
Anocectal lesions	Rectal pain on defecation; history of hemorrhoids; blood on stool, on toilet tissue, or in toilet	On rectal examination: hemorrhoids, fissures, tears, abrasions; increased sphincter tone	Anoscopy
Drug-induced constipation	History of chronic laxative use; history of taking medications that produce constipation	Normal rectal and abdominal examinations	None if resolved; consider colonoscopy or sigmoidoscopy, barium enema if not resolved
Colorectal cancer	Recent onset: pain and abdominal distention, stool leakage, urgency; late onset: weight loss, anorexia; rectal bleeding; increased incidence after age 40 yr; uncommon in children	Can have palpable abdominal mass or organomegaly	CBC, FOBT, FIT, fecal or stool DNA; colonoscopy

CBC, Complete blood count; *FIT,* fecal immunochemical test; *FOBT,* fecal occult blood test; *LLQ,* left lower quadrant.

11 Cough

Cough is one of the most common symptoms for which patients seek health care. Cough occurs when inspiration is followed by an explosive expiration, promoting clearance of secretions and foreign bodies from the airways. It is usually the result of a reflex initiated by stimulation of the sensory nerve endings beneath and between the epithelium of the larynx and tracheobronchial tree. There are three mechanisms that trigger cough: (1) rapidly adapting receptors activated by punctate mechanical stimuli, airway smooth muscle contraction, and gastric acid; (2) C-fibers that respond to various chemicals; and (3) cough receptors that are stimulated by mechanical stimuli such as postnasal drip.

The reflex stimulation follows the vagus nerve to the "cough center," which is located in the medulla oblongata of the brainstem. However, other anatomical locations can be stimulated and initiate the cough reflex, including the pleura, pericardium, ear canals, esophagus, and stomach. The cough reflex is absent in very young infants. Effective coughing may also be impossible in emaciated individuals, in patients whose respiratory musculature is weak or paralyzed, and in those with massive ascites.

Although most coughs are a symptom of minor upper respiratory infections (URIs), such as the common cold, a persistent cough can greatly affect a patient's quality of life and ability to sleep. Keep in mind, however, that a cough in a patient in acute distress can signal a life-threatening problem such as foreign body aspiration with occlusion of airway, severe asthma, escalating heart failure, or pneumonia.

DIAGNOSTIC REASONING: FOCUSED HISTORY

What type of cough is this?

Key Questions
- How long have you had a cough?

Duration

Cough can be characterized by the following three categories of duration: (1) acute, less than 3 weeks; (2) subacute, lasting 3 to 8 weeks; and (3) chronic, lasting more than 8 weeks. A cough of recent onset is most often the result of viral or bacterial infection in the respiratory system. Allergies can also precipitate acute onset of cough in both children and adults. Cough lasting a longer duration (>3 weeks) is more likely caused by chronic lung or heart disease such as chronic obstructive pulmonary disease (COPD), cystic fibrosis (CF), chronic bronchitis, asthma, heart failure, or an infectious process such as pertussis and chronic sinusitis. Gastroesophageal reflux disease (GERD) and a foreign body in the ear canal should also be considered as a possible cause of cough in both adults and children.

EVIDENCE-BASED PRACTICE *How Long Does a Cough Last Before a Patient Seeks Care?*

There is a mismatch between patient expectations and reality for the natural history of acute cough illness (ACI). Patient expectations are that ACI lasts 6 to 7 days, and they often seek care for antibiotics at 5 to 6 days. If they are prescribed antibiotics and begin to feel better 3 to 4 days later, the belief that antibiotics helped is reinforced. Yet in reality, the natural history of acute cough would resolve without antibiotic treatment within 10 days. This mismatch suggests that clinicians need to educate patients about the natural history of ACI to reduce the demand for inappropriate antibiotic use.

Reference: Ebell et al, 2011.

Key Questions

- Are you short of breath?
- Do you have a history of heart failure?
- Do you have a history of asthma?
- If a child: Have you noticed the child putting small objects in his or her mouth?

Shortness of Breath

Cough associated with shortness of breath (SOB) usually suggests a physical obstruction of the airway caused by a foreign body or the effects of acute asthma. Patients with heart failure report orthopnea, paroxysmal nocturnal dyspnea (PND), cough with possible frothy sputum, weight gain with swollen feet and ankles, and often a history of heart disease. Cardiac failure of any kind results in decreased lung compliance and cough.

History of Asthma

Acute exacerbation of asthma is characterized by an irritating nonproductive cough that can progress to tachypnea, dyspnea, wheezing, grunting, cyanosis, fatigue, and finally respiratory and cardiac failure. Other than viral infection, especially respiratory syncytial virus (RSV), common triggers are cigarette smoke, allergens, exercise, and cold air.

Foreign Body

Consider a foreign body aspiration (FBA) in a child. A child who has aspirated a foreign body can have a varied presentation; generally, the onset of cough is sudden and unexpected. The presentation of FBA depends on whether the event was witnessed, the age of the child, the type of object aspirated (size and composition), the elapsed time since the event, the degree of airway blockage, and the location of the object. A common presentation of lower airway FBA is a period of severe coughing, gagging, and choking followed by a quiet period with no coughing. This can last for hours, days, or even months. An FBA in the lower airway can produce air trapping and hyperinflation of the lung. A mobile FBA in the lower airway can also produce a paroxysmal cough, with cyanotic episodes and stridor

as a result of proximal migration and subglottic impaction.

An FBA in the esophagus can also produce airway obstruction, cough, and dysphagia to solid foods because the posterior trachea is compliant and adjacent to the anterior esophagus. Coins are the most frequently found foreign bodies.

Key Questions

- Do you have nasal congestion or a sore throat?
- Do you have or have you had a fever? Do you have chills?
- Do you have a headache?

Nasal Congestion

Nasal congestion occurs as a result of a cascade of events. First, the offending organism invades the epithelial cells of the upper respiratory tract. Inflammatory mediators are released, resulting in altered vascular permeability, edema, and nasal stuffiness. Stimulation of cholinergic nerves in the nose and upper respiratory tract leads to increased mucus production (rhinorrhea) and occasionally to bronchoconstriction, which causes cough. It is hypothesized that cellular damage to the nasopharynx is probably the cause of a sore and scratchy throat.

Runny nose with cough and mild fever, followed by a persistent cough, clear to off-white mucus that is greater in the morning and lasts more than 1 week, suggests bronchitis.

Nasal congestion or a sensation of postnasal discharge, especially associated with facial pain or pressure, suggests sinusitis. A history of bloody nasal discharge can also be present.

Infants with nasal congestion 3 days to 8 weeks after birth who have a cough but are afebrile could have *Chlamydia trachomatis,* contracted from the mother during childbirth. Older children, adolescents, and adults with a sore throat, fever, headache, and malaise progressing to a cough could have mycoplasma pneumonia.

Fever

In both adults and children, the most common signs and symptoms of a viral infection are a low grade temperature that is less than 38.3°C (101°F), small amounts of clear to yellow sputum production, nasal congestion, sore throat, and generalized malaise. Acute cough of a more serious nature (e.g., bacterial pneumonia) is usually accompanied by a temperature of greater than 38.3°C (101°F), chest pain, SOB, and purulent or dark sputum. Persistent fever, loss of appetite, and ill appearance are associated with a bacterial infection. Acute cough resulting from noninfectious processes (heart failure or pulmonary embolism) lacks signs such as fever, chills, and purulent sputum.

Headache

Headache pain can signal sinusitis as the cause of the cough (see Chapter 25).

What does the nature of the sputum tell me?

Key Questions
- Do you cough up sputum?
- Does it have an odor?
- How much have you coughed up?
- What color is the sputum?

Malodorous sputum suggests anaerobic infection of the lungs and sinuses. Very thick, tenacious, dark sputum is characteristic of bronchiectasis. Cloudy, thick sputum suggests lower respiratory tract infection but can also reflect an increase in the number of eosinophils from an asthmatic process. Viral bronchitis rarely causes more than 2 tablespoons of mucopurulent sputum per day. Bacterial bronchitis, however, is frequently associated with purulent sputum, often more than 2 tablespoons per day. Clear, mucoid sputum indicates allergic disorder. Hemoptysis, uncommon in children, usually indicates a more serious disease such as bacterial pneumonia, an acute inflammatory bronchitis, tumor, or a foreign body.

Children tend to swallow rather than expectorate sputum. Occasionally, emesis will have mucus in it and can be used to identify the sputum. A child with a persistent cough and purulent sputum is likely to have an infectious lung disease unless he or she has CF.

What does the nature of the cough tell me?

Key Questions
- Is the cough getting worse or more frequent?
- What time of day is the cough most bothersome?
- If a child: Did the child have an episode of severe cough, gagging, and choking recently?
- What type of work do you do?
- What does the cough sound like?

Severity and Progression of Cough

A cough in children or adults that becomes progressively worse can indicate pertussis. Pertussis has three stages. The first stage presents with a mild cough, rhinorrhea, conjunctivitis, and low-grade fever for 1 to 2 weeks. In the next stage, the cough becomes severe and comes in short paroxysms. There is a "whoop" on the inspiration effort at the end of the paroxysm. In the convalescent stage, the coughing and paroxysmal whooping decrease, but the cough can persist in a milder form for 3 months. Young infants and older adults with pertussis do not "whoop."

A cough in children that begins with a history of mild URI followed in 2 to 3 days with a cough that sounds like the barking of a seal can indicate croup. The cough is usually worse at night. Symptoms escalate as the viral agent (usually parainfluenza) compromises the upper airway. Obstruction increases, stridor becomes continuous, and there is nasal flaring and suprasternal, infrasternal, and intracostal retraction. The child is agitated and sits up. In most children, recovery occurs within a few hours. The Westley Croup Score is used to measure the severity of croup. Total score is the sum of points (0–17) based on five indicators: level of consciousness, cyanosis, stridor, air entry, and retractions. Any intensification of symptoms of respiratory obstruction requires hospitalization. Persistent nocturnal paroxysmal coughing is often associated with asthma.

Timing of Cough

Coughs that awaken people at night are frequently associated with respiratory problems in which bronchial irritation is a factor, such as asthma or chronic bronchitis, or with nonrespiratory conditions such as GERD or heart failure. A hallmark of asthma is coughing at night, usually between midnight and 2:00 AM, and is caused by the low level of cortisol or glucocorticoids in the body at this time. A severe cough in the early morning indicates postnasal drip, CF, or bronchiectasis. Secretions accumulate through the night, and fits of coughing are followed by bronchorrhea. Cough that is worse at night indicates croup, postnasal drip, lower respiratory tract infection, and allergic reaction. A cough that disappears with sleep is a habit cough.

History of Choking Episode

Consider FBA in a child with a cough lasting longer than 3 weeks. Frequently, the caregivers report an episode of severe coughing and choking 1 to 3 weeks before a persistent cough appears, with a period of absence of cough (because the level of obstruction is in a lobar or segmental bronchus) followed by a sudden recurrence of coughing. This period of absence of cough can last for hours, days, or even months. The cough can reappear when irritation of the foreign body or reaction to the foreign body occurs.

Occupation

An occupational and hobby review is warranted. Asbestos or coal dust exposure increases a person's risk of lung disease, including lung cancer and silicosis. Aerosol sprays, insecticides, chemical exposures, and sawdust can cause cough.

Nature of the Cough

A throat-clearing cough is indicative of postnasal drip caused by irritation of the cough receptors in the pharynx, which are sensitive to mechanical stimulation such as secretions. A dry, brassy cough indicates pharyngeal or tracheal irritation, allergy, or habit. A loose or moist cough can indicate lung disease such as CF or asthma.

A paroxysmal cough is seen with asthma, pertussis, CF, and occasionally after inhalation of a foreign body. A barking, croupy cough indicates an irritation in the glottic and subglottic area. A sudden, short burst of a cough in infants, called a staccato cough, is indicative of *C. trachomatis*. A harsh, dry cough caused by airway compression from enlarged nodes in the perihilar or paratracheal region seems to occur with tuberculosis (TB) or fungal infection.

A loud, bizarre cough that seems to be attention seeking can have a psychogenic origin. The cough usually is vibrating, throaty, and dry. The severity can range from occasional clearing of the throat to spells lasting several minutes. The cough usually follows a respiratory tract infection. The cough disappears with sleep or when the child is distracted.

Is the cough related to any event that would help me narrow down the cause?

Key Questions
- Does eating affect your cough?
- Does your cough get worse during certain times of the year?
- Does exercise affect your cough?

Eating

Aspiration into the tracheobronchial tree can occur as a result of lack of esophageal motility, GERD, with regurgitation into the pharynx, or central nervous system and neuromuscular disorders. In children, difficulty with sucking, swallowing, coughing, or choking during eating is highly suggestive of an underlying disorder, such as congenital malformations, congenital heart disease, or pneumonia.

In adults, GERD probably causes cough through the direct stimulation of cough receptors by gastric acid or through inflammation from aspiration of stomach contents into the airway.

Season

Chronic cough during winter months suggests viral infections. Exacerbation of cough during seasonal changes is suggestive of allergic disease with increased pollen counts. Croup occurs most commonly in the fall from the parainfluenza virus type 1. Smaller peaks of croup are seen with influenza B outbreaks in the winter months. RSV is common in infants during the winter months. In the warmer months, parainfluenza type 3 is the agent frequently isolated.

Exercise

The hyperpnea of exercise causes bronchospasm because of heat loss from the airway surface and is more pronounced in cold, dry air. Asthma attacks are frequently exercise related, as is cough resulting from heart disease or airway compression.

Is this something that is going around?

Key Questions
- Is anyone else at home ill?
- Is anyone else ill in daycare, school, or the workplace?

Exposure to respiratory viruses is very common in daycare, school, and the workplace. Viruses that cause the common cold are shed in nasal secretions. Contacts acquire the virus by being sneezed on or by touching a sneezed-on object and then touching their own noses or conjunctivae. The incubation period is 2 to 5 days. *Mycoplasma pneumoniae* tends to spread through school or households slowly because the incubation period is 21 days.

Is there anything that would lead me to suspect allergies or reactive airway disease?

Key Questions
- Does smoke, pollen, dust or exposure to animals trigger a cough?
- Does anyone in your family have allergies or asthma?
- Is there anything you do or take to relieve the cough?
- Is the cough getting better or worse?

Environmental Exposure

Frequently the patient notices that the cough occurs after exposure to certain environmental irritants, such as smoke, pollen, dust, or animals. The cough can resolve spontaneously with withdrawal from these irritants. Ingestion of antihistamines or inhalation of bronchodilators can relieve a cough associated with allergies or asthma.

Chronic cough is common in people who smoke. Smoke exposure can trigger cough in people with allergies or asthma.

Family History

Allergy-prone individuals are at increased risk for coughs associated with postnasal drip and asthma. Allergy-prone adults and children are those with a personal or family history of atopic dermatitis, asthma, and allergic rhinitis. Pets residing in the household are frequently the source of the allergen, especially cats and dogs.

Self-Management of Cough

Most individuals self-treat cough symptoms with over-the-counter medications that act as cough suppressants, expectorants, decongestants, and antihistamines. Environment conditions that trigger symptoms help to identify the trigger and allow an individual to minimize or reduce exposures.

Getting Better or Worse

A change in the chronic cough of a smoker can indicate the development of a new and serious underlying problem such as pneumonia, pulmonary edema, atelectasis, or cancer.

Does the patient have any risk factors for systemic disease that could present with cough?

Key Questions
- Do you have any chronic health problems?
- Do you have human immunodeficiency virus (HIV) infection, heart disease, or high blood pressure?
- Are you being treated for cancer?
- Have you ever been exposed to TB?
- Have you been immunized for pneumonia or whooping cough?

Chronic Health Problems

Chronic lung and heart disease can present with cough, indicating an exacerbation or complication of the disease. In addition, information about chronic health problems can indicate which medications patients take that may place them at risk for cough. Angiotensin-converting enzyme (ACE) inhibitors can be given to treat hypertension, heart failure, and diabetes. A cough may indicate exacerbation of heart failure. An ACE inhibitor–induced dry, hacking cough can be eliminated by stopping the medication. In addition, a medication history can reveal use of drugs that treat or cause immunocompromise.

Immunocompromise

Cancer therapy, HIV, and administration of steroids should raise suspicion of immunocompromise. Adults and children who are immunocompromised are at high risk for infectious lung problems.

Tuberculosis

Inquiry should be made about potential exposure to TB. Family history of TB, incarceration, international travel, and living in poor socioeconomic locations put individuals at risk for TB.

Immunization

A complete course of immunization against *Bordetella pertussis* is 80% to 85% effective. The Centers for Disease Control & Prevention (CDC) recommends a booster shot of DTaP (diphtheria, tetanus, and pertussis) between 12 to 18 years of age because of the lessening effect of the initial series. Adults may be reservoirs for the disease, and study results suggest repeated immunization. Pneumococcal vaccine (PCV13 followed by PPSV23) is recommended for persons 65 years and older.

DIAGNOSTIC REASONING: FOCUSED PHYSICAL EXAMINATION

Note General Appearance

When a patient appears to be in acute distress with manifestations of oxygen deprivation, dehydration, and is febrile, think first of bacterial pneumonia. If a patient has significant oxygen deprivation that is not accompanied by fever, consider FBA, acute heart failure, or pulmonary embolism.

The setting in which the patient is encountered will influence your response to the situation of acute distress. In most instances, oxygen is started immediately. If obstruction by a foreign body is strongly suspected, emergency personnel should be summoned for removal of the object if you are unable to accomplish this. Emergency chest radiographs may be needed to look for pulmonary infiltrates or foreign bodies, and pulse oximetry assesses oxygen saturation. Adults and children in acute respiratory distress require specialized care by health care professionals, and their assistance should be requested immediately.

Patients with viral respiratory tract infections or chronic cough from postnasal drainage, GERD, and chronic bronchitis appear less acutely ill and are able to participate in the interview process without difficulty. Those whose cough is caused by bronchospasm can exhibit varying degrees of distress.

Assess Mental Status

Diminished level of consciousness, confusion, and restlessness are manifestations of hypoxia in the patient experiencing respiratory problems. Frequently, the patient with a pulmonary embolus expresses a sense of impending doom.

Restlessness and agitation in the child can indicate hypoxemia. A lethargic and somnolent child can have carbon dioxide (CO_2) retention.

Take Vital Signs

An elevated pulse rate and temperature can signal bacterial or viral infection.

Respiratory rate is the best indicator of pulmonary function in young infants. The respiratory rate and tidal volume together produce adequate alveolar ventilation. For any given level of alveolar ventilation, there is an optimum respiratory rate at which the muscular work of breathing is at a minimum. Airway resistance increases at higher flow rates. In children with decreased compliance (e.g., pneumonia, pulmonary edema), respirations are very rapid and shallow. Children with increased airway resistance (e.g., asthma) have respirations that are relatively slow and deep to minimize the high-resistance work. The most reliable and reproducible respiratory rate is the sleeping respiratory rate.

Weigh the Patient

Children with a cough from a chronic disease can present with failure to thrive.

Examine the Head and Neck

Erythema of upper respiratory tract mucous membranes, accompanied by enlarged anterior cervical nodes, is a common finding in a URI.

Observe the neck for jugular venous distention; this can be a sign of heart failure.

Oral pharyngeal reflexes mediated by the auricular branch of cranial nerve X is a rare cause of chronic cough. Careful examination of the ears, with removal of cerumen and any hairs in contact with the tympanic membrane or the opposite wall of the external auditory canal, should be done.

A cobblestone appearance of the posterior pharynx is caused by lymphoid hyperplasia secondary to chronic stimulation by postnasal drip.

Inspect the Chest for Shape, Symmetry, and Use of Accessory Muscles

To inspect the chest, have the patient assume a sitting position. Note if the patient has to lean forward or sit up to breathe comfortably. Also observe the patient in a supine position to note if cough or respiratory symptoms change with position. Some respiratory abnormalities are unilateral or localized, such as pulmonary embolus. Compare findings on one side of the body with those on the other. Also compare front to back.

Upper airway obstruction causes suprasternal and supraclavicular retractions. Intercostal retractions and subcostal retractions occur with lower airway obstructive disease. Severe obstruction of either upper or lower airways causes retractions of all the accessory muscles. Retractions occur when an increase in the work of breathing requires an increase in the negative pressure within the chest. Remember that the pediatric airway is much

smaller in diameter than that of the adult, and because resistance to flow is related inversely to the fourth power of the radius, decreased diameter of this airway causes enormous increases in resistance. The chest wall is pliable, and the softest parts of the thorax are pulled inward on inspiration, causing retractions of the intercostal, suprasternal, and infrasternal spaces. The degree of retraction is proportional to the negative pressure generated within the thorax and therefore correlates with the severity of the problem.

Normally, the anteroposterior (AP) diameter is approximately one-third to one-half of the lateral diameter. If the AP diameter is equal to the lateral diameter, the condition known as barrel chest is evident and indicates probable COPD in adults. Children with chronic cough because of CF or severe asthma can have an increase in the AP diameter. In children up to 6 months of age, the head circumference is larger than the chest circumference. After 6 months of age, the chest circumference is larger than the head circumference.

Observe Respirations

Next, observe the rate, rhythm, and depth of the patient's breathing. The normal respiratory rate in adults is 12 to 20 breaths/min; in older adults, it is 16 to 25 breaths/min. Children younger than 12 years may have respiratory rates up to 30 to 40 breaths/min. The only way an infant or child can increase oxygen uptake is to increase the ventilation rate. The depth and pattern of respiration change; the infant's breaths are shallower and more frequent.

Exhalation normally lasts about twice as long as inhalation, but in patients with COPD, it can take up to four times longer. Note any abnormal breathing patterns (see Box 14.1).

Listen to the Cough

Note whether the cough is dry or moist. Listen also for the quality of the cough, such as whooping or honking.

Palpate the Chest

Palpate the entire chest for tenderness, depressions, bulges, and crepitus. Assess for chest symmetry by measuring diaphragmatic excursion and chest expansion. As the patient takes a deep breath, each hand should move the same distance out from the spine. With COPD, less movement will be seen. Pneumonia and partial paralysis of the diaphragm will result in a reduction in expansion of one side of the chest wall.

Assess for vocal fremitus (the vibrations transmitted to the chest wall during speech) by placing the ulnar side of the hand lightly on the chest and asking the patient to repeat the words "ninety-nine." Evaluate the intensity of the vibration over all lung fields, comparing side to side. Dense tissue conducts sound better than air does; thus, such conditions as pneumonia, heart failure, and tumors can increase fremitus. Fremitus is diminished in pneumothorax, asthma, and emphysema.

Percuss the Chest

Percuss systematically at 3- to 5-cm intervals, starting just above the scapulae and moving downward from side to side. Note any differences in volume and pitch. Resonance is a long, low-pitched sound that can normally be heard over most lung fields. Hyperresonance is an abnormally long, low-pitched sound that can signal emphysema or pneumothorax. Dullness or flatness can be heard with pleural effusion, pneumonia, or large tumors. Perform diaphragmatic excursion by percussing for resonance to dull with full inspiration and again in full exhalation to assess symmetry and adequate diaphragmatic movement.

Auscultate Breath Sounds

Instruct the patient to breathe through the mouth slowly and deeply. Determine the presence, type, and location of both normal and abnormal breath sounds (see Chapter 14).

Most children know what a stethoscope is, and you should use this to your advantage. Infants see the shiny parts; have older children listen to their own chests. Some clinicians begin by listening to the child's leg or hand first. Ensure that the stethoscope is warm before you place it on the chest. Infants are in good position when supine, toddlers should be on the parent's lap, and older children should be sitting or standing.

Auscultate Heart Sounds

Note the location of normal and abnormal heart sounds, the location of their greatest intensity, and the heart rate and rhythm. Also note any murmurs and their location, grade, and radiation. Incompetent heart valves could be the cause of heart failure. In patients with COPD, lung hyperinflation can muffle heart sounds. Poor tissue oxygenation or fever can result in tachycardia.

Examine the Skin and Extremities

Note the presence of cyanosis of the oral cavity (central cyanosis). Central cyanosis is associated with low arterial saturation and can result from inadequate gas exchange in the lungs or from cardiac shunting. Mucous membranes in dark-skinned patients can appear gray with central cyanosis. This can also be seen in individuals with COPD. Bluish color of the extremities (peripheral cyanosis) can be observed in whites and is associated with low venous saturation, resulting in vasoconstriction, vascular occlusion, or reduced cardiac output.

Clubbing is a loss of the angle between the skin and nail bed. Clubbing is a manifestation of chronic tissue hypoxia, which occurs frequently with chronic lung disease but may occur for other reasons or may be an individual variation. Edema of the lower extremities can be a sign of increased right-heart filling pressure, caused by primary lung disease or left ventricular failure.

Examine the Abdomen

Epigastric tenderness to palpation can be elicited in the patient with GERD, or the abdominal examination results might be entirely normal. If heart failure is the cause of cough, ascites or hepatojugular reflex may be present. To test for hepatojugular reflex, position the patient so that jugular pulsation is evident in the neck. Exert firm and sustained pressure with the hand over the patient's right upper quadrant for 30 to 60 seconds. An increase in the jugular venous pressure of more than 1 cm during this maneuver is abnormal.

LABORATORY AND DIAGNOSTIC STUDIES

Some clinical guidelines suggest all patients with a cough lasting longer than 3 weeks have a chest radiograph. If the radiograph has abnormal findings, consistent with infectious or noninfectious inflammatory disease or malignancy, the health care provider should order expectorated sputum studies, computed tomography (CT) of the lungs, or bronchoscopy. If the history, physical examination, and radiography suggest heart failure, an electrocardiogram, echocardiogram, or both are indicated (see Chapter 8).

If the patient's history and physical examination findings are strongly suggestive of a specific etiology (i.e., postnasal drip, asthma, GERD), appropriate treatment should be initiated. Keep in mind that there can be more than one cause of the cough. For patients whose history and physical examination findings are suggestive of chronic symptoms, sinus radiography or CT scan of the sinuses may be indicated. Also consider allergy testing for individuals whose history indicates that allergens precipitated the syndrome.

In situations in which investigation of signs and symptoms leads to a diagnosis of asthma or if no probable cause is identified, a spirometry test (see Chapter 14) should be performed. If the result is normal but asthma is still suspected, a methacholine challenge test can be done. This test is performed in the laboratory and involves administering methacholine chloride by nebulizer and then repeating the spirometry test. If the patient's cough is related to reactive airways disease, the patient exhibits a 20% decrease in FEV_1 (forced expiratory volume in 1 second), and a methacholine challenge is done to reverse airway resistance.

Complete Blood Count

A complete blood count (CBC) can provide evidence of acute infection with an elevated white blood cell count. Eosinophilia can be caused by a variety of allergic diseases such as bronchial asthma, allergic rhinitis, and atopic dermatitis.

Esophageal Probe

Gastroesophageal reflux disease is best diagnosed with 24-hour esophageal pH probe monitoring. A barium swallow is less sensitive, and a gastroscopy will verify ulcerative disease but not mild reflux.

Sputum Culture

Sputum culture is important for the diagnosis of a specific infectious agent in the pulmonary system. A sputum specimen must originate from deep within the bronchi. Coughing usually enables the patient to produce a satisfactory specimen. Examination includes macroscopic appearance, cellular composition, and bacterial count.

Sweat Test

A result of more than 60 mEq/L of chloride is considered diagnostic of CF.

Tuberculin Skin Testing

The Mantoux test is used to detect TB. A Mantoux test result is considered to be positive at three different levels (≥ 5, ≥ 10, and ≥ 15 mm) of induration (diameter transverse to the long axis of the arm measured and recorded) and depends on the individual's degree of risk for TB. In adults, a diameter of less than 5 mm is considered negative, a 5- to 9-mm diameter is considered weakly positive, a 10- to 14-mm diameter is considered intermediately positive, and a 15-mm or more diameter is considered a strongly positive. In a child who has no known risk factors for TB, only a large reaction (≥ 15 mm) is considered to be positive. If a child is very young (younger than 4 years old), has other medical risk factors, or has some environmental exposure to TB, then an intermediate reaction (≥ 10 mm) is considered to be positive. If a child is at high risk (e.g., a child who lives in a household with someone who has TB), then a small reaction (≥ 5 mm) is considered to be positive.

Nasal Swab for Pertussis and Polymerase Chain Reaction

Culture is the gold standard for diagnosis. It has excellent specificity (100%), but sensitivity in clinical practice is only 30% to 60%. Factors that reduce the sensitivity of culture include the nature of the organism, prolonged duration of illness by the time a specimen is collected, recent antibiotic use, prolonged transport time to the laboratory, and delayed specimen plating. Nasopharyngeal secretions for culture should be obtained using a calcium alginate or Dacron-tipped swab. The swab is inserted into the posterior nasopharynx and gently rotated for a minimum of 15 seconds and optimally for 1 minute. Throat swabs are not acceptable for the diagnosis of pertussis.

Polymerase chain reaction (PCR) is rapidly replacing nasal swab cultures for *B. pertussis*. This is a rapid, specific, and sensitive diagnostic test that will indicate abnormal findings late into the course of the illness.

Polymerase chain reaction is not affected by previous antibiotic use, and results are typically available within 1 to 2 days. Compared with culture, PCR may increase the diagnostic yield three- to fivefold. Disadvantages to PCR include its relatively high cost and lack of availability to many clinicians as well as the potential for false-abnormal results. The CDC recommends use of PCR together with culture for diagnosis of pertussis.

Rapid Influenza Testing

Rapid influenza testing is used to detect a virus in nasal or throat secretions. It can help differentiate influenza from other viral and bacterial infections with similar symptoms. Rapid influenza tests are best used within the first 48 hours of the onset of symptoms. The positive and negative predictive values vary considerably depending on the prevalence of influenza in the community. Testing is most effective when flu prevalence is high.

Chest Radiograph

Obtaining a chest radiograph is suggested in patients whose cough with accompanying fever persists longer than 3 days or who present with an unusual clinical course. If a foreign body is suspected, an expiratory film can identify the object (see Chapter 41).

DIFFERENTIAL DIAGNOSIS

Life-threatening causes of cough must be considered initially when arriving at a differential diagnosis. See Chapters 8 and 14 to review those conditions associated with cough.

Common Cold (Nasopharyngitis)

The common cold is a self-limiting viral infection of the upper respiratory tract that is generally caused by a rhinovirus. The virus invades the mucous membranes of the upper respiratory tract and causes swelling and hypersecretion of mucus. Associated symptoms include a low-grade fever, mild sore throat, and rhinorrhea of clear to yellow mucus. Hypersecretion of mucus causes coughing, especially at night when secretions pool in the nasopharyngeal cavity. Physical examination findings can include red and swollen nasal mucosa with secretions present, mild pharyngeal erythema, and enlarged cervical lymph nodes. Other physical examination findings are normal. The patient is advised to return if the cough persists for more than 3 weeks or if additional symptoms develop, such as temperature of more than 38.3°C (101°F), chest pain, or SOB.

Chronic Obstructive Pulmonary Disease Exacerbation

Chronic obstructive pulmonary disease is a condition primarily consisting of emphysema and chronic bronchitis. It is almost always a condition of heavy smokers but can also occur in patients with α_1-antitrypsin deficiency.

Acute exacerbations of COPD include three clinical findings: worsening dyspnea, increase in sputum purulence, and increase in sputum volume. Patients will have a chronic cough associated with a barrel chest, tachypnea, and distant breath sounds on physical examination. Chest radiography will show hyperexpansion of the lungs, and spirometry will indicate airflow obstruction when emphysema is present. Acute COPD exacerbations can also be associated with a URI, fever without a known cause, increased wheezing or cough, a 20% increase in respiratory rate, and a heart rate above baseline.

Bordetella Pertussis Infection

Pertussis (whooping cough) is an acute infection of the respiratory tract caused by *Bordetella pertussis*. It is a condition primarily seen in children younger than the age of 2 years and in individuals who have not had adequate diphtheria, tetanus toxoid, and pertussis (DTP) vaccination. Pertussis infection has occurred among adolescents who become susceptible approximately 6 to 10 years after childhood vaccination. It begins with a prodromal stage of malaise, cough, coryza, and anorexia. The cough then becomes more severe and ends in a high-pitched inspiratory "whoop." Vomiting and cyanosis may also be present. Physical examination can be within normal limits. Pertussis is associated with extremely high absolute lymphocytosis (>10,000 cells/mm^3).

Bacterial Pneumonia

Pneumonia is usually associated with dyspnea, pleuritic chest pain, cough with greenish or rusty-colored sputum, fever, and chills. Infants and young children will not produce sputum. Anorexia, malaise, and posttussive vomiting are seen. Objective manifestations of pneumonia include fever, tachycardia and tachypnea, inspiratory crackles, asynchronous breathing, tactile fremitus, dull percussion sound over the area of consolidation, and bronchophony. Pneumonia can be confirmed by chest radiography, CBC, and sputum and nasal bacteria cultures.

Fever is frequently absent in older adults with pneumonia, and thus a new onset of cough, especially when accompanied by either tachypnea or altered mental status, should suggest pneumonia.

The majority of pediatric pulmonary infections are viral and usually caused by RSV, parainfluenza viruses, or influenza viruses. In infants and young children, acute nonbacterial pneumonia presents after a 1- to 2-day history of coryza, decreased appetite, and low-grade fever. Increasing fretfulness, respiratory congestion, vomiting, cough, and fever can occur. Objective manifestations include tachypnea, tachycardia, nasal flaring, and retractions.

Viral Upper Respiratory Infection

Viral agents include a vast number of serotypes. Cough, nasal congestion, sore throat, fever, chills, and myalgias are the most common symptoms. Most symptoms of URIs, including local swelling, erythema, edema, secretions, and fever, result from the inflammatory response of the immune system to invading pathogens and from toxins produced by pathogens. An initial nasopharyngeal infection can spread to adjacent structures, resulting in sinusitis, otitis media, epiglottitis, laryngitis, tracheobronchitis, and pneumonia. Influenza (flu) caused by the family of influenza viruses typically produces more severe symptoms and has more serious sequelae. Fever is usually higher, and stuffy nose and sneezing may be absent. Because flu cannot be distinguished from other URIs on symptoms alone, rapid flu testing can be useful during flu outbreaks.

Mycoplasma Pneumoniae

Mycoplasma pneumoniae is the most common cause of infection of the lower respiratory tract in children and young adults. There is a slow onset of symptoms with fever (39°C or 102.2°F), a cough that is usually dry at the onset, headache, malaise, and sore throat. The child does not look particularly ill, but on auscultation, rales and rhonchi are frequently present. The white blood cell count is usually normal, and cold agglutinin titer can be elevated during the acute presentation in more than half of patients with this infection. A titer of 1:32 or higher supports the diagnosis.

Chlamydial Pneumonia

Chlamydial pneumonia is a pulmonary disease caused by *C. trachomatis* and is transmitted during delivery. It also occurs in young adults. In infants 3 to 11 weeks of age, it is one of the most common causes of interstitial pneumonitis and presents with tachypnea and a characteristic staccato cough in an afebrile child. In adults, infection is associated with upper respiratory tract symptoms followed by fever and a nonproductive cough. Fine rales, usually without wheezes, are heard on auscultation. Chest radiographs show hyperinflated lungs with diffuse interstitial or alveolar infiltrates.

Bronchiolitis

Respiratory syncytial virus is mainly responsible for bronchiolitis in children younger than 2 years old. The infection is associated with 1 to 2 days of fever, rhinorrhea, and cough followed by wheezing, tachypnea, tachycardia, and respiratory distress. Nasal flaring and retractions with accessory muscle use are seen along with shallow, rapid respirations. Cough increases as inflammation increases. The infant appears lethargic and has circumoral cyanosis. Wheezes are predominant, with a long expiratory phase. Crackles and rhonchi can also be heard diffusely throughout the lung fields. The chest radiograph shows hyperinflation with mild interstitial infiltrates. Viral isolates from sputum, throat swabs, or nasal washings are used for diagnosis.

Acute Bronchitis

Inflammation of the large airways causes bronchitis that begins with a dry, nonproductive cough, usually seen in winter. Continued cough and nasal congestion produce a productive cough and fever. Chest pain can accompany the cough. Lung auscultation reveals diffuse rhonchi on expiration. The white blood cell count is normal or mildly elevated.

Croup (Acute Laryngotracheobronchitis)

Inflammation or edema of the subglottic area causes obstruction of the airways of the larynx, trachea, or bronchi. Parainfluenza virus causes the most inflammation. Generally, the onset occurs after a few days of a URI. Hoarseness, inspiratory stridor, and a barking cough are usually worse at night. A low-grade fever can be present. Inspiratory stridor, suprasternal and intercostal retractions, and an increased respiratory rate are seen. Lateral neck radiographs in croup show a normal epiglottis, subglottic narrowing, and ballooning of the hypopharynx. The posteroanterior neck view shows a steeple sign (narrowing of the air column at the top).

Subacute and Chronic Cough

Upper airway cough syndrome

Upper airway cough syndrome is the most common cause of chronic cough. The cough results from stimulation of the afferent limb of the cough reflex in the upper respiratory tract. Causes of postnasal drip include allergic response, secondary infection after an upper respiratory tract illness, environmental irritants, vasomotor rhinitis, or sinusitis. Both children and adults report dry cough, throat clearing, sensation of something in the back of the throat, and nasal congestion. Physical examination can reveal mucus in the posterior pharynx or a cobblestone appearance of the posterior pharynx. Sinus radiographs, CT scan of the sinuses, and allergy testing can be indicated if this syndrome is suspected to be the cause of the cough.

Asthma

Asthma is the most common cause of chronic cough in children. It initially produces a dry cough, commonly worse at night, characteristically exercise related, and often triggered by respiratory tract infections. Physical examination findings depend on the severity of the disease. The prolonged expiratory phase of respiration can be heard. Lungs can have crackles that clear with coughing, and overt or latent wheeze can be produced with forced expiration. Use of neck muscles to facilitate inspiration (called tracheal tugging or chin lag) can be seen. A chest radiograph can show hyperinflation during acute attacks. Pulmonary function testing and reversibility of airway resistance after a methacholine challenge can confirm a diagnosis of asthma.

Gastroesophageal Reflux Disease

Gastroesophageal reflux disease should be considered when patients report heartburn, a sour taste in the mouth, or a history of esophagitis. Often people with GERD are cigarette smokers, overuse alcohol, and are overweight. Microaspiration into the airways or reflux of acid into the esophagus occurs. Young infants can also experience reflux with their cough, which could be the only symptom. This symptom usually worsens after feeding. A recurrent, effortless vomiting with failure to gain weight and irritability can also occur. The physical examination findings of patients with GERD are most often normal. The diagnostic test of most significance is esophageal pH monitoring; values outside the normal physiological range indicate reflux.

Chronic Bronchitis

Chronic bronchitis should be considered when the patient expectorates sputum almost daily during a period spanning at least 3 consecutive months and such periods have occurred for more than 2 successive years. In addition, exposure to smoke, irritating dust, or fumes is highly likely. Cigarette smoke as well as fumes and dust stimulate the afferent limb of the cough reflex as irritants, inducing inflammatory changes in the mucosa of the respiratory tract, causing hypersecretion of mucus and slowing of mucociliary clearance. People with chronic bronchitis exhibit a rasping, hacking cough, possible rhonchi that clear with coughing, resonant to dull chest, possible barrel chest, prolonged expiration, and possible wheezing. Chest radiography and pulmonary function tests are indicated.

Angiotensin-Converting Enzyme Inhibitor–Induced Cough

This cough occurs hours to months after beginning an ACE inhibitor. The patient reports a nonproductive cough associated with an irritating, tickling, or scratching sensation in the throat. Physical examination results are normal. The cough resolves within days to weeks after the drug is discontinued.

Bronchogenic Carcinoma

A risk factor for lung cancer is smoking; however, bronchogenic cancer does occur in nonsmokers. Hemoptysis as well as weight loss and SOB are frequent health concerns reported by a patient with bronchogenic cancer. Physical findings can include enlarged supraclavicular nodes, dull chest percussion over the tumor, and increased breath sounds distal to the tumor. Hemoptysis should be evaluated with a chest radiograph and a CT scan if indicated.

Cystic Fibrosis

A chronic cough is associated with CF. The cough is productive, and the child has signs of failure to thrive with poor weight gain. The child could have a family history of the disease. The cough is initially dry and hacking but eventually becomes loose and produces purulent material. Physical examination often shows an increased AP diameter of the chest. Scattered or localized coarse rales and rhonchi are audible. Digital clubbing is often present. The sweat chloride test shows abnormal findings.

Foreign Body Aspiration

Foreign body aspiration occurs most frequently in children and older adults. A child or adult who aspirates a foreign body can have a varied presentation. Generally, the onset of cough is sudden and unexpected. A brief period of severe coughing, gagging, and choking occurs. If the foreign body does not completely obstruct the airway, an asymptomatic period ensues. This period can last for hours, days, or even months. A foreign body in the lower airway can present with air trapping or hyperinflation because of the ball-valve phenomenon or can occur as a complete distal atelectasis created by absorption of the trapped gas. A mobile foreign body in the lower airway can produce a paroxysmal cough, with cyanotic episodes and stridor because of proximal migration and subglottic impaction. A foreign body in the esophagus can cause airway obstruction and cough, as well as dysphagia for solid foods because the posterior trachea is compliant and opposed to the anterior esophagus. Coins are the most common FBA. Obtain a chest radiograph to determine the location.

Allergic Rhinitis

Upper airway allergy and vasomotor rhinitis can cause a reflex cough secondary to postnasal drip and irritation of the cough receptors. Such a cough is generally seasonal in nature with a history of sneezing. Allergic shiners, allergic salute, and eczema can be present. Rhinorrhea with clear, watery drainage is seen. Skin testing for allergies can confirm that allergens are present.

Chronic Sinusitis

Chronic sinusitis produces a recurrent cough that is especially worse at night because of trickling of infected mucus from the nasopharynx down the posterior pharyngeal wall.

Involvement is usually in the maxillary sinuses. History reveals coldlike symptoms that become persistent or recurrent. Noisy breathing and snoring during sleep may also be present. Physical examination reveals clear to mucopurulent secretions in the posterior throat. Purulent rhinorrhea can be present. Sinus tenderness is less frequently present than in acute sinusitis. A radiograph using the Waters view of the head reveals abnormal findings.

Tuberculosis

Brassy cough is the most common symptom of TB, but it is often ascribed to smoking, a recent cold, or a bout of influenza several weeks before. At first, it is minimally productive of yellow or green mucus, usually on arising in the morning. As the disease progresses, the cough becomes more productive. In adults, a multinodular infiltrate above or behind the clavicle (the most characteristic location) is suggestive of the recurrence of an old TB infection. In younger people in whom recent infection is more common, infiltration can be found in any part of the lung, and unilateral pleural effusion is often seen. In sputum examination, the finding of acid-fast bacilli in a sputum smear is strong presumptive evidence of TB. A definitive diagnosis is made only on results of a culture.

Smoking

Smoking is most prevalent in female adolescents, and many smoke in closed rooms, increasing their respiratory irritation. History of a mildly productive hacking cough can be indicative of smoking. Infants exposed to passive cigarette smoke inhalation have increased bronchial reactivity. Physical examination can reveal yellow stains on the fingers, teeth, or tongue. Mild chronic conjunctivitis can also be present. Chest radiography can be positive with interstitial markings.

Psychogenic Origin

Psychogenic or habit cough is a rare cause of cough and can be misdiagnosed in a patient with postnasal drip syndrome. School-age children or adolescents with a history of a loud, brassy, disturbing cough that is nonproductive and explosive can indicate a psychogenic etiology. The child usually has missed many school days. The cough is not heard while sleeping, and the child is afebrile with no weight loss. The physical examination findings are normal.

> ## DIFFERENTIAL DIAGNOSIS OF *Common Causes of Recent Onset of Cough*

CONDITION	HISTORY	PHYSICAL FINDINGS	DIAGNOSTIC STUDIES
Nasopharyngitis	Acute-onset, low-grade fever, rhinorrhea, cough, especially at night	Nasal mucosa red and swollen, pharynx mildly red; otherwise normal	None
COPD exacerbation	Worsening dyspnea, increased wheezing or coughing, smoker	Purulent sputum, fever, and increased respiratory and heart rates	Chest radiograph, spirometry
Pertussis	Persistent hacking cough; can have inspiratory whoop, vomiting	Fever absent, coryza	Nasopharyngeal aspirate abnormal, PCR abnormal, chest radiograph to rule out pneumonia

> **DIFFERENTIAL DIAGNOSIS OF** *Common Causes of Recent Onset of Cough—cont'd*

CONDITION	HISTORY	PHYSICAL FINDINGS	DIAGNOSTIC STUDIES
Pneumonia[a]	Noisy cough, dyspnea, pleuritic chest pain, sputum production (yellow, green, red color), chills; in children also see poor feeding and irritability	Fever, tachycardia, tachypnea, inspiratory crackles, asynchronous breathing, tactile fremitus, percussion dull or flat over area of consolidation, bronchophony, egophony	Chest radiograph, CBC, sputum and nasal cultures, O_2 saturation, blood cultures
Viral URI	Cough, nasal congestion, sore throat, fever, chills, myalgias	Fever, pharyngitis, enlarged anterior cervical lymph nodes, normal TMs, nasal mucosa erythema, normal chest examination	None. Rapid influenza testing during outbreaks
Mycoplasma pneumoniae	Child or young adult: dry cough, headache, malaise, sore throat	Fever, rales and rhonchi on auscultation	Cold agglutinin, chest radiograph
Chlamydial pneumonia	Paroxysmal staccato cough in infant age 4–12 wk	Afebrile, conjunctivitis in 50% of infants, tachypnea of 40–80 breaths/min, crackles, no wheezing	Radiograph shows hyperexpansion of lungs with diffuse interstitial infiltrates
Bronchiolitis (RSV)[a]	Grunting, sneezing, cough, anoxia, exposure to passive smoke	Fever, wheezing on auscultation, prolonged expiratory phase, tachypnea of 60–80 breaths/min, tachycardia >200 beats/min	WBC 5000–24,000/mm³ with increased PMNs; chest radiograph shows hyperinflation; infants younger than 2 mo, refer; progressive respiratory distress, refer
Acute bronchitis	Duration <3 mo, winter months, URI for 3–4 days; loose, hacking cough that becomes productive, afebrile	Coarse, fine crackles on auscultation; low-grade fever or afebrile	Chest radiograph shows normal findings
Croup (acute laryngotracheobronchitis)[a]	History of URI; brassy, barking cough usually at night	Low-grade fever, inspiratory stridor, flaring of nares, prolonged expiratory phase, can see retraction of accessory muscles, breath sounds diminished	None

[a]Because of the possible rapid changes in condition in infants and children, nonemergent causes of cough can become emergent.

COPD, chronic obstructive pulmonary disease; *PCRs,* polymerase chain reaction; *PMNs,* polymorphonuclear neutrophils; *RSV,* respiratory syncytial virus; *TM,* tympanic membrane; *URI,* upper respiratory infection.

▶ **DIFFERENTIAL DIAGNOSIS OF** *Common Causes of Chronic Cough*

CONDITION	HISTORY	PHYSICAL FINDINGS	DIAGNOSTIC STUDIES
UACS	Dry cough, sore throat, frequent throat clearing	Mucoid secretions in posterior pharynx, cobblestone appearance of posterior pharynx, tenderness to palpation of sinuses, normal chest examination	Sinus radiographs, sinus CT scan, allergy testing
Asthma	Dry, hacking cough, especially at night, and with feeding and laughter	End-expiratory wheeze, prolonged expiratory phase	Pulmonary function testing, chest radiography, O_2 saturation, bronchoprovocation, allergy testing
GERD	Cough worse at night, sour taste in mouth, heartburn, history of esophagitis, cigarette smoker, alcohol abuse, overweight; in children 0–18 mo: failure to thrive, dysphagia, cough after eating and lying down, vomiting	Normal chest examination, normal upper respiratory tract examination, possible epigastric pain with palpation or normal abdominal examination	Esophageal pH monitoring, blood count for anemia, radiograph for aspiration pneumonia; endoscopy if no response to therapy; manometry
Chronic bronchitis	Cough, mild dyspnea, history of COPD, history of cigarette smoking, yellow sputum	Hacking, rasping cough; normal breath sounds or rhonchi that clear with coughing; resonant to dull chest, possible barrel chest, prolonged expiration, possible wheezing	Chest radiograph, pulmonary function tests
ACE inhibitor–induced cough	Begins hours to months after starting ACE inhibitor; nonproductive, dry cough; scratching sensation in throat	Normal examination	Trial of ACE inhibitor
Bronchogenic carcinoma	Cough with hemoptysis; history of cigarette smoking, weight loss, shortness of breath	Enlarged supraclavicular nodes, dull chest percussion over tumor, increased breath sounds distal to tumor	Chest radiograph, CT scan of chest
Cystic fibrosis	Failure to thrive, chronic cough, bulky stools, family history	Nasal polyps, clubbing of fingernails, sputum	Sweat test abnormal findings
Foreign body in ear canal	Cough	Cerumen in ears, hairs in contact with TM or opposite wall of external auditory canal	None

► DIFFERENTIAL DIAGNOSIS OF *Common Causes of Chronic Cough—cont'd*

CONDITION	HISTORY	PHYSICAL FINDINGS	DIAGNOSTIC STUDIES
Foreign body aspiration	History of environmental hazard, choking episode	Asymmetrical physical findings of decreased breath sounds, wheezing	Asymmetrical radiograph with forced expiratory view
Allergic rhinitis	History of sneezing, cough	Allergic shiners, allergic salute, rhinorrhea clear and watery	Chest radiograph negative, allergy testing positive
Chronic sinusitis	Rhinorrhea >7–10 days	Mucopurulent rhinorrhea	Waters radiograph
Mycoplasma pneumonia	School-age child, gradual onset, headache, malaise, sore throat, hacking cough	Reddened pharynx, slightly enlarged lymph nodes, rales often fine and crackling	Radiograph shows interstitial pneumonia; cold agglutinins present, ESR elevated, CBC, O_2 saturation, sputum cultures, blood cultures
Tuberculosis	History of exposure, high-risk group, weakness, malaise, weight loss	Brassy cough, weight loss, can have fever, night sweats	Mantoux test, chest radiograph shows abnormalities in apical and hyaline, sputum culture positive for *M. tuberculosis*
Smoking (passive or active)	History of smoking or being around a smoker	Yellow teeth, fingers; odor of smoke, productive sputum	Radiograph can have abnormal findings, with interstitial markings
Psychogenic origin	School age or adolescent; dry, hacking cough present only during waking hours	None	As indicated to rule out other causes

ACE, angiotensin-converting enzyme; *CBC,* complete blood cell count; *COPD,* chronic obstructive pulmonary disease; *CT,* computed tomography; *ESR,* erythrocyte sedimentation rate; *GERD,* gastroesophageal reflux disease; *UACS,* upper airway cough syndrome.

Next to respiratory disease, acute gastroenteritis is the most common illness in families in the United States. Most cases are of viral origin and are self-limiting. In children, 50% are of viral origin, 25% are of bacterial origin, and 25% are of undetermined cause. Diarrhea can be classified according to the pathophysiological pattern (osmotic, secretory, exudative, or motile), cause (infectious or noninfectious), or duration (acute or chronic).

Osmotic or malabsorptive diarrhea occurs when nonabsorbable, water-soluble solutes remain in the bowel and retain water. This can occur through damage to the intestinal microvillus membrane. The result is malabsorption of luminal solutes with osmotic loss of free water into the gut lumen. This is the most common cause of chronic diarrhea in children. Lactose intolerance is an example of this kind of diarrhea. Ingestion of large amounts of sugar substitutes in diet foods, drinks, candies, and chewing gum can cause osmotic diarrhea through a combination of slow absorption and rapid small bowel motility.

Secretory diarrhea occurs when the balance between fluid secretion and absorption across the intestinal mucosa is altered. When there is a change in this balance, produced by physiological causes, diarrhea occurs. The loss of water and electrolytes can be rapid and massive. Traveler's diarrhea and diarrhea caused by *Vibrio cholerae* are examples.

Exudative diarrhea occurs in the presence of mucosal inflammation or ulceration, which results in an outpouring of plasma, serum proteins, blood, and mucus. The consequence is an increase in fecal bulk and fluidity. Many mucosal diseases, such as regional enteritis, ulcerative colitis, and carcinoma, can cause this exudative enteropathy.

Diarrhea from abnormal intestinal motility (either increased or decreased) results in an alteration in contact between the luminal contents and the mucosal surface. Examples include irritable bowel syndrome (IBS) and laxative use.

Infectious agents can be viral, bacterial, or parasitic.

DIAGNOSTIC REASONING: FOCUSED HISTORY

What does this patient mean by "diarrhea"?

Key Questions
- How frequent are the stools?
- What is the volume of stools?
- Are the stools formed or liquid?
- At what intervals does the diarrhea occur?

Frequency of Stools

In the United States, typical bowel frequency ranges from one to three times a day to two or three times per week and varies considerably from person to person. Changes in stool frequency, consistency, or volume can indicate disease.

Stool Volume and Consistency

Processes involving the small bowel tend to produce large-volume watery stools that are relatively infrequent. Large bowel involvement, usually resulting from a bacterially induced inflammatory process, tends to produce more-frequent, less-watery, and smaller-volume stools. The Bristol Stool Form Scale can help patients identify stool consistency (see Chapter 10, Fig. 10.1).

Intervals

A history of acute diarrhea followed by continuous or intermittent episodes of loose stools suggests malabsorption commonly caused by lactase deficiency exacerbated by the ingestion of lactose in milk or milk products. Intermittent diarrhea alternating with constipation can indicate a type of IBS.

Proximal Colon Symptoms

Proximal colon symptoms include large-volume, less-frequent, more-homogeneous stools, without urgency or tenesmus (painful defecation), and suggest food intolerance or infectious or inflammatory disease.

Distal Colon Symptoms

Symptoms of small volume, frequency, urgency, tenesmus, incontinence, and mucus suggest proctocolitis, colon cancer, diverticular disease, or IBS.

If this is an infant, is there a risk of dehydration?

Key Questions
- How many wet (urine) diapers has the infant produced in the past 24 hours?
- Does the infant seem thirsty?
- Does the infant have tears when crying?

Wet Diapers

Dehydration in infants and young children can occur quickly and with fatal consequences, especially in infants. Diagnosis and treatment must be done in a timely manner. A general rule of thumb to determine signs of dehydration in infants is fewer than six wet diapers over 24 hours or a period longer than 4 hours without urination.

Thirst

Infants demonstrate their thirst with irritability, crying, and eagerness to drink fluid that is offered to them. Test for thirst by offering fluids either in a bottle or on a spoon. The child with mild dehydration will exhibit increased thirst; the moderately dehydrated child will be very thirsty; and, with severe dehydration, the child will continue to be very thirsty. If left untreated, a child can become stuporous and unresponsive and therefore unable to manifest thirst.

Tears

In mild dehydration, tears are present; in moderate dehydration, tears are or are not present; and in severe dehydration, no tears are present.

If this is an adult, is there risk for dehydration?

Key Questions
- How many times have you urinated in the past 24 hours?
- Are you thirsty?
- Do you have a dry mouth or dry eyes?

Dehydration

Symptoms of dehydration in an adult are more related to the rate of fluid loss than to the absolute degree of fluid loss. The degree of dehydration can be estimated by symptoms of thirst, dry mouth, or dry eyes, and by the frequency, volume, and color (concentration) of urination. Patients can also experience weakness.

Is this an acute or chronic problem?

Key Questions
- How long have you had diarrhea?
- Have you had this problem before?

Acute Diarrhea in Adults

An acute onset of diarrhea in a previously healthy patient without signs or symptoms of other organ involvement is suggestive of an infectious cause. Acute diarrhea in adults is commonly viral in origin. The viral illnesses are self-limited, and an aggressive diagnostic workup is not indicated. Acute diarrhea in adults usually has an abrupt onset and lasts less than 2 weeks. Most of the disorders cause some combination of abdominal pain, diarrhea, nausea, vomiting, fever, and tenesmus.

Acute Diarrhea in Children

Acute diarrhea in children is characterized by loose or liquid stools. A large quantity of fluid and electrolytes that become pooled in the intestinal lumen is lost as stool is expelled. The number of stools is usually increased, but this is not an essential manifestation. Severe or protracted diarrhea can lead to metabolic acidosis, dehydration, azotemia, and oliguria. Diarrhea in a neonate or young infant is considered more serious than that in an older child because of lower tolerance to fluid shifts and the greater likelihood of associated infection or congenital anomaly.

Chronic Diarrhea in Adults

Diarrhea is chronic when it lasts more than 2 weeks. Unless the diarrhea is bloody or the patient has a systemic illness, the most common causes of chronic diarrhea are parasites, medications, IBS, lactose intolerance, and inflammatory bowel disease (IBD).

Chronic Diarrhea in Children

Chronic diarrhea in children is defined as diarrhea for longer than 3 weeks. The major causes of diarrhea change with age. In an infant, formula protein intolerance is the most common cause. Toddler's diarrhea (irritable colon of infancy), protracted enteritis after a viral infection, and infection with *Giardia lamblia* are the common causes in a toddler. In children and adolescents, malabsorption disorders are the most common causes. The diarrhea is the result of the ingestion of solutes that cannot be digested or absorbed, such as lactose products or excessive intake of sorbitol. Another cause of diarrhea in this age group is IBD (ulcerative colitis and Crohn disease).

Does the presence or absence of blood help me narrow the cause?

Key Questions
- Is there any noticeable blood in the stool or tissue? How much?
- What color is the blood?
- What color are the stools?

Blood in the Stools

Bright red blood limited to small spots on the toilet tissue is suggestive that the source of bleeding is from hemorrhoids and not from a diarrheal process higher in the gastrointestinal (GI) tract. Because diarrhea and repeated cleansing of the rectum produce local irritation, minor bleeding from hemorrhoids is not uncommon and must be distinguished from true blood in the stool. Reports of blood in the stool in acute diarrhea are suggestive of a bacterial pathogen, notably *Shigella* species. The blood is red.

In infants and children, blood in the stool is most commonly caused by intolerance of cow's milk or by anal fissures. In a newborn, blood in stools can be a result of hemorrhagic disease of the newborn, thought to be caused by a lack of vitamin K. Premature infants or infants who are of low birth weight are at risk for necrotizing enterocolitis presenting with red or maroon stools (hematochezia), vomiting, and abdominal distention.

In adults and children, chronic bloody diarrhea can indicate IBD, dysentery, colitis, or an invasive organism. Blood that is red usually indicates lower GI tract bleeding, whereas dark or black, tarry stools (melena) typically indicate upper GI tract bleeding. However, bleeding from the small bowel or right colon can also produce melena.

Color of Stools

Some patients believe they have blood in their stool based on stool color. Sources of black stools are blood, iron, charcoal, bismuth, licorice, huckleberries, and lead. Sources of red or pink stools include blood, food (beets, cranberries, tomatoes, peppers), food coloring (breakfast cereals, gelatin), and drugs (anticoagulants, salicylates, rifampin, phenazopyridine hydrochloride (pyridium), diazepam syrup, phenolphthalein in alkaline stool). Green-black stools can be caused by grape-flavored drinks and iron. Dark gray stools occur with cocoa and chocolate ingestion. Pale gray or white stools can be caused by cholestasis, obstructive jaundice, malabsorption, excessive milk ingestion, and antacid ingestion. Green stools are produced by bile salts and chlorophyll-containing vegetables, such as spinach.

What does the presence or absence of pain tell me?

Key Questions
- Are you having any pain or gas with the diarrhea?

- Where is the pain?
- What does the pain feel like?
- Is the pain constant or does it come and go? Is it relieved by passage of gas?
- Does the pain awaken you at night?
- Does the pain interfere with your activities (e.g., working, sleeping, eating)?

Occurrence of Pain

Diarrhea with abdominal pain and flatulent stools in an afebrile patient is characteristic of a malabsorptive process. Most self-limiting viral diarrheas cause some combination of abdominal pain, diarrhea, nausea, vomiting, fever, and tenesmus.

Abdominal pain is common when diarrhea is caused by infective bacteria in the colon, such as ingestion associated with food poisoning. *Giardia lamblia*, introduced through the ingestion of contaminated water or by the orofecal route, produces crampy abdominal pain and is frequently seen in children and diapered infants in day care where handwashing is not done between diapering.

Location of Pain

Generalized abdominal pain is produced by diffuse inflammation of the GI tract, which occurs with IBD, or abdominal cramping from infective diarrhea. The pain from ulcerative colitis may occur over the entire abdomen or may be localized to the lower quadrants. The pain associated with IBS is usually confined to the lower quadrants or to the sigmoid colon. Whereas large intestine pain is felt in the lower abdominal quadrants, small intestine pain is felt in the epigastric and umbilical areas.

Severity of Pain

Self-limited diarrhea usually presents with cramping but not severe abdominal pain. Other causes of abdominal pain should be investigated (see Chapter 3).

Sleep-Related Pain

Persistent diarrhea that awakens the patient from sleep usually indicates a serious organic disease, such as diabetes enteropathy or human immunodeficiency virus (HIV) enteropathy. The symptoms associated with IBS occur during the waking hours.

What do associated symptoms tell me?

Key Questions
- Do you have any fever? Did you take your temperature?
- Do you have any vomiting?
- What occurred first: the diarrhea or the vomiting?

Fever

Patients often report having a "fever" when they have such symptoms as facial flushing, chills, headache, malaise, muscle aches, or a sensation of warmth. These symptoms are usually not validated by measuring body temperature with a thermometer. Fever is a cardinal manifestation of disease. GI tract and respiratory tract infections are responsible for 80% of febrile illnesses. Generally, low-grade fever occurs with viral causes of diarrhea, although high fevers are more often associated with bacterial causes.

Vomiting

Vomiting is often present early in the course of viral gastroenteritis (especially the Norwalk virus), food poisoning, and food-borne bacterial infection. Vomiting is one of the main causes of dehydration in acute diarrhea. Small bowel processes commonly associated with viral agents cause delayed gastric emptying and luminal distention, which often induces vomiting before the onset of diarrhea.

Occurrence of Vomiting and Diarrhea

When diarrhea occurs before the vomiting, suspect a bacterial etiology.

Could this be caused by exposure to others or to contaminated food?

Key Questions
- If a child: Does the child attend day care?
- If a child: Are any of the other children in day care ill?
- If older adult: Do you attend or live in a congregate setting such as assisted living, personal care home, nursing home, or adult day care?
- Have you been around others who have similar symptoms?

Day Care Attendance

Children who attend day care are at greater risk of acquiring many bacterial infections transmitted through orofecal contamination and diapering.

Adult Congregate Living

Older adults who attend or live in congregate settings are at greater risk for diarrhea associated with *Clostridium difficile* infection. Outbreaks associated with viral causes of diarrhea have also been reported.

Others with Similar Symptoms

It is common for foodborne infections to be acquired at social gatherings where food is served; in this case, others at the gathering can become ill with similar symptoms. However, patients do not always know if others became ill, especially when the onset of diarrhea occurs 1 to 2 hours after food ingestion.

Could this be the result of exposure to animals?

Key Questions
• What pets do you have?
• Have you had contact with or have you handled dogs, cats, or turtles?

Exposure to Infectious Agents Through Animal Contact

Campylobacter jejuni infection can be acquired from infected dogs or cats. Infected turtles are a source of *Salmonella* organisms.

Could this be caused by exposure to contaminated water?

Key Questions
• Have you traveled recently? Where?

Recent Travel

Travel outside of the United States carries the potential to acquire enterotoxigenic *Escherichia coli*, or less commonly, *G. lamblia*, *Salmonella* spp., *Shigella* spp., *C. jejuni*, or *Entamoeba histolytica*. Camping exposes individuals to *Giardia* and *Campylobacter* spp. through untreated water. Outbreaks of diarrhea caused by *Cryptosporidium* organisms

have been linked to contaminated water in urban areas of the United States. Diarrhea caused by the norovirus has been linked to cruise ship travel.

Could sexual activities explain the diarrhea?

Key Questions
• Do your sexual practices include anal sex? Suspect *Shigella* infection in patients who engage in anal sex, particularly homosexual men. Accompanying pain, tenesmus, and the passage of mucus indicate the presence of proctitis.

Could this be the result of an immune problem?

Key Questions
• Have you been diagnosed with an immune system problem?
• Do you have frequent colds or other illnesses?
• Are you receiving chemotherapy?

Immunocompromised Host

Immunoglobulin A (IgA) and immunoglobulin G (IgG) deficiencies are frequent causes of chronic diarrhea in children. Patients with a compromised immune system from acquired immunodeficiency syndrome (AIDS) or chemotherapy often develop enteropathy.

Could this be caused by medications?

Key Questions
• Have you taken any antibiotics recently? Which one(s)?
• What prescription medications are you taking?
• What over-the-counter medications or preparations are you currently using?

Recent Treatment with Antibiotics

Pseudomembranous enterocolitis caused by *C. difficile* has been reported in individuals who have been recently treated with antibiotics, most commonly ampicillin, clindamycin, or cephalosporins. Pseudomembranous enterocolitis is a serious disorder that can lead to paralytic ileus. More often, antibiotics disturb the normal flora of the gut, leading to diarrhea.

Medications

Diarrhea can be caused by antacids that contain magnesium, and medications such as antibiotics, methyldopa, digitalis, β-blockers, systemic antiinflammatory agents, colchicine, quinidine, phenothiazine, high-dose salicylates, laxatives, and acetylcholinesterase inhibitors.

Could this be related to a surgical procedure?

Key Questions
- Have you had recent surgery?

Recent Gastrointestinal Surgery

Gastrointestinal surgery can result in dumping syndrome after the ingestion of meals. Inadequate mixing and digestion take place in the stomach, resulting in rapid transit and diarrhea. Anatomical derangement from surgery can also cause stagnant loops of bowel. This stagnation leads to bacterial overgrowth and results in diarrhea. Extensive bowel resection can produce short bowel syndrome, which results in diarrhea from malabsorption.

Is this diet related?

Key Questions
- How much fruit juice or soda do you drink in a day?
- Do you drink milk or eat milk products?
- Do you eat wheat products?
- What have you eaten in the past 3 days?

Excessive Intake of High-Carbohydrate Fluids

The ingestion of large amounts of apple juice or nonabsorbable fillers, such as sorbitol, can lead to malabsorptive diarrhea. Bacterial contamination of nonpasteurized apple juice can cause diarrhea.

Lactose Intolerance

The ingestion of specific disaccharides, such as lactose, produces a malabsorptive osmotic diarrhea in people with lactose intolerance.

Cow's Milk Protein or Soy Protein Hypersensitivity

The symptoms of diarrhea, vomiting, colic, occult blood in stool, grossly bloody stools, and white blood cells within the stool may be caused by protein hypersensitivity if they begin within 2 to 3 weeks after starting either cow's milk or soy formulas.

Celiac Sprue (Gluten Enteropathy)

Gluten enteropathy is manifested by increasing stool frequency, looseness, paleness, and bulkiness of stool that occurs within 3 to 6 months of dietary intake of wheat, rye, barley, or oat products. Patients have a hypersensitivity reaction to the protein in these grains. A gluten-free diet will alleviate symptoms.

Starvation Stools

The history of this condition includes diarrhea that persists for 2 to 3 weeks. Stools are loose because the liquid low-fiber diet used to ease the symptoms of acute diarrhea is continued for too long. Health care providers can neglect to tell patients or parents to resume a regular diet when acute diarrhea begins to resolve. New guidelines recommend feeding soon after rehydration has been achieved.

Could this be caused by food preparation problems?

Key Questions
- Have you recently eaten raw or undercooked poultry, seafood, or beef?
- Have you recently ingested unpasteurized milk?
- Do you prepare poultry or beef on the same surface as other foods?
- Is anyone else you know ill with similar symptoms?

Dietary Exposure to Infectious Agents

Undercooked poultry is a potential cause of Salmonella or *C. jejuni* diarrhea. Undercooked beef and unpasteurized milk are food sources that contain *E. coli* O157:H7. Raw shellfish is a potential source of Norwalk virus. Food can be contaminated through bacteria that remain on incompletely cleaned food preparation surfaces.

Other Ill People

Food poisoning should be considered if diarrhea develops in two or more individuals after ingestion of the same food. Such multiple occurrences suggest ingestion of infected food or toxic substances (e.g., lead, mercury).

Is there any family predisposition that can point to a cause?

Key Questions

• Have you or anyone in your family been diagnosed with cystic fibrosis?
• Does anyone in your family have a history of chronic diarrhea, ulcerative colitis, or IBD?

Family History of Cystic Fibrosis

Cystic fibrosis (CF) is the most common genetic disease in the white population. It has an autosomal recessive mode of inheritance. The condition leads to fat malabsorption and produces fatty, foul-smelling diarrhea.

Family History of Diarrheal Illnesses

Inflammatory bowel disease is genetically linked.

DIAGNOSTIC REASONING: FOCUSED PHYSICAL EXAMINATION

Inspect General Appearance

Observe the patient's general appearance. Diarrhea should be considered a symptom in all instances, and principal attention should be directed to determine and correct the cause.

Assess Hydration Status

Assessment of hydration status is the most important aspect of physical examination in the child. Dehydration in otherwise healthy adults is uncommon unless the diarrhea is very severe (Table 12.1). Hydration is also an important consideration in older adults, chronically ill people, and individuals who cannot replace fluid losses with oral intake. In the presence of hypernatremia, the state of dehydration might be greater than suggested by physical examination because extracellular fluid volume tends to be preserved, at the expense of intracellular volume.

Indicators of Hydration Status

Mucous membranes

The earliest clinical sign of dehydration is dryness of mucous membranes. Hyperventilation

---

| Table 12.1 | **Determining Hydration Status**[a] | | |

SIGNS OR SYMPTOMS	MILD DEHYDRATION	MODERATE DEHYDRATION	SEVERE DEHYDRATION
Estimated fluid deficit (% of body weight)	<5	>6–9	10
Estimated fluid deficit (mL/kg)	30–50	60–90	>100
Thirst	Increased	Marked increase	Very marked increase
Blood pressure	Normal	Postural drop only	Low or not measurable peripherally
Pulse (peripheral)	Normal	Rapid	Rapid, thready
Heart rate	Mildly elevated	Elevated	Greatly elevated
Mucous membranes	Thick saliva	Dry	Very dry
Eyes	Normal	Sunken	Deeply sunken
Tears when crying	Present	Absent	Absent
Skin turgor	Normal	Tenting	None
Fontanel	Normal	Sunken	Very sunken
Urine output	Mildly decreased	Decreased	Markedly decreased or absent
Affect/sensorium	Normal	Restlessness/irritability	Lethargy/coma

[a]Percent body weight loss = ([Normal weight − Present weight] ÷ Normal weight) × 100.

with mouth breathing can dry the mucous membranes of the mouth in the absence of dehydration. Recent vomiting makes the mucous membranes appear moist. The patient may also have halitosis.

Tissue turgor

Turgor reflects the amount of fluid in the interstitial spaces and is best assessed on the thigh, chest, and abdomen. Abdominal testing alone can be misleading because distention can mask the loss of turgor. Obese children often do not appear to have loss of skin turgor because of the elasticity of their skin.

Fontanel

The fontanel, if still open, is best assessed with the child in an upright position. The normal fontanel can feel tense in the infant who is supine. In a crying child, physiological bulging occurs only during expiration; this bulging disappears when the child relaxes or inspires. The fontanel will be sunken in a dehydrated state.

Peripheral perfusion

Blanching of the nail bed (using the sternum in the infant) with pressure and quick refill of capillary blood in less than 2 seconds is a normal finding. In dehydration, it takes longer for the blood to reappear in the tissue.

Measure urine output and specific gravity

In a mildly dehydrated child, the output decreases with a slight increase in specific gravity. In a moderately dehydrated child, the urinary output is decreased, and the specific gravity is increased. In a severely dehydrated child, the urinary output is decreased to oliguria, and the specific gravity is markedly increased, up to 1.030. Specific gravity is also the best indicator for dehydration in the older adult population.

Measure Temperature

An elevated temperature increases insensible water loss and can lead to more rapid dehydration. The presence of a fever in a patient with acute diarrhea indicates viral or bacterial infection. Fever in a patient with chronic diarrhea points to inflammatory causes.

The generally accepted normal basal body temperature is 37°C (98.6°F) determined orally or 0.6°C (1°F) or higher determined rectally. Fever is generally accepted as any oral temperature above 37.8°C (100°F).

Weigh Patient and Note Persistent or Involuntary Weight Loss

Lactose intolerance, CF, intestinal malabsorption, infectious diarrhea, and IBD can cause weight loss. Patients with these conditions have adequate or even increased food intake, but they cannot absorb sufficient nutrients to sustain normal nutrition. In children, this can cause failure to thrive and interruption of growth. In adults, colonic neoplasm can cause partial obstruction and diarrhea, and weight loss can be evident.

Observe Abdominal Contour

Abdominal distention can be associated with an ileus, as in enteritis, or with gaseous dilation resulting from malabsorption. A scaphoid abdomen can be seen in children with severe dehydration.

Auscultate the Abdomen

The major objective is to detect the presence of bowel sounds anywhere in the abdomen. Listen in all four quadrants. The absence of bowel sounds is established only after 5 minutes of continuous listening. Bowel sounds that are high pitched are heard with peristaltic rushes found in enteritis and secretory diarrhea. Bowel sounds are diminished or absent with necrotizing enterocolitis.

Palpate the Abdomen for Tenderness

Peritonitis can cause diarrhea as a result of inflammation and local enteric irritation. Signs of peritoneal irritation include a rigid abdomen, rebound tenderness (Blumberg sign), and abnormal findings on the following tests: iliopsoas muscle test, obturator muscle test, and heel jar test (Markle sign) (see Chapter 3). Tenderness is uncommon in self-limiting diarrhea. Localized right-lower-quadrant tenderness in a "sick" patient with acute diarrhea can indicate appendicitis, Crohn disease, right-sided diverticulitis, or carcinoma. Localized left-lower-quadrant tenderness suggests diverticulitis, fecal impaction, colon cancer, and various causes of proctocolitis. Localized pain in chronic diarrhea can also occur with IBS.

Perform a Digital Rectal Examination

Assess for fissures, hemorrhoids, and lacerations and feel for impacted stool. Impacted stool can be felt as a puttylike mass that fills the rectum and extends upward. Also obtain a stool sample for occult blood testing and laboratory studies. Observe stool on finger for color and the presence of blood.

Palpate Lymph Nodes

Evidence of systemic disease should be assessed. Chronic diarrhea in patients who have lymphadenopathy is associated with lymphoma and AIDS.

LABORATORY AND DIAGNOSTIC STUDIES

Laboratory or diagnostic studies are not necessary if the patient appears to have a viral or toxigenic bacterial infection because the disease is usually mild and self-limiting. Reserve stool cultures and examine for ova and parasites in patients who appear relatively ill, patients with signs of invasive or persistent diarrhea, and those who have a history of suspected parasite infection.

Fecal Leukocytes

Fecal leukocyte detection is an easy and inexpensive test that is 75% specific for bacterial diarrhea. Leukocytes are found in inflammatory diarrheal disease and are present in bacterial infections that invade the intestinal wall (*E. coli, Shigella* spp., and *Salmonella* spp.). Leukocytes are also present in diarrhea from ulcerative colitis, Crohn disease, and antibiotic use. Leukocytes are not seen in viral gastroenteritis, parasitic diarrhea, *Salmonella* carrier states, or enterotoxigenic bacterial diarrheas. Obtain a small fleck of mucus or stool. Do not allow the specimen to dry.

Place the specimen on a slide, add 2 drops of Löffler alkaline methylene blue stain, and wait 2 minutes. Microscopic white and red blood cells indicate the presence of Shigella, enterohemorrhagic *E. coli*, enteropathogenic *E. coli, Campylobacter* spp., *C. difficile,* or other inflammatory or invasive diarrhea.

Fecal Occult Blood Testing

Fecal occult blood testing (FOBT) is used to test for occult blood in the stool. Red blood cells often appear in diarrhea caused by enteropathic bacteria or protozoa. A 3-day series of stool samples is used to screen for colon cancer. Ingestion of red meats during the testing period can produce a false abnormal finding.

Fecal Immunochemical Test

Also called immunochemical FOBT (iFOBT), fecal immunochemical test (FIT) uses antibodies to human hemoglobin to detect a specific portion of a human blood protein in the stool. Immunochemical FOBTs are more specific for lower GI tract bleeding, as they target the globin portion of hemoglobin, which does not survive passage through the upper GI tract. Vitamins or foods do not affect the fecal immunochemical test, and some forms require only one or two stool specimens.

Fecal Fat

A 72-hour fecal fat analysis is done by instructing the patient to have a daily dietary intake of 100 g of fat for 3 days before and during a 72-hour period of stool collection. In children, a fat retention coefficient is determined. An abnormal result is greater than 6 g/day in the stool on an 80- to 100-g/day diet of fat and indicates a malabsorption syndrome.

D-Xylose Absorption Test

The d-xylose absorption test is used to determine whether diarrhea is caused by malabsorption or maldigestion. Blood is taken before the patient ingests the d-xylose. The patient is then asked to drink a fluid containing 25 g of d-xylose. Repeat venipuncture to obtain blood is performed in 2 hours for adults and 1 hour for children. Urine is collected approximately 5 hours after ingestion of the fluid. Blood and urine levels are subsequently evaluated. An abnormal result is found if less than 4.5 g of the d-xylose is excreted in a 5-hour urine collection, and blood levels are less than 25 to 40 mg/dL in adults (30 mg/dL in children). The abnormal result indicates the diarrhea is caused by malabsorption.

Stool pH

The pH of the stool specimen is determined by using litmus strips. A pH value of 5.5 indicates lactose or other carbohydrate malabsorption. Normal stool pH is neutral or weakly alkaline.

Wet Mount

Wet mounts are useful to assess for trophozoites, cysts, ova, and certain helminth larvae. Obtain a sample of feces on a wooden applicator stick, mix with 1 drop of saline, and add iodine contrast to view and examine under a microscope. *V. cholerae* can be identified by using dark-field microscopy. The characteristic darting motility of vibrios can be recognized in fresh wet preparations.

C. difficile Toxin Assay

This assay detects *C. difficile* toxin in the stool, which is diagnostic of clostridial enterocolitis. The clostridial bacterium releases a toxin that causes necrosis of the colonic epithelium.

Stool Culture

Stool culture is used to detect common bacteria such as *Enterococcus* spp., *E. coli, Proteus* spp., *Pseudomonas* spp., *Staphylococcus aureus, Candida albicans, Bacteroides* spp., and *Clostridia* spp. Special enriching techniques or media are necessary to look for some agents. Pathogenic bacteria are *Salmonella* spp., *Shigella* spp., *Campylobacter* spp., *Yersinia* spp., *E. coli, Staphylococcus* spp., and *C. difficile.*

Stool for Ova and Parasites

Stool can be tested for the presence of ova and parasites. Fresh stool is required to preserve the trophozoites of some parasites. Common parasites are *Ascaris lumbricoides* (hookworm) and *Strongyloides* spp. (tapeworm).

Giardia Antigen Test

Giardia antigen test is a solid phase immunoassay used for the detection of Giardia-specific antigen 65. Only one stool specimen is required, and the test result is available within 1 day.

Indirect Hemagglutinin Assay

The indirect hemagglutinin assay (IHA) detects antibodies to *E. histolytica.* An abnormal finding is a titer greater than 1:128.

Tissue Transglutaminase Antibody

Tissue transglutaminase antibody (tTG) IgA is the primary test ordered to screen for celiac disease. Elevated tissue transglutaminase immune globulin A (TTG IgA) antibody is sensitive and specific for celiac disease.

Molecular Testing

Molecular testing can be used to test for a variety of pathogens in the stool (see Differential Diagnosis table). The tests are both sensitive and specific.

Complete Blood Count with Differential

A complete blood count with differential should be obtained in severely ill or dehydrated patients to screen for infection. Infection is indicated with increased leukocytes. Microcytic hypochromic anemia (mean corpuscular hemoglobin concentration [MCHC] <30 g/dL; mean corpuscular volume [MCV] >85 fL) can indicate the presence of chronic disease. Most bloody diarrhea produces an elevated platelet count as an acute-phase reactant in an inflammatory process. In hemolytic uremic syndrome (HUS), the platelet count can be normal or low.

Peripheral Blood Smear

A peripheral blood smear is an examination of the cellular contents of the blood under a microscope using a variety of stains. Hemoglobin can be estimated by the depth of staining present. This quantitative analysis assists in characterizing a number of conditions, including hemolytic anemia associated with HUS. In HUS, the peripheral smear shows characteristic schistocytes.

Blood Urea Nitrogen and Creatinine

The blood urea nitrogen and creatinine tests are indicated in severely ill or dehydrated patients to ascertain adequate kidney functioning. Dehydration is a cause of prerenal failure. HUS will cause impaired renal function.

Endoscopic Studies

Further endoscopic diagnostic studies such as flexible sigmoidoscopy or colonoscopy should be considered when the cause of diarrhea is not determined or when the diarrhea lasts for longer than 1 month. Duodenal biopsy is indicated in patients with a high likelihood of celiac disease.

DIFFERENTIAL DIAGNOSIS

Acute Diarrhea

Viral gastroenteritis

Viral gastroenteritis presents with an explosive onset of diarrhea, vomiting, low-grade fever, anorexia, and myalgia. Symptoms last for 1 week or less. Norwalk virus is a major causative agent and is usually seen in school-age children and in adults. Rotavirus is the most common cause of diarrhea in children ages 6 to 24 months and is usually seen in the winter.

Shigella

Infection with *Shigella* organisms presents with acute diarrhea that contains mucus and blood. The patient has up to 7 days of watery diarrhea; then toxins are produced that result in ulceration, mucosal irritability, and frequent bowel movements. Stools are yellow or green and contain undigested food, mucus, and blood. Leukocytes and red blood cells are seen in the stools. It is the second most common cause of diarrhea in children ages 6 to 10 years old and is common in day-care settings. Symptoms of upper respiratory tract infection can also be present.

Cryptosporidium

This is one cell parasite found in the small intestine producing watery diarrhea that may last up to 2 weeks. In immunocompromised patients, the condition could be life threatening.

The parasite is found in water supplies, swimming pools, and lakes.

Giardia

Similar to *Cryptosporidium*, *Giardia* is a parasite that is found in areas of poor sanitation and in lakes and streams. Symptoms are abdominal bloating, cramps, and bouts of watery diarrhea. Giardia can be transmitted in food and person to person.

Food poisoning with staphylococci or Bacillus aureus

Food poisoning from staphylococci or *Bacillus aureus* causes explosive diarrhea 2 to 6 hours after eating. High attack rates are seen among people who have eaten contaminated food (improperly stored meats or custard-filled pastries). Cramping and vomiting in addition to diarrhea are present. There usually is no fever. The diarrhea lasts 18 to 24 hours, and the person recovers quickly. However, the condition could be life threatening in older adults and in those with other serious illness.

Food poisoning with Clostridium perfringens

Infection with *C. perfringens* causes severe diarrhea 8 to 20 hours after eating. The patient reports crampy abdominal pain and diarrhea. The stool is watery and nonbloody. Nausea, vomiting, and fever can be present but are less common. The diarrhea usually lasts for less than 3 days.

Salmonella

Infection with *Salmonella* organisms causes severe diarrhea and fever. It is seen more often in patients with AIDS, sickle cell disease, or reticuloendothelial dysfunction. The incubation period is 3 to 40 days with an insidious or abrupt onset. The patient has fever, anorexia, and weight loss. GI symptoms occur first followed by fever, abdominal cramps, and vomiting. Stools are green, loose, and slimy and have the odor of spoiled eggs. Rarely is blood present.

Campylobacter

Campylobacter infection causes fever, headache, and myalgia for 12 to 24 hours; then diarrhea develops. Roughly two-thirds of patients have watery diarrhea, and one-third have bloody dysentery. The incubation period is 2 to 5 days. The patient has abdominal cramping, pain, and fever, and the diarrhea contains mucus and blood. The condition can mimic appendicitis because of mesenteric lymphadenitis. Toxic megacolon and colonic hemorrhages can occur, especially if antimotility agents have been used.

Vibrio cholerae

V. cholerae infection causes severe watery diarrhea without a preceding illness. It usually occurs in epidemics. The onset is acute, usually 8 to 18 hours after the ingestion of contaminated seafood, water, or food prepared in contaminated water. Diarrhea resolves in 3 to 5 days. The essential element in cholera is the speed at which fluid is lost. This quick loss of fluid and dehydration can lead to death within hours. Red and white blood cells are not seen on stool examination.

Enterotoxic E. coli

E. coli causes moderate amounts of nonbloody diarrhea. This develops acutely 8 to 18 hours after the ingestion of contaminated food or water and typically lasts for 24 to 48 hours. The patient experiences cramping and abdominal pain with the diarrhea. The organism (gram-negative rod) is transmitted via the orofecal route. It is spread through contaminated water or incompletely cooked food that was rinsed in contaminated water, or through incompletely cooked beef, especially ground hamburger meat. Enterotoxic *E. coli* is the leading cause of traveler's diarrhea. The diagnosis can be confirmed with fecal leukocytes or stool culture.

Entamoeba histolytica

A patient with diarrhea caused by this parasite presents with large amounts of bloody diarrhea, abdominal cramping, and vomiting that develop acutely 12 to 24 hours after the ingestion of contaminated food or water. The diagnosis is confirmed through molecular testing or an IHA. Antibodies to *E. histolytica* are formed; a positive titer is greater than 1:128.

Antibiotic-induced diarrhea

This condition produces a mild, watery diarrhea and is caused by taking antibiotics, especially ampicillin, tetracycline, lincomycin, clindamycin, and chloramphenicol. The patient often reports crampy abdominal pain. Diagnosis is made through history and clinical findings.

Pseudomembranous colitis

Pseudomembranous colitis is caused most often by *C. difficile*. This diarrhea is induced by antibiotics, most commonly ampicillin, clindamycin, or cephalosporins. An acute inflammatory bowel disorder occurs, with symptoms that range from transient, mild diarrhea to active colitis with bloody diarrhea, abdominal pain, fever, and leukocytosis. Symptoms usually begin during a course of antibiotic therapy but can begin 1 to 10 days after treatment is completed. The diagnosis is established with sigmoidoscopy or colonoscopy. The diagnosis is confirmed with *C. difficile* toxin assay, stool culture, or molecular testing.

Necrotizing enterocolitis

Necrotizing enterocolitis is an inflammatory bowel condition that occurs in newborns. The patient is usually a premature or low-birth-weight infant who presents with feeding intolerance; vomiting; abdominal distention; lethargy; and loose, bloody stools containing mucus. It is the most common cause of death in the second week of life for low-birth-weight infants. Radiography shows pneumatosis intestinalis, indicating air within the subserosal bowel wall, which is the radiologic hallmark used to confirm the diagnosis.

Hemorrhagic disease of the newborn

Hemorrhagic disease of the newborn is caused by a deficiency in coagulation factors dependent on vitamin K. Most newborns do not have adequate levels of vitamin K, but bleeding problems develop in only a few. GI bleeding occurs 2 to 3 days postnatally. Laboratory studies typically show markedly elevated prothrombin time and partial thromboplastin time and depressed levels of vitamin K–dependent factors. The routine use of prophylactic vitamin K prevents most cases.

Hemolytic uremic syndrome

Hemolytic uremic syndrome is seen in children and is usually preceded by a GI illness. The leading bacterial cause of HUS in the United States is now *E. coli* O157:H7. The patient presents with a history of bloody diarrhea, fever, and irritability. Initially, laboratory blood values are essentially normal except that the platelet count is normal or low. The stool culture result is negative. A peripheral blood smear reveals schistocytes, confirming the diagnosis. Molecular testing confirms the pathogen. Fragmented red blood cells are often seen on the peripheral smear before complications of renal involvement occur. The child may have a sudden onset of acute renal failure. Renal function test results will be altered.

Chronic Diarrhea

Irritable bowel syndrome

Irritable bowel syndrome is commonly seen in young and middle-aged women with a history of intermittent diarrhea. The patient may report abdominal pain in the left lower quadrant, although it can occur anywhere. The pain seldom occurs at night, does not awaken the patient, and is commonly present in the morning. The patient can have rectal urgency or abdominal distention. There is no weight loss, the patient is afebrile, and the colon can be tender on palpation. IBS is a diagnosis of exclusion, and sigmoidoscopy or proctoscopy is used to rule out other disorders. The Rome IV criteria to diagnose IBS include abdominal pain associated with defecation or a change in bowel habits present at least 1 day per week on average during the preceding month.

Ulcerative colitis

Ulcerative colitis is an IBD that causes proctitis with rectal bleeding, tenesmus, and the passage of mucus. Abdominal cramping is common, but abdominal pain and tenderness are not common. The greater the extent of colon involvement, the greater the likelihood that the patient will have diarrhea.

Crohn disease

Crohn disease is an IBD that presents with abdominal cramping, tenderness, rectal bleeding, and diarrhea. The disease can produce chronic, bloody diarrhea and cause failure to thrive in children. The patient may have a fever. Weight loss is common because of malabsorption or a reduced intake of food used to minimize postprandial symptoms. Diagnosis is made through colonoscopy and biopsy.

 EVIDENCE-BASED PRACTICE *The Utility of Symptoms in Diagnosing Irritable Bowel Syndrome*

A systematic review was conducted on the accuracy of symptoms in diagnosing irritable bowel syndrome (IBS). In six studies evaluating 1077 patients, symptoms of lower abdominal pain, mucus per rectum, incomplete evacuation, loose or frequent stools associated with pain, pain relieved by defecation, and patient-reported abdominal distention were reviewed. Each of these symptoms had limited accuracy in diagnosing IBS. Lower abdominal pain had the highest sensitivity (90%) but poor specificity (32%); patient-reported visible abdominal distention had the highest specificity (77%) but low sensitivity (39%).

Reference: Ford et al, 2008

Carbohydrate malabsorption and lactose intolerance

Malabsorption or lactose intolerance causes the patient to experience diarrhea, bloating, and increased flatus. The ingestion of specific disaccharides, such as lactose or sorbitol, exacerbates the episodes of diarrhea. A trial of elimination of offending foods often confirms the clinical diagnosis.

Fat malabsorption

Fat malabsorption is seen with patients who have CF or vitamin A, D, or K deficiency. Patients with CF have foul, pale, bulky diarrhea that is greasy, oily, and consistent with steatorrhea. The diarrhea usually precedes lung involvement. Laboratory testing for fat malabsorption includes a 72-hour fecal fat analysis.

Toddler's diarrhea

Toddler's diarrhea is described as the occurrence of abnormal amounts of formless stools with mucus in children ages 1 to 3 years. Symptoms rarely persist beyond age 4 to 5 years. The diarrhea is chronic and nonspecific, with three or four stools per day, some containing mucus. Physical examination and growth are within normal limits for the child's age. This is a diagnosis of exclusion, and other causes of chronic diarrhea must first be ruled out.

Celiac sprue or protein hypersensitivity

This diarrhea causes increasing stool frequency and loose, pale, and bulky stool, 3 to 6 months after dietary intake of wheat, rye, and other grains. Patients have a hypersensitivity reaction to the protein in wheat, rye, barley, and oats. Children appear lethargic, irritable, and anorexic. Serologic testing for antibodies is useful in excluding the diagnosis in individuals at low risk. Those at moderate to high risk should have both serologic testing and small bowel biopsy to confirm diagnosis.

Giardia spp.

Infection with *Giardia* spp. is the leading parasitic cause of chronic diarrhea in children in the United States and can be contracted through travel both inside and outside of the country. Patients experience watery, foul-smelling diarrhea, abdominal pain, distention, and gas.

Cryptosporidium spp. and Isospora belli

Cryptosporidium spp. and *Isospora belli* are parasites that produce recurrent episodes of nonbloody diarrhea with varying amounts of water. The volume can be massive. The organisms are transmitted via the fecal–oral route and are spread through the ingestion of contaminated water or direct orofecal contact.

Postgastrectomy dumping syndrome

This syndrome occurs after GI surgery. The condition can occur whenever the pyloric mechanism is disrupted by pyloroplasty, gastroduodenostomy, or gastrojejunostomy. The diarrhea occurs after meals because of increased transit of food through the colon. Patients can experience associated symptoms, including diaphoresis and tachycardia.

Diabetic enteropathy

Diabetic enteropathy occurs in patients with diabetes. Patients can experience nocturnal diarrhea, postprandial vomiting, and fatty stools from malabsorption. The condition is a diagnosis of exclusion in people with diabetes.

HIV enteropathy

HIV enteropathy has an insidious onset and is recurrent. Patients have large amounts of nonbloody diarrhea and mild to moderate nausea and vomiting. It is caused by direct infection of mucosa and neuronal cells in the GI system. Patients will demonstrate other HIV-related symptoms and lymphadenopathy.

Medication-induced diarrhea

Diarrhea can occur as a result of taking prescription or over-the-counter drugs; the most common ones are antacids that contain magnesium, antibiotics, methyldopa, digitalis, β-blockers, systemic antiinflammatory agents, colchicine, quinidine, phenothiazine, high doses of salicylates, and laxatives.

> **DIFFERENTIAL DIAGNOSIS OF** *Common Causes of Acute Diarrhea*

CONDITION	HISTORY	PHYSICAL FINDINGS	DIAGNOSTIC STUDIES
Viral gastroenteritis (e.g., Norwalk or rotavirus viral agents)	Abrupt onset 6–12 hr after exposure; nonbloody, watery diarrhea; lasts <1 wk; nausea or vomiting, fever, abdominal pain, tenesmus	In children, can see severe dehydration; hyperactive bowel sounds, diffuse pain on abdominal palpation	Molecular testing
Shigella (gram-negative rod; fecal–oral transmission; common in day-care setting)	Acute onset 12–24 hr after exposure; lasts 3–7 days; large amounts of bloody diarrhea with abdominal cramping and vomiting	Lower abdominal tenderness, hyperactive bowel sounds, no peritoneal irritation	Fecal leukocytes, positive stool culture; molecular testing
Staphylococcus aureus food poisoning (gram-positive cocci; from improperly stored meats or custard-filled pies)	Acute onset 2–6 hr after ingestion; lasts 18–24 hr; large amounts of watery, nonbloody diarrhea; cramping and vomiting	Hyperactive bowel sounds	Fecal leukocytes, negative stool culture; molecular testing
Clostridium perfringens food poisoning (gram-positive rod; from contaminated food)	Acute onset 8–20 hr after ingestion; lasts 12–24 hr; large amounts of watery, nonbloody diarrhea; abdominal pain and cramping	Hyperactive bowel sounds, diffuse pain on abdominal palpation	Fecal leukocytes, negative anaerobic culture of stool; molecular testing
Salmonella food poisoning (gram-negative bacilli; ingestion of contaminated food, poultry, eggs)	Acute onset 12–24 hr after ingestion; lasts 2–5 days; moderate to large amounts of nonbloody diarrhea; abdominal cramping and vomiting	Fever of 38.3°–38.9°C (101°–102°F) common; hyperactive bowel sounds, diffuse abdominal pain	Fecal leukocytes, positive stool culture, WBC count normal; molecular testing
Campylobacter jejuni (gram-negative rod; fecal–oral transmission; household pet)	Acute onset 3–5 days after exposure; lasts 3–7 days; moderate amounts of bloody diarrhea	Fever, lower quadrant abdominal pain	Fecal leukocytes, positive stool culture; molecular testing

► DIFFERENTIAL DIAGNOSIS OF *Common Causes of Acute Diarrhea—cont'd*

CONDITION	HISTORY	PHYSICAL FINDINGS	DIAGNOSTIC STUDIES
Vibrio cholerae (gram-negative rod; fecal–oral transmission; ingestion of contaminated water, seafood, or food)	Acute onset 8–24 hr after ingestion of contaminated food; lasts 3–5 days; large amounts of non-bloody, watery, painless diarrhea; can be mild or fulminate	Cyanotic, scaphoid abdomen, poor skin turgor, thready peripheral pulses, voice faint	Fecal leukocytes, negative stool culture; molecular testing
Enterotoxic *Escherichia coli* (gram-negative rod; fecal–oral transmission; ingestion of contaminated water or food)	Acute onset 8–18 hr after ingestion of contaminated food/water; lasts 24–48 hr; moderate amounts of non-bloody diarrhea; pain, cramping, abdominal pain; adults in United States generally do not develop illness from enterotoxic *E. coli*	No fever; dehydration is major complication	Fecal leukocytes, positive stool culture; molecular testing
Entamoeba histolytica parasite (cysts in food and water, from feces)	Acute onset 12–24 hr after ingestion of contaminated food or water; large amounts of bloody diarrhea; abdominal cramping and vomiting	Right lower quadrant abdominal pain; in small number of cases hepatic abscess forms	IHA: antibodies to *E. histolytica*; positive titer is >1:128; molecular testing
Antibiotic-induced diarrhea (begins after taking antibiotics)	Mild, watery diarrhea; crampy abdominal pain	Diffuse abdominal pain on palpation, fever absent	Usually not needed
Pseudomembranous colitis (antibiotic-induced *Clostridium difficile*)	Induced by antibiotics, most commonly ampicillin, clindamycin, or cephalosporins; symptoms range from transient mild diarrhea to active colitis with bloody diarrhea, abdominal pain, fever	Lower quadrant tenderness, fever	CBC: leukocytes; sigmoidoscopy/colonoscopy; *C. difficile* toxin assay or stool culture; *C. difficile* toxin; molecular testing
Hemolytic uremic syndrome (HUS) (primary cause of HUS in United States is *E. coli* O157:H7)	Children age <4 yr with history of gastroenteritis; history of bloody diarrhea, fever, and irritability	Fever, irritability; can have oliguria or anuria	CBC, platelet count, renal function tests, peripheral blood smear; negative stool culture; molecular testing

Continued

▶ **DIFFERENTIAL DIAGNOSIS OF** *Common Causes of Acute Diarrhea—cont'd*

CONDITION	HISTORY	PHYSICAL FINDINGS	DIAGNOSTIC STUDIES
Necrotizing enterocolitis	Premature or low-birth-weight infant who presents with feeding intolerance	Vomiting, abdominal distention, lethargy, loose stools with blood and mucous	Refer
Hemorrhagic disease of the newborn	GI bleeding 2–3 days postnatal; history of lack of vitamin K injection; history of mother on anticonvulsants prenatally	Bruising, ecchymoses, mild to moderate bleeding	Laboratory studies typically show markedly elevated PT and PTT with depressed levels of vitamin K–dependent factors

CBC, complete blood count; *IHA*, indirect hemagglutinin assay; *PT*, prothrombin time; *PTT*, partial thromboplastin time; *WBC*, white blood cell.

▶ **DIFFERENTIAL DIAGNOSIS OF** *Common Causes of Chronic Diarrhea*

CONDITION	HISTORY	PHYSICAL FINDINGS	DIAGNOSTIC STUDIES
Irritable bowel syndrome (IBS)	IBS-D: loose stools >25% of the time and hard stools <25% of the time IBS-M: both hard and soft stools >25 of the time Mucus with stool; seldom occurs at night or awakens patient; commonly present in morning; can have rectal urgency; episodes often triggered by stress or ingestion of food; affects women three times as often as men	Tender colon on palpation; can have abdominal distention; no weight loss; afebrile	Diagnosis of exclusion; sigmoidoscopy, proctoscopy
Ulcerative colitis (distal colon is most severely affected and rectum is involved)	History of severe diarrhea with gross blood in stools, no growth retardation; few reports of pain; age of onset second and third decades with small peak during adolescence; positive family history	Overt rectal bleeding; initially no fever, weight loss, or pain on palpation of abdomen; moderate colitis: weight loss, fever, abdominal tenderness	CBC shows leukocytosis or anemia, ESR elevated; stool cultures to rule out other causes of diarrhea; colonoscopy

DIFFERENTIAL DIAGNOSIS OF *Common Causes of Chronic Diarrhea—cont'd*

CONDITION	HISTORY	PHYSICAL FINDINGS	DIAGNOSTIC STUDIES
Crohn disease (associated with uveitis, erythema nodosum)	History of chronic bloody diarrhea with abdominal cramping, tenderness, and rectal bleeding; in children a history of growth retardation, weight loss, moderate diarrhea, abdominal pain, and anorexia	Weight loss; rare gross rectal bleeding; fistulas common	Colonoscopy with biopsies
Carbohydrate malabsorption	Bloating, flatus, diarrhea exacerbated by ingestion of certain disaccharides (e.g., lactose, milk, milk products); can follow viral gastroenteritis	Diffuse abdominal pain	Trial elimination of offending foods
Fat malabsorption	Greasy, fatty, malodorous stools; associated with deficiencies of vitamins K, A, and D; cystic fibrosis	Rectal prolapse, poor weight gain, abdominal distention	72-hr fecal fat, sweat test
Toddler's diarrhea	Three or four stools/day; some contain mucus; rare past age 4–5 yr	Physical examination and growth normal	Clinical diagnosis
Celiac sprue or protein hypersensitivity (reaction to protein in wheat, rye, barley, and oats)	Increased stool frequency, looseness, paleness, and bulkiness of stool within 3–6 mo of dietary onset; children are lethargic, irritable, and anorectic; peak frequency 9–18 mo	Failure to thrive, abdominal distention, irritability, muscle wasting	IgA anti tTG antibodies Clinical findings, improvement on gluten-free diet, CBC, anemia, folate deficiency, radiography, biopsy
Giardia spp. parasite (primary cause of chronic diarrhea in children)	Watery, foul diarrhea; common in day care, among travelers	Low-grade fever, weight loss; chronic form: fatigue, growth retardation, steatorrhea	Giardia antigen test; molecular testing
Cryptosporidium spp. or *Isospora belli* protozoan parasites (fecal–oral transmission; ingestion of contaminated water or direct oral–anal contact)	Recurrent episodes; variable amounts watery, nonbloody diarrhea; amounts can be massive	Weight loss, severe right upper quadrant abdominal pain with biliary tract involvement	Stool for O&P Antigen Test; molecular testing

Continued

DIFFERENTIAL DIAGNOSIS OF *Common Causes of Chronic Diarrhea—cont'd*

CONDITION	HISTORY	PHYSICAL FINDINGS	DIAGNOSTIC STUDIES
Postgastrectomy dumping syndrome	After GI surgery, diarrhea occurs after meals because of increased transit of food through colon	Diaphoresis and tachycardia	Upper GI series
Diabetic enteropathy	Nocturnal diarrhea, postprandial vomiting, fatty stools from malabsorption	Findings associated with diabetes	Diagnosis of exclusion in diabetic people
HIV enteropathy (direct infection of mucosa and neuronal cells in GI system)	Insidious onset, recurrent large amounts of non-bloody diarrhea, mild to moderate nausea or vomiting	Findings associated with HIV infection	Testing for HIV
Medication-induced diarrhea	Mild to moderately severe nonwatery, nonbloody diarrhea	No specific findings related to diarrhea	Usually none needed

CBC, complete blood count; *ESR*, erythrocyte sedimentation rate; *GI*, gastrointestinal; *HIV*, human immunodeficiency virus; *O&P*, ova and parasites.

13 Dizziness

Dizziness is a symptom of a variety of conditions, including vertigo, lightheadedness, and loss of balance. In children, the symptom is frequently a new sensation and is usually poorly defined. Family members often state that the child has trouble walking or is irritable or that the child's behavior is different. Older children, like adults, tend to categorize everything from lightheadedness and unsteadiness to spinning and falling as dizziness. This chapter is limited to the discussion of vertigo. Patients with vertigo have the sensation of either their body moving (subjective vertigo) or their environment moving around them (objective), usually described as a spinning or rotary motion.

The sensation of balance depends on interconnections among the visual, vestibular, and sensory systems. Vertigo can be thought of as a disruption of one of these three systems. Vertigo can be central, involving the brainstem or cerebellum; be peripheral, involving the inner ear or vestibular apparatus; or result from systemic causes.

Central vertigo is generally either neoplastic or vascular in origin, although any central nervous system disorder, such as multiple sclerosis, that disrupts the pathway between the vestibular apparatus and the brain can result in dizziness. Common vascular causes include recurrent intermittent vascular insufficiency, transient ischemic attack, or stroke. Migraine headache is a vascular-related central cause of vertigo.

Peripheral vertigo is typically produced by disruption of the inner ear or vestibular apparatus. Common causes include idiopathic etiologies, canalithiasis (tiny crystals of calcium carbonate migrate from their usual position to the semicircular canals), vestibular nerve inflammation, inner ear inflammation or infection, or tumor. Systemic origins include psychogenic, cardiovascular, and metabolic causes. Mixed or other causes include trauma and ototoxicity.

DIAGNOSTIC REASONING: FOCUSED HISTORY

What does the patient mean by dizziness?

Key Questions
- Can you describe how you feel when you are dizzy?
- Do you feel yourself or the room spinning?
- Do you feel your balance is off?
- Do you feel like you are about to faint?

Sensation

Vertigo produces the sensation of either the patient spinning or the environment spinning around the patient. Some patients describe a sensation of their body moving forward or accelerating.

Patients can also report loss of equilibrium accompanying the vertigo. Neoplasms and progressive vestibule loss typically produce a change in vestibular function that is slow in onset and manifested as imbalance.

Loss of balance and lack of coordination in the absence of vertigo can be the result of degenerative, neoplastic, vascular, or metabolic disorders. With these symptoms, look for other nervous system abnormalities. Imbalance can also occur in adults as a result of impaired sensory input, either visual or kinetic, such as occurs with peripheral neuropathy.

When interviewing children, using words such as *swinging* or *being on a merry-go-round* helps give them ways to describe the feeling. Children who have a vague sense of unsteadiness can have peripheral neuropathy or a dysfunction of the vestibular or cerebellar system, but children who report a feeling of motion are more likely to have an abnormality of the vestibular system.

In contrast to dizziness and imbalance, lightheadedness is the feeling that one is about to faint (near syncope). Some patients describe it as a generalized weakness and the feeling that they are about to pass out if they do not lie down. True syncope, or a sudden transient loss of consciousness, with concurrent loss of postural tone, always has a spontaneous recovery (see Chapter 33).

Orthostatic hypotension is a frequent cause of lightheadedness and is most common in older patients, occurring as a result of abnormal regulation of blood pressure. Neurologic causes of orthostatic hypotension are less common and are usually accompanied by neurologic findings.

In both children and adults, a report of lightheadedness can accompany anemia, hypoglycemia, or hyperventilation syndrome.

Is the vertigo from a systemic cause?

Key Questions
- What other health problems do you have?
- Would you describe yourself as anxious or nervous?
- Do the episodes occur with any specific activity or movement?

Other Health Problems

Cardiovascular problems are a common cause of vertigo that is systemic in origin. The mechanism of vertigo can include vasomotor instability that decreases systemic vascular resistance, venous return, or both; severe reduction in cardiac output that obstructs blood flow within the heart or pulmonary circulation; or cardiac dysrhythmia that leads to transient decline in cardiac output. Patients with hypertension can experience vertigo while taking antihypertensives, potassium-depleting medications, or as a result of postural hypotension.

Anxiety

Psychogenic dizziness is one of the most common causes of vertigo. Symptoms tend to be vague and can include other symptoms

such as fatigue, fullness in the head, lightheadedness, and a sense of feeling apart from the environment. Patients may describe themselves as anxious or nervous. Patients can also have other psychiatric diagnoses. Stressors and tensions affecting children, such as divorce, custody battles, and day care, can cause vertiginous-like symptoms in an older child. Anxiety with hyperventilation can cause lightheadedness in a child, who then reports the symptom as dizziness.

Relationship to Activity or Movement

Dizziness when turning, especially when rolling over in bed, is usually caused by vertigo. However, unsteadiness while walking is considered to be disequilibrium, which can be caused by many factors. Dizziness on standing can be the result of decreased cerebral perfusion.

In children, episodes of dizziness that occur with sudden changes of posture can be the result of hypotension, vascular disease, or positional vertigo.

Is the vertigo central (brainstem or cerebellar) or peripheral (vestibular) in origin?

Key Questions
- Do you have migraine headaches?
- Do you have other symptoms that bother you?
- Do you have nausea and vomiting?
- When do the episodes occur?

Headaches

Headache is a vascular-related cause of central vertigo. Approximately one-third of patients with migraine headaches experience vertigo. The vertigo can appear as an aura occurring during the headache or separately. Patients with vestibular-type migraine headaches often experience photophobia, phonophobia, and visual aura during the episodes of vertigo. Patients with basilar-type migraines can have other symptoms consistent with vertebrobasilar vascular abnormalities such as visual changes, tinnitus, decreased hearing, ataxia, or paresthesia. Migraine, both with and without headache, is recognized as a source of dizziness in children.

Other Symptoms

Patients with central vertigo nearly always have neurologic symptoms such as double vision, facial numbness, and hemiparesis.

Cerebellar causes can produce other symptoms, such as loss of balance, that closely resemble those of a peripheral disorder; therefore neurologic examination findings are important in differentiating the two. Pay particular attention to reports of motor dysfunction or lack of coordination.

Vertigo that is peripheral in origin does not produce additional neurologic signs or symptoms. If the patient has nausea and vomiting, suspect a peripheral vestibular apparatus problem rather than a central cause. Nausea and vomiting are common with vestibular neuronitis and labyrinthitis and occur less often with brainstem lesions.

Timing

Vertigo that occurs on first arising in the morning is usually the result of a vestibular disorder. Vertigo that occurs while turning over in bed is characteristic of benign paroxysmal positional vertigo (BPPV).

What do characteristics of the episodes tell me?

Key Questions

• How long do the episodes of dizziness last?
• Is the onset sudden or gradual?
• Do you have any hearing loss?
• Do you have ringing in your ears?

Duration of Episodes

Episodes that last a few seconds are typically caused by BPPV and are usually elicited by rapid head movement. Episodes lasting minutes to hours can be caused by Ménière disease or recurrent vestibulopathy.

Episodes that last days or weeks are commonly produced by vestibular neuronitis. Patients usually feel better when they lie completely still. Stroke can also produce long-lasting episodes. The two can be differentiated based on medical history and physical examination findings.

Sudden onset of prolonged dizziness (lasting ≥60 minutes) suggests central causes such as infection, brainstem infarction, inflammation, or vestibular hemorrhage. Trauma can also produce prolonged dizziness.

The child with chronic recurrent dizziness (episodes lasting <30 minutes) can have central causes such as seizure problems or migraine headache. The cause can also be peripheral, such as BPPV. Chronic persistent episodes can indicate brainstem lesions, anemia, diabetes, thyrotoxicosis, or a psychosomatic disorder.

Onset

A gradual onset of dizziness is typical of an acoustic neuroma or other neoplastic process that is slow-growing. BPPV can also have a gradual onset.

Acute or sudden onset of vertigo is characteristic of labyrinthitis, Ménière disease, stroke, or vertebrobasilar causes.

Recurrent episodes are typical of BPPV, vertebrobasilar causes, and Ménière disease.

Hearing Loss and Tinnitus

A classic triad of symptoms—vertigo, hearing loss, and tinnitus—defines Ménière disease. Patients can also report a sensation of fullness in the ears. The hearing loss can be unilateral or bilateral. Patients with secondary or early tertiary syphilis can have symptoms identical to those of Ménière disease. Tinnitus, hearing loss, and ear pain point to lesions in the inner ear or acoustic nerve (cranial nerve [CN] VIII).

Patients with labyrinthitis and perilymphatic fistulas may also experience hearing loss but without tinnitus. An acoustic neuroma will produce unilateral hearing loss with tinnitus. Patients with recurrent vestibulopathy usually do not report hearing loss.

What else should I consider?

Key Questions

• What medications are you taking?
• Are you now or have you recently been ill?

- Have you had any recent injury to your head? Did you have dizziness before the head injury?
- Have you had any previous ear surgery?

Medications

Mediations that are salt-retaining or ototoxic can produce vertigo, lightheadedness, or unsteadiness. Salt-retaining drugs include steroids and phenylbutazone. Ototoxic medications include ethacrynic acid, streptomycin, gentamicin, aminoglycosides, aspirin, and furosemide.

Psychotropic drugs can also produce vertigo. Antihypertensive drugs can cause hypotension leading to lightheadedness. Sedatives, alcohol, and anticonvulsants can cause a sense of disequilibrium.

Current or Recent Illness

Vestibular neuronitis is associated with recent viral infection, often an upper respiratory tract infection. If a patient is currently ill, consider labyrinthitis because it is frequently associated with concomitant bacterial and viral infection. Current ear or sinus infection can produce dysfunction of the vestibular apparatus, resulting in vertigo. Recent abnormalities of middle ear ventilation and middle ear effusion are the most common cause of balance disturbance in childhood. In balance disturbance, transmission of pressure gradients through the labyrinthine windows to the inner ear fluids and the vestibular sensory receptors is altered.

History of Head Trauma

Trauma to the head or ear can cause disturbance of both peripheral and central balance mechanisms. Certain traumas can cause acute destruction of the inner ear and produce vertigo. Direct trauma can occur to the labyrinth from a temporal bone fracture. A blow to the head or a whiplash injury can also produce a concussive effect on the labyrinth. Children who have a history of head trauma can present with vertigo caused by labyrinthine damage.

Vertigo often occurs as a residual symptom and usually gradually improves over the course of a year. Trauma can also produce a fistula between the middle and inner ear, causing tympanic membrane (TM) damage and ossicle disruption.

Previous Otology History and Procedures

Patients with cholesteatoma usually have a history of chronic middle ear infection, otorrhea, and conductive hearing loss. Prior surgical procedures of the ear can produce peripheral vertigo through disruption of the vestibular apparatus or through formation of a perilymph fistula.

DIAGNOSTIC REASONING: FOCUSED PHYSICAL EXAMINATION

Take Vital Signs and Note Blood Pressure

Assess orthostatic blood pressure to rule out postural hypotension as the cause of vertigo. Assessment is made by measuring the blood pressure in both the supine and standing positions. A drop in arterial blood pressure of at least 30 mm Hg systolic and 20 diastolic mm Hg when the patient changes from the supine to the standing position indicates orthostatic hypotension.

Note General Appearance

In a patient who is currently ill, suspect labyrinthitis. In a patient who is acutely nauseated and vomiting, suspect vestibular neuronitis.

Have the Patient Hyperventilate and Perform Valsalva Maneuver

Perform this testing if you suspect psychogenic vertigo because the maneuver can reproduce the vertigo in these patients. Ask the patient to perform a Valsalva maneuver and to breathe in and out or blow vigorously for 1 to 3 minutes.

Perform Vision Examination

A recent change in visual acuity or new corrective lenses can cause transient episodes of imbalance.

Perform Ear Examination

Look for the presence of effusion or infection that signals serous otitis or otitis media. Look for the presence of a cholesteatoma. It will appear as a shiny, white, irregular mass; foul-smelling discharge can also be present. Note the integrity of the TM; trauma can sometimes cause its disruption. Perform pneumatic otoscopy (see Chapter 15), which will enable you to determine whether changes in pressure trigger an episode of vertigo. If the patient has a fistula, changes in pressure transmitted directly to the inner ear will cause a sudden episode of vertigo.

Perform Screening Hearing Tests

Perform Rinne (air conduction [AC] greater than bone conduction [BC]) and Weber (lateralization) tests. Expect sensorineural loss with Ménière disease, labyrinthitis, perilymph fistula, and acoustic neuroma. In sensorineural loss, the sound lateralizes to the unaffected ear. With sensorineural hearing loss, bone and air conductions are both reduced in Rinne tests but the ratio remains the same (AC greater than BC). Patients with a cholesteatoma, serous otitis, or otitis media may have conductive hearing loss (see Differential Diagnosis table).

Assess Nystagmus

A test for nystagmus assesses the function of the vestibular branch of the acoustic nerve (CN VIII). The presence and characteristics of nystagmus are important in determining central versus peripheral causes of vertigo. Nystagmus is defined by the axis on which it occurs (horizontal, vertical, rotary, or mixed) and by the direction in which it occurs. Nystagmus is composed of quick and slow components that can be observed. With the eye fixated, a slow drift away from the position of fixation is corrected by a quick movement back to the original position. The direction of the nystagmus is determined by the quick component because it is easier to see. The quick component depends on the interaction between the vestibular system and the cerebral cortex and represents the compensatory response to vestibular stimulation. The slow component moves in the direction of the movement of the endolymph, a clear fluid within the membranous labyrinth of the inner ear.

Fixed nystagmus, which always beats in the same direction, occurs with peripheral disorders of BPPV, Ménière disease, vestibular neuronitis, or labyrinthitis. Vestibular nystagmus typically consists of a horizontal-rotary, jerk motion of both the slow and fast components. The nystagmus associated with central causes can be horizontal, vertical, rotary, or inconsistent. Pronounced rotary, unidirectional upgaze or downgaze nystagmus always arises from central processes. Nystagmus that is equally rapid in both directions is characteristic of central causes. In vertigo of peripheral origin, nystagmus generally resolves on fixation within 24 to 48 hours, whereas nystagmus associated with central vertigo does not. See Table 13.1 for a comparison of characteristics.

Perform Positional Nystagmus Testing or Provoking Maneuvers

If the patient does not have nystagmus at rest, perform position testing or provocation maneuvers.

Table 13.1   Comparison of Nystagmus in Central and Peripheral Vertigo

CHARACTERISTICS	CENTRAL	PERIPHERAL
Severity	Can be disproportionate to vertigo	Proportionate to vertigo
Axis	Horizontal, vertical, rotary; unidirectional upgaze or downgaze	Horizontal, rotary
Consistency of direction	Can be inconsistent	Consistent; always beats in same direction
Type	Irregular or rapid in both directions	Has both slow and quick components

Positional maneuver (Dix-Hallpike maneuver)

To determine the origin of vertigo and accompanying nystagmus, seat the patient on the table with the patient's head turned to the left or right at 45 degrees. Holding the head in this position, quickly lower the patient to a lying position with the head 20 to 30 degrees lower than the table edge so that the ear faces the floor. Repeat with the head turned to the other side and then again with the head in the midline. The maneuver produces intense vertigo in patients with vestibular problems and can cause mild vertigo in patients with central causes. The patient's eyes should be kept open to observe the duration and direction of nystagmus. The nystagmus associated with peripheral causes has a 3- to 10-second delay in onset, lessens with repetition, and is in a fixed direction (see Evidence-Based Practice box). In contrast, the nystagmus associated with central causes begins immediately, does not fatigue with repetition, and can occur in any and changing directions. With inner ear damage, the rapid phase of nystagmus is always in the same direction regardless of the direction of gaze. For a demonstration of the maneuver, see http://www.youtube.com.

Provocation maneuvers

In patients who experience vertigo associated with position changes or rapid movement of the head, provoke nystagmus and vertigo by having the patient assume the positions that cause the vertigo. Provocation assists in the diagnosis of BPPV. If you suspect a perilymph fistula, perform pneumatic otoscopy. The pressure applied to the middle ear can provoke nystagmus and vertigo.

Assess the Vestibular Ocular Reflex

Assessment of the vestibular ocular reflex (VOR) is useful in confirming a vestibular origin of vertigo and in determining which labyrinth is abnormal. This is demonstrated when the head is moved in the direction of the damaged labyrinth (or vestibular nerve). Assess the VOR using the head impulse (head thrust test) (Fig. 13.1). The test

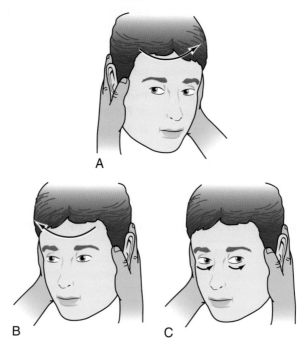

A

B   **C**

FIGURE 13.1 Vestibular ocular reflex or head thrust test. (From Cameron MH, Monroe LG: *Physical rehabilitation: Evidence-based examination, evaluation, and intervention,* St. Louis, 2007, Saunders.)

EVIDENCE-BASED PRACTICE *Dix-Hallpike Maneuver to Diagnose Benign Paroxysmal Positional Vertigo*

In this systematic review, the authors conclude that the reference standard for benign paroxysmal positional vertigo (BPPV) is a positive Dix-Hallpike maneuver (intense vertigo and fixed nystagmus with a 3- to 10-second delay in onset). The conclusion is based on randomized trials that demonstrate the success of canalith repositioning procedures in patients with no focal neurologic findings or central nervous system disease, whose diagnosis of BPPV is confirmed with the Dix-Hallpike maneuver. The randomized trials demonstrated that within 1 month of treatment, patients with a positive Dix-Hallpike maneuver benefit from the repositioning procedures with symptom resolution and that the Dix-Hallpike maneuver result returns to normal.

Reference: David et al, 2009.

assesses horizontal semicircular canal function. Hold the patient's head and ask him or her to fixate on your nose. Then very quickly thrust the patients head to one side. In healthy patients, the VOR is intact, and when the head is rotated, the eyes will remain fixed on your nose regardless of the head position. If the VOR is unilaterally impaired, when the head is rotated, the patient's eyes will momentarily move with the head and lose their fixation on your nose. Look for one or more catch-up corrective eye movements directed back toward your nose. This quick corrective eye movement is the abnormality. Carry out several trials in each direction, in no recognizable pattern. In a patient with a labyrinthine abnormality, the eyes will move with the head when turned to the side of the abnormality.

Perform Neurologic Examination

Look for brainstem or cerebellar dysfunction, which could cause abnormal neurologic findings. Specifically test CNs, looking for sensory and motor deficits. With the exception of hearing loss, CN function should be normal in patients with peripheral vertigo. Patients with brainstem dysfunction typically have diplopia and changes in sensory and motor function.

Test cerebellar function. Testing gait differences while the patient is blindfolded can be helpful. Whereas ataxia from bilateral vestibular loss is worsened by loss of visual input, ataxia from cerebellar disease remains about the same. The sensitivity of gait testing is increased by watching tandem gait (heel to toe). When trying to walk a straight line, a patient with a cerebellar lesion will tend to fall toward the side of the lesion. However, gait disturbances can also be present with peripheral vertigo.

Test the patient's ability to perform rapid alternating movements (RAMs) either through pronation-supination or through touching thumb to fingers sequentially. Movements should be smooth and rhythmic, and the patient should be able to gradually increase speed. Stiff, slowed, or jerky movements indicate cerebellar dysfunction.

Perform the past-pointing test. Have the patient sit with one arm extended forward and the index finger pointed while you sit in the same position facing the patient. The tips of your fingers should touch. Then ask the patient to close the eyes, raise the arm above the head, and bring the arm and finger back to the same position. In patients with central lesions or unilateral vestibular abnormalities, the arm will deviate toward the side of the lesion.

Test sensory and motor function. Look for focal deficits that can occur with central vertigo. Many patients with vertigo also report generalized weakness; therefore, it is important to distinguish between generalized weakness and focal motor impairment caused by brainstem disorder.

> **EVIDENCE-BASED PRACTICE** *Romberg Test to Assess Balance?*
>
> This study of 103 patients assessed the sensitivity, specificity, and positive and negative predictive value of the Romberg Test of Standing Balance on Firm and Compliant Support Surfaces (RTSBFCSS) for the identification of patients with vestibular system impairments. The criterion standards were the caloric test and the cervical vestibular evoked myogenic potential (cVEMP) test. Sensitivity ranged from 55% to 61%, and specificity ranged from 58% to 64%. Positive and negative predictive values ranged from 39% to 55% and 64% to 78%, respectively. The authors concluded that the RTSBFCSS is a test of balance, not vestibular function, and should not be used as a screening measure for vestibular impairment.

Reference: Jacobson et al, 2011.

Perform Cardiovascular Evaluation

Note the heart rate and rhythm and attempt to detect dysrhythmias. Auscultate carotid and temporal arteries for bruits that can alert you to a cardiovascular cause for the vertigo.

Congenital heart disease can produce episodes of syncope that might be falsely interpreted as vertiginous episodes (see Chapter 33).

LABORATORY AND DIAGNOSTIC STUDIES

Audiometry

Audiometry is used to quantify hearing loss. The patient is tested at specific frequencies (pure tones) and specific intensities. Hearing loss is measured in decibels. Audiometry is used anytime the patient presents with both vertigo and hearing loss (i.e., Ménière disease, acoustic neuroma, labyrinthitis, perilymph fistula, or use of ototoxic medications) (see Chapter 15).

Electronystagmography

Electronystagmography electronically detects nystagmus that cannot be detected visually. Vestibular function is evaluated using gaze testing, positional changes, and caloric stimulation. Eye movements are recorded electronically. Caloric stimulation is produced by ear irrigation with warm and then cool water.

Electronystagmography is most useful in diagnosing chronic peripheral disorders (i.e., Ménière disease and persistent BPPV) to determine the degree and progression of the vestibular deficit. It can also be useful in patients with psychogenic vertigo to provide reassurance that no organic disease is present.

Magnetic Resonance Imaging

Magnetic resonance imaging (MRI) of the brain is indicated when the history and physical examination point to acoustic neuroma or a central cause of the vertigo. Consider urgent MRI if vertigo is of sudden onset; is accompanied by severe headache, direction-changing nystagmus, or neurologic signs or if the patient has risk factors for stroke.

Computed Tomography

Computed tomography (CT) scanning of the brain is indicated whenever there is persistent vertigo and in all cases with additional signs of neurologic disturbance. In patients with medical conditions such as renal failure, hypertension, or a hematologic malignancy and who have sudden onset of vertigo, CT scanning is used to look for hemorrhage into the cerebellum, brainstem, or labyrinth.

Electroencephalography

An electroencephalogram should be obtained for patients who have vertigo associated with alterations of consciousness.

Cardiac Monitoring

An electrocardiogram or Holter monitoring can provide confirmatory information on cardiovascular causes of vertigo.

Hematology and Urinalysis

Complete blood count (CBC) can reveal anemia, which can cause presyncopal lightheadedness. Urine or serum glucose levels will detect diabetes mellitus, which can produce vertigo. Urine testing and blood urea nitrogen (BUN) level can reveal renal failure, which can also be associated with vertigo.

Serologic Testing for Syphilis

Because secondary syphilis or early tertiary syphilis can produce the same symptoms that occur in Ménière disease, screening high-risk individuals is advocated to rule out syphilis as a cause.

DIFFERENTIAL DIAGNOSIS

Central Causes

Brainstem dysfunction and cerebellar dysfunction

Central vertigo produced by disorders of the brainstem and cerebellum is usually caused by neoplastic or vascular processes, including recurrent intermittent vascular insufficiency, transient ischemic attack, and stroke. Neoplasms are usually slow growing; therefore, vestibular dysfunction is of gradual onset and usually manifests as a problem with equilibrium.

Vascular causes are more common and can produce acute-onset, long-lasting, or recurrent transient episodes of vertigo. Patients usually manifest other neurologic deficits. With brainstem disorders, patients can have reports of diplopia, dysarthria, dysphagia, and paresthesia. They can demonstrate sensory and motor deficits. Cerebellar dysfunction usually results in gait disturbance and difficulties in fine motor coordination, including RAMs and finger-to-finger testing.

Multiple sclerosis

Multiple sclerosis can produce a range of neurologic symptoms. Vertigo occurs in up to 50% of patients with multiple sclerosis. Disease onset is usually in the third or fourth decade of life. MRI shows characteristic demyelinating plaques.

Migraine headache

Approximately 30% of people with migraine headaches have vertigo. It can be present before the headache begins, during the headache, or independent of the headache. Patients with vestibular-type migraine headaches often experience photophobia, phonophobia, and visual aura during the episodes of vertigo. Patients with basilar-type migraine may have other symptoms consistent with vertebrobasilar vascular abnormalities such as visual changes, tinnitus, decreased hearing, ataxia, or paresthesia. Diagnosis is usually made on the basis of the history.

Peripheral Causes

Benign paroxysmal positional vertigo

Episodes of BPPV are characterized by acute onset of vertigo associated with rapid head movement or position changes. Many women report dizziness with position change around the time of their menses. The episodes are brief, lasting a few seconds. Nystagmus can be elicited by the Dix-Hallpike maneuver. Testing positional changes can provoke the vertigo. There is no hearing loss. Diagnosis is made on the basis of the history and clinical findings. This is one of the most common causes of vertigo, especially in older adults. In patients with BPPV, tiny crystals of calcium carbonate (otoliths) in the inner ear that monitor head position relative to gravity become dislodged and migrate into one of the semicircular canals. When the head moves, the gravity-dependent movement of the otoliths in the affected semicircular canal causes endolymph displacement and a sensation of vertigo.

Benign paroxysmal vertigo of childhood

Benign paroxysmal vertigo of childhood occurs most often in children 2 to 3 years old. The disorder tends to be recurrent with one to four episodes per month. The episodes occur suddenly and are often associated with vomiting, pallor, sweating, and nystagmus. The neurologic and audiologic examinations produce normal findings. Some children can have a hypoactive or absent response to caloric testing (ear irrigation with warm and then cool water).

Ménière disease

Ménière disease is characterized by a classic triad of symptoms: vertigo, hearing loss, and tinnitus. A sensation of ear fullness can also be present. The attacks are abrupt and recurrent and last for minutes to several hours. The interval between attacks can be weeks or months. Between episodes, the patient is asymptomatic. On physical examination, sensorineural hearing loss is present in the affected ear, or it can be bilateral. Nystagmus is lateral or rotary. The visual ocular reflex will lateralize to the symptomatic ear.

Vestibular neuronitis

Vestibular neuronitis is frequently preceded by an acute viral infection. These patients usually present with severe vertigo, nausea, and vomiting. The vertigo lasts for days to weeks. Remaining completely motionless can help alleviate the symptoms. Auditory function is not affected. Physical examination reveals nystagmus that intensifies in amplitude when the gaze is directed away from the affected ear. Visual fixation minimizes the nystagmus. The visual ocular reflex will lateralize to the affected side.

Labyrinthitis

Frequently associated with a concurrent viral or bacterial illness, labyrinthitis produces severe vertigo that lasts for several days. Labyrinthitis can be a complication of otitis media or meningitis. This condition is distinguished from vestibular neuronitis by the accompanying hearing loss that occurs as a result of destruction of the inner ear. The visual ocular reflex will lateralize to the affected side.

Acoustic neuroma

Also called a vestibular schwannoma, acoustic neuroma is a benign tumor that originates most often in the vestibular portion of the acoustic nerve (CN VIII). It usually causes unilateral sensorineural hearing loss, tinnitus, and loss of equilibrium. The neuroma grows slowly; therefore loss of equilibrium is more often a symptom than is vertigo. Acoustic neuroma can also occur in the trigeminal nerve (CN V) with symptoms of paresthesia consistent with the nerve distribution. Large tumors of the abducens nerve (CN VI) can compress the brainstem.

Perilymph fistula

Fistula formation can occur as a result of ear trauma, from a direct blow, secondary to otologic surgery, or indirectly from straining, coughing, or pressure changes. In this condition, there is leakage of perilymph from either the round or the oval window into the middle ear. Sensorineural hearing loss and vertigo are frequently present. The fistula will often heal spontaneously but sometimes can require surgery.

Sinusitis and otitis

Serous otitis, otitis media, and sinusitis can cause disruption of the vestibular apparatus, producing vertigo. History and physical examination findings will be consistent with the specific disorder (see Chapters 15 and 25).

Cholesteatoma

Collection of squamous debris, often associated with chronic middle ear infection, can form a cholesteatoma, which enlarges and destroys structures in its way. On physical examination, the cholesteatoma will appear as a shiny, white, irregular mass. Foul-smelling discharge may be evident, and there may be visible bone destruction. Conductive hearing loss can be present.

Systemic Causes

Psychogenic

Psychogenic causes of vertigo are common. Patients often describe themselves as anxious or nervous and may have psychiatric diagnoses (see Chapter 4). Their symptoms are vague and imprecise. Neurologic examination findings are normal. No nystagmus is present or elicited. The vertigo can be reproduced with hyperventilation. MRI can be useful to provide reassurance.

Cardiovascular

Orthostatic hypotension and cardiac dysrhythmias can produce vertigo. Postural hypotension can be diagnosed by taking orthostatic blood pressure readings. The diagnosis of cardiac conditions can involve CBC, blood chemistry, ECG, cardiac stress testing, and echocardiography.

Neurosyphilis

Secondary or early tertiary syphilis can present with symptoms similar to those of Ménière disease. The patient demonstrates various clinical symptoms, including papilledema, aphasia, monoplegia or hemiplegia, CN palsies, pupillary abnormalities, or focal neurologic deficits. The Argyll Robertson pupil, which occurs almost exclusively in neurosyphilis, is a small irregular pupil that reacts normally to accommodation but not to light. Serological testing will be positive for syphilis.

Other Causes

Ototoxic drugs and drugs causing salt retention

Medications that are ototoxic, salt-retentive, or psychotropic can produce vertigo, lightheadedness, or unsteadiness. Drugs causing salt retention include steroids and phenylbutazone. Ototoxic medications include aspirin, ethacrynic acid, streptomycin, gentamicin, aminoglycosides, and furosemide. Psychotropic drugs can also produce vertigo. Ototoxic drugs can produce a sensorineural hearing loss. Audiometry should be performed with any noted hearing loss.

Trauma

Injury to the head or ear from labyrinthine concussion, temporal bone fracture, or perilymph fistula can produce disturbance of the vestibular apparatus and result in vertigo. Head trauma can also produce cerebral concussion involving the anterior tip of the temporal lobe. Trauma from otologic procedures can also cause vertigo.

▶ **DIFFERENTIAL DIAGNOSIS OF** *Common Causes of Dizziness*

CONDITION	HISTORY	PHYSICAL FINDINGS	DIAGNOSTIC STUDIES
CENTRAL CAUSES			
Brainstem dysfunction or cerebellar dysfunction	Older adult; acute onset; recurrent vertigo; tinnitus; hearing OK	Symptoms of brainstem or vertebrobasilar vascular abnormality: ataxia, double vision; lack of coordination; sensory or motor deficits; vertical, lateral, rotary nystagmus; hearing normal; cerebellar: impaired RAM, finger-to-finger testing	MRI
Multiple sclerosis	Onset is often in third or fourth decade of life	Can have no other findings or can have other neurologic symptoms	MRI
Migraine headache	Headache history; other migraine symptoms	Can have symptoms of vertebrobasilar vascular abnormalities, as above	None

Continued

▶ **DIFFERENTIAL DIAGNOSIS OF** *Common Causes of Dizziness—cont'd*

CONDITION	HISTORY	PHYSICAL FINDINGS	DIAGNOSTIC STUDIES
PERIPHERAL CAUSES			
Benign paroxysmal positional vertigo (BPPV)	Adults: associated with positional changes; recurrent episodes; lasts seconds to minutes; some relief if motionless	Lateral or rotary nystagmus; no tinnitus or hearing loss	Provoke nystagmus and vertigo by position that causes response; Dix-Hallpike maneuver; ENG
Benign paroxysmal vertigo of childhood	Children: usually 2–3 yr old; sudden onset with crying by child	Vomiting, pallor, sweating, and nystagmus common; no loss of consciousness; neurologic and audiologic examination can be normal	Can have hypoactive or absent response to caloric testing
Ménière disease	Sudden onset; lasts hours, recurrent; tinnitus and fullness in ears	Lateral or rotary nystagmus; fluctuating hearing loss: low tones; sensorineural	Positional maneuvers, positive VOR test, audiometry, ENG
Vestibular neuronitis	Sudden onset; antecedent viral infection	Nausea and vomiting; nystagmus; no hearing loss, loss of equilibrium always to the same side	Positional maneuvers; positive VOR test
Labyrinthitis	Sudden onset, lasts hours to days	Can currently be ill; lateral nystagmus; hearing loss; rarely tinnitus; nausea and vomiting can be present	Positional maneuvers, positive VOR test, audiometry
Acoustic neuroma	Adults; gradual onset; mild vertigo; persistent tinnitus; facial numbness, weakness	Unilateral hearing loss, poor speech discrimination	MRI; audiometry
Perilymph fistula	History of trauma; hearing loss	Nystagmus and vertigo with pneumatic otoscopy; sensorineural hearing loss	Audiometry
Otitis/sinusitis	Pain in ear or face; history of ear or sinus infections; gradual onset of vertigo	Serous otitis, otitis media; tenderness over sinuses; purulent nasal discharge; no nystagmus	See Chapters 15 and 25
Cholesteatoma	History of chronic middle ear infections	Shiny, white, irregular mass on otoscopic examination; foul-smelling discharge can be present; bone destruction can be visible; conductive hearing loss can be present	Audiometry

> **DIFFERENTIAL DIAGNOSIS OF** *Common Causes of Dizziness—cont'd*

CONDITION	HISTORY	PHYSICAL FINDINGS	DIAGNOSTIC STUDIES
SYSTEMIC CAUSES			
Psychogenic	Vague symptoms; recurrent; can describe self as anxious; can have other psychiatric diagnoses	Normal neurologic and auditory examinations	Hyperventilation to reproduce the vertigo
Cardiovascular	Cardiovascular history; antihypertensive medications	Orthostatic blood pressure; dysrhythmias; carotid or temporal bruits	Depends on client condition and symptoms
Neurosyphilis	Vertigo, tinnitus, fullness in ears	Various clinical symptoms; papilledema, aphasia, monoplegia or hemiplegia, central nervous palsies, pupillary abnormalities, Argyll Robertson pupil; focal neurologic deficits	Serology for syphilis
OTHER CAUSES			
Ototoxic and salt-retaining drugs	Medication history: steroids, phenylbutazone, ethacrynic acid, aspirin, streptomycin, gentamicin, aminoglycosides, furosemide, psychotropic drugs	Sensorineural hearing loss	Audiometry
Trauma	History of trauma to head or ear	Depends on nature and location of injury; can exhibit peripheral or central symptoms	MRI or CT

BPPV, benign paroxysmal positional vertigo; *CT,* computed tomography; *ENG,* electronystagmography; *MRI,* magnetic resonance imaging; *RAM,* rapid alternating movements.

14 Dyspnea

Dyspnea, or shortness of breath (SOB), is a subjective sensation of air hunger that results in labored breathing. True dyspnea results from three general causes: (1) an increased awareness of normal breathing, such as with hyperventilation; (2) an increase in the work of breathing, such as in airway obstruction or restricted volume; and (3) abnormalities in the ventilatory system, such as in neurologic disorders, diseases of the muscles, and chest wall abnormalities. In disease states, it is usually a result of pulmonary or cardiac pathology. When eliciting the history, it is helpful to determine if this is new-onset acute dyspnea, chronic progressive dyspnea, or chronic recurrent dyspnea. Carefully directed questioning will provide essential clues for identifying the differential diagnosis. In children younger than 3 years, who usually cannot express the sensation, caregivers can observe tachypnea, retractions, stridor, nasal flaring, or feeding difficulty.

DIAGNOSTIC REASONING: FOCUSED HISTORY

Is this an emergency?

Severe dyspnea is a medical emergency. If not treated immediately, respiratory failure and death can occur. Assess the adequacy of the airway first. Emergency measures should be instituted to establish ventilation. When the patient is stabilized, search for the underlying cause of the dyspnea.

Key Questions
- Did this occur suddenly, or has it been developing gradually? Over what period of time (hours, days, weeks) has it developed?
- What were you (or the child) doing just before having difficulty in breathing?
- Do you (or the child) have other symptoms such as itching or swelling?

Onset

New-onset acute dyspnea in a patient in respiratory distress can signal a life-threatening problem. In a patient with no previous history of heart or lung disease, dyspnea can indicate several conditions that require immediate treatment such as aspiration of a foreign body, anaphylaxis, pulmonary embolism (PE), and pneumonia. A common cause of acute-onset dyspnea is left ventricular dysfunction.

Acute upper or lower airway obstruction in children has the greatest potential to cause serious morbidity or mortality and therefore must initially be ruled out. The most serious problem is hypoxemia caused by the inability to transport oxygen past a blocked upper airway, such as with epiglottitis, croup, or a foreign body.

Acute dyspnea requires immediate assessment of the airway and ventilatory status with oxygen and cardiac monitoring. Often this must occur before a definitive diagnostic evaluation has been completed.

Acute epiglottitis in children is caused by *Haemophilus influenzae*. Inflammation of the epiglottis causes edema that obstructs the tracheal airway. The onset is sudden, and the course of the disease is rapid. The patient's presenting symptoms usually include drooling, dysphonia, dysphagia, and respiratory distress with inspiratory stridor. The child looks anxious and sits up and forward with the jaw open to assist in air intake.

Status asthmaticus is a progressive bronchospasm from an increase in airflow resistance in children who are having an asthma event that does not respond to pharmacologic intervention. Fever can be present, and pulse rate and respirations are increased. The use of accessory respiratory muscles is seen. Sometimes wheezing is not heard because of lack of air movement. The combination of hypoxia, hypercapnia, and acidosis can result in cardiovascular depression and cardiopulmonary arrest.

Foreign Body Aspiration

An adult patient with foreign body aspiration (FBA) reports that dyspnea occurred while eating solid foods or drinking large amounts of alcohol. Children who put small objects in their mouths are at risk for aspiration of the object into the airway and subsequent airway obstruction. The patient or the care provider gives a history of sudden onset of choking, coughing, or wheezing without preceding upper respiratory tract infection. Often the child has been playing on the floor or outside at the time of the onset of symptoms.

Anaphylaxis

Anaphylaxis can follow insect bites or the ingestion of medication or other potential allergens (e.g., shellfish, peanuts). Primary symptoms include flushing, generalized pruritus, anxiety, faintness, and sneezing. An allergic response can lead to shock, cardiac arrhythmia, laryngeal edema, and death within minutes. Generally the sooner the symptoms occur, the more severe the reaction.

Is the dyspnea caused by a secondary obstruction in the lower respiratory tract?

Key Questions
- Have you had a cough or recent cold?
- Do you have a history of asthma?
- Is there a family history of asthma?

Cough

Secondary partial airway obstruction caused by small airway disease contributes to hypoxemia via intrapulmonary shunting. The pulmonary obstruction can be intraluminal (distal foreign objects, asthma), intramural (edema, bronchomalacia, bronchiolitis), or

extramural (compression from tumor, lymph nodes). The narrowing increases both airway resistance and turbulence of airflow. The imbalance between pulmonary ventilation and perfusion affects oxygen exchange. This causes the patient to work harder to maintain adequate ventilation, resulting in dyspnea.

History of Asthma

Both adults and children can experience airway obstruction caused by reactive airways disease or asthma. Personal or family history of asthma increases the risk of dyspnea from acute bronchospasm.

Is the dyspnea caused by trauma to the chest?

Key Question
- Have you experienced any trauma to the chest?

Trauma

Limitation of motion of the thoracic cage because of pain or trauma can be associated with severe alveolar hypoventilation and subsequent dyspnea.

Pneumothorax occurs most frequently in young people during strenuous activity. Spontaneous pneumothorax results in sudden loss of lung volume, hypoxia, hypercapnia, and significant SOB. Blunt chest trauma can be caused by a fall or motor vehicle accident.

Is the dyspnea caused by a pulmonary embolus?

Key Questions
- Have you recently been confined to bed or been sitting for a long period of time?
- Have you had recent surgery?
- Have you recently sustained a fracture?
- Are you taking birth control pills or estrogen?
- Have you had any pain in your legs?
- Do you have a history of deep vein thrombosis?
- Do you have a family history of clotting disorders?

- Do you smoke?
- What medications are you taking?
- Are you feeling anxious or scared?

The person with PE is usually in acute distress and reports significant SOB, localized pleuritic chest pain, apprehension, bloody sputum production, diaphoresis, fever, and history of conditions that increase risk for emboli. These risk factors include age older than 60 years, pulmonary hypertension, congestive heart failure, chronic lung disease, ischemic heart disease, stroke, and cancer. Predisposing factors that can contribute to thrombus formation include (1) venous stasis, (2) hypercoagulability, and (3) endothelial injury with inflammation to the vessel lining. Trauma, muscle spasm, or clot dissolution can cause the thrombus to dislodge, creating an embolus. Emboli circulate in the blood to the right side of the heart and enter the lungs via the pulmonary artery. If the clot is not dissolved within the lungs, it occludes the pulmonary artery and obstructs blood flow and perfusion of the lungs. Patients with suspected PE are referred for emergency pulmonary or vascular consultation.

Confinement, Surgery, and Fracture

People with a history of deep vein thrombosis or prolonged immobility are at greater risk for PE. Vascular lung disease is characterized by a decrease in the size of the pulmonary vascular bed. When emboli reach the pulmonary artery, the reduced blood flow through the lungs results in arterial hypoxemia and hypercapnia. Hypoxemia and hypercapnia lead to symptoms of dyspnea. Dyspnea resulting from PE is usually accompanied by fever, chest pain, and restlessness.

Family History of Clotting Disorders

Antiphospholipid syndrome, occurring either as an isolated disorder or as a part of systemic lupus erythematosus, can lead to abnormal clotting. This has a hereditary component and can occur as a spontaneous mutation.

Trauma to the Leg

There is an increased risk of PE in individuals who have sustained traumatic injury to their lower limbs.

Anxiety

People with PE often express a sense of impending doom. Significant oxygen deprivation can contribute to this symptom.

Oral Contraceptives or Estrogen

The estrogen in oral contraceptives causes increased coagulation of red blood cells, which increases the risk for PE. In addition, the risk of PE increases with the combination of smoking and oral contraceptives, especially in patients older than age 35 years.

Medications

A complete medication history can provide clues to a possible hypercoagulability state. Patients who are taking anticoagulants and are underdosed can be at risk for PE. Patients taking medication for heart failure, such as digitalis or angiotensin-converting enzyme inhibitors, are at risk because of chronic heart failure. Serum estrogen receptor modulators (tamoxifen, raloxifene) increase the risk for PE.

> *Is the dyspnea related to a preexisting disease?*

Key Questions

- Do you have a history of heart problems, lung problems (asthma), or anemia?
- Do you have any numbness or tingling in your body? Where?
- Have you noticed any other symptoms?

Past History of Disease

History of coronary artery disease (CAD), heart failure, valvular heart disease, chronic obstructive pulmonary disease (COPD), or asthma should raise the level of suspicion for recurrence or complications of that disease. Myocardial infarction (MI) can cause sudden dyspnea in individuals with or without a prior history of CAD. Careful questioning regarding associated symptoms and risk factors can reveal characteristics of probable MI (see Chapter 8).

Progressively increasing SOB is frequently a symptom of worsening COPD. It is often associated with cough that is worse in the morning, clear to yellow color sputum, exercise intolerance, and fatigue. Chronic progressive dyspnea in the patient with a history of heart failure or cardiac valve disease is most frequently a symptom of heart failure. Associated symptoms include peripheral edema, ascites, cough (possibly with frothy sputum production), chest pain, and fatigue. Orthopnea (difficulty breathing when lying flat) and paroxysmal nocturnal dyspnea (PND) (a sudden onset of SOB when lying flat) are most often associated with heart failure.

In children with heart disease, dyspnea occurs because of insufficient blood being pumped to the lungs as a result of congenital structural anomaly or pump failure or secondary to pulmonary hypertension. Simple respiratory tract infections can cause severe respiratory insufficiency in the child who has cardiopulmonary disease. Associated symptoms include retractions (including abdominal muscles), tachypnea, nasal flaring and grunting, peripheral edema, ascites, cough, and fatigue.

Chronic progressive dyspnea because of lung involvement can also be present in patients with a history of systemic illnesses such as sarcoidosis, rheumatological disease (rheumatoid lungs), cystic fibrosis, or Goodpasture syndrome (a rare syndrome of progressive glomerulonephritis, hemoptysis, and hemosiderosis); fibrotic lung disease such as scleroderma, silicosis, asbestosis; and in progressive neurologic disorders such as myasthenia gravis, amyotrophic lateral sclerosis (ALS), and multiple sclerosis.

Periodic recurrent dyspnea is most often the result of bronchospasm and inflamed bronchi caused by asthma. People with asthma can be relatively symptom free between episodes and can often identify the cause of their SOB with little prompting. Symptoms are frequently associated with recent respiratory tract infection, exercise, or exposure to allergens. The patient or parent may report audible wheezes, decreased exercise tolerance, and frequent cough. Wheezing is extremely unusual in the neonatal period and implies intrathoracic airway obstruction caused by intraluminal obstruction, fixed airway narrowing, variable narrowing, or external compression. All of these factors lead to turbulent expiratory flow and audible wheeze.

Hematologic diseases can affect the oxygen-carrying capacity of the blood, resulting in tissue hypoxia and a decrease in arterial pH, which stimulates the central nervous system (CNS) to produce the symptom of dyspnea. Severe anemia from any cause can result in this reaction. Dyspnea can occur whenever the oxygen-carrying capacity of the blood is decreased because of the inability of hemoglobin to bind oxygen. Carbon monoxide poisoning, cyanide poisoning, and methemoglobinemia are examples.

The progressive dyspnea of anemia is usually associated with fatigue, palpitations, lightheadedness, or dizziness.

Hyperventilation

Hyperventilation syndrome, a nonemergent but frightening experience, is usually accompanied by paresthesias around the mouth and of the distal extremities. Anxiety-related dyspnea should not be diagnosed until more serious causes have been ruled out.

When dyspnea is caused by pulmonary or cardiac conditions, the SOB worsens with increasing activity and improves with rest. Dyspnea caused by anxiety does not improve, and can worsen, with rest.

What factors precipitate or aggravate the dyspnea?

Key Questions

- What activities are associated with SOB?
- Do you take any medication?
- Do you have any known allergies (to trees, dust, pollen, animals)? Have you been exposed to these recently?
- Is there anything you can do to help yourself feel less short of breath, such as sit up, stay indoors, lie down, or use medication?

Precipitating Factors

Chronic dyspnea of pulmonary origin is most frequently precipitated and aggravated by exposure to smoke. This is true for both progressive and recurrent dyspnea. Progressive dyspnea manifested in COPD is often exacerbated by exertion and is alleviated or improved with rest. As the disease progresses, less and less intense exercise, even talking, and respiratory tract infection can result in increased SOB. Exercise-induced asthma will cause dyspnea related to activity and is relieved with rest or use of bronchodilators.

Medication Use

The dyspnea related to asthma may be relieved by use of bronchodilator agents and steroids.

Allergies

Exposure to cold or allergens, exercise, and viral respiratory tract infections frequently precipitate chronic recurrent dyspnea associated with asthma.

Recumbence, missed medications, high sodium intake, and exertion often precipitate chronic dyspnea associated with heart failure. This applies to both progressive and recurrent chronic dyspnea.

Alleviating Factors

Alleviating factors for dyspnea include sitting upright, taking diuretic medications, using bronchodilators, and resting for a prolonged period.

Is the dyspnea caused by a neuromuscular problem?

Key Questions
• Are your immunizations up to date?
• If a child: Has the child eaten any honey?
• Do you live on a farm?
• If a child: Is the child at risk for lead poisoning?
• Do you have a headache, muscle weakness, or other symptoms?

Immunizations

Lack of childhood or adult immunizations for poliomyelitis or tetanus can lead to paralysis or tetany of the respiratory musculature, resulting in dyspnea and subsequent respiratory distress.

Honey

Honey is a common source of contamination of *Clostridium botulinum,* which can cause respiratory distress in infants and small children.

The incubation period is only a few hours. Nausea, vomiting, and diarrhea result followed by cranial nerve involvement, diplopia, weak suck, facial weakness, and absent gag reflex. Generalized hypotonia and weakness then develop and can progress to respiratory failure.

Farm Residence

Exposure to organophosphate chemicals that are commonly used as insecticides can cause a myasthenia-like syndrome in children. Children who reside on farms are most at risk.

Lead Poisoning

In children, some causes that affect the primary respiratory center are myopathies, insecticide poisoning, and lead poisoning. Children younger than 6 years are most vulnerable. Major sources of lead poisoning are from flaking lead-based paint or lead contaminated dust, water, air, and soil. In adults, certain occupational exposures increase risk.

Neuromuscular Effects

Abnormalities of neural or neuromuscular transmission to the respiratory muscles can result in paresis or paralysis, leading to alveolar hypoventilation. Direct involvement of the respiratory muscles affected by systemic musculoskeletal diseases can lead to a reduction of vital capacity and total lung capacity and result in hypercapnic hypoventilation and dyspnea. Examples of neuromuscular health problems leading to dyspnea include infections, such as poliomyelitis, tetanus, and CNS insult such as ALS. Urge incontinence can be an early sign of multiple sclerosis; easy fatigability can be associated with myasthenia gravis.

Secondary Causes

Diseases that affect the CNS and produce respiratory distress include meningoencephalitis, seizures, and CNS lesions.

Does the patient have any pertinent risk factors that will point me in the right direction?

Key Questions
• Do you smoke? Have you ever smoked? Are you regularly exposed to cigarette smoke?

- What type of work do you do?
- Have you had a recent weight gain?
- Have you ever had eczema?

Risk Factors

Individuals at risk for developing dyspnea are those with a history of pulmonary or heart disease, cigarette smokers and those subjected to passive exposure or secondhand smoke, people exposed to noxious environmental pollutants, and individuals with a predisposition to allergies or asthma.

Work

Occupational exposures to asbestos, silicon, paint and chemical fumes, and coal dust place the patient at risk for lung disease with resultant dyspnea.

Obesity

Physically deconditioned people and people who are obese report dyspnea on exertion more frequently than their physically active and nonobese counterparts. A person with obesity may report dyspnea, especially during exercise. This is caused by an increase in the metabolic requirement for a given amount of work. In addition, the diaphragm moves against increased abdominal pressure, and the chest wall is heavier, resulting in more energy required to maintain ventilation. Obesity hypoventilation syndrome is when severely obese individuals may fail to breathe rapidly enough or deeply enough to avoid low oxygen and higher CO_2 levels.

Eczema History

Asthma occurs in 20% to 40% of children with a history of atopic dermatitis.

DIAGNOSTIC REASONING: FOCUSED PHYSICAL EXAMINATION

Note General Appearance and Observe Posture

Patients who appear in acute distress with manifestations of severe oxygen deprivation require emergent evaluation and treatment. Assess vital signs immediately. Tachypnea and hypopnea are critical clues to impending respiratory failure. Use of accessory muscles to breathe, posturing, and chest retraction all point to severe dyspnea. The severity of the dyspnea almost always correlates with the severity of the problem. In such situations, consider PE, anaphylaxis, FBA, pneumothorax, status asthmaticus, and severe heart failure. Patients presenting with symptoms of COPD, anemia, mild asthma, and mild heart failure appear less acutely ill.

Determine if the patient has to lean forward or sit up to breathe comfortably. With severe respiratory distress or upper airway obstruction, an infant can adopt a posture of hyperextension of the trunk and neck. A child with epiglottitis prefers to sit up and lean forward.

A child who is in acute respiratory distress, sitting forward, and perhaps speaking with a muffled voice or drooling may have epiglottitis, and immediate assistance should be secured. Do not attempt to lay the child down or inspect the throat because this can occlude the airway.

Assess Level of Consciousness

Diminished level of consciousness, confusion, and restlessness are manifestations of hypoxia in a patient experiencing respiratory problems. Frequently, the patient with a PE expresses a sense of impending doom.

An acutely ill child can have an alteration in level of consciousness, restlessness, mouth breathing, and flaring of the nostrils.

Observe Chest Movement

Place the patient in a sitting or side-lying position with the chest exposed. The chest cannot be adequately viewed through clothing. Many respiratory abnormalities are unilateral or localized. Compare findings on one side of the body with those on the other. Also compare front to back. Pneumothorax and PE can cause unequal expansion of the chest.

Inspect the Shape and Symmetry of the Chest

Cardinal features of restrictive pulmonary disease are deformities of the chest wall and reduction in lung volume and pulmonary compliance secondary to pathological changes in the lung parenchyma or pleura. Examples of deformities that cause decreased lung volume include kyphosis, scoliosis, and kyphoscoliosis. Decreased volume necessitates an increase in respiratory rate to maintain a normal volume. The work of breathing must be increased to overcome the reduced compliance.

Kyphoscoliosis is associated with marked structural abnormality of the thoracic cage, leading to abnormal positioning and functioning of the respiratory muscles. The lungs are compressed by the thoracic deformity, leading to a small lung volume. Breathing entails a high work and energy cost, and dyspnea can appear.

An increased anteroposterior (AP) diameter indicates air trapping. This is a frequent finding in individuals with COPD. Other musculoskeletal chest abnormalities to note include pectus excavatum and pectus carinatum. These conditions can contribute to chest infection and respiratory failure because of decreased lung volume and ability to cough. Bronchomalacia, a softening of the bronchial tissue, is an abnormality associated with pectus excavatum. Pectus carinatum is associated with chronic lung disease such as asthma or with cystic fibrosis, heart disease such as mitral valve prolapse, Marfan syndrome, and idiopathic scoliosis. Harrison sulci are exaggerated grooves running parallel to the subcostal margins, produced by prolonged diaphragmatic traction, and are associated with chronic airway disease or rickets.

In the presence of neuromuscular disease, chest movement in children should be examined in both the supine and sitting positions. Diaphragmatic weakness leads to paradoxical abdominal movements in the supine position, which can be missed if the child is examined only in the sitting position.

Respiratory distress triggered by placing the child in the supine position can be the only subtle abnormality in older children with mediastinal compression of the trachea.

Look for Retractions

In normal breathing, inspiration is the work necessary to overcome the elastic forces of the lung, the tissue viscosity of the lung and chest wall, and airway resistance. When there is a problem with any of these, the accessory muscles (sternocleidomastoid, serratus anterior, and external intercostal) are recruited. Contraction of these muscles causes forceful expansion of the thorax, resulting in increased negative pressure that draws in the soft tissues of the chest wall and results in retractions. Retractions begin in lower intercostal spaces and then move up to the higher spaces. In an infant, head bobbing in time with respiration reflects use of the accessory muscles of respiration.

Observe the Rate, Rhythm, and Depth of Respiration for 1 Full Minute

In children, the respiratory rate should be counted while the child sleeps, if possible.

Tachypnea is an early sign of most pulmonary, parenchymal, cardiac, or systemic causes of respiratory distress. Hyperventilation can occur secondary to acidosis or CNS disease. CNS depression can lead to hypoxemia and shock; systemic infection can lead to metabolic acidosis and trigger hyperventilation.

Exhaling should take about twice as long as inhaling, but in patients with COPD, it can take up to four times longer. Rhythm should be even, with occasional sighs. Shallow respirations, which are rapid, indicate that restrictive forces must be overcome. Box 14.1 describes abnormal breathing patterns.

Listen for Stridor

Stridor is caused by extrathoracic, inspiratory, dynamic narrowing of the airway in the oropharynx, glottis, subglottic region, or midtrachea. Any condition that causes further decrease in the lumen of the airway will obstruct airflow and produce stridor. Inspiratory stridor usually indicates a supraglottic obstruction. If the obstruction varies or is extrathoracic (above the vocal cords), inspiration is affected more because the negative intra-airway pressure during inspiration tends to collapse the extrathoracic airway. If the obstruction varies and affects the intrathoracic airways, expiration is prolonged because the positive intrathoracic pressure tends to collapse these airways during expiration.

| Box 14.1 | **Abnormal Breathing Patterns** |

Cheyne-Stokes respirations are manifested by rhythmic increase and decrease in depth, punctuated by regular episodes of apnea. This can be a sign of severe heart failure or neurologic disease.

Tachypnea is rapid breathing with no change in depth and can be caused by hypoxia, pain, fever, or anxiety. Consider pulmonary embolism, foreign body aspiration, anaphylaxis, pneumothorax, heart failure, asthma, or pneumonia.

Asymmetrical chest movement with respirations can be observed in lobar pneumonia, pleural effusion, or any condition that affects just one side of the chest.

Use of accessory muscles indicates respiratory distress. Observe for bulging or retraction of the intercostal, sternocleidomastoid, or trapezius muscles. Nasal flaring is an objective manifestation of hypoxia.

Expiratory or biphasic respiratory stridor generally indicates an obstruction at or below the larynx.

With severe narrowing of the air passage, stridor can be audible on both inspiration and expiration but is worse during inspiration. Biphasic or expiratory stridor alone usually indicates a more significant obstruction. Supraglottic stridor is usually quiet and wet and is associated with a muffled voice, dysarthria, and a preference to sit. Subglottic lesions produce a loud stridor, often causing a hoarse voice, barky cough, and possibly facial edema. Inspiratory stridor can be a sign of incomplete obstruction of the airway by a foreign body.

Infants younger than 6 months who present with stridor can have an underlying anatomical abnormality that may be symptomatic secondary to an acute illness. Common anomalies that predispose infants to upper airway obstruction are anomalous vascular rings, laryngeal webs, laryngomalacia, or tracheomalacia. Stridor in older children can indicate FBA, infection, inflammation, trauma, or tumor.

Listen for Audible Wheeze

Expiratory wheezing is a high-pitched musical sound caused by partial airway obstruction. It is commonly associated with disorders of the lower respiratory tract that cause inflammation, infection, or bronchoconstriction such as asthma and bronchitis.

Increased inspiratory effort suggests disease in the upper airways, but increased expiratory effort suggests disease in the smaller airways or lower respiratory tract.

Listen for Voice Changes

Voice changes can occur in association with upper airway obstruction. Paralysis of the vocal cords results in dysphonia. Subglottic stenosis results in decreased volume of the voice because a much smaller column of air is making the vocal cords vibrate. Involvement of the supraglottic area, proximal to the vocal cords, can result in hyponasality or muffled voice such as in tonsillitis and epiglottitis. A normal voice with stridor can indicate a subglottic or tracheal lesion (see Chapter 21).

Take Pulse, Temperature, and Blood Pressure

Palpate the radial, femoral, popliteal, and pedal pulses for rate and quality.

Tachycardia increases cardiac output. It occurs either as a result of primary heart disease or as a secondary process in response to oxygen deprivation because of PE, pneumonia, fever, and/or heart failure. Tachycardia and drowsiness can indicate metabolic acidosis. Bradycardia is usually seen late in respiratory disease.

Tachycardia can occur with an irregular pulse, signaling heart failure from atrial fibrillation or heart block. Diminished peripheral pulses indicate possible atherosclerotic vessel disease or decreased cardiac output.

Fever can indicate epiglottitis or any other upper or lower respiratory tract infection.

Orthostatic hypotension can be secondary to dehydration associated with pneumonia or status asthmaticus. Anaphylaxis is also manifested by severe hypotension. Pulsus paradoxus, an inspiratory drop in systolic blood pressure of more than 10 mm Hg, is caused by greater inspiratory effort from increased airway resistance. Negative intrathoracic pressure is associated with increased afterload and low systolic blood pressure. In heart failure, decreased stroke volume reduces the systolic blood pressure. Compensatory vasoconstriction maintains a constant diastolic pressure and, along with the decreased systolic pressure, can produce a decreased pulse pressure.

Inspect the Oral Cavity

First observe the oropharyngeal cavity for any evidence of a foreign body obstructing the airway. Evidence of vomitus can indicate possible aspiration. Note the color of the tongue and mucous membranes for signs of central cyanosis.

Inspect the posterior pharynx for peritonsillar cellulitis, retropharyngeal abscess, or other intraoral pathology that might be causing obstruction. Lift the jaw forward. Obstruction of the airway associated with micrognathia, depressed airway reflexes, or an enlarged tongue will diminish with this maneuver because the tongue will be lifted off the posterior pharynx. If epiglottitis is suspected, do not examine the oral cavity.

Inspect the Nose

Assess the patency of the nares. Fifty percent of airway resistance comes from the nose. Check for nasal flaring. An infant who has nasal flaring is using a compensatory mechanism to decrease airway resistance. Noisy, difficult breathing in an infant, especially while feeding, can signal choanal atresia. A deviated septum compromises the patency of one side of the nose when there is mucosal swelling.

Palpate the Neck

Neck masses caused by intraoral, paratracheal, or intrathoracic malignant disease can cause respiratory distress. Inspect the position of the trachea. To assess the trachea for lateral displacement, position your index finger first on the right side of the suprasternal notch and then on the left. If the trachea has shifted to the side, you will feel the wall on one side but only soft tissue on the other. This is most likely to occur with pneumothorax. Observe the neck for jugular venous distention; this is a sign of heart failure.

Examine the Skin and Extremities

Note cyanosis. Bluish color seen in the lips and mucous membranes of the mouth (central cyanosis) is associated with low arterial saturation and can result from inadequate gas exchange in the lungs or from cardiac shunting. Cyanosis implies more than 5 g/100 mL of desaturated hemoglobin, but its absence does not imply that hypoxemia is not present. Dark-skinned patients' mucous membranes can appear gray with central cyanosis. Central cyanosis can also be seen in people with COPD. Bluish color of the extremities (peripheral cyanosis) may be observed in white individuals and is associated with low venous saturation, resulting from vasoconstriction, vascular occlusion, or reduced cardiac output.

Pallor of sclera or nail beds can be a manifestation of severe anemia.

Note clubbing, which is characterized by the loss of the angle between the skin and nail bed. Clubbing is a manifestation of chronic tissue hypoxia that occurs with lung cancer and other chronic lung diseases but can also be idiopathic. It is uncommon in children other than those with cystic fibrosis, cyanotic congenital heart disease, thyrotoxicosis, and in celiac disease. Clubbing develops rapidly with infective endocarditis.

Test for peripheral edema. Edema of the lower extremities can be a sign of increased right-heart filling pressure caused by primary lung disease or left ventricular failure. Make note of how high the edema extends up the extremity. In children, the location of peripheral edema is age dependent. In young infants, edema occurs as hepatomegaly and periorbital or flank edema. In older children, lower extremity edema can occur.

Note any angioedema. The presence of generalized or local urticaria is objective evidence of probable anaphylaxis.

Check skin perfusion by pressing on the skin of a finger or sole of a foot and saying "capillary refill" after removing the pressure. In a normal finding, the color returns to the skin in 2 seconds or before you can finish saying the words.

Feel the skin for diaphoresis. When respiratory muscles are working at their maximum level to overcome increased resistive and elastic forces, the child will sweat, especially on the forehead and above the lip.

Palpate the Chest

Using the palmar surface of the hands, palpate the entire chest for tenderness, depressions, bulges, and crepitus (presence of air in the subcutaneous tissues). Crepitus can indicate a chest injury, pneumothorax, or cutaneous emphysema.

Pneumothorax, atelectasis, pneumonia, and partial paralysis of the diaphragm will result in reduced expansion of one side of the chest wall, and chest wall motion will be decreased.

Assess for Tactile Fremitus

Fremitus is diminished in pneumothorax, asthma, emphysema, and other conditions that trap air in the lung. Tactile fremitus intensity can be increased in pneumonia, heart failure, and tumor, all conditions that increase the lung density.

Percuss the Chest

Sounds produced by percussion indicate the density of lung tissue (see Chapter 11). In children, transmission of a percussion note and assessment of the quality of transmitted sound are useful to reveal an area of consolidation or effusion that would be difficult to auscultate with an uncooperative child.

Auscultate Breath Sounds

Auscultation of bronchial or bronchovesicular breath sounds over the peripheral lungs can indicate consolidation, which occurs when lungs fill with exudate. Young children normally have bronchovesicular sounds because of the thinness of their chest walls.

If breath sounds are diminished over all lung fields, suspect shallow breathing, lack of air movement, neuromuscular diseases, obesity, or COPD. Breath sounds will be inaudible in areas of pneumothorax.

Abnormal lung sounds are superimposed on normal sounds and can be auscultated over any area of the lung field during inspiration or expiration. Documentation of abnormal lung sounds should include type of sound, location where it is heard, and the phase(s) of respiration in which it is noted. In small children, it can be difficult to distinguish upper and lower airway sounds. Listening with the stethoscope over the nose or mouth and then returning to the lungs can help to identify the findings.

Crackles or rales are discontinuous popping sounds heard most often during inspiration. They are caused by the explosive equalization of gas pressure between two compartments of the lung when a closed section of the airway that separates them suddenly opens. They indicate the presence of fluid, mucus, or pus in the smaller airways. Fine crackles are soft and high pitched. Medium crackles are louder and lower pitched. Coarse crackles are moist and more explosive.

EVIDENCE-BASED PRACTICE *Physical Examination Techniques to Detect Pleural Effusion*

A systematic review was conducted to review the evidence regarding the accuracy of the physical examination in assessing the thorax for pleural effusion. Eight physical examination techniques were evaluated: manual percussion; auscultatory percussion (tapping on the manubrium and listening to the posterior chest with a stethoscope simultaneously) for decreased resonance; auscultation for breath sounds, crackles, and pleural friction rubs; chest expansion; tactile vocal fremitus; and vocal resonance. Dullness to manual percussion increased the likelihood of pleural effusion. However, chest radiography is necessary to confirm a diagnosis. If tactile fremitus is not decreased in a patient at low risk for pleural effusion, chest radiography may not be necessary. In summary, dullness to percussion and tactile fremitus are the most useful findings when evaluating a patient for pleural effusion.

Reference: Wong et al, 2009.

The frequency and timing of crackles are the important parts of assessment. In resolving pneumonia, crackling is heard on inspiration caused by a mix between the aerated and nonaerated alveoli and bronchioles. In airways that are swollen and narrowed, such as in asthma or bronchiolitis, generalized medium or coarse crackles are heard throughout both phases of respiration. Early inspiratory crackles are heard in COPD. Mid to late inspiratory crackles are more likely a sign of interstitial lung disease or heart failure. Crackles can be heard over the site of a pulmonary embolus.

Wheezing is frequently described as a whistling sound and may be heard during inspiration, expiration, or both. The sound is high pitched and musical. Wheezing indicates that there is fluid in the large airways such as in severe heart failure or, more often, heralds bronchospasm, as seen in asthma. In addition, localized wheezing can accompany incomplete obstruction of the airway by a foreign body.

A wheeze of fixed pitch occurring with inspiration and expiration suggests a localized abnormality. Wheezes of varying pitch occurring predominantly throughout expiration reflect the narrowing of airways of different calibers.

Rhonchi are continuous, deep-pitched, coarse breath sounds usually heard during expiration. Rhonchi are frequently present when the patient has bronchitis or pneumonia.

Pleural friction rub is a grating or squeaking sound usually heard in the lateral lung fields during inspiration and expiration. It indicates that parietal and visceral pleural linings are inflamed and are rubbing together as can occur with pneumonia, pleural effusion, pleuritis, and tumors. It is often accompanied by limited chest expansion because of pain.

If abnormal lung sounds are detected, additional auscultation for bronchophony, egophony, and whispered pectoriloquy is indicated. Consolidation will produce abnormal findings for each of these tests. To test for bronchophony, instruct the patient to say "ninety-nine." The words are heard louder and clearer than usual. In egophony, instruct the patient to say "ee." This sound is transmitted as "ay" if consolidation is present. To test whispered pectoriloquy, instruct the patient to whisper a sentence. Whispered sounds are louder and clearer than normal.

Auscultate Heart Sounds

In COPD, lung hyperinflation can muffle heart sounds. Poor tissue oxygenation can result in tachycardia. In children, muffled heart sounds can indicate pericarditis.

In heart failure, the first and second heart sounds (S_1 and S_2) can equal the peripheral pulse rate. If the peripheral pulse rate is less than the heart rate, this pulse deficit is a sign of decreased cardiac output. S_3 (ventricular gallop) is an early sign of heart failure and is heard best at the apex of the heart. S_4 (atrial gallop) in children typically indicates a stressed heart and heart failure. In adults, it can be the result of hypertension, MI, or CAD causing heart failure. A summation gallop can also occur with heart failure; this is the result of S_3, S_4, and rapid rate.

Listen for the presence of any murmurs and note their location, grade of loudness, timing, or radiation. Incompetent heart valves can be the cause of heart failure.

LABORATORY AND DIAGNOSTIC STUDIES

Diagnostic tests are indicated in almost all initial evaluations of the patient presenting with SOB. Posteroanterior (PA) and lateral chest radiographs, hemoglobin level, and spirometry are useful preliminary tests.

Transcutaneous Pulse Oximetry

Oximetry measures the fraction of oxygen carried in hemoglobin and provides noninvasive information about the delivery of oxygen from the atmosphere to the pulmonary capillaries. The partial pressure of oxygen in arterial blood (PaO_2) in healthy adults ranges from 80 to 103 mm Hg, and more than 95% saturation of hemoglobin is considered normal. In children, a pulse oximetry reading of 95% to 98% is normal, 90% to 95% is mild hypoxia, 85% to 90% is moderate hypoxemia, and less than 85% is severe hypoxemia.

Chest Radiography

Chest radiographs are essential in the diagnosis of dyspnea and can show pneumothorax, pneumonia, malignant disease, pleural disease, foreign body, or pulmonary edema. They can also provide clues to other causes of dyspnea such as cardiomegaly, deformities of the chest bones and musculature, and the position of the diaphragm. When a foreign body is suspected, both inspiratory and expiratory chest radiography can be helpful.

Electrocardiography

An electrocardiogram (ECG) can provide important information about myocardial ischemia, arrhythmias, pericarditis, or the presence of pulmonary disease. Cardiopulmonary exercise testing can be done if the severity of the dyspnea is disproportionate to objective tests, there are coexisting cardiac and pulmonary causes, or if deconditioning, obesity, or psychological factors are suspected.

Echocardiography

An echocardiogram is performed when cardiac disease is suspected; this test can define the cause of dyspnea related to heart chamber size, valves, pericardial disease, and ventricular function.

Hemoglobin and Hematocrit

Significantly below-normal hemoglobin and hematocrit levels suggest anemia as a possible cause of dyspnea. Erythrocytosis can indicate chronic hypoxia resulting from a number of causes including COPD, carbon monoxide (CO) poisoning, and smoking.

Spirometry

Spirometry is indicated if the dyspnea is related to obstructive or restrictive lung disease. Spirometry measures forced vital capacity (FVC), forced expiratory volume in 1 second (FEV_1), the FEV_1/FVC ratio, and the peak expiratory flow rate (PEFR). In obstructive lung disease (i.e., asthma and COPD), the FEV_1 and the FEV_1/FVC ratio are less than predicted. In restrictive lung disease (i.e., pneumonia, pneumothorax, pleural effusion), the FVC is reduced, and the ratio is normal or elevated. Spirometry that indicates restrictive disease or mixed obstructive restrictive disease should have follow-up studies to test for lung volumes with either helium dilution, body plethysmography, or diffusion capacity.

Additional Testing

Additional diagnostic tests may be indicated after the initial data gathering and can include the following:

- Computed tomography (CT) provides more detailed assessment of mass lesions.
- Computed tomography pulmonary angiography (CPTA) confirms PE.
- A D-dimer assay can help diagnose thrombosis. Normal findings rule out thrombosis; abnormal findings may indicate thrombosis but do not rule out other potential causes. It is used to exclude thromboembolic disease where the probability is low.
- Wells criteria can be applied to arrive at a score to estimate the probability of PE.
- Complete blood count including white blood cell count with differential is used to determine the presence of bacterial infection.
- Blood urea nitrogen and creatinine levels help assess renal function. Renal insufficiency frequently presents with dyspnea as a result of the combined effects of volume overload and anemia.
- Arterial blood gases (ABGs) should be determined in an acutely ill patient with dyspnea or tachypnea.
- If sputum is present, a sputum culture should be obtained to determine the presence of an infectious agent.

DIFFERENTIAL DIAGNOSIS

When a patient reports severe dyspnea and manifests significant oxygen deprivation, emergent assessment and referral are indicated. The following health problems can be the cause of the emergent situation.

Emergent Conditions Manifested by Dyspnea

Pulmonary embolus

A patient reporting severe dyspnea, cough, fever, hemoptysis, chest pain, history of deep vein thrombosis, or history of recent immobilization should be evaluated for possible PE (see Chapter 8). The Wells risk score can be used to assess the probability of PE.

Foreign body aspiration

Foreign body aspiration occurs most frequently in children and older adults. If the event was witnessed, history of aspiration is usually clear. If the person is found after the event, the history cannot be as revealing. Generally, the onset of cough is sudden and unexpected. If the foreign body is obstructing the airway, the patient is in acute respiratory distress, and immediate intubation or bronchoscopy is indicated to remove the foreign body and open the airway. Partial obstruction of the airway can cause stridor, cyanosis, labored respirations, or wheezing. Lateral neck and chest radiographs can reveal the location and size of the obstructing object (see Chapter 11).

Anaphylaxis

Anaphylaxis is an emergent situation. History can include insect bite, drug ingestion, or recent meal containing exposure to known allergens. Early symptoms include pruritic rash, feeling of warmth, wheezing, fatigue, lightheadedness, and dyspnea. On examination, patients in anaphylaxis manifest angioedema, tachypnea, clammy skin, hypotension, wheezes, and tachycardia. Immediate treatment and support of ventilation is necessary.

Pneumothorax

History of blunt chest trauma, often seen after a motor vehicle accident or a fall, can cause pneumothorax, hemothorax, or pulmonary contusion. Cystic fibrosis can cause a spontaneous pneumothorax from rupture of subpleural blebs located at the apex of the upper lobe or in the superior segment of the lower lobe. Spontaneous pneumothorax can also occur, with the highest incidence in tall, thin boys and men between the ages of 15 and 30 years. There is sudden severe chest pain and dyspnea aggravated by normal respiratory movement. Absent or decreased breath sounds are found on the side of the pneumothorax. Chest radiography can be diagnostic.

Croup

Croup, or laryngotracheobronchitis, is a parainfluenza infection that is usually preceded by symptoms of an upper respiratory tract infection. The illness is usually gradual in onset and includes a hoarse, seal-bark cough and fever. The degree of respiratory distress is variable.

Acute epiglottitis

Acute epiglottitis is a serious, life-threatening bacterial infection caused primarily by *H. influenzae*. It typically has a rapid onset with stridor, high fever, drooling, muffled voice, and sore throat. A child will appear anxious and may be sitting forward. Parents should be asked if the child has received an *H. influenzae* B or Hib immunization. This condition is rare in children who have been immunized.

Bacterial tracheitis

Bacterial tracheitis is usually a secondary infection caused by *Staphylococcus aureus* or *H. influenzae* that inflames the trachea after a viral infection. It is a subglottic lesion and mimics croup; however, a high fever and toxic appearance are present. Frequently, there is a copious amount of purulent sputum present.

Status asthmaticus

Acute bronchoconstriction in a patient with asthma can develop as a result of a respiratory tract infection, exposure to allergens, inhalation of fumes or other airway irritants, or environmental factors. Airway obstruction is caused not only by bronchial smooth muscle constriction but also by mucosal edema and excessive mucus production. Predominant symptoms include breathlessness, wheezing, and coughing. Absence of wheezing in a child with asthma can indicate severe airway obstruction with poor air exchange.

Botulism

Botulism poisoning can occur after ingestion of the toxin in inadequately cooked or improperly canned food. Infant botulism is caused by ingestion of the spores of *C. botulinum* rather than the exotoxin. It occurs before the first year of life, and honey has been implicated in 20% of patients. Symptoms occur within hours after ingestion of contaminated food. Weakness and respiratory dyspnea and failure often accompany visual problems. Infant botulism begins with constipation, and the infant becomes weaker and listless. Respiratory arrest can be sudden.

Nonemergent Conditions Manifested by Dyspnea

Chronic progressive dyspnea is most often caused by COPD, heart failure, and obesity. It is seen less often in severe anemia and carcinoma of the pulmonary system. These patients report gradual onset of SOB over days or weeks.

Chronic obstructive pulmonary disease

Chronic obstructive pulmonary disease is associated with frequent cough that is worse in the morning, sputum production that is clear to yellow in color, decreasing exercise tolerance, and mild to moderate fatigue. History of smoking is present in most instances. Exposure to asbestos, coal dust, and other significant environmental pollutants may also be reported. Objective manifestations of COPD include rapid, shallow respirations; reddish complexion; increased AP diameter; use of accessory muscles to breathe; pursed-lip breathing; decreased tactile fremitus; decreased respiratory excursion bilaterally; hyperresonant lungs; distant breath sounds; prolonged expiration; occasional wheezes; and muffled heart sounds. Chest radiography, pulmonary function tests, and possible exercise tests are indicated to confirm the diagnosis of COPD.

Heart failure

Individuals reporting a history of heart disease or heart valve disease, dyspnea, orthopnea, PND, peripheral edema, weight gain, cough with frothy sputum, fatigue, and palpitations must be further assessed for acute heart failure. Physical examination findings can include altered level of consciousness, anxiety, jugular venous distention, tachypnea, rales, rhonchi, tachycardia, displaced point of maximum impulse, S_3, S_4, and possible ascites. Symptoms in children also include sweating on the forehead or upper lip. An ECG and chest radiograph will show increased heart size, oximetry will reveal a decreased arterial PO_2, and an echocardiogram will display a significantly reduced ejection fraction.

Anemia

Patients reporting dyspnea (especially on exertion), fatigue, lightheadedness, palpitations, and possible a history of chronic disease should have blood tests to measure the oxygen-carrying capacity of their blood (hemoglobin and hematocrit levels). Hematologic diseases affect the oxygen-carrying capacity of the blood, with resulting tissue hypoxia. Hypoxia from anemia leads the patient to hyperventilate to try to get more oxygen, which leads to respiratory alkalosis or an increasing pH. Objective signs of anemia include tachycardia and pallor.

Poor physical conditioning

Poor physical conditioning can cause a patient to experience SOB with exertion. Associated symptoms may include cardiac palpitations, history of excessive weight, and a sedentary lifestyle. The physical examination is often normal except for tachycardia and possible obesity. Exercise stress tests can be done for an adult with cardiovascular risk factors or a history of cardiovascular disease.

Asthma

Asthma is the most frequent cause of recurrent dyspnea. People usually report a history of asthma and possibly allergies and can be taking prescribed inhaled bronchodilators or inhaled steroids. Paroxysmal cough and an audible wheeze often accompany dyspnea. They can report recent respiratory tract infection, exposure to known allergens, or strenuous exercise. Objective manifestation on physical examination includes restlessness, tachypnea, use of accessory muscles to breathe, intercostal retraction, decreased tactile fremitus, decreased breath sounds, and inspiratory and possible expiratory wheezes. Pulse oximetry and spirometry testing will assist in the diagnosis of asthma. ABGs are indicated in the patient manifesting acute oxygen (O_2) deprivation or carbon dioxide (CO_2) retention, and chest radiographs are indicated if a lower respiratory tract infection is suspected. If the patient does not have a history of asthma and the spirometry test result has normal findings, a methacholine challenge test can be diagnostic.

The lessening or absence of wheezes in a person with asthma can indicate mucus plugging and an impending episode of status asthmaticus.

Pneumonia

Pneumonia is usually associated with dyspnea, pleuritic chest pain, cough with greenish or rust-colored sputum, fever, and chills. In children, irritability, feeding problems, and lack of playfulness can also be seen. Objective manifestations of pneumonia include fever, tachycardia, tachypnea, inspiratory crackles, asynchronous breathing, tactile fremitus, dull percussion sound over area of consolidation, and bronchophony. Pneumonia can be confirmed by chest radiography and sputum cultures.

Hyperventilation syndrome

Hyperventilation syndrome is a common cause of recurrent faintness without actual loss of consciousness. Dyspnea, lightheadedness, palpitations, and paresthesias (perioral and extremities) occur. Restlessness, anxiety, and a normal cardiovascular examination are present. Recumbency does not relieve the symptoms. Chest radiographs show normal findings.

Bronchomalacia

Bronchomalacia is the most common cause of persistent stridor in infancy. Onset of the stridor is almost always within the first 4 weeks of life, commonly in the first week (with preterm neonates who were on ventilation at high risk). Occasionally, parents become aware of the condition when a respiratory tract infection is present. Stridor is predominantly inspiratory, and the sound can be altered with change in position of the infant. The cry and cough are normal. Direct visualization of the larynx is performed for diagnosis.

Vascular ring

Tracheal compression from vascular anomalies can cause stridor and dyspnea in infants. The main symptom is soft inspiratory stridor with expiratory wheeze. Frequently, a brassy cough and difficulty swallowing may be present. Barium swallow followed by echocardiography is done to establish the diagnosis.

> **DIFFERENTIAL DIAGNOSIS OF** *Emergent Conditions Manifested by Dyspnea*

CONDITION	HISTORY	PHYSICAL FINDINGS	DIAGNOSTIC STUDIES
Pulmonary embolus	Acute-onset dyspnea, cough, mild to severe chest pain, sense of impending doom; hemoptysis; history of DVT, recent surgery, oral contraceptive, smoker, hypercoagulability states	Restlessness, fever, tachycardia, tachypnea, diminished breath sounds, crackles, wheezing, pleural friction rub	CTPA, ABGs, chest radiograph, ECG, ventilation/ perfusion scans, D-dimer, Wells score
Foreign body aspiration	Acute-onset dyspnea; history of drinking large amounts of alcohol; in children, history of putting small objects in mouth; possible cough	Apnea or tachypnea, restlessness, suprasternal retractions, intoxication, inspiratory stridor, localized wheeze	Lateral neck radiograph, chest radiograph, bronchoscopy

DIFFERENTIAL DIAGNOSIS OF *Emergent Conditions Manifested by Dyspnea—cont'd*

CONDITION	HISTORY	PHYSICAL FINDINGS	DIAGNOSTIC STUDIES
Anaphylaxis	Acute-onset dyspnea; history of insect sting, ingestion of drug, or allergen	Angioedema, tachypnea, clammy skin, hypotension, bilateral wheezes, tachycardia	None; emergency measures necessary
Pneumothorax	Acute-onset dyspnea; sharp, tearing chest pain; pain can radiate to ipsilateral shoulder	Tachycardia, diminished breath sounds, decreased tactile fremitus, hyperresonance of lung area affected; possible hypertension and tracheal shift	Chest radiograph, ABGs
Croup	History of upper respiratory tract infection	Hoarse, seal-bark cough, fever (variable)	None initially; if respiratory distress increases, pulse oximeter and referral
Acute epiglottitis	Positional sitting forward; sore throat, anxious, toxic child	High fever, drooling, stridor, muffled voice	None; emergency measures for airway support
Bacterial tracheitis	Recent viral infection	Fever, stridor, purulent sputum	Radiography of airway, WBC count increased, tracheal culture
Status asthmaticus	Recent URI, exposure to allergens, breathlessness	Wheezing, coughing, tachycardia, tachypnea	Peak flows, chest radiograph, ABGs
Botulism	Honey ingestion in infant, contaminated food ingestion	Hypoventilation, drooling, weak cry, ptosis, ophthalmoplegia, loss of head control	Pulmonary function testing, chest radiograph, fluoroscopy, stool culture

ABG, arterial blood gas; *DVT,* deep vein thrombosis; *ECG,* electrocardiogram; *WBC,* white blood cell.

DIFFERENTIAL DIAGNOSIS OF *Nonemergent Conditions Manifested by Dyspnea*

CONDITION	HISTORY	PHYSICAL FINDINGS	DIAGNOSTIC STUDIES
Pneumonia	Dyspnea, cough, sputum production (green, rust, or red), pleuritic chest pain, chills; in infants and children: irritability and feeding problems	Fever, tachycardia, tachypnea, inspiratory crackles, asynchronous breathing, vocal fremitus, percussion dull or flat over area of consolidation, bronchophony, egophony	Chest radiograph, sputum cultures, ABGs, WBC count
Hyperventilation syndrome	Dyspnea, lightheadedness, palpitations, paresthesias (perioral and extremities)	Restlessness, anxiety, normal CV examination	Chest radiograph, TSH

Continued

> **DIFFERENTIAL DIAGNOSIS OF** *Nonemergent Conditions Manifested by Dyspnea—cont'd*

CONDITION	HISTORY	PHYSICAL FINDINGS	DIAGNOSTIC STUDIES
Bronchomalacia	Neonate, infant: history of stridor, history of URI	Inspiratory stridor; normal cough, cry	Refer for visualization of larynx
Vascular ring	Infant: dyspnea, brassy cough, difficulty swallowing	Inspiratory stridor with expiratory wheeze	Barium swallow, echocardiography
Heart failure	Chronic progressive dyspnea, cough, frothy sputum, fatigue, lightheadedness, syncope, weight gain, ankle swelling, palpitations, PND, orthopnea, history of heart disease; in children: chronic progressive dyspnea, sweating above lip and forehead, especially while eating	Altered level of consciousness, restlessness, jugular venous distention, tachypnea, use of accessory muscles to breathe, rales, rhonchi, wheezes, tachycardia, decreased peripheral pulses, cool extremities, displaced PMI, S_3, S_4, ascites, liver enlargement	ECG, chest radiograph, ABGs, echocardiogram
Anemia	Dyspnea on exertion, fatigue, palpitations, lightheadedness, history of chronic disease	Pallor, tachypnea, cool dry skin of extremities, possible orthostatic hypotension	CBC, iron studies
Poor physical conditioning	Dyspnea on exertion, weight gain, palpitation on exertion, sedentary lifestyle, cigarette smoker	Overweight, tachycardia	Cardiac stress test
Asthma	Dyspnea, paroxysmal cough, audible wheeze, history of asthma or allergies	Restlessness, tachypnea, use of accessory muscles to breathe, intercostal retractions, decreased vocal fremitus, decreased breath sounds, inspiratory and possibly expiratory wheezes	Spirometry followed by a methacholine challenge, chest radiograph, ABGs
COPD	Chronic progressive dyspnea, dyspnea on exertion, persistent cough, minimal sputum, easy fatigue, history of smoking	Rapid shallow respirations, reddish complexion, increased AP diameter of thorax, use of accessory muscles to breathe, pursed-lip breathing, decreased tactile fremitus, decreased respiratory excursion bilaterally, lungs hyperresonant, distant breath sounds, prolonged expiration, occasional wheezes, possible tachycardia, muffled heart sounds	Chest radiograph, spirometry, exercise tests, ABGs

ABG, arterial blood gas; *AP*, anteroposterior; *COPD*, chronic obstructive pulmonary disease; *CPTA*, computer tomography pulmonary angiography; *CV*, cerebrovascular; *ECG*, electrocardiogram; *PMI*, point of maximal impulse; *PND*, paroxysmal nocturnal dyspnea; *TSH*, thyroid-stimulating hormone; *URI*, upper respiratory tract infection; *WBC*, white blood cell count.

CHAPTER

15 Earache

Otalgia, or ear pain, is a common problem in both children and adults and is generally caused by an inflammatory process. In children, inflammation most commonly occurs in the middle ear. Adults more often have an earache from external ear conditions or from referred pain from other head and neck structures. Acute otitis media (AOM) refers to any inflammation of the middle ear and encompasses a variety of clinical conditions. Otitis media with effusion is a collection of fluid in the middle ear. This condition is also known as serous otitis media, secretory otitis, or nonsuppurative otitis. External or middle ear disorders can often be distinguished after a brief history and physical examination. If the physical findings are normal, referred pain is a likely cause. About 50% of referred pain is caused by dental problems, although other causes may include temporomandibular joint (TMJ) disorder, parotitis, pharyngitis, and cervical, mouth, or facial disorders. The most serious, although least common, cause of referred pain is nasopharyngeal cancer, a condition more common in people of Asian descent. Figure 15.1 illustrates the structures of the ear.

DIAGNOSTIC REASONING: FOCUSED HISTORY

Is this an acute infection?

Key Questions
- How old are you?
- Have you had a fever?
- Have you had a recent upper respiratory infection?
- Have you had a recent ear infection?
- Is there a family history of ear infections?

Age
The occurrence of AOM declines significantly after age 6 years. Increased age raises the likelihood of secondary otalgia caused by disorders of the head, face, and neck; by sinus or periodontal disease; by chronic reflux; and by malignancy.

Fever
Fever is present in 60% of all children with AOM. In infants younger than 2 months, fever with AOM is uncommon. A high fever accompanying otitis is more likely to indicate a systemic illness such as pneumonia or meningitis.

Upper Respiratory Infection
An upper respiratory infection (URI) occurs when the mucous membranes of the nasopharynx or sinuses become infected and organisms are forced up the lumen of the eustachian tube. Inflammation of the mucosa or enlarged adenoids obstruct the eustachian opening so that the air in the middle ear is absorbed and replaced by mucus. This mucus creates a mechanical obstruction and can serve as a medium for bacterial growth.

Previous Infections
Infants younger than 3 months who have their first AOM run a high risk of recurrence. Up to 71% of children younger than age 3 years have had at least one episode, and one-third have had an average of three episodes. Chronic otitis media can result in anatomical changes to the tympanic membrane (TM) and middle ear ossicles, which may predispose the patient to additional ear infections.

Family History
Having a sibling or parent with chronic otitis media makes it twice as likely for the illness to develop in the child. The presence of chronic otitis media may also be related to child care practices such as bottle propping or environmental exposures such as secondhand cigarette smoke.

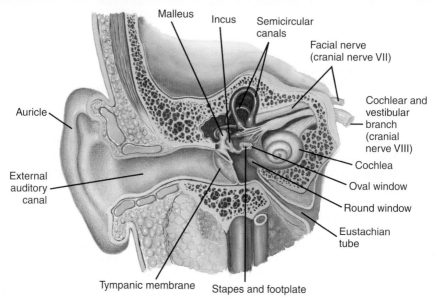

FIGURE 15.1 External auditory canal, middle ear, inner ear. (From Barkauskas VH, Baumann L, Darling-Fisher C: *Health and physical assessment,* ed. 3, St. Louis, 2002, Mosby.)

What environmental conditions might suggest increased risk?

Key Questions
- Does anyone around you smoke? Do you smoke?
- If a child: Does the child attend day care?
- If a child: Does the infant take a bottle lying down?
- Have you been swimming recently?
- Have you recently been in an airplane or been scuba diving?

Smoke Exposure
Secondhand cigarette smoke exposure has been associated with a two- to threefold increased risk of otitis media. Cigarette smoking leads to functional eustachian tube obstruction and decreases the protective ciliary action in the tube.

Attending Day Care
Attending a day care with other children is associated with an increased incidence rate of otitis media because of exposure to organisms.

Bottle Propping
In very young children, lying supine while drinking from a bottle has been associated with AOM. It is postulated that swallowing while lying down allows nasopharyngeal fluid to enter the middle ear, with subsequent infection.

EVIDENCE-BASED PRACTICE *What Is the Risk of Secondary Smoke Exposure for Otitis Media?*

A systematic review and meta-analysis of 61 epidemiological studies were done to examine the association between secondhand tobacco smoke (SHTS) and middle ear disease (MED) in children. Results showed that living with a smoker was associated with an increased risk of MED in children. Both maternal smoking and smoking by any household member increased risk of MED with an odds ratio (OR) of 1.62 (95% confidence interval [CI], 1.33–1.97) for maternal smoking and an OR of 1.37 (95% CI, 1.25–1.50) for any household member smoking. Maternal postnatal smoking and paternal smoking increased the risk of surgery for MED almost twofold.

Reference: Jones et al, 2012.

Swimming

Repeated or prolonged immersion in water results in loss of protective cerumen and chronic irritation, with maceration from excessive moisture in the canal. This leads to an increased occurrence of otitis externa, also called swimmer's ear.

Airplane Travelers and Divers

Barotrauma is a cause of acute serous otitis related to pressure changes from flying or scuba diving. This is often aggravated by recent upper respiratory tract infection (URI) or nasal congestion. Failure of the eustachian tube to open and equilibrate during descent results in a collection of serosanguineous fluid in the middle ear. This may be felt as ear pressure that can lead to pain, tinnitus, and temporary deafness. Swallowing, chewing, or blowing out the nose with the mouth and nose occluded can relieve symptoms.

Could this be related to another organ system?

Key Questions
- Do you have diabetes?
- Do you have any other health conditions you are being treated for?
- Have you ever had dermatitis, eczema, or psoriasis?
- If a child: Does the child have a cleft palate that is not repaired?

Diabetes Mellitus

Diabetes mellitus predisposes adults to malignant otitis externa, which is cellulitis involving the ear and surrounding tissue. People with diabetes are also at increased risk for otitis media, mastoiditis, and osteomyelitis of the skull base.

Immunosuppression

Patients being treated for cancer or HIV/AIDS may be on immunosuppressive medications and are at increased risk for malignant otitis externa.

History of Seborrheic Dermatitis or Psoriasis

The etiology of debris in the external canal in seborrheic dermatitis and psoriasis is the result of the increased desquamation associated with these two disorders, and in the case of psoriasis hyperkeratosis, thickening of the epidermis with desquamation. Chronic inflammatory dermatitis can result as a reaction to wearing a hearing aid. Overproduction of sebum in the external canal can cause otitis externa.

Cleft Palate

Anomalies that are not repaired anatomically predispose a child to otitis media because of functional obstruction of the eustachian tubes.

What does the presence of pain tell me?

Key Questions
- Where specifically is the pain felt?
- Is the pain in one or both ears?
- What does the pain feel like?
- How severe is the pain?
- Does it interfere with sleeping, eating, or other activities?
- How long have you had this pain?
- Is the pain constant or intermittent? If intermittent, how long does it last?
- Does the pain travel (radiate) to other areas?

Location of the Pain

Pain of otitis externa is described as tenderness around the outer ear or the opening to the ear canal that worsens with manipulation of the pinna. Mastoiditis is often associated with severe pain or tenderness over the mastoid bone. Bilateral pain occurs with otitis externa. Referred pain or pain of AOM is usually unilateral. Ramsay Hunt syndrome is more common in older adults and produces a painful rash with vesicles in, on, or around one ear; facial weakness may appear on the same side. Infants cannot assist in location of the ear pain; instead, they exhibit behavioral changes that may indicate pain, such as irritability, malaise, poor appetite, vomiting, and diarrhea. Young children may pull or tug at their ears.

Quality of the Pain

The pain of AOM is often described as a deep pain or a blockage of the ear. Serous otitis is often painless or may be described as a bubbling, popping, or stuffy sensation in the ear. Otitis externa involves a tenderness of the outer ear or ear canal that can be accompanied by itching. A cerumen impaction creates a milder pain or vague discomfort of stuffed ears.

Quantity and Severity of the Pain

The pain of AOM is severe enough to interfere with sleep and may be suddenly relieved if the eardrum perforates. Chronic ear pain that is unresponsive to treatment may indicate a tumor.

Onset, Timing, and Duration of the Pain

Temporomandibular joint pain is often described as severe pain lasting a few minutes and recurring three or four times per day, sometimes associated with headache. It is worse in the morning because nighttime teeth grinding is associated with this condition. The pain is intermittent but can be acute and is related to trauma or overextension of the mouth. Chronic pain may be related to dental malocclusion or rheumatoid arthritis.

Crying when sucking is often an infant's only indication of pain with compression and increased pressure in the ears. Nocturnal onset of otalgia from a developing infection is caused by increased vascular pressure in the reclined position, which causes the TM to bulge and to stimulate pain sensation.

What does the presence of discharge or itching tell me?

Key Questions
- Do you have any itching in the ear?
- Do you have any discharge from the ear?

Itching or Drainage

Itching or drainage from the ear usually indicates an infection or inflammation of the external canal. Itching can also be a precursor to herpes zoster of the trigeminal nerve (cranial nerve [CN] V), which can cause paroxysmal pain of the face and jaw, and hyperalgesia to minimal stimulation such as tooth brushing, cold air, or grimacing. The prodrome for herpes zoster consists of itching, burning, or tingling before vesicular eruption. The facial nerve (CN VII) is also involved in ear pain. Itching may be related to allergic rhinitis, especially when patients describe a deep itching in the ears.

Drainage may also be present after the TM ruptures from increased middle ear pressure,

as exudate from otitis externa or malignant otitis externa, or it may be from exudate secondary to mastoiditis. Cholesteatoma is an epidermal inclusion cyst of the middle ear or mastoid. A perforation of the TM and associated foul-smelling discharge may occur.

What does a history of trauma or injury tell me?

Key Questions
- Have you had any recent trauma to the ear?
- Have you had any head trauma?
- How do you clean your ears? Do you use cotton-tipped swabs?
- Do you have a history of excessive earwax?
- If a child: Does the child have a history of putting objects in the ears?
- Have you had any recent insect bites around the ear?
- Have you been exposed to any loud noise?

Ear Trauma

Perforation of the eardrum can be caused by blunt or penetrating trauma. Blunt trauma might include a slap to the ear or barotrauma. Penetrating trauma to the canal or TM may be self-induced with cotton-tipped swabs or other sharp objects used to remove cerumen or to scratch the canal.

Head Trauma

Direct injury to the inner ear by fracture of the petrous temporal bone, located at the base of the skull, also destroys the inner ear.

Cerumen Impaction

Cerumen is a naturally wet, sticky, honey-colored wax that lubricates and protects the external ear canal. In some individuals, it occurs in a dark, scaly form and accumulates in the ear canal. This accumulation may cause hearing loss, tinnitus, pressure sensation, vertigo, and infection. Self-cleaning practices can produce trauma to the canal, and cerumen-softening solutions can cause chemical irritation to the canal tissue.

Foreign Bodies

Foreign bodies such as feathers, beads, and insects (especially cockroaches) can produce ear pain and inflammation. Children often insert objects into the ear canal.

Insect Bites

Insect bites can lead to acute pain and tenderness of the external canal and may develop into a secondary infection.

Loud Noise

Exposure to high-pitched and loud noise for a prolonged period of time destroys the cochlear hair cells. Exposure to noisy work environments, to the operation of heavy machinery, and to loud music increases the risk of injury and eventual hearing loss.

Is hearing loss a clue?

Key Questions

- Do you have any difficulty in hearing?
- What is your age?
- Do you have any dizziness?
- Do you have any ringing in the ear?
- If a child: Do you think the child can hear normally?
- If a child: Does the child turn his or her head to listen?
- If a child: Does the child seem to focus on your mouth when listening to you?

Difficulty in Hearing

Reports of hearing loss or "difficulty hearing" can indicate blockage of the ear canal by cerumen or a foreign body, inflammation of the middle or inner ear, or a neoplasm. The most frequent cause is conductive hearing loss caused by blockage of the external canal, usually by cerumen. Chronic otitis media is usually a condition of adults who have a chronic infection that may destroy the ossicles and spread to the mastoid, labyrinth, and intracranial structures, causing hearing loss. Chronic ear pain is often associated with hearing loss and ear discharge secondary to a perforated nonhealing TM.

Age-Related Hearing Loss

Age-related hearing loss (presbycusis), affects adults after 65 years. The onset is gradual and bilateral. The cause is related to changing structures in the ear and changes in neural pathways and exposures to loud noise.

Hearing Loss in Children

Chronic otitis media with effusion causes a conductive hearing loss in children. This loss may be caused by negative middle ear pressure, the presence of an effusion in the middle ear, or structural damage to the TM or ossicles.

Dizziness and Ringing in the Ear

Hearing loss associated with dizziness, vertigo, or tinnitus may indicate a serious inner ear condition such as acoustic neuroma or Ménière disease. Abnormal middle ear ventilation and middle ear effusion are the most common causes of balance disturbance in children. These symptoms are caused by reestablishment of aeration in the middle ear cavity as the effusion clears.

DIAGNOSTIC REASONING: FOCUSED PHYSICAL EXAMINATION

A correct diagnosis of ear pain requires a good view of the TM and external ear canal. Cerumen obstruction should be removed through lavage or by separating an impaction with an ear curette so that irrigation fluid can penetrate behind the impaction. The curette must be manipulated cautiously because trauma to or inflammation of the sensitive perichondrium, which lies immediately below a thin layer of epithelium in the ear canal, elicits excruciating pain and bleeds easily.

Lavage should not be performed if the medical history suggests perforation of the TM. Without visualization of the TM, however, otitis media cannot be ruled out. Lavage solution helps to soften the cerumen and can be purchased commercially in kits, or a solution can be made of hydrogen peroxide and water (1:1 ratio).

Note Behaviors in Children

Otitis media is the most common childhood disorder. Young infants may exhibit nonspecific signs of irritability, poor feeding, congestion, and fever. Older infants and young toddlers are irritable, may pull on the painful ear, or bang their head on the affected side. Older children will report an earache.

Inspect the External Ears

General inspection should begin with the pinna and condition of the skin around the ear, face, and scalp. Hemorrhage over the mastoid bone (Battle sign) may occur with a basal skull fracture. Eczema, seborrheic dermatitis, or psoriasis manifests as redness and scaling of the skin that can extend into the external ear canal. Pain in the opening of the ear canal and inflamed skin may be suggestive of a bacterial infection. Fungal and yeast infections appear as white or dark patches. Furuncles or lesions secondary to trauma or irritation appear as localized areas of tenderness or swelling. A hot, swollen, and erythematous ear and surrounding skin indicate cellulitis. Redness and painful swelling over the mastoid process is a sign of infection in the mastoid air cells.

Palpate the External Ears

Palpate the pinna and tragus for tenderness. In mastoiditis, the pinna is displaced forward, and swelling may be present behind the ear. Palpation of the mastoid process elicits severe tenderness. Otitis externa is associated with pain on manipulation of the pinna and tragus. With referred pain, the structures will appear normal, although palpation over the TMJ may elicit tenderness, and movement of the jaw may create a clicking sound.

Palpate the preauricular and postauricular areas on the right and left simultaneously to elicit pain. Palpate the anterior and posterior cervical lymph nodes and the area over the mastoid process. Preauricular nodes may be enlarged in AOM and otitis externa. Postauricular swelling may indicate extension of infection into the mastoid cavity.

Inspect the Ear Canals

With the otoscope, observe for the patency of the canal, the condition of the skin of the ear canal, and the presence of cerumen. With cerumen impaction, no structures can be visualized. A foreign body is easily visualized. Vesicles on the external ear canal and auricle may indicate herpes zoster (Ramsay Hunt syndrome).

Visualize any discharge, noting color, consistency, and odor. Discharge is usually indicative of an active infection. However, cranial trauma with cerebrospinal fluid leakage must be kept in mind. Cheesy, green-blue, or gray discharge can be seen with otitis externa.

Inspect the Tympanic Membranes

Visualize the TM, noting light reflex and anatomical structures. A normal TM is translucent and pearly gray in color. Mild diffuse redness can occur from crying or coughing. Mild vascularity is sometimes seen in the normal eardrum, especially on the handle of the malleus. Localized redness is a sign of inflammation. Scarring and effusion can cause whitening and opacification of the TM.

The contour of the normal TM is somewhat concave. Fullness or bulging indicates either increased air pressure, or more commonly, increased hydrostatic pressure within the middle ear. Fullness of the eardrum is seen first around the periphery of the TM. As pressure increases, central fullness becomes visible. Concavity or retraction of the eardrum is associated with negative middle ear pressure or postinflammatory adhesions. As the eardrum retracts, the handle of the malleus short process becomes more visible.

Myringitis is a red, inflamed eardrum without effusion. Bullous myringitis describes an extremely painful condition of small blisters on the TM caused by bacterial otitis media. Figure 15.2 illustrates the usual landmarks of a normal right TM. Chronic otitis media can lead to cholesteatoma, or a cyst-like mass behind the eardrum caused by the proliferation of squamous epithelium. The mass can grow to cause necrosis of the ossicles. Examination will reveal a collection of white granulation tissue with perforation of the TM. A series of videos that show the examination of the TM when otitis media with effusion is present is available at https://www.aap.org/en-us/about-the-aap/Committees-Councils-Sections/Section-on-infectious-diseases/Pages/VideoHighlights.aspx.

Perform Pneumatic Otoscopy (Insufflation)

The normal eardrum is suspended from its margins and responds to slight pressure changes. Insufflation tests the mobility of the TM. It can be an insensitive test for otitis media if poor technique fails to create a seal. Properly performed, however, it is more reliable than visualization alone.

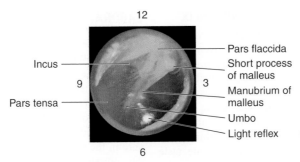

12

Incus

9

Pars tensa

3

Pars flaccida

Short process of malleus

Manubrium of malleus

Umbo

Light reflex

6

FIGURE 15.2 Usual landmarks of the right tympanic membrane with a "clock" superimposed. (From Barkauskas VH, Baumann L, Darling-Fisher C: *Health and physical assessment,* ed. 3, St Louis, 2002, Mosby.)

To perform insufflation, a large speculum is needed to create a seal. A normal finding elicits a slight motion of the TM when air is insufflated. This movement is compared with the opposite ear. A TM that has been retracted as a result of negative middle ear pressure or adhesions does not move with inflation, but rebound mobility is seen when the bulb is released. Any accumulation of liquid in the middle ear (e.g., effusion) or scarring of the TM inhibits movement when air is insufflated.

Test Hearing Acuity

Hearing acuity is tested using the whisper test and the tuning fork for the Rinne and Weber tests. The sensory function of the acoustic nerve (CN VIII) should be tested to determine whether air or bone conduction loss is present with ear pain.

The Weber test is performed with a 512-hertz (Hz) or higher frequency tuning fork. To perform the test, firmly place the vibrating tuning fork on a midline point of the skull. If there is unilateral conductive hearing loss, sound will lateralize to the ear with the loss because the better ear will be distracted by ambient noise. Alternately, if the patient has unilateral sensorineural loss, the sound will lateralize to the better ear because the neural pathway will be interrupted on the affected side. Equal perception of vibration can indicate normal hearing or bilateral hearing loss. The Rinne test compares air conduction (AC) with bone conduction (BC); the ratio should be 2:1 AC greater than BC. A 20- to 30-decibel (dB) conductive loss would result in better sound transmission through bone than through air. Conductive hearing loss results when sound transmission is impaired through the external or middle ear. Sensorineural hearing loss results from a defect in the inner ear. Findings of both the Weber and Rinne tests must be considered for optimal diagnosis. Sensorineural loss in the right ear lateralizes to the left with both the Weber and Rinne, and AC is greater than BC in both ears. With a conduction loss in the right ear, the Weber lateralizes to the right and BC is greater than AC on the right; if BC is greater than AC in both ears, there is a mixed defect.

Examine Related Body Systems

Examine other regional body systems of the head and neck, including inspection of the conjunctiva; examination of the mucosa and patency of the nose; percussion and palpation of the frontal and maxillary sinuses for tenderness; and inspection of the posterior pharynx for lymphedema, color, and presence of exudate. Inspection of the condition of the oral mucosa (teeth and gums) will provide information about possible causes of referred pain. A focused physical examination for head and neck symptoms should include palpation of cervicofacial lymph nodes, especially the preauricular and postauricular nodes.

Perform an Intraotic Manipulation

If referred pain is suspected, conduct a more extensive neurologic examination and assess for TMJ disorder. TMJ pain can be replicated by instructing the patient to open the mouth wide. Face the patient, insert a single fingertip in each ear and pull the patient toward you as the patient is instructed to open and close the mouth. Pain will be elicited in 90% of patients with TMJ disorder.

Evaluate Cranial Nerves V, VII, and IX

To evaluate the trigeminal nerve (CN V), observe jaw and facial muscle movement for symmetry and strength by palpating over the masseter muscles and ask the patient to bite and clench the teeth. Assess intactness of sensation to pain and light touch using a sharp and dull stimulus over the three branches of CN V. Both CN VII (anterior two-thirds) and CN IX (posterior one-third) innervate taste sensation to the tongue as well as sensation to the external ear. Have the patient protrude the tongue and apply sweet and salty substances separately to each half of the tongue to test CN VII and apply bitter and sour substances to test CN IX.

LABORATORY AND DIAGNOSTIC STUDIES

Tympanometry

Tympanometry involves inserting a probe into the external ear canal while continually changing pressure against the eardrum to assess the mobility of the TM. The tympanogram provides an indirect measure of pressure in the middle ear. Under normal middle ear pressure, the TM absorbs the sound energy waves and produces a bell-shaped pattern that peaks when sound pressure is introduced. With positive or negative middle ear pressure, the tympanogram results in a flat pattern or an early peak pressure. Figure 15.3

Pneumatic otoscopy				Middle ear status		Tympanograms
Tympanic membrane position		External canal pressure		Content	Pressure	Jerger's classification
		Pos	Neg			
1. Neutral	Ext. canal / Middle ear	2+	3+	Air	Normal	Type A
2. Neutral monometric		3+	4+	Air	Normal	Type A
3. Neutral	Air	1+	2+	Air and liquid	Normal	Type A
4. Retracted slightly		1+	3+	Air	Low negative	Peaked Type C / Gradual
		0	2+	Air and liquid		
5. Retracted markedly		0	2+	Air	High negative	Peaked / Gradual Type C
		0	1+	Air and liquid		
6. Retracted		0	0	Liquid	Indeterminate	Type B / Type C
7. Full		1+	0	Liquid and air	Positive or indeterminate	Type A+ / Type B
8. Bulging	Liquid	0	0	Liquid	Indeterminate	Type B
						−400 −200 0 +200

FIGURE 15.3 Middle ear evaluation with pneumatic otoscopy and impedance tympanograms. (From Daeschner CW Jr: *Pediatrics: An approach to independent learning,* New York, 1983, John Wiley & Sons.)

illustrates examples of various tympanogram results.

Audiometry

Audiometry assesses both the frequency and the intensity of sound that can be perceived. An air conduction audiometer tests each ear separately via earphones and transmits a pure tone that has variable frequency and intensity settings. The goal of audiometry is to test the lowest decibel intensity that can be heard for each frequency tested. An individual trained in the proper technique will produce reliable, reproducible, and valid test results. A threshold of up to 20 dB is considered normal. At a higher level, hearing loss is graded as mild, moderate, moderately severe, severe, or profound.

Mastoid Process Radiography

Radiographs of the mastoid bone show clouding of the air cells when otitis media is present. Chronic mastoiditis may reveal decalcification of the bony wall between the mastoid air cells.

Computed Tomography Scanning

A computed tomography (CT) scan of the temporal bone is helpful in diagnosing cholesteatoma and congenital syndromes.

DIFFERENTIAL DIAGNOSIS

External Otitis

External otitis is more common in adults than in children and often presents as bilateral pain that worsens with manipulation of the pinna. The patient reports a stuffed ear, and occasionally conductive hearing loss occurs. Discharge and itching that occur 1 to 2 days after swimming may be associated with otitis externa. The affected canal may be swollen shut. Palpation will often disclose enlarged preauricular or postauricular nodes. Malignant otitis externa is a rare complication and involves infection and damage of the bones of the ear canal and at the base of the skull.

Acute Otitis Media

Acute otitis media most often occurs in children younger than 6 years and is associated with URI. It is an acute infection associated with ear pain and a bulging, red eardrum. The pain of otitis media is severe enough to interfere with sleep and may be suddenly relieved if the eardrum perforates. Swelling of the preauricular node is sometimes seen in children with AOM.

Otitis Media with Effusion

Otitis media with effusion commonly occurs in children and is by definition painless. It is caused by a mechanical process or eustachian tube blockage that leads to inadequate ventilation of the middle ear. On examination, a collection of fluid that resembles mucus, air bubbles, or a fluid level is seen. Associated conductive hearing loss is usually present. The TM may be injected and immobile, either bulging or retracted, as noted by the shape of the cone of light reflex and pneumatic otoscopy. Associated recent URI is a common finding in adults.

Cholesteatoma

Cholesteatoma is an epidermal inclusion cyst formation in the middle ear and mastoid cavity. It is often the sequelae of chronic otitis media. The formation occurs with chronic negative middle ear pressure, causing the migration of skin cells from the external ear canal through a perforation in the TM. After being established in the middle ear, the cells desquamate and form the cholesteatoma. This condition is life threatening if left untreated because it will continue to erode away medially to impinge on intracranial structures. A cholesteatoma can also occur congenitally. A cholesteatoma appears as a cyst or collection of granulation tissue on the TM, commonly located in the pars flaccida area in the superior anterior quadrant of the TM.

Mastoiditis

Mastoiditis is an infection of the soft tissue surrounding the air spaces in the mastoid bone and is connected to the middle ear space. Mastoiditis usually occurs with bacterial otitis media and is associated with fever. More advanced mastoiditis is manifested by swelling, erythema, and tenderness over the mastoid bone. Swelling can displace the position of the auricle. The swelling can extend to the facial nerve, causing paralysis, or to the labyrinth or cerebrospinal fluid, causing meningitis or brain abscess. Advanced mastoiditis requires immediate referral and surgical management.

Foreign Bodies

Foreign bodies are easily visualized on examination of the ear canal and can produce foul-smelling ear drainage secondary to infection or abscess.

Cerumen Impaction

Impaction of cerumen is likely if the patient reports a stuffed-up ear or decreased hearing acuity. An impaction may also produce pain if cerumen is pressed against the TM. Examination will reveal cerumen that occludes the external canal.

Barotrauma

Barotrauma produces an acute serous otitis that is caused by pressure changes (e.g., in divers or airplane travelers) and is often aggravated by a recent URI or nasal congestion. Serosanguineous fluid collects in the middle ear; during descent, this may be felt as ear pressure, pain, tinnitus, or temporary deafness. Swallowing, chewing, or blowing out the nose with the mouth and nose occluded can relieve symptoms.

Trauma

Blunt or penetrating trauma can perforate the TM. A hole in the TM is visible on examination, or the examiner may notice an absence of normal landmarks. A perforated eardrum does not significantly impair hearing or result in vertigo, and it usually heals within 4 to 6 weeks without sequelae. Assess the extent of other damage to the ear when perforation is identified.

Cervical Lymphadenitis

Anterior cervical lymphadenitis is a common cause of referred ear pain in children. This may be seen with strep throat, as well as in cases of mononucleosis with extensive cervical node swelling in adolescents or young adults.

Referred Pain from Cervical and Cranial Nerves

Cervical nerves II and III innervate the skin and muscles of the neck and include the great auricular nerve, which supplies the external canals and posterior auricular area. Pain is perceived in these areas. The ear examination will be normal.

Cranial nerves associated with referred ear pain include V, VII, IX, and X. The trigeminal nerve (CN V) supplies the anterior portion of the auricle and tragus, the anterior and superior auditory canal, and the anterior TM. The facial (CN VII), vagus (CN X), and glossopharyngeal (CN IX) nerves innervate the posterior portion of the TM and the external auditory canal. Inflammation of CN X is associated with lesions of the larynx, esophagus, trachea, and thyroid. With referred pain, the structures of the ear will appear normal.

Temporomandibular Joint Disorder

Temporomandibular joint disorder is a common secondary cause of ear pain. Diagnosis of the disorder is likely if palpation over the TMJ elicits tenderness and movement of the joint creates a clicking sound. Results of examination of the ear are normal. Pain also increases with intraotic manipulation. TMJ pain is often worse in the morning. The pain can be acute (related to trauma or overextension of the mouth) or chronic (related to dental malocclusion or rheumatoid arthritis).

▶ DIFFERENTIAL DIAGNOSIS OF *Common Causes of Ear Pain*

CONDITION	HISTORY	PHYSICAL FINDINGS	DIAGNOSTIC STUDIES
External otitis	More common in adults, especially those with diabetes, ear pickers, or swimmers; bilateral itching; pain	Discharge; inflamed, swollen external canal; pain with movement of pinna; TM normal or not visible	None
Acute otitis media	More common in children younger than 6 yr; those with smoke exposure, recent URI; severe or deep pain; unilateral; sensation of fullness	Red, bulging TM; fever; decreased light reflex; opaque TM; decreased TM mobility	None initially
Otitis media with effusion	More common in children but occurs in adults with recent URI; unilateral pain; sensation of crackling or decreased hearing	Fluid line or air observed behind TM; conductive hearing loss; decreased TM mobility	Pneumatic otoscopy, tympanogram
Cholesteatoma	Hearing loss; recent perforated TM	Pearly white lesion on or behind TM	Immediate referral
Mastoiditis	History of recent otitis media; chronic otitis pain behind ear	Swelling over mastoid process; fever, palpable tenderness, and erythema over mastoid process	Radiograph of mastoid sinuses reveals cloudiness; referral
Foreign body or cerumen impaction	Both children and adults have pain or vague sensation of discomfort; decreased hearing	Visualize foreign body or cerumen; may detect foul odor; conductive hearing loss	None
Barotrauma	History of flying, diving; severe pain; hearing loss; sensation of fullness; history of recent nasal congestion	Retraction or bulging of TM; perforation of TM; fluid in canal	Tympanogram
Trauma	History of blunt trauma, penetrating trauma	Perforation of TM	Radiography or CT scan as directed by injury
Cervical lymphadenitis	History of cervical node swelling; pain in ear common in children	Enlarged, tender, cervical lymph nodes; may see early onset of AOM in children and young adults	Throat culture if indicated; in adolescents Monospot if indicated
CNs II and III (referred pain)	Pain in skin and muscles of neck and in ear canal	Dermatome evaluation for cervical nerve involvement	None
CNs (referred pain)	History, depending on CN involved	Test function of CNs V, VII, IX, and X; ear examination normal	Radiography or CT scan, directed by CN involvement
TMJ disorder	More common in adults; 50% related to dental problems; discomfort to severe pain; unilateral; pain worse in morning	Malocclusion; bruxism; normal external and middle ear structures and function; jaw click; abnormal CN function; ear examination results normal	None

AOM, acute otitis media; *CN*, cranial nerve; *CT*, computed tomography; *TM*, tympanic membrane; *TMJ*, temporomandibular joint; *URI*, upper respiratory tract infection.

Fatigue, also called asthenia, is a constitutional symptom that can be the result of normal physiological consequences of exertion or a symptom of illness. It is a sensation of profound tiredness that is not relieved by rest or sleep and is without an objective finding of muscle weakness. Fatigue can result from any disruption of energy production. Anemia, decreased oxygenation of blood, or reduced blood flow limits the amount of oxygen available to cells. Other factors that contribute to fatigue interfere with restorative mechanisms provided by sleep and rest, nutritional state, and mechanisms to remove or regulate wastes of metabolism. When fatigue is associated with cardiovascular or respiratory symptoms, clues are present that may point to the cause. However, most patients who report fatigue have normal physical examination results, and psychological factors are often a contributing cause.

Fatigue is classified as physiological, psychological, and acute or chronic. Physiological fatigue is the result of normal activities that lead to overwork or exhaustion. Psychological fatigue is often related to a stressful event. Organic causes can produce acute or chronic fatigue. Acute fatigue lasts less than 6 months and is often a prodrome to other illnesses, most often infections such as endocarditis, hepatitis, or other acute bacterial or viral illnesses. However, fatigue can also indicate a disease state, most often related to hyperthyroidism, hypothyroidism, heart failure, anemia, chronic obstructive pulmonary disease (COPD), sleep apnea, autoimmune disorder, or cancer.

Chronic fatigue lasts longer than 6 months, and its onset is usually slow and progressive. Chronic fatigue may be an indication of depression, chronic infection, or systemic disease, or it may be secondary to alcohol or medication use. Chronic fatigue syndrome is a distinct clinical entity characterized by fatigue that is persistent or relapses, is not alleviated with rest, and affects the patient's ability to function.

Fatigue is uncommon in very young children; the younger the child, the more likely the cause is organic. Most cases of fatigue in school-age children are related to acute infection. Fatigue is common in adolescents and in older adults because of lifestyle factors, especially insufficient hours of sleep.

DIAGNOSTIC REASONING: FOCUSED HISTORY

Is this really fatigue?

Key Question
- Can you tell me what you mean by fatigue?
- How old are you?
- Do you notice other symptoms with feelings of fatigue?

Fatigue versus Weakness

It is important to discriminate between weakness and fatigue. Often, patients describe muscle weakness when speaking about fatigue such as, "I am tired all the time, and I feel weak." In children with weakness, parents will say the child is floppy or "doesn't run in gym like the other children." An individual tends to tire easily with metabolic or neuromuscular diseases such as hypothyroidism or myasthenia gravis.

Young children tend not to vocalize fatigue; often it is the caregiver who brings the child to seek treatment. The caregiver may state "the child is lying around," "I can't get the child to do anything," or "the child just doesn't have any energy." Adolescents will say they are "always" tired.

Fatigue versus Frailty

Frailty is a distinct health condition associated with age and is present in more than 10% of adults older than 65 years and in more than 25% of adults older than 85 years. Frailty can be measured based on the presence of five symptoms: unintentional weight loss, slow mobility, weakness, decreased reduced activities, and fatigue. Presence of frailty increases the risk for falls.

Is the fatigue physiologic?

Key Questions

- Tell me about your lifestyle habits (e.g., exercise and diet).
- What is your sleep pattern?
- Do you require naps? How often?
- Do you feel rested when you wake up in the morning?
- When was your last menstrual period?

Lifestyle Habits

A history of the patient's daily living and working habits may reveal a physiological cause for exhaustion. Erratic eating patterns, dieting, and missed meals may result in undernutrition or overnutrition. High levels of caffeine can affect the amount of energy a person has as well as the sleep cycle, causing fatigue. Academic stress, athletic participation, high-intensity training, and employment further contribute to fatigue in adolescents.

Sleep Pattern

Lack of adequate amounts of sleep is often the cause of fatigue (see Chapter 31). Adults need at least 6 to 8 hours of sleep for adequate rest; adolescents, 8 to 9 hours; and children, 10 hours. Patients with sleep apnea, which is more common in men older than 45 years, may report waking up and not feeling refreshed. Heart failure causes postural nocturnal dyspnea, leading to difficulty breathing at night and disturbed sleep. Early-morning wakening is a symptom of depression, as is excessive sleeping during the day. Men over 50 years of age may have nocturia associated with benign prostatic hypertrophy.

Last Normal Menstrual Period

Fatigue is an early sign of pregnancy, a symptom after childbirth, and a symptom associated with menopause. Perimenopausal adults may have fatigue as a result of disrupted sleep because of night sweats or hot flashes.

Do I need to consider an organic cause?

Key Questions

- Do you practice safe sex (if sexually active)?
- Have you ever had hepatitis?
- What medications do you take?
- Do you drink alcohol or use recreational drugs?

Exposure to Body Fluids

Fatigue may be the initial and most prominent symptom of hepatitis, human immunodeficiency virus (HIV) infection, or acquired immunodeficiency syndrome (AIDS). Hepatitis B can be sexually transmitted through semen or contracted from exposure to contaminated blood. Sexual practices that traumatize mucous membranes, such as anal intercourse, increase the risk of transmission of organisms. People with HIV/AIDS experience cognitive impairment that includes difficulty processing complex information. These impairments are correlated with the severity of fatigue.

Medications

Almost any drug may have fatigue as a side effect. The most common drugs that cause fatigue are antihypertensive drugs, cardiovascular medications, psychotropic medications, and opiates. Side effects also occur with drugs such as sedatives and antihistamines. Many drugs that cause fatigue are over-the-counter preparations.

Alcohol and Drug Use

Alcohol abuse and use of recreational drugs may be overlooked as a cause of chronic fatigue in adolescents and school-age children. This fatigue is due directly to the substance, usually alcohol or marijuana, and to secondary factors such as associated poor lifestyle habits related to sleep, rest, and nutrition. Family and friends may express the greatest concerns about fatigue that affects the patient's ability to function. The CAGE questionnaire is a useful screening tool to assess for alcohol abuse (see Box 4.3).

What other clues can help me rule out an organic cause?

Key Questions
- Have you noticed a change in appetite? Increased thirst?
- Have you had unintentional weight loss?
- Do you have any joint tenderness or pain?
- Have you noticed increased urination?
- What other symptoms have you experienced?

Appetite

An increased appetite may indicate hypoglycemia; increased thirst may indicate hyperglycemia. A decreased appetite may indicate an infectious process.

Weight Loss

Weight loss may indicate malignancy, infection, or poor nutrition related to depression or lack of information about a healthy and balanced diet. Unintentional weight loss is a loss of greater than 10 lb in the past year and may be associated with other signs and symptoms.

Joint Tenderness

In children with juvenile rheumatoid arthritis (JRA), severe fatigue that seems to be more than expected with the degree of joint involvement is seen. In young and middle-aged patients, chronic fatigue syndrome can involve multiple tender points on the body that are over joints.

Increased Urination

Diabetes mellitus, especially type 2, often presents with fatigue along with polydipsia, polyphagia, and polyuria.

Associated Symptoms

Psychological fatigue is often associated with nonspecific and multiple symptoms, such as muscle aching, abdominal pain, and general lethargy. Organic causes of fatigue are associated with a few specific symptoms that worsen over time, such as dry skin and nails with hypothyroidism, or shortness of breath with exertion or when lying flat, as seen in congestive heart failure.

Could this have an environmental cause?

Key Questions
- Where do you work?

- Have you been exposed to any toxins?
- Have you been camping?

Occupational Exposure

Heavy metals and pesticides may cause fatigue and other neurologic symptoms. Soldiers returning from combat zones may develop unrelenting fatigue from an unknown cause.

Camping

Lyme disease is carried by the deer tick. The patient may present with a history of weeks of malaise and chronic fatigue before any skin manifestations appear.

What else do I need to know about the fatigue?

Key Questions
- Describe the onset and pattern of your fatigue.
- When did you first notice this?
- How severe is the fatigue?
- What makes the fatigue better or worse?
- Have you had a fever?
- Have you had any bleeding?

Onset and Pattern

The onset of psychological fatigue is often related to a stressful event and may have a sudden onset. Fatigue associated with metabolic causes may have a slow and progressive onset. Significant fatigue is considered to last longer than 2 weeks and is experienced by about 25% of adults. Fatigue may be an early sign of pregnancy.

Severity

Clinically significant fatigue may vary throughout the day but never completely disappears. Children with Lyme disease and JRA experience severe fatigue that is in excess of the degree of disease involvement. The patient may need to limit social functioning and recreational activities as a result of fatigue, which may then exacerbate mood disturbances and, in turn, contribute to fatigue.

Aggravating and Alleviating Factors

Psychological fatigue is usually worse in the morning, and physical activity may relieve the fatigue. Organic fatigue is not associated with intensity or duration of activity and is not relieved with rest or sleep.

Fever

Fever generally accompanies infectious diseases, which are common causes of fatigue (see Chapter 17). Prolonged fever may indicate chronic infection, inflammatory disease, or malignancy.

Bleeding

Heavy menstrual flow may lead to anemia (see Chapter 36). Other sources of bleeding, such as gastrointestinal (GI) ulcers, polyps, or cancer of the bowel, may result in occult blood loss and fatigue.

If I suspect a psychological cause, what else do I need to know?

Key Questions

- What is your stress level and how do you cope with stress in your life?
- Are you a caregiver?
- Have you recently had a stressful event in your life?
- Do you or does anyone in your family have a problem with anxiety or depression?
- How are you doing in school?

Stress

Stressful life events increase the risk of depression in some adolescents and adults. In the presence of organic disease, stress may be secondary to pain or discomfort that may disrupt sleep and rest patterns. Deconditioning secondary to muscle atrophy with inactivity or bed rest can lead to fatigue (see Chapter 4).

Caregiver Role

Individuals who are caregivers to children or adults can experience physical and emotional stress or burnout. They are more likely to report fatigue, anxiety, and depression. Those caring for a person with dementia experience high level of stress.

Anxiety and Depression

Children who have family members with depression are at a greater risk for depression. Generally, the first episode of major depression occurs between the ages of 20 and 30 years and affects women and transgender individuals more often than men. Major depressive disorder may have a genetic component. Diagnostic criteria will point to depression or anxiety as a cause.

School Performance

Decreased academic performance and decreased productivity may be an early sign of low self-esteem and early depression. Children also may overachieve academically to compensate for their lower self-esteem and to hide their depression.

DIAGNOSTIC REASONING: FOCUSED PHYSICAL EXAMINATION

A general physical examination, including psychological screening for depression and anxiety, is needed to make a differential diagnosis of fatigue. The majority of patients will have a normal physical examination, but clues can be found for the presence of systemic disease.

Note General Appearance

Observe the patient entering the examination room to note any abnormality of gait that may indicate neurologic involvement or generalized weakness. Observe the patient's demeanor and appearance for signs of neglect or a facial expression that might indicate depression or generalized anxiety. In the presence of organic disease, the patient will appear ill; with psychological stress, the patient may appear depressed or anxious. Children may appear sad or irritable.

Take Vital Signs

The presence of fever suggests inflammation or infection. Blood pressure reading, pulse rate, and respiratory rate reflect the function of the cardiorespiratory system. An elevated pulse rate may be associated with anxiety, anemia, dehydration, and hyperthyroidism. Evaluate the patient for orthostatic hypotension or neutrally mediated hypotension. Weigh and measure the patient to obtain the body mass index (BMI); a BMI outside the normal range can indicate poor nutritional status as well as cardiovascular risk.

Inspect Skin, Hair, and Nails

Observe for signs of thyroid dysfunction. Hypothyroidism is associated with coarse, dry hair and skin and thickening of nails. Hyperthyroidism is characterized by fine, limp hair and warm skin. Look for skin lesions or rashes that may indicate infection or inflammation. A faint maculopapular rash is sometimes associated with mononucleosis. Lyme disease is associated with a macular lesion with a clear center. Atrophic skin of the lower extremities is an indication of arterial insufficiency and underlying arteriovascular disease. Venous stasis can lead to swelling of the ankles, varicose veins, and skin ulcers. Patients with anxiety disorders may bite their nails or self-inflict excoriation lesions, usually over the face and extremities.

Examine the Nose, Eyes, Mouth, and Throat

Inspect for any signs of infection or inflammation secondary to an allergic response. Petechiae on the palate may be seen with mononucleosis. Palpate for cervicofacial nodes. Lymphadenopathy is seen with HIV, malignancy, and mononucleosis. Inspect mucous membranes for lesions and moisture. Dry, cracked, and ulcerated mucosa can indicate a nutritional deficiency or dehydration.

Conduct a Cardiovascular Examination

Palpate the anterior thorax for the location of the point of maximal impulse (PMI) and for lifts or heaves. Listen for carotid and thyroid bruits. Auscultate the heart, listening carefully for rate, rhythm, and murmurs, especially a late systolic murmur heard loudest over the mitral area, which may indicate mitral prolapse. Audible third or fourth heart sounds (S_3 or S_4) in an adult may indicate heart failure.

Examine the Lungs

First, observe the patient for ease of breathing and respiratory rate. Note the anteroposterior (AP)/lateral diameter of the thorax. An increased AP diameter indicates COPD. Test for egophony and palpate and percuss the anterior and posterior thorax to listen for resonance (normal) or consolidation. Tactile fremitus will increase over areas of consolidated lung. Listen for rales and wheezes. Bilateral basilar rales may indicate congestive heart failure; most pneumonia is unilateral. Barely audible breath sounds are associated with COPD.

Examine the Abdomen

Begin the examination by observing the abdomen (see Chapter 3). Observe the intactness and condition of the skin. A rigid abdomen suggests peritoneal irritation. Generalized symmetrical distention may occur with obesity, enlarged organs, fluid or ascites, and gas. Dehydration or malnutrition may present as a concave contour of the abdomen.

Listen for bowel sounds. Anxiety, GI irritation, and hunger can increase the frequency and loudness of bowel sounds. Depression can decrease bowel sounds.

Perform general light palpation to assess the skin and abdominal musculature. Note the patient's response to the examination. Perform deep palpation over the liver and spleen. Fist palpation over the posterior thorax tests for kidney tenderness associated with pyelonephritis, renal calculi, or stenosis.

Perform a Musculoskeletal Examination

Observe and palpate joints for inflammation and swelling. Bilateral tenderness of at least 11 of 18 tender points is diagnostic of fibromyalgia. An informative example of how to examine for tender points can be found at http://www.youtube.com/watch?v=08qtNhsTXHQ. Test stamina by asking the patient to perform certain musculoskeletal movements or to walk a certain distance to evaluate changes in fatigue level.

Conduct a Neurologic Examination

Assess both cognitive and physical function to evaluate attention span, judgment, memory, and affect. Abnormalities may suggest a psychiatric disorder or brain pathology. Dementia is also seen in patients with HIV/AIDS. Test cranial nerves. A change in deep tendon reflexes may indicate thyroid dysfunction. Cerebellar and motor testing will rule out weakness or any associated neurologic pathology.

LABORATORY AND DIAGNOSTIC STUDIES

Complete Blood Count with Indices and Differential

A complete blood count (CBC) with indices will provide information about the degree and cause of anemia. Hematocrit and hemoglobin levels reflect the degree of anemia, and the indices point to a cause. Microcytic hypochromic anemia reflects chronic blood loss, whereas normocytic normochromic anemia suggests an acute blood loss.

A white blood cell (WBC) count of greater than 12,000/μL indicates inflammation or infection. Normally the circulating neutrophils are in a mature form, called segs because the cell nuclei are segmented. Immature neutrophils are called bands. Infection will increase the total number of neutrophils, with an increase in the number of immature cells or bands.

Ferritin

Ferritin is a protein that stores iron in bone marrow, and the ferritin level most accurately reflects total body iron stores. The ferritin level is low in a patient with iron deficiency anemia. In contrast, the ferritin level may be elevated or normal in a patient with anemia caused by chronic disease or a patient with a thalassemia caused by a reduced life cycle of red blood cells (RBCs). The bone marrow fails to compensate for the loss by increasing RBC production.

Total Iron-Binding Capacity

Iron is transported in plasma bound with transferrin, a serum protein synthesized in the liver. Total iron-binding capacity (TIBC) of serum is an indirect measure of transferrin. This capacity may be increased in iron deficiency anemia because although the capacity to bind with iron is high, hemoglobin is decreased, and both mean corpuscular volume and mean corpuscular hemoglobin concentration are decreased (e.g., hypochromic microcytic anemia). TIBC

is normal or low in patients with a chronic disease, often because of the shorter life cycle of an RBC and the body's inability to compensate.

Urinalysis

Dipstick urinalysis can rule out or point to infection or systemic disease if incontinence is present. Hematuria, pyuria, bacteruria, and the presence of leukocyte esterase or nitrites indicate urinary tract infection. Glycosuria or proteinuria is suggestive of infection, cardiovascular disease, diabetes mellitus, or renal disease. The presence of bacteria or WBCs on microscopic examination indicates urinary tract infection; RBC casts may indicate nephropathy (see Chapter 35).

Erythrocyte Sedimentation Rate

An increased erythrocyte sedimentation rate (ESR) is a general indication of an inflammatory process and does not identify the source. The ESR is often elevated as a result of acute or chronic infection and inflammatory conditions such as rheumatoid arthritis, temporal arteritis, or any other injury causing an inflammatory response.

Fasting Blood Glucose

A fasting blood glucose level of 126 mg/dL or higher points to a diagnosis of diabetes mellitus. Prediabetes is indicated when the fasting blood glucose level is between 100 to 125 mg/dL. Unless changes in lifestyle behaviors and weight occur, the person will most likely develop diabetes.

Hemoglobin A1c

Hemoglobin A1c or glycated hemoglobin measures the average blood glucose over 3 months. A normal value is 4–5.6%.

▧ EVIDENCE-BASED PRACTICE *Can Prediabetes Be Reversed?*

The Diabetes Prevention Program (DPP) is the largest diabetes prevention trial conducted in the United States. It had more than 3800 participants with impaired glucose tolerance randomly assigned to one of four conditions: (1) intensive lifestyle adjustments or standard lifestyle plus one of these treatment arms: (2) placebo, (3) metformin, or (4) troglitazone. The troglitazone arm was discontinued early because of adverse drug effects. After 2.8 years of follow-up (the study was discontinued early because of an observed significant benefit to the intervention group), both metformin and intensive lifestyle adjustment were found to reduce the risk of developing diabetes by 31% and 58%, respectively. The DPP showed that both metformin and intensive lifestyle modifications can effectively delay or prevent the development of diabetes.

Reference: Ratner, 2006.

Hepatic Function

Obtain aspartate aminotransferase and alanine aminotransferase values to assess for general inflammation of the liver associated with hepatitis.

Thyroid-Stimulating Hormone

A serum thyroid-stimulating hormone (TSH) level identifies hyper- or hypothyroidism.

HIV Infection

Antigen/antibody tests, HIV antibody tests and molecular tests, can be used to rule out HIV infection as a cause. The Centers for Disease Control and Prevention recommends a three-step process of testing (see https://stacks.cdc.gov/view/cdc/45930).

Tuberculin Skin Testing

A Mantoux test is used to test for tuberculosis antibodies but is being replaced with the QuantiFERON-TB Gold (QFT) test. QFT is highly specific and sensitive: a positive result is strongly predictive of infection with *M. tuberculosis*. However, the QFT cannot distinguish between active tuberculosis disease and latent tuberculosis infection.

Monospot

The Monospot is a rapid slide test that detects heterophil antibody agglutination. It is not specific for Epstein-Barr virus (EBV). It is most sensitive 1 to 2 weeks after symptoms appear and remains positive for up to 1 year. If chronic fatigue syndrome is being considered as a differential diagnosis, specific EBV antibody tests should be considered.

Chest Radiography

A chest radiograph can reveal the presence of pneumonia, a lesion in the lungs, heart size, or the presence of fluid in the lungs as a result of congestive heart failure.

DIFFERENTIAL DIAGNOSIS

Physiological Causes

Poor sleep and rest

In general, total sleep time is greatest during infancy, decreases in childhood, may increase again during parts of adolescence, remains relatively stable during the adult years, and declines during the late years of adulthood (see Chapter 31).

Total sleep time for a newborn is 14 to 18 hours a day. As the child matures, the sleep cycle increases in length, and the total sleep time decreases. Sleep patterns of 8 to 10 hours develop during childhood. Many adolescents need increased amounts of sleep.

Most healthy adults spend 7 to 9 hours sleeping each day. Older adults sleep less and may experience more frequent awakenings during the night; some need to compensate for this with rest periods during the day.

Poor nutritional status

Assessment of nutritional risk is determined by data from the history and physical examination, food recall data, BMI (BMI <18.5 = underweight; BMI 18.5 to 24.9 = healthy weight; BMI 25 to <30 = overweight; BMI >30 = obesity), and waist circumference (WC). A WC greater than 35 inches in women and 40 inches in men is a risk factor for heart disease.

The 2015 to 2020 Dietary Guidelines for Americans provide five overarching principles that encourage healthy eating patterns, recognize that individuals will need to make shifts in their food and beverage choices to achieve a healthy pattern, and acknowledge that all segments of society have a role to play in supporting healthy choices. These principles are:

1. **Follow a healthy eating pattern across the lifespan.** All food and beverage choices matter. Choose a healthy eating pattern at an appropriate calorie level to help achieve and maintain a healthy body weight, support nutrient adequacy, and reduce the risk of chronic disease.

2. **Focus on variety, nutrient density, and amount.** To meet nutrient needs within calorie limits, choose a variety of nutrient-dense foods across and within all food groups in recommended amounts.

3. **Limit calories from added sugars and saturated fats and reduce sodium intake.** Consume an eating pattern low in added sugars, saturated fats, and sodium.

Cut back on foods and beverages higher in these components to amounts that fit within healthy eating patterns.

4. **Shift to healthier food and beverage choices.** Choose nutrient-dense foods and beverages across and within all food groups in place of less healthy choices. Consider cultural and personal preferences to make these shifts easier to accomplish and maintain.

5. **Support healthy eating patterns for all.** Everyone has a role in helping to create and support healthy eating patterns in multiple settings nationwide, from home to school to work to communities.

Psychological Causes

Depression

About 30% of primary care patients will have symptoms of depression. An adult patient will most often present with a loss of interest in usual activities, feelings of worthlessness and guilt, and thoughts of suicide for more than 2 weeks' duration. The practitioner must assess the risk of suicide and intervene, or refer to a mental health specialist (see Differential Diagnosis box in Chapter 4).

Other symptoms include sleep and appetite disturbances, malaise, and decreased libido. Patients with bipolar disease may have a history of a manic episode associated with increased activity, increased libido, and feelings of grandiosity. The physical examination is usually normal.

Children will appear sad, angry, or irritable. They may have somatic complaints or low self-esteem and have problems with school performance. Adolescents may exhibit euphoria, hypersomnia, and lack of interest in activities.

Anxiety

Diagnostic criteria for anxiety (*Diagnostic and Statistical Manual of Mental Disorders,* ed 5, text revision [DSM-V-TR]) will guide the diagnosis of anxiety disorder or panic attack. The patient may report a sense of doom and fear of losing control, dyspnea and chest discomfort, fatigue, restlessness, and sleep disturbance. Physical findings include tachycardia, palpitations, and diaphoresis (see Differential Diagnosis table in Chapter 4).

Organic Causes of Acute Fatigue

Infection

The prodrome stage of many viral infections may produce fatigue before other symptoms such as sore throat, nasal congestion, and myalgia appear. Acute hepatitis A and B can cause fatigue before symptoms of jaundice or abdominal discomfort appear. Endocarditis, an infection of the heart valves, can cause fatigue.

Drugs

Alcoholism is one of the most common causes of acute fatigue related to organic causes. Chronic alcohol abuse is associated with undernutrition, a contributing factor to fatigue.

Anemia

The fatigue associated with anemia is secondary to the body's compensation to increase oxygen in blood that is oxygen-deprived because of the abnormal size or quantity of RBCs. The body compensates by increasing the heart rate but may not be able to make up for this deficit, which leads to increased breathlessness with activity. A diet history may show inadequate dietary intake of iron; a general history may reveal heavy menstrual bleeding. Early symptoms are fatigue, weakness, and shortness of breath. A CBC will identify the cause of anemia. Serum iron, serum ferritin, and transferrin levels may also support the diagnosis of anemia.

Hypothyroidism (Myxedema)

Patients report cold intolerance, constipation, weight gain, hoarseness, depression, and fatigue. Physical examination reveals bradycardia, dry skin, generalized edema, and delayed recovery of deep tendon reflexes. An elevated TSH level is present in primary hypothyroidism.

Hyperthyroidism (Graves disease)

This disorder is associated with increased sweating, heat intolerance, weight loss, irritability, disturbed sleep, and menstrual irregularity. The physical examination may disclose tachycardia, atrial fibrillation, tremor, warm moist skin, and lid lag. Graves disease is associated with exophthalmos. Radioiodine uptake scan will differentiate Graves disease, toxic nodule, and thyroiditis.

Organic Causes of Chronic Fatigue

Sleep apnea

Sleep apnea most often affects middle-aged and older adults. Risk factors include obesity and hypertension. Patients describe excessive daytime fatigue, morning headaches, and erectile dysfunction. Bed partners of patients report restless sleep, loud snoring, and periods of apnea for at least 30 seconds during the night.

Medication

Antihypertensive medications such as β-blockers are often associated with fatigue. Fatigue is a side effect of some pain medications, antihistamines, and many other medications.

Heart failure

Heart failure is associated with dyspnea, orthopnea, paroxysmal nocturnal dyspnea, peripheral edema, weight gain, cough with frothy sputum, palpitations, and fatigue (see Chapter 11). People with a history of heart disease or valvular disease are at greater risk. Physical examination may reveal an altered level of consciousness, anxiety, jugular venous distention, tachypnea, rales and rhonchi, and a displaced PMI. An S_3 and S_4 can be heard on cardiac auscultation. Chest radiographs will disclose basilar consolidation and increased heart size. An echocardiogram shows a reduced ejection fraction.

Cancer

Lymphoma and leukemia may first be detected by unexplained fatigue that increases with activity and worsens over time. A CBC with differential will show blood dyscrasias. GI cancer may produce occult blood loss that leads to anemia and fatigue.

Mononucleosis

Mononucleosis is often a disease of young adults that is caused by EBV in 90% of cases. History discloses a gradual onset of low-grade fever, mild sore throat, posterior cervical lymphadenopathy, fatigue, and malaise. Splenomegaly occurs in 50% of cases, and palatine petechiae are a less common sign. The diagnosis can be confirmed with a positive Monospot test and a CBC that shows greater than 50% lymphocytosis. Ten percent of patients may also have concurrent β-hemolytic streptococcal pharyngitis.

Hepatitis

Fatigue is generally associated with hepatitis. Patients will report a history of malaise, fatigue, flulike symptoms, abdominal pain, arthralgia, and an aversion to smoking. A health history will reveal risky sexual behavior, exposure to body secretions through blood transfusion or injectable drug use, or exposure to contaminated food or water. Physical findings may include jaundice, fever, and an enlarged and tender liver. Hepatitis serology for hepatitis A, B, and C will determine the causative agent.

Fibromyalgia

Fibromyalgia occurs most often in women 20 to 50 years old. It is associated with chronic pain and stiffness of the trunk and extremities, especially the neck, shoulders, low back, and hips. Patients report fatigue, headaches, sleep disturbance, and symptoms of bowel irritability. To diagnose fibromyalgia, 11 of 18 bilateral tender points must be confirmed by physical examination.

Chronic fatigue syndrome

There is no single pathological mechanism to explain this condition. It appears as an infectious or autoimmune disorder and has neurologic, affective, and cognitive symptoms. Chronic fatigue syndrome is severe fatigue lasting longer than 6 months in association with (1) impaired memory or concentration, (2) sore throat, (3) tender cervical or axillary lymph nodes, (4) muscle pain, (5) multiple joint pain, (6) new-onset headaches, (7) nonrestorative sleep, and (8) postexertional malaise.

▶ DIFFERENTIAL DIAGNOSIS OF *Common Causes of Fatigue*

CONDITION	HISTORY	PHYSICAL FINDINGS	DIAGNOSTIC STUDIES
PHYSIOLOGICAL CAUSES			
Poor sleep and rest	Adolescent and younger adult; history of over-work, psychological stress, disturbed sleep, poor sleep hygiene	Normal examination	None
Poor nutritional status	Depression, decreased appetite, lack of balanced nutrient intake, excessive alcohol intake	BMI reflecting under-weight or overweight	Hematocrit increased or decreased, low serum ferritin
PSYCHOLOGICAL CAUSES			
Depression: children	Feeling sad, angry, irritable Decrease in academic performance Somatic complaints	Normal examination	DSM-PC
Depression: adults	Loss of interest in usual activities Feelings of worthlessness Sleep problems	Depressed affect, normal examination	Depression screening instrument
Anxiety	Numerous somatic com-plaints, breathlessness	Tachycardia, palpita-tions, diaphoresis	None
ORGANIC CAUSES: ACUTE FATIGUE			
Infection	Sudden onset; history of exposure; recent viral illness	Fever; lymphadenopa-thy, localized signs of erythema, edema	CBC, ESR, Monospot
Drugs and alcohol	History of smoking, alcohol use, antihistamines, analgesics, antihyperten-sive medications	Bilaterally enhanced or depressed DTRs, pupillary changes, reduced attention span, poor judgment	CAGE alcohol screening
Anemia	Breathlessness with exertion, menstruating or postpartum female, recent surgery	Increased pulse rate, pale mucosa, smooth red tongue	CBC with indices, serum iron, ferritin, transferrin
Hypothyroidism (myxedema)	Poor appetite, fatigue, weight gain, cold intolerance	Decreased pulse rate; dry skin, coarse dry hair; thyroid possibly enlarged, hoarseness	T_4 low, T_3 low, TSH elevated
Hyperthyroidism (Graves disease)	Hyperactivity, heat intolerance, sleep problems	Lid lag, fine thinning hair, tachycardia	T_4 increased, T_3 increased, TSH depressed

Continued

► **DIFFERENTIAL DIAGNOSIS OF** *Common Causes of Fatigue—cont'd*

ORGANIC CAUSES: CHRONIC FATIGUE			
Sleep apnea	Male, middle-age or older; partner reports periods of no breathing during sleep; fatigue	Hypertension, obesity, narrowed upper airway	Sleep studies
Medications	History of allergies treated with antihistamines, medications for hypertension, heart disease, chronic pain	Nasal congestion, cough, injected conjunctiva	Evaluate medication choices
Heart failure	Dyspnea, weight gain, fatigue, cough	Anxiety, jugular venous distention, displaced PMI, rales	ECG, chest radiography, ABGs
Cancer	Fatigue, unexplained weight loss	Observe, palpate, and percuss all systems for lumps, lesions, or consolidation; physical examination may be normal	CBC to rule out anemia; leukocyte count
Mononucleosis (Epstein-Barr virus)	Young adult; slow onset of malaise, low-grade fever, mild sore throat	Palatine petechiae, posterior cervical lymphadenopathy, splenomegaly	Positive Monospot; CBC with differential; >50% leukocytes
Hepatitis	Jaundice, anorexia, fatigue, abdominal pain, fever	Jaundice, weight loss, arthralgia, skin rash	Bilirubin increased; hepatitis panel
Fibromyalgia	Female 20–50 yr; history of depression, sleep disturbance, chronic fatigue, general muscle and joint aches	Palpation of tender points will produce pain; normal physical examination	None
Chronic fatigue syndrome	Fatigue lasting longer than 6 mo; sudden onset of flulike symptoms that persist or recur	Physical examination may be normal; cervical and axillary lymphadenopathy	CBC, ESR

ABG, arterial blood gas; *BMI,* body mass index; *CBC,* complete blood count; *Diagnostic and Statistical Manual for Primary Care* 4th ed (DSM-PC), American Psychiatric Association, Washington DC, 1995. *DTR,* deep tendon reflex; *ECG,* echocardiogram; *PMI,* point of maximal impulse; T_3, triiodothyronine; T_4, thyroxine; *TSH,* thyroid-stimulating hormone.

CHAPTER

17 Fever

Fever, also known as pyrexia, is an elevation of temperature above the normal daily variation of 37°C (98.6°F) and is a sign of an underlying process. A body temperature is generally not considered a fever until it is greater than 38°C (100.4°F), although there is no consensus on a specific number. The most common cause of fever is infection; however, noninfectious processes may present with fever. Fever of unknown origin (FUO) occurs in a small percentage of cases when a specific cause has not been identified. A meticulous history and physical examination supported by laboratory investigation are necessary to find the origin of the fever.

There are three types of fevers, each caused by a specific pathophysiological process. The first involves the raising of the hypothalamic set point. The receptors in the area of the hypothalamus regulating body temperature are triggered to reset at a higher core body temperature. This results in an elevation of the helper T-cell production and an elevation in the effectiveness of interferon. Infection, collagen disease, vascular disease, and malignancy are commonly responsible for these fevers.

A second type of fever is a result of heat production exceeding heat loss. Here the set point is normal, and heat loss mechanisms are active. Fever occurs either because the body raises its metabolic heat production or because the environmental heat load exceeds normal heat loss mechanisms. Aspirin overdose, malignant hyperthermia, hyperthyroidism, or hypernatremia may cause this type of fever.

A third type of fever is caused by a defective heat loss mechanism that cannot cope with normal heat load. Heat stroke, poisoning with anticholinergic drugs, ectodermal dysplasia, and burns are causes of this kind of fever.

For the first type of fever, antipyretics are given to lower the hypothalamic set point. Antipyretics are ineffective for the second and third types of fever.

DIAGNOSTIC REASONING: FOCUSED HISTORY

Is this really a fever?

Key Questions
- How do you know you have a fever?
- Have you taken your temperature?
- How did you measure your temperature?

Occurrence of Fever

Fever is a common presenting problem and a cardinal manifestation of disease. Patients often report a subjective fever (i.e., symptoms such as flushing, chills, shaking chills, headache, malaise, muscle aches) that is assumed by the patient to be a fever but not validated with a thermometer. Nevertheless, the absence of fever in a single patient visit does not eliminate a febrile illness.

Measurement of Temperature

Many people use touch to determine whether a fever is present. Although not a precise indication, touch can signal a high fever. During the early stages of fever, perfusion to the skin is decreased, and skin temperature falls. In later stages, when temperature within the muscles has risen significantly, increased body temperature is reflected by increased skin temperature. In children, hands and feet should not be used to gauge a fever because there may be circulatory vasoconstriction causing them to feel cold. An accurate temperature should be measured orally, rectally, or in the axilla using a thermometer; a special thermometer is used for the ear; thermosensitive strips are used on a dry forehead. Because of the diurnal variation in normal body temperature and the effect of physiological factors and body rhythms, frequent recordings throughout the day are needed to monitor fever.

Should sepsis or meningitis be of concern?

Key Questions

- Have you had any recent head trauma?
- Do you have recurrent ear infections?
- Have you had contact with anyone who has been ill?
- Have you had a headache, lethargy, confusion, or a stiff neck?
- If an infant: How old is the baby?

Head Trauma, Otitis Media, and Contact

Recent head trauma, especially at the base of the skull, may provide an entrance for infectious organisms. Children with recurrent or chronic otitis media may have mastoiditis spreading to the meninges. Contact with anyone with meningococcal disease or *Haemophilus influenzae* places the individual at risk for contracting the disease.

Headache, Vomiting, Lethargy, or Stiff Neck

Headache, fever, lethargy, confusion, vomiting, and a stiff neck characterize meningitis. However, the presentation is highly variable. Any patient with even minimal neurologic signs and symptoms should be evaluated for meningitis.

Infant

Fever in children younger than 2 months of age is uncommon but must be viewed as serious. Generally, neonates and young infants are less able to mount a febrile response; when they do, it is a significant finding. Fever can be viral or bacterial in nature. Fevers in a neonate may also be an indication of an underlying anatomical defect. Urinary tract infection (UTI) and bacteremia are often the first indications of a structural abnormality of the urinary tract. Also, infants with galactosemia may present in the first weeks to 1 month of life with gram-negative sepsis. Occasionally, infants present with sepsis associated with delivery (prolonged rupture of membranes); acquired from instrumentation

used during delivery, such as scalp electrodes; or from a procedure performed in a neonatal intensive care unit.

All infants younger than 2 months with fever are considered to have sepsis or meningitis until proven otherwise.

What does the pattern of fever tell me?

Key Questions

- How long have you had the fever?
- What has been the highest temperature reading?

Duration of Fever

In adults, fevers from an acute process usually resolve in 1 to 2 weeks. Fevers that last 3 weeks or longer, that exceed temperatures of 38.4°C (101.1°F), and that remain undiagnosed after 1 week of intensive diagnostic study are classified as FUOs.

Fevers in children can be grouped into three categories: short-term fever, fever without localizing signs, and FUO. Short-term fever is defined as a fever of short duration, readily diagnosed, and that resolves within 1 week. Fever without localizing signs is a fever of brief duration (usually <10 days) that is not explained by findings on history or physical examination. FUO is a fever usually greater than 38.5°C (101.2°F) that lasts longer than 2 weeks on more than four occasions.

Height of Fever

Dehydration and seizures are related to the height of the fever. Generally, body temperatures greater than 41.1°C (106 F) are seen in heat illness, central nervous system (CNS) disease, and infection. The higher the fever, the greater the likelihood of bacteremia.

Is the Fever Caused by a Localized Infection?

Key Questions

- Do you have frequency, burning, or urgency with urination?
- Are you having unusual vaginal or penile discharge?
- Do you have face or sinus pain?
- Do you have nasal discharge? If so, what color is the discharge?

- Do you have a cough? Is it productive? What color is the sputum?
- Do you have ear pain?
- Is your throat sore?
- Do you have any sores (aphthous ulcers) in your mouth?
- Are you having any nausea, vomiting, or diarrhea?
- Do any of your joints hurt?

Location of Symptoms

Localizing symptoms will point to the site of the infection. These diagnostic clues include headache, sinus pain, purulent nasal discharge, ear pain, toothache, sore throat, breast tenderness, chest pain, cough, dyspnea, abdominal pain, flank pain, dysuria, vaginal discharge, genitourinary (GU) pain, joint pain or stiffness, pain or heat, skin lesions, rashes, or focal neurologic deficits (see appropriate chapters).

Genitourinary Tract

Upper UTI in adults commonly produces systemic symptoms with flank pain and fever (see Chapters 18, 34, and 35). Fever with cystitis is uncommon in adults, but children with UTIs present with systemic rather than localized signs and symptoms. UTI is the most common infection in girls younger than 2 years who present with a high fever and in all infants younger than 90 days with fever. Pelvic inflammatory disease (PID) may cause fever as well as an increased amount of vaginal discharge and bleeding after intercourse. Acute UTIs are rare in patients with male genitalia and often present with chills, high fever, urinary frequency and urgency, perineal pain, low back pain, and penile discharge.

Ear, Nose, and Throat Symptoms

Viral upper respiratory tract infections are common and usually produce fever (see Chapters 15, 25, and 32). Otitis media is common in children. Fever may accompany both viral and bacterial pharyngitis. Pharyngitis is frequently manifested only by fever, with the infection localizing 1 or 2 days later. Acute sinusitis can produce a fever. Aphthous ulcers with pharyngitis and cervical lymphadenopathy are seen in children with periodic fevers.

Respiratory or Gastrointestinal Symptoms

Most febrile illnesses are caused by viral upper respiratory infection (URI), lower respiratory infection (LRI) (see Chapters 11 and 14), or gastrointestinal (GI) tract infection (see Chapter 3). Localized symptoms can help pinpoint the cause of the fever. Vomiting occasionally signals pneumonia, especially in children.

Joint Pain

Joint pain may indicate connective tissue disorders in adults and in children more than 6 years of age (see Chapters 22 and 23). Osteomyelitis or septic arthritis may also produce fever. Symptoms of polymyalgia rheumatica, an inflammatory disorder, include upper body aches and stiffness, usually bilateral, headache, and a mild fever. This condition affects northern Europeans and females more often and occurs almost exclusively in adults older than 65 years. Psoriatic arthritis begins as a skin disorder and progresses to cause joint pain and swelling.

> *Can I narrow the diagnostic possibilities or eliminate a cause?*

Key Questions
- Have you noticed a rash?
- Do you ache all over?

Skin Rash

The prodromal period of a rash is an important historical clue to diagnosis (see Chapter 28). Fever and rash usually appear together 1 to 5 days after infection. Common eruption periods are as follows:

- Varicella, rubella, erythema infectiosum: 1 day
- Scarlet fever: 2 days
- Rocky Mountain spotted fever: 3 days
- Measles: 4 days
- Roseola infantum: 5 days
- Hand, foot and mouth: 3 days

Muscle Aches

Fevers localized to a site without general body manifestations are often bacterial in nature. Fevers accompanied by muscle aches (myalgias), malaise, or respiratory symptoms are often viral in nature.

Does the patient have an increased risk for complications?

Key Questions
- Do you have any chronic health problems?
- Have you had recent surgery?
- Have you been diagnosed with an infectious disease recently?
- Are you sexually active? If so, how many partners do you have?
- Have you had any recent immunizations?
- Do you or anyone in your family have tuberculosis (TB) or hepatitis?

Chronic Disease

Chronic conditions and systemic disorders (e.g., diabetes mellitus, chronic obstructive pulmonary disease [COPD], human immunodeficiency virus [HIV], malignancies, neutropenia, and sickle cell anemia) compromise host resistance and increase susceptibility to infection. Prosthetic devices, such as heart valves or joint prostheses, also increase susceptibility to infection.

Health Problems, Surgery, and Recent Infection

Current health problems, recurrent infection, or incomplete treatment of infection may be the cause of fever. Such risk factors as diabetes mellitus, neutropenia, HIV or other immune system disorders, and sickle cell anemia heighten the likelihood of bacterial infection. Patients with a past history of infection may be prone to recurrence. Recent surgical procedures can provide a locus for occult infection; however, a surgical procedure can also induce an inflammatory response, which causes a fever without infection.

Sexual Activity

High-risk sexual activity may raise the index of suspicion for HIV or hepatitis B infection and for PID.

Immunizations

Tuberculosis or hepatitis exposure

Exposure to populations with a high incidence of TB or viral hepatitis increases the risk of infection. Inquire further about constitutional symptoms such as cough, night sweats (TB), malaise, and abdominal discomfort (hepatitis).

Does the parent report a behavior change in the child?

Key Questions
- Is the child sleepier than normal?
- Is the child more irritable?
- How is the child's behavior?

In infants and children, behavior changes may be the only indication that the child is ill. Mildly ill infants may act alert, be active, smile, and feed well. Moderately ill infants may be fussy or irritable but continue to feed, be consolable, and may smile. Severely ill infants appear listless, cannot be consoled, and feed poorly or not at all.

Could the fever be caused by something acquired while traveling?

Key Questions
- Have you been out of the country recently?
- Have you spent time in the woods or been camping recently?

Travel

Patients can be exposed to an emerging infectious disease based on their travel activities. A history of travel out of the country presents the possibility of infection with amebiasis, malaria, schistosomiasis, typhoid fever, or hepatitis A and B. Dengue is the most common vector-borne disease worldwide and is a differential diagnosis for acute febrile illnesses in patients who live or have recently traveled to the tropics or subtropical areas of the United States. Epidemiologic surveillance data continually provide updates on patterns of occurrence of infections such as severe acute respiratory syndrome (SARS), avian influenza or "bird flu," and West Nile virus (Box 17.1).

Camping

Camping or exposure to wooded areas may indicate exposure to ticks, Q fever, tularemia, Rocky Mountain spotted fever, *Giardia,* or Lyme disease.

Box 17.1 **Emerging Infectious Diseases Associated with Fever[a]**

AVIAN INFLUENZA

A highly pathogenic strain of avian influenza A virus, H5N1, infects birds and mutates rapidly to acquire genes from viruses infecting other animal species. Avian influenza is transmitted to humans usually through the slaughtering and processing of infected birds. Symptoms of infection can range from flulike symptoms (e.g., fever, cough, sore throat, muscle aches) to pneumonia and severe respiratory distress. Suspect infection in people showing flulike symptoms, such as high fever and cough, and have confirmed contact with birds in an area where confirmed outbreaks have occurred. Clinical deterioration is rapid over 4 to 13 days. Laboratory findings include leukopenia, thrombocytopenia, and elevated levels of aminotransferases. Although avian influenza is a rare disease, more than half of reported cases have been fatal, and there is great potential for this virus to evolve into a world pandemic.

EBOLA VIRUS DISEASE

Ebola is viral infection that is spread through contact with body fluids, infected objects, or infected animals, including contact with someone who has died from Ebola. A person is infectious when symptoms are present. Symptoms can appear from 2 to 21 days after exposure and include fever, headache, diarrhea, vomiting, stomach pain, muscle pain, and unexplained bleeding or bruising. The earliest indication of potential infection is history of travel to infected regions, predominately West Africa. A person is also at risk who has had close contact with someone who has recently traveled to an Ebola-affected area or someone who is symptomatic. Recovery from Ebola depends on good supportive clinical care and the patient's immune response. People who recover from Ebola infection develop antibodies

that last for at least 10 years. In 2014, the world experienced the largest Ebola outbreak to date that originated in West Africa.

SEVERE ACUTE RESPIRATORY SYNDROME

Severe acute respiratory syndrome (SARS) is a febrile, severe lower respiratory tract illness that is caused by infection with SARS-associated coronavirus (SARS-CoV). From 2002 through 2003, the World Health Organization received reports of more than 8000 cases and nearly 800 deaths. No specific laboratory test distinguishes SARS-CoV from other febrile respiratory illness. Lymphopenia and elevated levels of hepatic transaminases, creatinine, and C-reactive protein have been seen in some patients. The diagnosis is based on clinical features (e.g., fever, difficulty breathing, pneumonia) and epidemiologic history of exposure either to a SARS patient or to a setting in which the SARS-CoV transmission is occurring.

WEST NILE VIRUS

West Nile virus (WNV) is a potentially serious illness caused most often by the bite of an infected mosquito. It occurs mostly in summer and fall in North America. Symptoms develop 3 to 14 days after being bitten. Approximately 80% of people who are infected with WNV will not show symptoms; however, up to 20% have symptoms called West Nile fever, characterized by fever, headache, fatigue, truncal rash, lymphadenopathy, and eye pain lasting from days to several weeks. People older than 50 years of age are more likely to develop serious symptoms. A positive immunoglobulin M antibody test of serum or cerebrospinal fluid is needed to confirm the disease. The test result is positive in most patients within 8 days of onset of symptoms.

[a]The most current information on these diseases can be found online at the websites of the Centers for Disease Control and Prevention (http://cdc.gov) and the World Health Organization, (http://who.int).

Could the fever be medication related or caused by poisoning?

Key Questions

- Have you recently taken any new medications?
- Can you tell me what foods you have eaten in the past 3 days?
- Could the child have eaten a poisonous plant?

Medications

Medications may hide an occult infection. Many drugs (e.g., penicillin, atropine, sulfonamides, streptomycin, diphenylhydantoin) can induce fever in predisposed individuals. The fever starts about 7 days after the drug is taken for the first time, or soon after the first dose in a patient previously sensitized. Any patient who is taking immunosuppressive agents is at a higher risk for infection. Some medications interfere with thirst recognition (e.g., sedatives, haloperidol) or sweating (e.g., anticholinergics, phenothiazines).

Aspirin overdose can also cause fever. The earliest signs are vertigo and tinnitus, but fever can occur shortly thereafter and may be the only symptom that patients recognize.

Food Poisoning

Food poisoning fevers may occur up to 72 hours after ingestion of contaminated food.

Plants

Plants containing the alkaloid atropine (deadly nightshade, jessamine, and thornapple) cause dilated pupils, flushed skin, and fever because they interfere with the normal heat loss mechanism.

Could exposure to animals explain the fever?

Key Questions
- Has a cat scratched you recently?
- Do you have any pets or have you been around other animals?

Cat-Scratch Disease

Cat-scratch disease, or toxoplasmosis, is a bacterial infection transmitted by cats. The etiologic agent is a gram-negative bacillus. Exposure may occur when changing kitty litter boxes. Single-node or regional adenopathy is the dominant clinical feature. A low-grade fever is also present.

Animal Exposure

Also possible are brucellosis and leptospirosis from dogs; tularemia from rabbits; ornithosis, histoplasmosis, or psittacosis from birds; and lymphocytic choriomeningitis from hamsters or cats. Exposure to infected animals can produce infection and fever in humans. Occupational exposure to pathogens, such as brucellosis, should be investigated in patients who work with animals or animal products.

Could the fever be caused by heat exposure?

Key Questions
- Were you overdressed? If an infant: Is the infant swaddled or overbundled?

- Do you have air conditioning or windows that open?
- How warm is (are) the room(s) in which you live or sleep?

Overdressing

Classic heatstroke occurs when the person is unable to dissipate the environmental heat burden and is characterized by hyperthermia and change in level of consciousness. Heat illness is a milder form. Caregivers may inadvertently overdress children or cover them in blankets; older people may not be able to get out of bed when hot. Obese people have extra adipose tissue that insulates the body, preventing loss of heat. Some cultures treat illnesses with bundling, which can cause high fevers.

Air Conditioning and Room Temperature

During heat waves, people may become overheated in homes without air conditioning or with windows that will not open or are not opened because of safety concerns. The high ambient temperatures in those homes produce elevations in core body temperature that cannot be compensated for, leading to hyperthermia. Older people, those with impaired mobility, and individuals such as athletes physically exerting themselves in hot weather are most at risk.

DIAGNOSTIC REASONING: FOCUSED PHYSICAL EXAMINATION

Most fevers have an obvious cause, so look initially for localizing symptoms or clusters of symptoms that point to the cause. Remember that in both children and adults, bacterial and viral URIs, LRIs, and GI tract infections are the most common causes of fevers. Look for and rule out the common causes before investigating more unlikely causes. Boxes 17.2 and 17.3 list the common causes of fever in children and adults.

Fever in a Child Younger than 2 Months Old

The younger the child, the greater is the cause for concern in the presence of fever. Neonates and young infants are less able to

Box 17.2	Common Causes of Fever in Children

ACUTE FEVER
- Upper respiratory tract disorders
  - Viral respiratory tract diseases
  - Otitis media
  - Sinusitis
- Lower respiratory tract disorders
  - Bronchiolitis
  - Pneumonia
- Gastrointestinal disorders
  - Bacterial gastroenteritis
  - Viral gastroenteritis
- Musculoskeletal infections
  - Septic arthritis
- Osteomyelitis
- Cellulitis
- Urinary tract infections
- Bacteremia
- Meningitis

FEVER OF UNKNOWN ORIGIN
- Infectious diseases (localized and systemic)
- Collagen/inflammatory diseases
- Neoplastic diseases
- Miscellaneous disorders
  - Drug fever
  - Factitious fever
  - Kawasaki disease
  - Inflammatory bowel disease
  - Immunodeficiency
  - Central nervous system dysfunction

Box 17.3	Common Causes of Fever in Adults

ACUTE FEVER
- Upper respiratory tract infections
  - Tonsillitis
  - Sinusitis
  - Pneumonia
- Gastrointestinal disorders
  - Bacterial gastroenteritis
  - Viral gastroenteritis
  - Acute abdomen
- Urinary tract infection
- Pelvic inflammatory disease
- Prostatitis
- Drug reactions
- Alcohol withdrawal

FEVER OF UNKNOWN ORIGIN
- Infectious disease
- Neoplasm
- Collagen/vascular; other multisystem disease
- Drug fever
- Factitious fever

mount a febrile response and therefore are more vulnerable to meningitis and other hematogenous complications. The infrequency of high fever in this age group relates to innate differences in the ability to mount a febrile response. Fever in the first 2 to 3 months of life is relatively uncommon, but when it does occur, it is usually significant and often ominous.

Observe the Patient

General appearance is a most important aspect of physical examination. Note how the patient looks: do they appear acutely ill, look dehydrated, seem lethargic, and respond appropriately?

Responsiveness in children older than 2 months has been used to identify febrile children with serious illness. The Yale Observation Scale for severity of illness in children is commonly used to quantify observations. The scale has six general areas related to the child's appearance and behavior. Two thirds of children with acute illness have scores of less than 10, and of these, only 3% were found to have serious illness. Scores greater than 10 predicted serious illness, and a score of 16 was associated with serious illness 92% of the time.

Is there a cluster of clinical features, or red flags, that indicate the presence of a serious infection in a child?

A systematic review of 30 studies was done to determine what, if any, cluster of clinical features, or red flags, could assist clinicians in identifying a critically ill child. The studies were evaluated using the Quality Assessment of Diagnostic Accuracy Studies criteria. Clinical features with a positive likelihood ratio greater than 5 were rapid breathing, poor circulation, petechial rash, and cyanosis. Clinician judgment and parental concern also had a positive likelihood ratio as warning signs. The authors note that the Yale Scale of Observation had limited usefulness in determining a serious infection. Instead, the results of the review suggest that individual red flags can instead be used to exclude serious infection.

Reference: Van den Bruel et al, 2010.

Take Vital Signs and Note Temperature

The incidence of bacteremia, as well as specific infections, increases with the magnitude of fever. A temperature greater than 40°C (104°F) is the marker for occult bacteria. However, many patients with high fever do not have major diseases. In adults, take an oral temperature; in infants and younger children, a rectal or ear temperature is more reliable.

Most infectious diseases produce temperatures between 37.2° and 41°C (99° and 106°F, respectively). However, some patients with infectious diseases remain afebrile; these include neonates, immunocompromised hosts, patients with chronic renal insufficiency, and the elderly. Extreme pyrexia (i.e., temperatures exceeding 41.5°C) rarely occurs with an infectious disease. Conditions in which extreme pyrexia is seen include drug fevers, CNS injury, malignant hyperthermia, heat stroke, and HIV.

Hypothermia is always an unfavorable prognostic sign in the presence of infectious disease. This condition is seen with overwhelming sepsis (most common in older adults and neonates), uremia, cold exposure, and hypothyroidism.

Observe Skin and Mucous Membranes

A macular/papular rash may indicate a viral exanthema, an infectious disease, or a drug sensitivity reaction (see Chapter 28). Vesicular rashes occur with viral infection. A petechial skin rash indicates meningococcemia, Rocky Mountain spotted fever, or anticoagulation treatment that is outside therapeutic ranges. Petechial eruptions on the hard and soft palate may indicate mononucleosis. Splinter hemorrhages found in the nail beds and petechiae of the conjunctivae indicate endocarditis.

The presence of a petechial skin rash indicates a serious infection that requires immediate referral and hospitalization.

This systematic review examined normal body temperature values in people 60 years of age and older to determine differences in temperature, depending on the noninvasive measurement site and measurement device used and depending on the degree and extent of temperature variability according to time of day and time of year.

Twenty-two papers met inclusion criteria. Studies were included that focused on temperature measurement, sampled people 60 years of age and older, collected data from noninvasive temperature measurement sites, and used a prospective study design. Results showed that normal temperature values by site were rectal, 37.1°C (98.8°F); ear based, 36.8°C (98.3°F); urine, 36.5°C (97.6°F); oral, 36.3°C (97.4°F); and axillary, 36.2°C (97.1°F). Temperature exhibited a 0.4°C (0.7°F) diurnal and 0.1°C (0.2°F) circannual variation. Synthesis of data indicated that normal body temperature values in older people by sites were consistently lower than adults' acceptable values reported in the literature.

Reference: Lu et al, 2009.

Examine the Head and Neck

Percuss the sinuses and transilluminate for evidence of sinusitis (see Chapter 25). Examine and palpate the teeth for abscesses. Palpate the salivary glands for tenderness. Examine the throat and tonsils for signs of infection, specifically enlarged or red tonsils, lymphadenopathy, or tonsillar or pharyngeal exudate. Examine the mouth for aphthous ulcers.

Inspect the ears and tympanic membrane for effusion, erythema, fluid, or purulent secretion. Inspect the optic fundi for changes associated with infectious endocarditis (i.e., Roth spots: small, pale retinal lesions with areas of hemorrhage that have white centers, usually located near the optic disc).

In an infant, feel for a tense or bulging anterior fontanel. This is best noted if the patient is in the sitting position. The normal fontanel may feel questionably tense if the infant is supine. Tenseness may be noted in the crying child but only during expiration; this physiological bulging disappears when the patient relaxes or inspires.

Palpate the Lymph Nodes

Palpate all lymph nodes for enlargement and tenderness.
- Anterior cervical: Suspect viral or bacterial pharyngitis.
- Preauricular or postauricular: Suspect ear infection.
- Submental and submandibular: Suspect tooth abscess.
- Posterior cervical: Suspect mononucleosis.
- Supraclavicular: Suspect neoplasm.
- Axillary: Suspect breast inflammation, local infection, or neoplasm.
- Inguinal: Suspect a sexually transmissible infection (STI).
- Localized lymphadenopathy: Suspect local infectious process.
- Generalized lymphadenopathy: Suspect immunosuppression, such as being HIV positive, or neoplasm.

Examine the Heart, Lungs, and Chest

Auscultate the heart to listen for new murmurs that could indicate endocarditis. Percuss and auscultate the lungs (see Chapters 11 and 14). Adventitious sounds, decreased breath sounds, or areas of consolidation may indicate lower respiratory infection or pneumonia.

Examine the sputum for color, consistency, and presence of blood or odor.
- Yellow/green sputum: Suspect bacterial infection.
- Brown sputum: Check smoking history.
- Blood-streaked sputum: Suspect URI or bronchitis.
- Hemoptysis: Suspect tumor, trauma, pneumonia, TB, or pulmonary embolism.
- Clear: Suspect COPD or emphysema without infection.

Palpate the Breasts if Indicated

Observe for symmetry. Inspect the breasts for signs of inflammation (see Chapter 6), dimpling, or skin changes. Palpate for masses, tenderness, and discharge. Palpate the axillary lymph nodes for the presence of tenderness.

Examine the Abdomen if Indicated

Check for abdominal tenderness associated with intraabdominal infections or inflammatory bowel disorders as well as to check for hepatosplenomegaly seen in conditions with FUO.

Examine the Genitourinary System if Indicated

Palpate for suprapubic tenderness, which may indicate PID or UTI, and for costovertebral angle (CVA) tenderness, which suggests pyelonephritis (see Chapters 27, 35, and 37). Perform a pelvic examination on patients with a uterus who have no other obvious source of fever. Cervical motion tenderness, discharge, adnexal tenderness, and lower abdominal tenderness may indicate PID. In patients with a penis, examine for discharge, suggestive of an STI, UTI, or prostatitis.

Perform a rectal examination to evaluate for tenderness and discharge, which may indicate rectal abscess or infection as well as retrocecal appendicitis.

Perform a prostate examination in patients with a prostate who have no other obvious source of fever because prostatitis may be the cause. If you suspect prostatitis, do not perform a vigorous examination or massage the prostate because this can release bacteria and produce septicemia.

Examine the Musculoskeletal System if Indicated

Examination may suggest inflammation and infection of bones or joints if there is swelling, increased warmth, or tenderness (see Chapters 22 to 24). Infants may present with poor feeding, irritability, fever, or vomiting. Examination should reveal decreased mobility of the affected bone or joint area, increased heat, tenderness, and swelling.

Examine the lower extremities for asymmetrical swelling, calf tenderness, or palpable vessels as an indicator of deep vein phlebitis.

Osteomyelitis may occur in young children, most commonly between 3 and 10 years of age. Septic arthritis can occur in children under the age of 3 and in young women who are sexually active.

Perform Neurologic or Mental Status Examination

Evaluate for signs of meningeal irritation (see Chapters 13 and 19). Inflammation of the meninges from infection or blood evokes reflex spasm in the paravertebral muscles. In the cervical area, this manifests as neck stiffness. Normally, the chin can be flexed passively to touch the chest. If neck stiffness is present, this maneuver is not possible. With the patient supine, attempts to flex the neck cause the knees and hips to rise from the bed (Brudzinski sign) to reduce the pull on the meninges. In the lumbar region, meningeal irritation also causes spasm and can be demonstrated by passive movement of the lower limbs. Attempts to extend the knee joint when the hip joint is flexed are resisted, and the other limb may flex at the hip (Kernig sign). Neck stiffness (nuchal rigidity) or resistance to neck flexion or rotation is a late sign and not a true sign of meningitis in infants younger than 3 months old, very old people, or severely obtunded patients. Vomiting, headache, and photophobia may also be present.

Note the presence of focal deficits, which suggests vascular occlusion or abscess formation. Assess for disturbances in mentation, irritability, lethargy, somnolence, or coma, which indicates increased intracranial pressure. Seizures occur in 20% to 30% of children with meningitis.

A seizure in a febrile infant younger than 6 months old is suggestive of meningitis rather than a simple febrile seizure. Benign febrile seizure is uncommon in very young infants.

LABORATORY AND DIAGNOSTIC STUDIES

Laboratory studies can be used selectively to confirm or negate the clinical diagnosis, especially if the history and physical examination findings provide strong indication of a particular infectious process. In patients with obvious viral URI, no studies are necessary. Patients with a sore throat may require a throat culture, Monospot, or rapid strep test, depending on the clinical findings. In patients with urinary symptoms, a urinalysis (U/A) and culture may be sufficient unless clinical findings indicate an upper UTI, which would warrant further diagnostic testing such as radiography, ultrasonography, or intravenous pyelography.

Also see appropriate chapters for specific presenting problems and discussion of diagnostic tests.

Complete Blood Count

Leukocytosis with a left shift suggests a bacterial infection. Atypical lymphocytes are characteristic of systemic viral infection. Immature neutrophils suggest leukemia.

Anemia may be seen in inflammatory conditions such as juvenile arthritis, malaria, and parvovirus B19 infections. Low platelet counts may be associated with Epstein-Barr virus infection, histoplasmosis, TB, or spirochetal infections or may be drug induced. Thrombocytosis is common in Kawasaki disease (an acute febrile illness in children that resembles scarlet fever) and some viral infections.

Erythrocyte Sedimentation Rate

An elevated erythrocyte sedimentation rate (ESR) indicates an inflammatory condition. However, the test is nonspecific and does not indicate the source or cause of inflammation.

Antistreptolysin Titer

An increase in the antistreptolysin titer is detectable by comparing two blood samples more than 2 weeks apart (see Chapter 32). An elevated titer indicates immunologic response of the host after exposure to streptococcal antigen.

HIV Testing

There are two major tests used to diagnose HIV infection. The enzyme-linked immunosorbent assay (ELISA) detects the presence of HIV-specific antibodies that the body produces in response to the virus. Rapid HIV antibody tests also use blood, oral fluid, or urine to detect HIV antibodies. It can take 10 to 20 minutes to obtain results for these tests. A positive test result needs to be confirmed by a second test, the Western blot. A polymerase chain reaction test (PCR) detects the genetic material of HIV itself and can identify HIV in the blood within 2 to 3 weeks of infection. The Centers for Disease Control and Prevention recommends that everyone between the ages of 13 and 64 get tested for HIV at once as part of routine health care.

Urinalysis

Use a dipstick U/A to screen for an upper or lower UTI, which would reveal the presence of nitrites and leukocyte esterase (see Chapter 35). Microscopic evaluation discloses the presence of cells (white and red blood cells) and blood casts.

Urine Culture and Sensitivity

Performed on a clean catch of urine, this test will confirm a diagnosis of UTI and isolate the organism(s) (see Chapter 35).

Stool for Leukocytes

The presence of white blood cells (WBCs) may be suggestive of invasive bacterial gastroenteritis (see Chapter 12).

Stool culture and sensitivity

Use stool culture and sensitivity to detect the presence of *Salmonella* spp., *Clostridium difficile,* or *Shigella* spp. (see Chapter 12).

Stool Sample for Ova and Parasites

Have the patient collect three stool samples over a 5-day period (see Chapter 12). The first morning stool is preferred, and it must be delivered to the laboratory in 30 minutes or less after defecation.

Sputum for Acid-Fast Bacilli

A sputum sample to test for acid-fast bacilli is used to diagnose respiratory TB (see Chapter 11). A smear is prepared from a series of three first-morning specimens collected on three separate days to catch the sporadic discharge of the bacilli from the tubercle.

Sputum for Gram Staining

A smear is prepared from a sputum sample and stained with Gram stain. Gram-positive organisms stain purple; gram-negative organisms stain red.
- Gram-positive cocci or diplococci indicate pneumococcal, staphylococcal, or streptococcal infections.
- Gram-negative cocci indicate meningococcal or gonococcal infections.
- Enteric gram-negative bacilli indicate *Escherichia coli, Proteus* spp., *Bacteroides* spp., *Klebsiella* spp., typhoid, *Salmonella* spp., or *Shigella* spp.
- Other gram-negative bacilli indicate *Haemophilus* spp., pertussis, chancroid, brucellosis, tularemia, or plague.

Sputum for Culture and Sensitivity

Use a sputum culture to isolate a specific organism (see Chapter 11). Have the patient rinse the mouth well with water without swallowing before coughing to produce a specimen; this decreases the amount of saliva present. Do not use mouthwash because this can kill the bacteria. An early morning sample is best. The sample must contain mucoid or mucopurulent material.

Cultures of Discharge

Cultures can be prepared from any source with a discharge (e.g., vaginal, urethral, wound). Place the culture in the transport medium indicated. Cultures are used to isolate causative organisms.

Collect a specimen of vaginal or penile discharge on a sterile swab and place in the medium provided. For penile discharge, use a sterile urethral swab to collect a specimen from the anterior urethra by gentle insertion and scraping of the mucosa. For wound culture, use a sterile swab or aspirate with a sterile needle and syringe from the moist area. Bacteria from the center of a wound may be nonviable; culture near the periphery.

Molecular Testing for Infectious Organisms

Polymerase chain reaction testing can be used to detect specific pathogens in the stool. PCR is also used for detecting the presence of *Borrelia* DNA in Lyme disease and dengue fever. A positive PCR result suggests presence of the specific organism. The tests are sensitive and specific. DNA probes and nucleic acid amplification tests (NAATs) are available to test for *Chlamydia trachomatis* and *Neisseria gonorrhoeae*. Single or dual organism tests are available.

Blood Cultures

Two culture specimens are obtained at two different venipuncture sites. If one culture produces bacteria and the other does not, the positive culture is likely from a contaminant and not the infecting agent. Culture specimens drawn through an intravenous catheter are frequently contaminated. All culture specimens should be obtained before initiation of antibiotics if possible. Most organisms require approximately 24 hours for growth in the laboratory, and a preliminary report can be given at that time. Often 48 to 72 hours is required for growth and identification of organisms. Blood cultures may be positive in bacteremia.

Lumbar Puncture

A lumbar puncture is indicated if you suspect meningitis (see Chapter 19). Laboratory data on cerebrospinal fluid (CSF) always include leukocytes, protein, glucose, Gram stain, cell count, and culture and sensitivity. In meningitis, expect cloudy CSF fluid with many polymorphonuclear cells containing bacteria. Glucose level in CSF is decreased compared with blood glucose level, protein is increased, and the culture will be positive.

Radiographic Imaging

Chest radiographs may detect infiltrates, effusions, masses, or nodes. Kidney, ureter, and bladder (KUB) and upright abdominal films can reveal air-fluid levels in the bowel. Computed tomography (CT) may be used to detect abscess or tumor. Radiographs are useful for detecting bone and joint involvement in osteomyelitis. Radionuclide scanning is also beneficial in detecting osteomyelitis.

DIFFERENTIAL DIAGNOSIS

Upper Respiratory Infection

Viral infections can occur in any age group and are more prevalent during winter months (see Chapter 11). The temperature is usually less than 38.7°C (101.5°F). Systemic symptoms are common. Known contact with others who have had similar symptoms or illness is typical but not necessary. The patient usually has a cough and nonpurulent sputum. Pharyngitis may be present with erythema of the oral pharynx.

Gastroenteritis

Nausea, vomiting, and diarrhea are the hallmarks of a GI infection (see Chapter 12). Fever is usually mild. Abdominal cramping may be present.

Urinary Tract Infection

Urinary tract infections are more common in patients with female GU anatomy (see Chapter 35). Localized urinary tract symptoms are common in adults; systemic symptoms are more common in children. CVA tenderness indicates upper UTI. The temperature associated with an upper UTI is likely to be a high fever, and the patient feels systemically ill. U/A can support a clinical diagnosis of UTI. Urine for culture and sensitivity usually confirms the diagnosis.

Pelvic Inflammatory Disease

Suspect PID in patients with a uterus who have a fever for which there is no other explanation (see Chapter 37). There may be vague reports of lower abdominal pain; suprapubic tenderness may be present on abdominal examination. Pelvic examination reveals cervical motion tenderness, discharge, or adnexal tenderness.

Prostatitis

In patients with a prostate who have no other obvious source of fever, suspect prostatitis (see Chapter 27). The prostate will be exquisitely tender to gentle palpation. The results from other system examinations will be normal.

Pharyngitis

The patient reports a sore throat. In children, fever may precede throat complaints by 1 or 2 days. The pharynx is red, and the tonsils may be enlarged or have exudate. For differential diagnosis of bacterial and viral pharyngitis, see Chapter 32. Mononucleosis occurs most often in young adults and may present with palatine petechiae, tonsillar exudate, posterior cervical lymphadenopathy, and splenomegaly.

Acute Sinusitis

Sinuses that are tender to percussion or do not transilluminate may indicate sinusitis, especially in the presence of purulent nasal discharge. Patients often report a frontal headache, which worsens as the patient leans forward (see Chapter 25), and upper incisor toothache. Patients sometimes experience a sore throat and cough from postnasal discharge, which may be apparent in the posterior pharynx.

Ear Infections

Otitis media is more common in children (see Chapter 15). The tympanic membrane will appear red and may bulge. The light reflex will be absent or diminished. Tympanic membrane mobility will be limited. The child may tug at the ear and act restless or irritable. The young child or infant may feed poorly. The temperature may be a high- or low-grade fever. Respiratory symptoms occur if the patient has a concomitant respiratory tract infection. Ear infections are commonly associated with other upper respiratory tract symptoms.

Meningitis

The signs and symptoms of meningitis are related to nonspecific findings associated with bacteremia or a systemic infection or to specific manifestation of meningeal irritation with CNS inflammation (see Chapter 19). Inspect the skin for petechiae, cyanosis, state of hydration, and peripheral perfusion. Nuchal rigidity, back pain, Kernig sign, Brudzinski sign, nausea, vomiting, and bulging fontanel (in infants) may be seen. Papilledema is rarely seen. If it is present, look for other processes, such as brain abscess or subdural empyema. Ataxia may be a presenting sign. Lumbar puncture confirms the diagnosis.

Osteomyelitis

Bone infection is usually caused by bacteria and may arise from a clinically evident infection or from general bacteremia (see Chapters 22 and 23). Patients report pain in the affected bone or joint and may exhibit soft tissue tenderness and swelling. Children demonstrate localized tenderness near the epiphysis. The diagnosis requires isolation of the responsible organism via blood cultures, pus from tissue abscesses, synovial fluid aspirate, or material from needle aspiration or bone biopsy. Radionuclide scanning, CT, or magnetic resonance imaging may be helpful in determining the extent of infection and destruction.

Kawasaki Disease

Kawasaki disease is an acute mucocutaneous lymph node syndrome that is classified as a vasculitic syndrome (of which fever is only one sign) affecting infants and young children younger than age 9 years (see Chapter 28). It is more common in males and often occurs in fall and spring. The etiology is unknown. Fevers are of a high-spiking remittent pattern in the range of 38° to 40°C (100.4° to 104°F) and persist despite the use of empiric antibiotics and antipyretics. Seizures may be present, and other neurologic causes must be ruled out. The febrile phase lasts from 5 to 25 days with a mean of 10 days. Because of the rash associated with the fever, Kawasaki disease resembles scarlet fever.

To make the initial diagnosis of Kawasaki disease, fever lasting at least 5 days with at least four of the following signs, in the absence of a known diagnosis or infection, must be present:
- Bilateral conjunctival hyperemia
- Mouth lesions: dry fissured lips and injected pharynx, or strawberry tongue

- Change in peripheral extremities, edema, erythema, desquamation of skin at 10 to 14 days
- Nonvesicular erythematous rash
- Cervical lymphadenopathy

Factitious Fever

A factitious fever is when the patient artificially produces a fever by manipulating the thermometer or ingesting a pyrogenic substance. Suspect this when there is a discrepancy between oral or rectal temperature and urine temperature. The pulse rate will be inconsistent with elevated temperature. The patient has no weight loss. Repeated monitored temperature taking does not support previous readings.

Roseola Infantum

Roseola infantum is the most common exanthema of children younger than 3 years of age. Symptoms include an irritable child who has high fever with rapid defervescence when the rash appears on day 3 or 4. The rash is maculopapular and lasts 1 to 2 days.

Fevers without Localizing Signs

Often examination fails to disclose any specific signs or symptoms other than the fever itself. Most children who have a fever without localizing signs have neither an unusual nor a serious disease. In many cases, the fever will clear within a few days without a specific diagnosis. However, the longer the child has a fever without localizing signs, the less likely the fever is the result of infectious disease. Viral illness or malignancy must be considered.

In the history and physical examination, always investigate any abnormal growth suggestive of a possible preexisting chronic disease. Morning stiffness may signify rheumatoid arthritis, weight loss or abdominal pain could indicate inflammatory bowel disease, and frequent respiratory tract infections may point to cystic fibrosis or immunodeficiency.

Enterovirus

All enteroviruses may cause a mild, nonspecific, febrile illness that lasts 2 to 5 days. Most are seasonal, occurring in late summer and early fall. Herpangina, nonexudative pharyngitis with or without lymphadenopathy, generally occurs.

Occult Bacteremia

Occult bacteremia is diagnosed in children older than 3 months who have positive blood cultures but do not have the usual clinical manifestation of sepsis or septic shock. *Occult* means hidden from view; the child looks well. The majority of children who look well and are playful are at low risk for bacteremia despite fever. Those who look ill or who are toxic are at significant risk. The primary concern is the small but important percentage of children who develop secondary complications from invasive bacterial disease (i.e., meningitis, bacterial sepsis, septic arthritis, pneumonia). Peak ages for bacteremia are between 6 and 24 months, with *Streptococcus pneumoniae* being the organism most commonly responsible.

Periodic Fever in Children

This condition is characterized by an abrupt fever that occurs in children 2 to 5 years of age on a regularly recurring basis, generally every 6 weeks. The fever lasts an average of 4 days. Besides the fever, the child has malaise, sore throat, cervical adenopathy, and aphthous stomatitis. The WBC count may be elevated ($13,000/mm^3$), as is the ESR. There are no associated diseases or other physical examination and laboratory findings. The child has normal growth and development.

▶ **DIFFERENTIAL DIAGNOSIS OF** *Common Causes of Fever*

CONDITION	HISTORY	PHYSICAL FINDINGS	DIAGNOSTIC STUDIES
URI	Any age group; systemic symptoms; often known contact with ill others	Fever <38.7°C (101.5°F); cough; nonpurulent sputum; erythema of pharynx; viral exanthema	None

▶ DIFFERENTIAL DIAGNOSIS OF *Common Causes of Fever—cont'd*

CONDITION	HISTORY	PHYSICAL FINDINGS	DIAGNOSTIC STUDIES
Gastroenteritis	Nausea, vomiting, diarrhea; abdominal cramping	Mild fever; abdomen may be diffusely tender	None
UTI	Females more than males; burning urgency; frequency in adults; systemic symptoms or bedwetting in children	CVA tenderness with upper UTI; fever with upper UTI	U/A; urine C&S; CBC if suspect upper UTI
PID	May have pelvic or lower abdominal pain	May have suprapubic tenderness; cervical discharge; CMT, adnexal tenderness	CBC; molecular testing
Pharyngitis	Sore throat; may or may not have other upper respiratory tract symptoms	Erythematous pharynx; may have pharyngeal or tonsillar exudates, or ulcers; may have palatine petechiae in mononucleosis; lymphadenopathy	CBC; culture; rapid strep test if suspect strep; Monospot if suspect mononucleosis
Prostatitis	Perineal discomfort, frequent urination, chills, and malaise	Prostate tender to palpation; fever	Segmental urine specimen; C&S of urine; C&S of prostate discharge
Acute sinusitis	Facial or sinus pressure or pain; headache	Purulent nasal discharge; sinuses tender to percussion; headache or pressure worsens on bending forward	Radiographs or CT scan of limited value
Ear infections	Earache, pain; may have upper respiratory tract symptoms; child tugs at ear	High- or low-grade fever; TM red, may bulge, landmarks absent; TM mobility impaired; child irritable or restless	Pneumatic otoscopy
Meningitis	Nonspecific symptoms; nausea, vomiting, irritability, headache	Petechiae, nuchal rigidity, positive Kernig and Brudzinski signs, petechiae; bulging fontanel in infant	Lumbar puncture
Osteomyelitis	Pain in affected bone or joint	Swelling or tenderness over affected area of joint	Culture; CBC; radionuclide scan, CT, MRI
Kawasaki disease	Younger than 5 yr of age; males more than females; fall and spring	High fever, spikes; persists despite antibiotic therapy; may have seizures; fever for 5 days with at least four of the following: bilateral conjunctival hyperemia, mouth lesions, edema, erythema, desquamation of skin, nonvesicular erythematous rash, cervical lymphadenopathy	WBC increased, shift to left; slight anemia; thrombocytosis; positive CRP; ESR increased; serum IgM, IgE increased

Continued

▶ **DIFFERENTIAL DIAGNOSIS OF** *Common Causes of Fever—cont'd*

CONDITION	HISTORY	PHYSICAL FINDINGS	DIAGNOSTIC STUDIES
Factitious fever	Vague or no symptoms	Normal physical examination findings; no weight loss; pulse rate normal (not consistent with temperature elevation)	Discrepancy between oral–rectal temperature and urine temperature; repeated monitored temperature taking does not support previous readings
Roseola infantum	Irritable child with fever for 4–5 days	Normal physical examination; when fever breaks, rash appears	None
Fevers without localizing signs	No other specific symptoms	Physical examination findings usually normal initially; repeat examination in 24 hr and as needed	U/A; urine C&S; chest radiography; WBC; rule out systemic disease, malignancy
Enterovirus	Mild, nonspecific febrile illness lasting 2–5 days; summer and early fall peaks	Nonexudative pharyngitis with or without lymphadenopathy frequently observed	None
Occult bacteremia	Fever in children older than 3 mo	No localizing signs; child appears well	Blood culture; WBC
Periodic fever in children	Abrupt fever on periodic basis (about every 6 wk); lasts about 4 days; children aged 2–5 yr; malaise	Cervical adenopathy, aphthous stomatitis	WBC and ESR elevated

C&S, culture and sensitivity; *CBC,* complete blood count; *CRP,* C-reactive protein; *CT,* computed tomography; *CVA,* costovertebral angle; *ESR,* erythrocyte sedimentation rate; *MRI,* magnetic resonance imaging; *PID,* pelvic inflammatory disease; *TM,* tympanic membrane; *U/A,* urinalysis; *URI,* upper respiratory infection; *UTI,* urinary tract infection; *WBC,* white blood cell.

Genitourinary Problems in Patients with Male Genitalia

Urinary tract problems in patients with male genitalia represent a range of conditions from infections, inflammation, and urinary outlet obstruction to congenital malformation, trauma, or neoplasm. Any part of the renal, urologic, or reproductive tract can be involved. Symptoms may be localized to a single site but can also be vague or be referred from the site of involvement.

Dysuria is most commonly caused by urethritis, prostatitis, cystitis, or mechanical irritation of the urethra. Inflammation of the lower urinary tract is infrequent in children and adolescents, and increases with age.

Cystitis results from ascending infection of the urethra or prostate or occurs secondary to urethral instrumentation. The most common cause of recurrent cystitis is chronic bacterial prostatitis. *Escherichia coli* is the usual gram-negative pathogen. *Chlamydia trachomatis* is the major cause of sexually transmitted prostatitis and nongonococcal urethritis in patients younger than age 40 years. Recurrent urinary tract infections (UTIs) may involve resistant gram-negative *Klebsiella* spp., *Enterobacter* spp., *Pseudomonas* spp., or *Proteus mirabilis,* or gram-positive *Enterococcus* spp. and *Staphylococcus aureus.* Infection may involve the kidneys and cause pyelonephritis. Secondary infection can occur as the result of urinary stones.

The patient with urinary problems may also have symptoms involving urinary flow. Urine flow may be altered by compression of the urethra as it passes through an enlarged prostate, obstructing the flow of urine and producing hesitancy, slowing of the urinary stream, dribbling, and nocturia. Benign prostatic hyperplasia (BPH) is common after age 50 years, with frequency as high as 80% of after age 80 years. Patients with BPH are more prone to UTIs and incontinence.

Urinary stones can occur anywhere in the urinary tract and are common causes of obstructive symptoms, bleeding, and pain.

Trauma to the urinary tract may be caused by penetrating, straddle, blunt, and crushing injuries or by surgery and instrumentation. Hematuria, oliguria, and pain are the most common symptoms.

Neoplasms occur more often in the male GU tract than in the female GU tract. Kidney, prostate, and bladder neoplasms are more common in older men. Kidney and bladder neoplasms often produce painless hematuria. Prostate cancer may produce symptoms of outlet obstruction.

Kidney problems can range from asymptomatic blood chemical changes to life-threatening abnormal renal function that could manifest in fluid–electrolyte and acid–base imbalances. Patients with renal insufficiency may present with nonspecific complaints such as fatigue, anorexia, or weakness. A discussion of renal insufficiency and renal failure is beyond the scope of this chapter.

DIAGNOSTIC REASONING: FOCUSED HISTORY

Could the symptoms be from an acute systemic cause?

Key Questions
- Have you had fever, chills, nausea, or vomiting?
- Are you positive for HIV infection or receiving chemotherapy?
- Have you been able to pass any urine?

Fever and Chills

The presence of fever or chills suggests a systemic inflammatory response and indicates that the patient may be acutely ill and should be aggressively treated. Specifically, suspect pyelonephritis, lithiasis of the upper urinary tract, prostatitis, orchitis, or epididymitis of the lower urinary tract.

Immunocompromised Patients

Immunocompromised patients are susceptible to overwhelming infections by both common and atypical organisms, and aggressive investigation is warranted.

Anuria

A sudden decrease in urinary output to less than 100 mL/day or nonpassage of urine may result from compromised renal blood supply (prerenal); damaged interstitia, glomeruli, or tubules (intrarenal); or obstructed urine flow (postrenal). Patients with prerenal failure usually have a history of volume depletion or a reduction in arterial blood volume such as in low cardiac output states. Patients with intrarenal failure may present with history of renal damage from nephrotoxic agents. Anuria may represent renal failure or obstruction. Postrenal failure is the least likely cause of anuria, but it should be ruled out first because when failure results from obstructive causes, mechanical intervention may reestablish kidney function before permanent nephron damage occurs. Patients at greatest risk for acute renal failure are older adults; have diabetes; and a have history of renal, heart, or liver disease.

extrarenal. A lesion of the bladder or lower urinary tract is demonstrated in more than 60% of patients. The most common causes of gross hematuria from the kidney are nephropathy and polycystic kidney disease. No cause for hematuria can be found in 10% to 15% of patients.

Timing

Initial hematuria becomes clear during voiding and is indicative of anterior urethral lesions such as urethritis, stricture, or meatal stenosis. Terminal hematuria begins with clear urine and then becomes bloody and is suggestive of prostatic lesions or lesions in the prostatic urethra. Total hematuria is usually characteristic of lesions in the kidneys and ureters. Bladder lesions may produce bleeding independent of micturition. Recent trauma to the kidneys can also produce hematuria. Gross hematuria is often transient but may continue microscopically.

Pain

Hematuria with pain usually indicates the passage of a stone or sloughed renal papilla, often with concurrent infection. Painless gross hematuria is consistent with upper or lower tract tumor, systemic coagulopathy, or excessive anticoagulant effect. Less common causes include acute necrosis or sloughing of a papilla. In older adults, painless hematuria may be a late-presenting sign of renal cancer.

Is there hematuria?

Key Questions
- Have you noticed blood or blood clots in your urine?
- Is there blood every time you urinate or just occasionally?
- Describe when you notice the blood (e.g., does the blood start with the beginning of urination, continue throughout urination, or occur only at the end of urination? Is there blood without urinating?).
- Do you have pain with the blood?

Hematuria

Blood can enter the urinary tract at any site. The most common source of isolated hematuria is

---

Can the symptoms be localized within the urinary tract?

Key Questions
- Do you have trouble with your urine stream (e.g., slow or weakened urinary stream, trouble starting, intermittent stream, dribbling)?
- Are you able to empty your bladder?
- Do you have low back, flank, or abdominal pain?
- Do you have pain in the scrotum or testicles?
- Do you have aching in the perineal area?
- Do you have suprapubic discomfort?
- Have you had urinary incontinence?
- Do you have frequency, urgency, painful urination, or penile discharge?

- Do you urinate at night?
- Do you have an excessive volume of urine?

Slow Urinary Stream, Hesitancy, Intermittency, or Dribbling of Urine

In men older than 50 years of age, the presence of slow urinary stream, hesitancy, intermittency, and dribbling of urine with a gradual onset over time indicates obstructive problems from benign prostatic hypertrophy. Have the patient complete the American Urological Association (AUA) Symptom Index (Table 18.1). Using the index, classify symptoms as mild (0–7), moderate (8–19), or severe (20–35).

Ability to Empty the Bladder

Urinary retention can be acute or chronic. Acute urinary retention is the sudden and often painful inability to void despite having a full bladder and is a medical emergency. Chronic urinary retention is the inability to completely empty the bladder. Causes of retention include obstruction, infection, inflammation, medications, trauma, and neurologic causes. The most common cause is obstruction from an enlarged prostate. In transgender women, the practice of tucking of the scrotal contents can cause retention (see Chapter 42). Patients can present with complete lack of voiding, incomplete bladder emptying, or overflow incontinence. Complications include infection and renal failure.

Low Back, Flank, or Abdominal Pain

Patient reports of low back, flank, or abdominal pain are often indicative of ureteral and kidney involvement. Renal tract pain may present with a constant dull ache in the costovertebral angle (CVA) area. Dislodged kidney stones will produce an acute ureteral pain that is colicky and cyclic in nature. Gross blood in the urine and infection may accompany the ureteral pain. The pain can radiate to the abdomen, testes, and penis. However, renal disorders do not frequently cause pain. True renal pain can originate from the calyces or renal pelvis. Pain can result from stretching of the kidney capsule, interstitial edema, or inflammation of the capsule.

Testicular or Scrotal Pain

Acute pain in the scrotum or testicles may indicate infection or a pathological condition of the scrotal contents, or it may be referred pain from other sites in the urinary tract. Pain in the scrotum or testicles is characteristic of inflammation of the testicles, epididymitis, or torsion of a testicle. A common cause of scrotal contents pain in transgender women is tucking of the testicles into the inguinal canal. Some may maintain this positioning even at night while sleeping. Resulting pain may be traumatic, mechanical, or neuropathic (see Chapter 42).

Aching in the Perineal Area

Prostate pain is often interpreted by the patient as a vague ache in the perineal area. The usual cause of perineal aching is infection; another cause may be prostatic stones with infection.

Suprapubic Discomfort and Urinary Incontinence

Whereas discomfort in the suprapubic area is indicative of bladder involvement, urinary incontinence is characteristic of bladder neck irritability caused by inflammation. Bladder pain is most often caused by infection; however, it can also be produced by obstruction and bladder distention as the result of a tumor or stones.

Penile Discharge with Frequency, Urgency, and Dysuria

Penile discharge with frequency, urgency, and dysuria is characteristic of anterior urethral irritation and of exposure to a sexually transmitted infection (STI) (see Chapter 27).

Nocturia

Primary bladder disease from infection, stones, or tumors can produce nocturia. Prostate enlargement characteristically produces nocturia. Most adults do not need to void during the night, but some may get up once during the night, depending on the amount and timing of fluid ingestion.

Patients who report daytime frequency without nocturia are usually free of organic disease.

Table 18.1	**The American Urological Association (AUA) Symptom Index[a]**

Patients rate their answers to each question on a scale of 0 to 5.

QUESTIONS	NOT AT ALL	LESS THAN ONE TIME IN FIVE	LESS THAN HALF THE TIME	ABOUT HALF THE TIME	MORE THAN HALF THE TIME	ALMOST ALWAYS
Over the past month, how often have you had a sensation of not emptying your bladder completely after you finished voiding?	0	1	2	3	4	5
Over the past month, how often have you had to urinate again less than 2 hours after you finished urinating?	0	1	2	3	4	5
Over the past month, how often have you found you stopped and started again several times when you urinated?	0	1	2	3	4	5
Over the past month, how often have you found it difficult to postpone urination?	0	1	2	3	4	5
Over the past month, how often have you had a weak urinary stream?	0	1	2	3	4	5
Over the past month, how often have you had to push or strain to begin urination?	0	1	2	3	4	5
Over the past month, how many times did you typically get up to urinate from the time you went to bed at night until the time you got up in the morning?	0	1	2	3	4	5

[a]AUA Symptom Score = sum of above circled numbers. Symptoms are classified as mild (0–7), moderate (8–19), or severe (20–35).
From Barry et al, 1992.

Polyuria

Polyuria is defined as a volume greater than 3 L/day of urine and depends on fluid intake and the patient's state of hydration. Polyuria may be an early indication of renal disease progression because of the kidneys' inability to concentrate urine. Taking a history of fluid intake is important to identify possible causes of polyuria. Pseudo polyuria results from increased fluid ingestion and may present with certain personality disorders or as a result of excessive water intake as part of a health regimen. Alcohol ingestion inhibits antidiuretic hormone; glycosuria promotes excess solute excretion. Diabetes insipidus may also be implicated. Nocturia can occur with the mobilization of fluid during sleep, secondary to congestive heart failure.

Are there any risk factors to point me in the right direction?

Key Questions

- Have you had this or similar problems before?
- Do you have a family history of kidney problems, prostatitis, prostate cancer, or diabetes?
- How old are you?
- Have you been confined to bed (especially if an older adult)?
- Are you sexually active? How many partners do you have?
- Do you ride a bicycle?

History of Similar Problems

Patients with previous urinary problems are at risk for chronic relapsing conditions such as unresolved infections, resistant strains of organisms, or reinfection. Recurrent infections, pyelonephritis, or complications warrant urologic referral for workup and evaluation.

Family History of Urinary Problems

A family history of renal problems or prostatitis places the patient at increased risk for urinary problems. Familial disorders that may be implicated in kidney disease include diabetes mellitus, hypertension, collagen vascular disease, nephrolithiasis, and polycystic kidney disease.

Age

The occurrence of UTIs in patients with male genitalia increases with age. Slow development of prostatic obstruction is common after age 50 years and is usually painless. Patients have difficulty starting the urine stream, the urine stream has decreased force, and urine often continues to dribble after voiding. Chlamydia is the major cause of prostatitis, epididymitis, and nongonococcal urethritis before 40 years of age. Adolescents who are sexually active are at particular risk for STIs.

Confinement to Bed

Older adult patients confined to bed are at an increased risk of infection. Likely mechanisms include urinary stasis and reflux.

Sexual Activity

Sexually active patients, especially those who engage in unprotected sex, are at risk for STIs, which can produce urethritis. The risk increases with multiple partners.

Bicycle Riding

On an upright bicycle, the design of the seat puts pressure on the ischial tuberosities and perineum of the rider. The hip and pedaling motion of the rider contribute to neural symptoms by stretching the pudendal nerve, especially if the seat is not correctly fitted to the rider. Perineal and penile numbness, without pain, are symptoms frequently reported by long-distance cyclists.

What else could this be?

Key Questions

- Have you had a recent urologic procedure or urinary catheter?
- Have you had a recent STI?
- If you've been recently diagnosed with an STI, have you been treated ?
- What drugs have you taken (prescription, over the counter, or recreational)?
- What is your occupation?
- What are your hobbies (toxic exposure)?
- Has there been any scrotal swelling?

Recent Procedure or Catheter Use

Recent instrumentation in the urinary tract places the patient at risk for infections. Patients with indwelling catheters are also at risk for infection.

Recent Sexually Transmitted Infection

Sexually transmitted infections can produce urethritis and urinary tract symptoms. Recent treatment for an STI may indicate treatment failure, a coinfection that was not covered by the prescribed drug, or a reinfection.

Drugs

The most prevalent nephrotoxic drugs include aminoglycosides, nonsteroidal antiinflammatory drugs, iodinated radiocontrast media, and angiotensin-converting enzyme inhibitors. Less prevalent are antibiotics (e.g., amphotericin B), chemotherapeutic agents, cocaine, H_2-receptor antagonists, phenytoin, sulfonamide diuretics, and volatile hydrocarbons. Drugs that can cause urinary retention include antiarrhythmics, anticholinergics, antidepressants, antihistamines, antihypertensives, antiparkinsonian agents, antipsychotics, hormonal agents, and muscle relaxants.

Toxic Exposures

Occupational hazards that may cause kidney problems include exposure to volatile hydrocarbons, benzene, aniline, xylene, heavy metals, and ionizing radiation.

Scrotal Swelling

Scrotal swelling may indicate a hernia or hydrocele. In infants, swelling increased with straining or crying may indicate a communicating hydrocele.

DIAGNOSTIC REASONING: FOCUSED PHYSICAL EXAMINATION

Note General Appearance

A patient who appears ill or who is in pain is likely to have acute prostatitis or an upper urinary tract problems such as pyrlonephritis or urolithiasis. Except for acute prostatitis, lower urinary tract problems usually do not present with sings of systemic involvement or fever, and patients generally appear well.

Obtain Vital Signs

Obtain a resting blood pressure as hypertension is seen in patients with nephritis. Fever may result in an increased heart rate.

Inspect Skin and Mucous Membranes

A pale skin color may suggest anemia caused by poor nutrition or chronic renal failure. Yellow-colored to brown-colored skin without scleral icterus may indicate severe chronic uremia. Other skin changes seen with renal problems may range from rash to purpura.

Palpate and Percuss for Flank Pain at the Costovertebral Angle

Pain that is reproducible is indicative of renal capsule distention and characterizes acute pyelonephritis or acute ureteral obstruction. Perinephric abscess may cause flank swelling and redness.

Auscultate the Abdomen

If the patient is hypertensive, auscultate the abdominal aorta and renal and iliac arteries for bruits, which could indicate a renovascular cause of the hypertension.

Palpate and Percuss the Abdomen

Abdominal distention suggests ascites or fluid collection in the bowel. Pain in the lower quadrant indicates lower ureter involvement. Perform deep palpation to identify kidney or other abdominal masses. Normal kidneys are usually not easily palpated. A distended bladder rises above the symphysis pubis and is characteristic of residual urine from incomplete bladder emptying. Palpation of an enlarged bladder may cause pain. Chronic bladder distention is usually painless and cannot always be determined by manual palpation alone.

Inspect and Palpate the External Genitalia

Inspect the skin and hair for inflammation, lesions, parasites, and dermatitis. Note the hair pattern distribution and level of development of structures for age. Palpate the shaft of the penis for strictures. Observe for phimosis, if uncircumcised, and retract the foreskin. Note inflammation or presence of smegma. Inspect the glans, corona, and frenulum areas for lesions. Note personal hygiene; phimosis or paraphimosis in uncircumcised patients; and presence of urine, discharge, and fecal stains on undergarments. Check the position of the urethral meatus. Strip or milk the penis from the base toward the glans or head of the penis. Note the color, consistency, and amount of any discharge.

Check the scrotum skin surfaces and testicles for tenderness or masses and check for epididymis, spermatic cords, and inguinal canals. In infants, palpate the scrotum to assess for undescended testicles. Holding a finger in the inguinal canal prevents the testicle from slipping into the canal when palpating the scrotum. The left scrotal sac usually hangs lower than the right. Elevation of an affected testicle may relieve discomfort (positive Prehn sign) and is characteristic of epididymitis. In testicular torsion, elevation fails to relieve pain (negative Prehn sign). A painful scrotal mass is usually associated with inflammation or testicular torsion.

Perform scrotal transillumination in a darkened room. Do not use a halogen light source because it may burn the patient. A solid mass prevents the passage of light and requires further examination. A hydrocele is a nontender collection of fluid in the scrotum. It will transilluminate but may make testicular palpation difficult. A spermatocele (a cystic swelling on the epididymis) is not as large as a hydrocele but does not transilluminate. A varicocele occurs from dilated veins in the scrotal sac and usually occurs on the left side. A varicocele is often more prominent when the patient is standing and regresses with the patient in the prone position. It is classically described as a "bag of worms."

Observe Voiding

Observing the patient urinating may be useful to check for hesitancy in initiating the urine stream, force of stream, and dribbling at end of micturition. Observe the abdominal force used during urination. Patients will use abdominal muscles to increase the intraabdominal pressure to force urine from the bladder while holding their breath.

Perform Digital Rectal Prostate Examination

Digital rectal examination (DRE) of the prostate is performed to identify irregularities of the prostate that are suggestive of cancer and to note any tenderness or inflammation. The size and consistency should be noted. The median sulcus and lateral margins should be palpated. Induration or firmness is characteristic of early prostate disease; a hard, stony gland suggests advanced prostatic carcinoma. The gland may feel soft because of inflammation or infection. If hypertrophied, the prostate gland will extend

into the rectal canal, and the median sulcus may be obliterated. Massaging the prostate in order to obtain prostatic fluid (known as EPS – expressed prostatic secretion) is useful when chronic prostatitis is suspected. Do not massage the prostate if acute prostatitis is suspected because of the possibility of spreading the infection. Document the amount of prostate extension into the rectum using an acceptable clinical scale such as the following:

- Grade I: protrudes less than 1 cm into the rectum
- Grade II: protrudes 1 to 2 cm into the rectum
- Grade III: protrudes 2 to 3 cm into the rectum
- Grade IV: protrudes more than 3 cm into the rectum

LABORATORY AND DIAGNOSTIC STUDIES

The history and the findings of the physical examination determine the extent of diagnostic investigation. The symptoms reported by the patient are taken into account when ordering diagnostic tests to corroborate or verify the diagnosis. General screening tests can be used to provide additional data for patients with urinary tract problems.

Specific tests for kidney function include urinalysis, screening blood chemistry tests (e.g., urea, nitrogen, and serum creatinine), and hematologic studies. Abnormal blood tests include elevated creatinine and blood urea nitrogen levels, hyperkalemia, and hypocalcemia.

Urine collected for urinalysis should be freshly voided and preferably midstream. If not examined immediately, the specimen should be refrigerated, as cells begin to hemolyze after 1 to 2 hours.

Urine Dipstick

Reagent strips can be used to screen urine in the clinical setting. A positive leukocyte esterase or nitrite test result is indicative of urethritis. Urine that tests positive for leukocyte esterase should also be tested for bacteria. Proteinuria may indicate kidney involvement. Suspect proximal renal tubular damage if urine glucose is elevated while serum glucose levels are normal. Blood in the urine could be caused by acute or chronic prostatitis, urethritis, hemorrhagic cystitis, renal stones, or tumors of the kidney, renal pelvis, ureter, bladder, prostate, and urethra. Hematuria with proteinuria usually suggests a renal origin. Isolated hematuria is usually produced by sites outside the kidneys.

Urinalysis with Microscopic Examination

Turbidity with a foul odor indicates infection. Color changes of the urine may result from various sources: hemoglobin from systemic red blood cell (RBC) lysis; myoglobin from damaged muscle cells or rhabdomyolysis; vegetable pigments from food, such as red beets; pigments from drugs, such as rifampin and phenazopyridine; and porphyrins from porphyria. RBCs indicate acute inflammatory or vascular disorders of the glomerulus. Casts indicate hemorrhage or conditions of the nephron. Red cell casts are characteristic of glomerular origin. The presence of abnormal cells, protein, hemoglobin, myoglobin, or other debris with a cast helps identify the type of renal disease. Whereas significant proteinuria results from glomerulopathies, tubular disorders cause little proteinuria. Therefore the sediment findings are helpful to correlate with the degree of proteinuria. Urinalysis is indicated for all patients with male genitalia presenting with lower urinary tract symptoms. EPS rarely shows bacteria but the presence of WBCs with clumping may be seen in chronic prostatitis.

Segmented Urine Collection (Meares-Stamey 4-Glass Test) for Gram Stain, Culture and Sensitivity, and Leukocyte Count

Segmented urine collection is the gold standard test for identifying the site along the urinary tract where the colonization of organisms is occurring. The method for specimen collection and labeling is the following:
- Voided bladder specimen 1 (VB 1): 5 to 10 mL of first-voided urine collected
- Voided bladder specimen 2 (VB 2): sterile midstream urine collected
- Expressed prostatic secretion (EPS): prostatic massage performed and prostatic secretion collected from meatal opening
- Voided bladder specimen 3 (VB 3): complete emptying of bladder; urine specimen collected

Another option is the premassage and postmassage urine test (PPMT) (see Evidence-Based Practice box: 4 Glasses or 2?). The following two urine samples are collected:
- A midstream urine specimen before prostatic massage
- A first-voided urine specimen immediately after prostatic massage

Label each of the specimens and perform culture and sensitivity or Gram staining. The presence of bacteria in VB 1 suggests urethritis. The presence of bacteria in VB 2 suggests cystitis. Bacteria present in EPS or VB 3 in the absence of bacteria in VB 1 and VB 2 specimens or a bacterial culture at least 10 times higher in VB 3 samples than in VB 1 and VB 2 samples is suggestive of bacterial prostatitis.

On microscopic analysis, increased numbers of leukocytes in the EPS and VB 3 are indicative of inflammation. The presence of white blood cells (WBCs) helps diagnose prostatitis and chronic pelvic pain syndrome (Box 18.1).

Box 18.1	**National Institutes of Health Classification of Prostatitis**
CLASSIFICATION	**DESCRIPTION**
I	Acute bacterial prostatitis (acute symptoms)
II	Chronic bacterial prostatitis (symptoms present for 3 months)
III	Chronic prostatitis/chronic pelvic pain syndrome (CPPS) (no bacterial cause)
IIIA	Inflammatory CPPS (WBCs found in semen, expressed prostatic secretions, or final voided specimen)
IIIB	Noninflammatory CPPS (no WBCs in semen, expressed prostatic secretions, or final voided specimen)
IV	Asymptomatic inflammatory prostatitis (no subjective symptoms; incidental detection of WBCs in expressed prostatic secretions or prostate tissue)

WBC, white blood cell.
Reference: Krieger et al, 1999.

EVIDENCE-BASED PRACTICE *4 Glasses or 2?*

The Meares-Stamey 4-glass test is the standard method of assessing inflammation and the presence of bacteria in the lower urinary tract in men presenting with chronic prostatitis. However, evidence suggests that the simpler 2-glass premassage and postmassage urine test (PPMT) may be sufficient to detect inflammation and bacteria. In a study of 353 men, the 2-glass PPMT was compared with the Meares-Stamey 4-glass test in detecting inflammation and bacteria in men with chronic prostatitis syndrome. The PPMT had strong concordance with the 4-glass test and predicted a correct diagnosis in more than 96% of participants.

Reference: Nickel et al, 2006.

Urodynamic Testing

Urodynamic studies can be used to determine diminished force of urination and obstruction. Flow rate is defined as the volume of fluid expelled from the urethra per unit of time and is expressed in milliliters per second. The patient must have a full bladder because urine flow rate depends on voided volume. The patient urinates into an insert in the toilet, which measures the flow rate of the urine. The normal flow pattern exhibits a rapid increase to maximal flow rate, within one third of the ultimate voiding time. After achieving maximal rate, the flow decreases more slowly; the average flow rate should be approximately 50% of the maximal urine flow rate.

Gram Stain

Gram stain of urethral exudate or spun urine should be performed to determine inflammation (WBCs) and the presence of either gram-negative or gram-positive bacteria. Gram-negative bacteria stain pink-red; gram-positive bacteria stain dark blue to purple. The nuclei of polymorphonuclear neutrophils (PMNs) (leukocytes) stain pink-red. A Gram stain with more than 4 PMNs/high-power field (HPF) is indicative of urethritis (defined by the presence of 5–10 PMNs/HPF). However, any number of WBCs is suggestive of urethritis. A symptomatic patient with risk factors but no abnormal laboratory results should be retested using the first voided urine of the day.

If the stain is positive for PMNs, examine the smear for gram-negative intracellular diplococci (GNICDCs). If GNICDCs are found, the smear is considered positive for gonococcal urethritis. A smear that is equivocal or atypical indicates a mixed gonococcal and nongonococcal urethritis. If there are no GNICDCs, nongonococcal urethritis is indicated. The Gram stain has 95% specificity in gonococcal urethritis, with nearly 100% sensitivity in urethritis.

Culture and Sensitivity

Culture and sensitivity should be performed on specimens to identify the causative organism and its sensitivity to antibiotics. This is especially important in populations at increased risk for resistant organisms.

Molecular Testing for Infectious Organisms

DNA testing using a sample taken from the urethra or first-voided urine provides rapid, sensitive, and specific results. DNA tests include DNA probes, nucleic acid amplification tests, and polymerase chain reaction tests. Tests are available for *C. trachomatis* and *N. gonorrhoeae* as well as other organisms.

Creatinine and Blood Urea Nitrogen

Serum creatinine and blood urea nitrogen levels are used to indicate kidney function.

Prostate-Specific Antigen

Tumor markers, such as prostate-specific antigen (PSA), may be used to detect or monitor prostate cancer. PSA results should be correlated with the DRE. For average-risk patients at ages 45 to 75, levels of 1 to 3 ng/mL are considered within reference range, levels greater than 3 ng/mL requires additional testing or biopsy. PSA levels of 10 ng/mL or greater are abnormal and are suggestive of malignant activity of the prostate. The threshold level for African Americans who are at risk may be lower than for other groups. The higher the PSA level, the more likely the presence of prostate cancer; however, patients with prostate cancer may have a normal or borderline PSA level. In patients taking finasteride, normal PSA is reduced by as much as 50%. A normal PSA level and a normal DRE make the presence of cancer unlikely.

Currently, the use of PSA testing to screen men for prostate cancer is variable (see Evidence-Based Practice box: Prostate Cancer Screening).

CT Scan

If microscopic hematuria is present and the patient is younger than 50 years of age, obtain a CT scan with and without contrast. If stones are suspected a non-contrast CT scan is the gold standard. Uric acid and cysteine stones are not visualized by radiograph (see Chapter 40).

Ultrasonography

Ultrasonography is noninvasive and provides information on the kidneys, ureters, bladder, vascular structures, prostate, testicles, and post-void residual. Renal ultrasound is a good first test to determine kidney size and contour and the presence of calculi. A urinary bladder sonogram is used to identify tumors of the bladder, thickening of the bladder wall, posterior masses behind the bladder, and obstruction of the lower urinary tract evidenced by residual urine. A scrotal sonogram is used to evaluate chronic scrotal swelling; it can be used to identify abscess, infected testes, tumor, hydrocele, spermatocele, adherent scrotal hernia, and chronic epididymitis. However, because it does not assess perfusion, it is less helpful in the initial examination of an acute condition of the scrotum. A Doppler blood flow imaging examination is more appropriate. Transrectal prostate ultrasound imaging can be used to evaluate the prostate for tumors or nodules and to determine the volume of the prostate. It is also useful in diagnosing prostatitis, benign prostatic hyperplasia, and cancer of the prostate.

▌EVIDENCE-BASED PRACTICE *Prostate Cancer Screening*

Evidence about mortality outcomes from prostate cancer screening varies. Results from a large-scale randomized clinical trial on prostate-cancer mortality showed no difference in mortality rates from prostate cancer between the screening group and the usual care group (Andriole et al, 2009). The mortality rate from prostate cancer was low in both groups. Screening provided no reduction in death rates at 7 years, and no indication of a benefit appeared with 67% of the participants having completed 10 years of follow-up. Extended follow-up over a median of 15 years continued to indicate no reduction in prostate cancer mortality for the screening arm, showing no benefit of organized screening versus opportunistic screening (Pinsky et al, 2017).

However, a European study (Schröder et al, 2009) reports contrary evidence. The study is a combination of seven European trials with different screening protocols and different ages of entry. The study demonstrated that the relative risk of death from prostate cancer was reduced by 20% in men aged 55 to 69 years who underwent serial prostate-specific antigen (PSA) screening. The absolute risk difference was 0.71 deaths per 1000 men. This means that 1410 men would need to be screened and 48 additional cases of prostate cancer would need to be treated to prevent one death from prostate cancer.

Conclusion: The decision to engage in prostate cancer screening is complex. Based on the evidence of the benefits and harms of the service and an assessment of the balance, the US Preventive Services Task Force (USP-STF, 2012) recommends against (D grade) routine PSA-based screening. Authorities agree that a PSA test or screening should not be done unless the individual being screened understands the uncertainties, risks, and potential benefits of prostate cancer screening and makes a personal decision that even a small possibility of benefit outweighs the known risk of harms. Most authorities agree that prostate cancer screening should include prostate examination and PSA testing.

References: Andriole G, et al, 2009. Pinsky et al, 2017; Schröder et al, 2009; and USPSTF, 2012.

Computed Tomography

Noncontrast helical (spiral) computed tomography (CT) is the gold standard for evaluating kidney stones. It has 95% sensitivity and 98% specificity.

Doppler Flow Studies

Doppler blood flow studies are used to measure blood flow to the scrotal structures. Color Doppler provides a color image depicting the direction of the flow and the velocity in shades of blue and red. It is useful in the differential diagnosis of testicular torsion and epididymitis. Doppler of testicular torsion demonstrates reduced or absent blood flow, and epididymitis will show blood flow.

Biopsy

Biopsy of the prostate is necessary for definitive diagnosis of cancer. Guided biopsy is performed using transrectal ultrasound.

DIFFERENTIAL DIAGNOSIS

Cystitis and Urethritis

Patients may have inflammation limited to the penile segment of the urethra. The history would include meatal burning and discharge. Classic symptoms are frequency, urgency, and dysuria. Nocturia with suprapubic or low back pain is common.

Screening can be done in most settings with urine dip strips. A positive leukocyte esterase and nitrate test indicates infection. Urine culture and sensitivity confirms diagnosis and identifies the causative organism(s). Urinalysis with microscopic examination can determine if 20 or more organisms/HPF are present, which is indicative of UTI. Less than 20 organisms/HPF merits further study, such as culture and sensitivity. Colonization has taken place if 103 or more organisms/mL are present in the culture.

Pyelonephritis

The patient with pyelonephritis has fever and chills, appears toxic, and reports back pain. Nausea and vomiting may be present. Some patients also report lower urinary tract symptoms, including frequency and dysuria. The patient feels and looks ill. On physical examination, CVA tenderness is usually present. The abdomen may also be tender. On microscopic examination, WBCs are usually present. White cell casts suggest pyelonephritis. Bacterial casts, although rare, are pathognomonic of pyelonephritis. Urine culture and sensitivity confirm the diagnosis and identify the pathogen, which is usually *E. coli, Klebsiella* spp., *Proteus mirabilis,* or *Enterobacter* spp.

Urolithiasis

Urinary stones can occur anywhere in the urinary tract and may produce symptoms of pain, hematuria, and secondary infection. Many calculi are "silent" and may only cause hematuria, either microscopic or gross. Renal calculi may occur when a stone obstructs the urinary tract. Typical symptoms of renal colic include severe flank pain that radiates along the pathway of the ureter to the scrotum or inner thigh. Chills, fever, and urinary frequency are common. The patient may have nausea, vomiting, and abdominal distention. There may be a history of hematuria. Painful hematuria is characteristic of a stone, and the pain is described as colicky. Evaluate if the hematuria occurs at the time of urine initiation, at termination of micturition, or throughout micturition. This may be helpful in localizing the stone.

The clinical diagnosis is supported by urinalysis and imaging findings. The urine test results may be normal; gross or microscopic hematuria is common. Pyuria (WBCs) with or without bacteria may be present. Crystalline structures might be present. Noncontrast helical (spiral) CT is the gold standard for evaluating kidney stones.

Acute Bacterial Prostatitis

The patient with acute prostatitis is obviously ill and presents with chills, high fever, urinary frequency and urgency, perineal pain, and low back pain. The patient may exhibit varying degrees of obstructive symptoms, dysuria or burning, nocturia, hematuria, arthralgia, and myalgia. On examination, the prostate gland is tender, swollen, indurated, and warm. Do not massage the gland because bacteremia can result from the expression of microorganisms. Urine or prostate secretion culture can confirm the diagnosis. The most common causative organism is *E. coli*. Other common organisms include species of *Klebsiella* spp., *Enterobacter* spp., and *Proteus* spp. (See Box 18.1 for the classification of prostatitis.)

Chronic Bacterial Prostatitis

Chronic prostatitis is a common cause of recurrent cystitis. The patient may present with recurrent UTIs. Chronic bacterial prostatitis is caused by the same pathogens seen in acute prostatitis. Patients may be asymptomatic. Common symptoms, if evident, include low back pain and perineal discomfort, urinary frequency, and painful urination. Traditionally, symptoms are present for at least 3 months for a diagnosis of chronic prostatitis. Infection can involve the scrotal contents, producing epididymitis. Palpation of the prostate may reveal no specific findings. It may be moderately tender and irregularly indurated or boggy. Copious secretion may be present. Diagnosis is made on the basis of clinical symptoms and by culture of prostatic secretion or positive bacteria culture from postmassage urine. WBCs will be present in EPSs and VB 3.

Chronic Prostatitis/Chronic Pelvic Pain Syndrome

The diagnostic criterion for chronic prostatitis/chronic pelvic pain syndrome (CPPS) is persistent or recurrent symptoms that that have been present for at least 3 of the preceding 6 months, with no other urogenital pathology. The four main symptom categories are urogenital pain, lower urinary tract symptoms (e.g., dysuria, urgency, frequency, with or without obstructive voiding symptoms), psychological issues, and sexual dysfunction. Inflammatory CPPS is characterized by the absence of bacteria and the presence of WBCs in the semen, EPS, or VB 3. This category was previously called nonbacterial prostatitis. Noninflammatory CPPS is characterized by the absence of both bacteria and WBCs in the semen, EPS, or VB 3. This condition was formerly called prostadynia.

The prostate may feel normal on clinical examination.

Asymptomatic Inflammatory Prostatitis

This condition is diagnosed in patients during the evaluation of another genitourinary (GU) problem, such as benign prostatic hypertrophy. These patients do not experience GU pain. WBCs are found in the expressed prostatic secretions.

Epididymitis and Orchitis

The patient with epididymitis or orchitis is usually a sexually active young patient, and pain is the likely presenting symptom. The patient may be febrile. The history usually indicates a slow onset of discomfort over hours or days compared with testicular torsion, which has a rapid onset of symptoms. Elevation of the affected testicle may reduce the discomfort. Swelling of the scrotum and testicle may be present. Palpable swelling of the epididymis is usually present. Doppler flow studies with color can locate hot spots and identify intact blood flow. Urethral discharge or an intraurethral swab specimen should be Gram stained for a diagnosis of urethritis. DNA testing using either a urethral specimen or first-void urine should be performed to test for *N. gonorrhoeae* and *C. trachomatis*.

Testicular Torsion

The patient with testicular torsion is usually an adolescent with previous episodes of testicular pain. The history indicates a rapid onset of acute pain. Nausea and vomiting may have occurred or be present. Doppler blood flow studies may support the diagnosis by identifying lack of blood flow to the affected testicle. This is an emergent condition, and intervention must take place within the first 4 to 6 hours to salvage the testicle from infarction.

Hydrocele, Spermatocele, and Varicocele

A hydrocele is a nontender firm mass in the scrotum that results from fluid accumulation. It will transilluminate but may make testicular palpation difficult. A spermatocele (a cystic swelling on the epididymis) is not as large as a hydrocele but does not transilluminate. A varicocele occurs from dilated veins in the scrotal sac and usually occurs on the left side. A varicocele is often more prominent when the patient is standing and regresses with the patient in the prone position. It is classically described as a "bag of worms."

Benign Prostatic Hyperplasia

Prostatic hypertrophy is common after age 50 years. Presenting symptoms include lower urinary tract symptoms (LUTS), including hesitancy, slow urine stream, dribbling, and nocturia. DRE reveals an enlarged prostate with a reduced or obliterated median sulcus. Induration or firmness is characteristic of early prostate disease, and a hard stony gland suggests advanced prostatic carcinoma. The gland may feel soft because of inflammation or infection. The AUA Symptom Index (Table 18.1) is useful in determining treatment options based on the severity of symptoms, ranging from mild to severe. DREs combined with PSA testing are recommended to differentiate between BPH and prostate cancer.

Prostate Cancer

Patients with prostate cancer often present with the same obstructive symptoms as BPH, but they may also be asymptomatic. Patients who report lower abdominal pain may have an extension of the cancer with metastasis. On examination, the prostate is stony hard and protrudes into the colon. PSA levels may be elevated, and TRUS indicates enlargement or nodules. An abnormal DRE or an elevated PSA level necessitates further evaluation to determine or rule out prostate cancer (see Evidence Based Practice box: Prostate Cancer Screening).

Bladder or Kidney Tumor

Silent hematuria in older patients is often a late-presenting indication of cancer. It is more common in men than women. Patients often have a history of smoking or alcohol abuse.

Perineal Compression Syndrome

Compression of the pudendal nerve in long-distance cyclists can result in genital numbness without pain. An ill-fitting bicycle seat may contribute to the problem.

> **DIFFERENTIAL DIAGNOSIS OF** *Common Causes of Genitourinary Problems in Patients with Male Genitalia*

CONDITION	HISTORY	PHYSICAL FINDINGS	DIAGNOSTIC STUDIES
Cystitis or urethritis	Frequency, urgency, dysuria; nocturia with low back pain	Discharge may be present; may have suprapubic tenderness	Urine dipstick: positive leukocyte esterase; hematuria; urinalysis with microscopic examination; segmented urine collection; Gram stain; C&S; urine molecular test
Pyelonephritis	Fever, chills, back pain, nausea and vomiting, toxic appearance; some patients also have frequency and dysuria	Feels and looks ill; temperature >101°F; CVA tenderness; abdomen may be tender	Microscopic examination: WBCs may have white cell casts or bacterial casts; urine C&S; blood cultures
Urolithiasis	Pain, hematuria; may have symptoms of secondary infection; renal colic; pain that radiates to inner thigh; nausea, vomiting	May have CVA tenderness; looks ill during periods of acute pain; may have abdominal distention	Urinalysis: gross or microscopic hematuria; WBCs with or without bacteria; crystalline structures may be present; radiographu or ultrasonography

Continued

> **DIFFERENTIAL DIAGNOSIS OF** *Common Causes of Genitourinary Problems in Patients with Male Genitalia—cont'd*

CONDITION	HISTORY	PHYSICAL FINDINGS	DIAGNOSTIC STUDIES
Acute bacterial prostatitis	Chills, high fever, urinary frequency; urgency; perineal pain and low back pain; varying degrees of obstructive symptoms, dysuria or burning, nocturia, hematuria, arthralgia, and myalgia	Temperature >101°F; prostate gland tender, swollen, indurated, warm; do not massage as can cause bacteremia	Urinalysis; urine culture; prostate secretion culture; molecular test
Chronic bacterial prostatitis	Common cause of recurrent cystitis; same pathogen as in prostate secretion; may be asymptomatic; commonly have low back pain and perineal pain, urinary frequency, and painful urination	Infection can involve scrotal contents, producing epididymitis; palpation of prostate reveals no specific findings; may be moderately tender and irregularly indurated or boggy; may have copious secretion	Culture prostatic secretion; culture postmassage urine; WBCs present in EPS and VB 3
Chronic prostatitis/chronic pelvic pain syndrome (CPPS); can be inflammatory or noninflammatory	Persistent or recurrent symptoms present for at least 3 of preceding 6 mo, with no other urogenital cause; the four main symptom categories are urogenital pain, lower urinary tract symptoms (e.g., dysuria, urgency, frequency, with or without obstructive voiding symptoms), psychological issues and sexual dysfunction, and pelvic pain	Normal prostate examination	Inflammatory: absence of bacteria and presence of WBCs in semen, EPS, or VB 3 Noninflammatory: absence of both bacteria and WBCs in semen, EPS, or VB 3
Asymptomatic inflammatory prostatitis	Symptoms of another genitourinary problem; no pain	Specific for another genitourinary disorder	WBCs found in expressed prostatic secretions
Epididymitis or orchitis	Abrupt onset over several hours; febrile; pain in scrotum or testicles	Tender, swollen epididymitis or testicles; elevation of affected testicle may lessen discomfort (+ Prehn sign); may have fever	Doppler blood flow studies with color

> **DIFFERENTIAL DIAGNOSIS OF** *Common Causes of Genitourinary Problems in Patients with Male Genitalia—cont'd*

CONDITION	HISTORY	PHYSICAL FINDINGS	DIAGNOSTIC STUDIES
Testicular torsion	Sudden onset of testicular pain that radiates to groin; may also have lower abdominal pain	Exquisitely tender testicle; testicle may ride high because of shortened spermatic cord; cremasteric reflex absent; elevation of affected testicle does not relieve pain (negative Prehn sign)	Scrotal ultrasonography; this is a surgical emergency
Hydrocele, spermatocele, varicocele	Swelling or mass in the scrotum	Hydrocele: nontender fluid accumulation that transilluminates Spermatocele: cystic swelling on the epididymis, does not transilluminate Varicocele: "bag of worms" in the scrotum, often on left side, more prominent in standing position	Usually diagnosed by clinical examination; ultrasound may be used
Benign prostatic hyperplasia	Hesitancy, slow urine stream, dribbling, nocturia	Prostate protrusion into rectum; median sulcus reduced; prostate boggy	TRUS; PSA
Prostate cancer	Hesitancy, slow urine stream, dribbling, nocturia; low back pain; may be asymptomatic	Prostate protrusion into rectum; prostate hard	TRUS; PSA; biopsy
Bladder or kidney tumor	Patients often have history of smoking or alcohol abuse	Usually no signs other than silent hematuria	U/A: hematuria
Perineal compression syndrome	Genital numbness without pain; increase in training, miles, change in bicycle equipment	Usually no visible signs	Rule out cauda equina syndrome or other neuropathy; refrain from biking for 3 weeks, refit bike saddle

C&S, culture & sensitivity; *CVA,* costovertebral angle; *EPS,* expressed prostatic secretion; *NAAT,* nucleic acid amplification test; *PSA,* prostate-specific antigen; *TRUS,* transrectal ultrasound; *U/A,* urinalysis; *VB 3,* voided bladder specimen 3; *WBC,* white blood cell.

Headache

Headache is a subjective feeling of pain caused by a variety of intracranial and extracranial factors. It is one of the most common complaints in adults and children, with most headaches being self-treated using an over-the-counter (OTC) analgesic. Most headaches are acute and self-limited and are not life threatening. One in 10 people will have a migraine, and fewer than 1% of headaches are caused by serious intracranial disease. The goals for the practitioner in evaluating a headache are to:

- Identify life-threatening causes of headache.
- Diagnose treatable disease associated with some headaches.
- Provide symptom relief.

To accomplish these goals, the practitioner needs to conduct a careful history and physical examination even though physical findings will be normal for the majority of patients who report a headache.

Pain from headache arises from stimulation of pain-sensitive structures of the head and brain caused by traction, inflammation, vascular dilation, muscle contraction, or dysregulation of ascending brainstem serotonergic systems (Fig. 19.1). Headaches can be categorized as primary or secondary. Primary headaches are characterized by the absence of structural pathology or systemic disease; they account for more than 90% of all headaches. Secondary headaches are attributed to an underlying disorder. Primary headaches are of four major types: migraine, tension-type headache (TTH), cluster headache or other trigeminal autonomic cephalalgias, and other primary headaches. Generally, pain arising from disordered function, damage, or inflammation of structures located anterior to, and above, the tentorium (the fold of dura mater separating the cerebellum from the cerebrum) is felt in the front of the head, but pain felt in the back of the head arises from structures located below the tentorium. Extracranial structures that are sensitive to pain include the skin, scalp, blood vessels, facial muscles, eyes, ears, teeth, nasal cavity, mucous membranes of the mouth and pharynx, and the temporomandibular joint (TMJ). Brain tissue itself is not sensitive to pain, but sensitive structures of the brain include the blood vessels, sensory nerves, and ganglia.

Cranial structures project pain to the surface close to the source of pain. Pain from extracranial structures is usually felt in the immediate region affected (Fig. 19.2). The head is innervated extensively from the first branch of the trigeminal nerve (cranial nerve [CN] V). It has significant anatomical connections to the upper cervical roots C1 to C3, which supply the posterior fossa and neck structures.

Headache has been divided by symptomatology into types using the diagnostic criteria revised in 2013 by the Headache Classification Committee of the International Headache Society (https://www.ichd-3.org).

Of the types classified, only a few are common (Box 19.1). Headaches can also be categorized into acute (new onset), subacute, or chronic. Acute headaches warrant close attention. The headache associated with subarachnoid hemorrhage (SAH) has an intense sudden onset. Subacute headaches are localized headaches preceding neurologic findings, often caused by a vascular disorder or a space-occupying lesion. Headaches of greatest concern to clinicians are those that are persistent, severe, sudden in onset, and different from the patient's usual headache. The major clue to assessment of chronic headache is a change in the usual pattern of occurrence. Clinicians can ask patients to keep a headache diary that

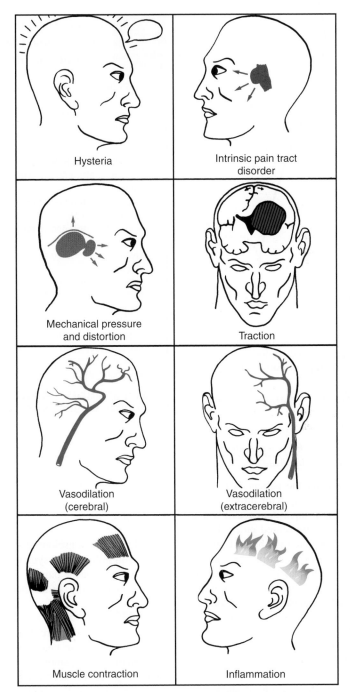

FIGURE 19.1 Mechanisms of cranial pain. (From Noble J: *Textbook of primary care medicine,* ed. 3, St. Louis, 2001, Mosby.)

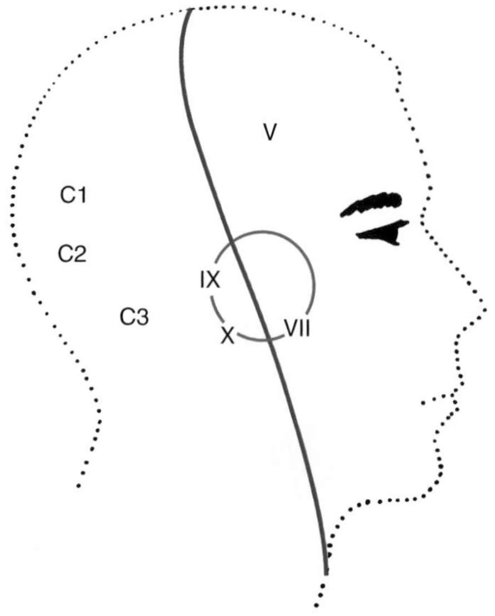

FIGURE 19.2 Sensory pathways for cranial pain.

includes notes on timing, frequency, and association with sleep, diet, emotional episodes, and other potential contributing factors.

DIAGNOSTIC REASONING: FOCUSED HISTORY

What clues indicate this is a potentially serious, life-threatening headache?

First assess whether the patient is fully oriented before proceeding with further history. The Mini-Cog is a three-item recall test for memory and a simple scored clock drawing that can be administered in about 10 minutes (https://www.alz.org/documents_custom/minicog.pdf). If the patient shows a mental status deficit, immediate evaluation with a head computed tomography (CT) scan and emergency treatment may be indicated.

Key Questions
• How did the headache begin?
• What is your age?
• Have you had this type of headache before?
• On a scale from 0 (no pain) to 10 (worst pain ever), how severe is the pain?
• Do you have a history of recent trauma to the head?

Box 19.1 First Level of the International Classification of Headache Disorders

PRIMARY HEADACHES
1. Migraine
2. Tension-type headache
3. Trigeminal autonomic encephalalgias
4. Other primary headaches

SECONDARY HEADACHES
1. Headache attributed to head or neck trauma
2. Headache attributed to cranial or cervical vascular disorder
3. Headache attributed to nonvascular intracranial disorder
4. Headache attributed to substance or its withdrawal
5. Headache attributed to infection
6. Headache attributed to disorder of homeostasis
7. Headache or facial pain attributed to disorder of cranium, neck, eyes, ears, nose, sinuses, teeth, mouth, or other facial or cranial structures
8. Headache attributed to psychiatric disorder

CRANIAL NEURALGIAS, CENTRAL AND PRIMARY FACIAL PAIN, AND OTHER HEADACHES
1. Painful cranial neuralgias and other facial pains
2. Other headache disorders

Data from the Headache Classification Committee of the International Headache Society: The International Classification of Headache Disorders, ed. 3, *Cephalalgia* 33:629-808, 2013.

• Did you lose consciousness?
• Do you notice other symptoms associated with the headache pain?
• Do you have any chronic health problems?

Onset and Severity

Sudden onset of a severe headache, without a history of chronic headache and with altered mental status, suggests an intracerebral hemorrhage (ICH) secondary to a ruptured aneurysm or vascular anomaly. Severity of headache is a very subjective measure and can sometimes be difficult to interpret. Headache of an ICH without a history of trauma is rare in children and adolescents, but the prevalence increases with age, especially in people older than 50 years with a history of uncontrolled hypertension or those being treated with anticoagulation therapy.

Onset of sudden severe headache with neurologic signs is an emergency; the patient needs immediate emergency treatment.

Subarachnoid hemorrhage is often precipitated by physical activity and is described as the "worst headache ever." Patients also report a stiff neck and may have a transient loss of consciousness, nausea and vomiting, photophobia, pupillary dilation, and seizure. Some patients, who have a leaking aneurysm, may report a headache for several days which will subsequently worsen with neurologic findings.

If SAH is suspected, the patient needs transport to an emergency center for a CT scan and possible surgical intervention because early diagnosis and treatment improve prognosis.

History of Trauma

Trauma to the head may cause subdural or epidural bleeding. Falls are a common cause of subdural bleeding in older adults. The patient may have a brief loss of consciousness followed by a period of lucidity that can last for minutes to days, with subsequent relapse and appearance of neurologic signs. In the older adults, especially after a fall, altered mental status may begin to manifest after 1 month. This delayed presentation results from the low-pressure leakage of blood from subdural veins. Epidural hematomas are more common in young adults and are often associated with skull fracture. The blood vessels that are ruptured in epidural bleeding are the middle meningeal artery or its dural branches. Because of the high arterial pressure, the mental status changes associated with epidural bleeds can be dramatic. A patient can go from a period of lucidity to a comatose state over a few hours.

Minor head trauma may result in headache because of soft tissue or extracranial injury. Pain is often localized to the site of injury and is self-limiting. Anyone who has experienced head trauma should be carefully observed for at least 24 hours for changing neurologic signs.

Associated Symptoms

The entry of infectious organisms, chemical agents, and drugs into the subarachnoid space causes inflammation of meningeal structures and associated blood vessels, resulting in a headache. Headache associated with infection presents with fever and possibly meningismus (stiff neck), which can indicate meningitis or encephalitis. Unilateral upper or lower extremity weakness with loss of manual dexterity is seen in children with hemiplegic migraine.

An ICH often presents as a sudden and severe "thunderclap" headache associated with confusion, vomiting, lethargy, and focal neurologic signs; it is caused by a ruptured vascular anomaly or an aneurysm. Drowsiness or confusion can be produced by increased intracranial pressure (ICP) secondary to meningitis or metabolic disorders.

Brain tumors in children, especially young children, are difficult to diagnose because of the child's inability to describe headache or diplopia until about 4 years of age. Signs are vague, and the developing skull in an infant may accommodate a pathological condition for some time. However, headache can be the initial manifestation of brain tumor if followed quickly by neurologic signs such as vomiting, recurrent morning headaches, reflex asymmetry, and papilledema.

Presence of Chronic Disease

Individuals with AIDS are at increased risk for cryptococcal meningitis, encephalitis, intracerebral abscess, and generalized sepsis. Patients being treated with anticoagulation therapy or older adults are at increased risk for headache from a serious cause such as an ICH or acute glaucoma.

Acute glaucoma caused by anticoagulation, a rare condition, may also occur with retinal detachment.

Headaches secondary to metabolic disorders can be the result of hyponatremia, hypercalcemia, uremia, hypoglycemia, and hypercapnia.

After determining that a headache is not serious, how can I narrow down the causes?

Key Questions

- What does it feel like?
- Where does it hurt?
- What makes it worse?
- How long have you had this headache?
- Can you tell when a headache is developing?

Characteristics of the Pain

A moderately intense, constant throbbing headache is associated with dilation of the cervical arteries. Severe pain associated with nausea, vomiting, and altered mental status indicates an expanding lesion such as a tumor, hematoma, edema, or enlargement of the ventricles secondary to hydrocephalus.

Migraine headache pain is caused by the production of various substances on dilated arteries that sensitize those arteries to pain. The patient usually has a high serum serotonin level early in the migraine headache. The pain is steady or throbbing and is usually limited to the same side. Migraine headaches are thought to result from an initial phase of intracranial or extracranial vasoconstriction followed by a longer interval of vasodilation. Frequently, the headache takes 3 to 4 hours to reach peak pain levels.

Cluster headaches (uncommon in children) are the result of an unknown vascular change that occurs within a period of 5 minutes. The serotonin level is unchanged in cluster headaches. The pain of cluster headaches is described as explosive and severe.

Tension (muscle contraction) headaches usually occur at school or work, generally when under a significant amount of pressure or stress, and often disappear on weekends and vacations and during periods of relaxation.

Location

Pain secondary to trauma or inflammation is perceived as near the site of insult such as the occipital area, nape of neck, bifrontal area, or generalized to the head. Noxious stimulation from any type of disease of the eye, ear, nose, or paranasal sinuses may spread to cause pain in the head.

Adults describe TTHs as a "hatband" distribution of pain; children describe a generalized headache or discomfort. Most patients describe a cluster headache as sudden severe pain beginning over one eye and spreading rapidly to the same side of the face.

Orbital pain is seen with increased intraocular pressure. Periorbital pain may be present with sinusitis, migraine, or trigeminal neuralgia, or it may be a sign of ocular disease. TMJ pain is located in the frontotemporal or temporal regions and may be unilateral or bilateral. Nonpulsatile headache in the occipital and paracervical regions is often caused by contraction of muscles of the head and neck.

Aggravating Factors

Triggers are present in many patients with migraine and include sound, odor, and estrogen fluctuations associated with the menstrual cycle. The most common food triggers are red wine, chocolate, and ripe cheese, which are foods high in tyramine or tryptophan. Migraine is usually worse with activity, but patients with TTHs are able to continue their usual routines. Stress can trigger any type of primary headache and must be considered a comorbid condition.

Duration

Most TTHs last less than 24 hours, a similar duration as migraine headaches. Cluster headaches usually last less than 3 hours and tend to occur in cycles. A subacute headache persists for days and weeks.

Aura and Prodrome

In migraine with aura, visual symptoms predominate and range from nonspecific blurring to scintillating scotomata with zigzag patterns, diplopia, and stars or flashes. Aura often precedes the onset or is simultaneous with headache. Prodromal symptoms include fatigue, depressed or euphoric mood, increased or decreased appetite, constipation or diarrhea, and yawning.

What does the chronicity of pain suggest?

Key Questions

- How often do you get a headache?
- Can you describe any pattern to the headache?

- How long does the headache last?
- Have you had this kind of headache before?
- Do you drink alcohol? Do you take any medications?

Frequency

A patient with a persistent headache for more than 3 months may demonstrate physical findings such as papilledema, bilateral or unilateral CN VI (abducens) palsies, gait or balance disturbances, or spasticity of the lower extremities. As a rule, in the absence of such symptoms, a recurrent headache of more than 3 months' duration is rarely related to structural or systemic findings. If a headache has been present continuously for more than 4 weeks, without accompanying neurologic signs or symptoms, it is most likely psychogenic in origin, especially if coupled with prolonged school or work absences, increased stress, and depression. This may be the case in a very small number of patients who present with complaints of headache.

Pattern and Duration of Headache

Headaches that occur throughout the day suggest a tension type. Sinus headaches occur after arising and worsen as the day progresses, especially when bending forward, and are less painful in the evening. Headaches associated with severe hypertension are not common and occur only with a diastolic blood pressure reading of 130 mm Hg or greater. These headaches are occipital, worse on arising, and lessen as the day progresses. Meningeal inflammation produces a pain that fluctuates throughout the day and night with no clear pattern. Migraine pain is episodic, occurring from several times a week to once a year. Cluster headache pain demonstrates a pattern of attacks that occur daily for several weeks with long periods of remission. The pain is short, often lasting less than 1 hour, but is intense.

Prior History of Headache

Headaches can be described as acute (new onset), subacute, or chronic. Acute-onset headaches must be evaluated for organic causes. Subacute and chronic headaches are usually caused by vascular inflammation or muscle tension. Chronic headaches are usually described as dull, bilateral, or bandlike. Chronic daily headaches may be mixed, produced by a combination of vascular and muscular causes.

Organic lesions may initially produce pain that is intermittent, but as the lesion progresses, the duration and frequency of the attack increase.

Psychogenic headache pain is daily, constant, diffuse, and difficult to describe.

Age of Patient at First Onset

The age of onset of migraines can be as early as 5 years old. Usually migraine headaches begin at ages 10 to 30 years. New onset of migraine headaches in adults older than age 50 years is unusual. Tension headaches have a usual first-onset age of 8 to 12 years. Cluster headaches have a usual first-onset age of 20 to 40 years.

 EVIDENCE-BASED PRACTICE *Association of Migraine Headache with Cardiovascular Disease*

A meta-analysis of studies and reviews published since 2009 was conducted to evaluate the association between migraine and cardiovascular disease, including stroke, myocardial infarction, and death caused by cardiovascular disease.

Migraine is associated with a twofold increase in risk of ischemic stroke only among people who have migraine with aura. There is a higher risk among women compared with men, and risk was further magnified for people with migraine who were younger than 45 years old, smokers, and women who used oral contraceptives. There was no association between a migraine and myocardial infarction or death caused by cardiovascular disease. Too few studies are available to reliably evaluate the impact of modifying factors such as migraine aura on these associations.

Reference: Schürks et al, 2009.

EVIDENCE-BASED PRACTICE *Prevalence of Headaches and Migraines in Children and Adolescents*

Migraine and headache are global disabling conditions causing impaired quality of life not only in adults but also in children and adolescents. This review covers epidemiological studies on migraine and headache in children and adolescents published in the past 25 years. A total of 64 cross-sectional studies were identified, published in 32 different countries. The estimated overall mean prevalence of headache was 54.4% (95% confidence interval [CI], 43.1–65.8), and the overall mean prevalence of migraine was 9.1% (95% CI, 7.1–11.1).

Reference: Wöber-Bingöl, 2013.

Lifestyle Habits and Medications

Alcohol is an important trigger for migraine and cluster headaches, although it may relieve a TTH. Smoking and secondhand smoke exposure can trigger headaches. Headaches may be a side effect of medications the patient is taking.

What other symptoms does the patient have?

Key Questions
- Do you have any nausea or vomiting?
- Do you notice any vision changes?
- Does light bother you?
- Are you dizzy?

Nausea and Vomiting

Whereas nausea and abdominal pain are more common in children with migraines, nausea and vomiting are more common in adults. Vomiting can be a sign of increased ICP. Headaches from tumors in the midline, cerebellar, and ventricular areas of the cranium obstruct the normal flow of the cerebrospinal fluid (CSF), producing hydrocephalus, headache, and early morning vomiting that usually occurs without nausea.

Vision Changes

Migraine headaches may have an aura that precedes them. A frequently reported visual aura is a scintillating scotoma, or twinkling spots of brightly colored lights. In children, visual scintillation is the most common aura of migraine and often limited to one eye.

Cluster headaches are associated with ipsilateral conjunctival injection, lacrimation, and edema of the eyelid.

Photophobia

Photophobia is often present with migraine headaches but is not present with tension headaches. Patients with meningitis often report photophobia.

Dizziness

Approximately one-third of patients with migraine headaches experience vertigo. The vertigo may appear as an aura, occur during the headache, or occur separately. A young child with vertigo may appear startled or have sudden ataxia.

What do the alleviating and aggravating factors suggest?

Key Questions
- Does anything make the headache better?
- Does anything make the headache worse?

Alleviating Factors

Patients with meningeal irritation obtain partial relief from being recumbent and lying quietly. Headaches that respond to mild analgesics are more likely to be tension headaches. Children obtain complete relief after a brief period of rest with a migraine headache, although rest does not affect a tension headache in children. Some adults experience migraine headache relief with sleep or rest, particularly in a dark, quiet environment.

Aggravating Factors

Increased headache with sneezing or coughing may indicate a benign headache, or it may be caused by a lesion at the level of the foramen magnum long before clinical signs are present. Migraine headaches are made worse with exertion. Patients with cluster headaches have worse pain when lying down. Headaches that are much worse in the early morning and improve on arising may indicate a tumor. Benign exertional headaches can occur during coitus. Trigeminal neuralgia pain can be triggered by stimulation of the affected nerve, produced by rubbing the face or chewing.

What does family history indicate?

Key Questions

- Does anyone else in the family have headaches?

Family History

Tension-type headaches have no family history. Migraines have a positive family history.

Is there anything else that would help narrow the cause or causes?

Key Questions

- Have you been ill recently?
- Are you taking any medications or vitamins?
- Could you have been exposed to carbon monoxide (CO)?
- Do you have working CO and smoke alarms in your home?

Recent Health History

Any substance introduced iatrogenically into the ventricular and lumbar fluid spaces can lead to chemical meningitis. Radiographic contrast media, antibiotics, and steroids can cause headache. Lumbar puncture (LP) can cause a severe headache in 25% of patients. A recent history of epidural anesthesia during childbirth or other epidural injections is also associated with headaches. The headache is eased by lying down and aggravated by sitting or standing. Chronic infection, including otitis media, mastoiditis, sinusitis, dental or pulmonary infection, cardiovascular lesions with shunting, or endocarditis, predisposes to development of a brain abscess. Half of all brain abscesses occur in children with cyanotic congenital heart disease. Penetrating skull fractures can also be a portal of entry for bacteria and contribute to the occurrence of brain abscess. Melanomas may metastasize years after excision and may first be indicated by neurologic changes.

History of Medications

Outdated tetracycline use can cause pseudotumor cerebri (increased ICP without an intracranial mass or hydrocephalus), as can an excessive intake of vitamin A and substances found in some topical acne preparations. Oral contraceptives and overuse of over-the-counter analgesics can cause headache. N-Methyl-D-aspartic acid or N-methyl-D-aspartate (NMDA) receptor antagonist drugs (i.e., memantine, amantadine, phencyclidine [PCP]), used to treat confusion in Alzheimer disease, as an anesthesia, and for the dissociative anesthesia or euphoriant properties as a recreational drug, can cause headaches.

Withdrawal from certain substances, such as caffeine or nitrates, can also produce headache.

Exposures

Carbon monoxide is a tasteless and odorless gas that contributes to many deaths each year.

Exposure to CO may cause a severe, throbbing, generalized headache. Hemoglobin values less than 10 g/dL may cause headache as a result of hypoxia. Home furnaces, hot water heaters, or gas dryers may cause CO exposure because of the incomplete breakdown of fossil fuel that does not have enough oxygen to produce carbon dioxide. Poor ventilation is usually the cause.

Assess occupational exposure to other toxins through an occupational history. A faulty kerosene or gas heater may cause headaches that occur during winter months.

DIAGNOSTIC REASONING: FOCUSED PHYSICAL EXAMINATION

Observe the Patient

Assess level of alertness and orientation to person, place, and time. Any patient who reports headache and exhibits an ataxic gait, uncoordinated movements, or reduced mental alertness should be immediately transported to an emergency center for neurologic evaluation.

A patient who appears ill or toxic is a suspect for meningitis. The patient is usually lying down with the lights off (photophobia) and may report chills. Most toddlers cannot communicate the characteristics of a headache but instead become irritable and cranky and rub their eyes and head.

Muscle spasm may cause tilting of the head or lifting of the shoulder when there is a posterior fossa tumor, cervical spine disease, or whiplash injury. Ptosis of the eyelid may accompany a cluster headache or brain tumor. Blinking and squinting of the eyes indicate photophobia.

Take Vital Signs and Obtain Growth Parameters

Take temperature, blood pressure, and pulse measurements. Fever may be the only sign of infection. Bradycardia and narrowing of pulse pressure are signs of increased ICP. In children, if the plotted height and weight chart is significantly below average, consider a hypothalamic neoplasm. Plot head circumference to assess for normal skull growth. Macrocephaly may indicate hydrocephalus or a brain tumor.

Palpate and Percuss the Skull

Palpate for symmetry of contour, tenderness, and lesions on the scalp, face, and neck. Palpate the temporal arteries for quality of pulse and tenderness. Focal tenderness and induration are seen in TTHs. Tenderness over nodular temporal arteries is a sign of temporal arteritis.

Brain abscesses cause pain by localized traction and produce tenderness on skull percussion over the area involved.

Auscultate the Cranium

Intracranial arteriovenous malformations may mimic migraine. Auscultate the orbit and skull to evaluate for cranial bruits.

Inspect the Ears, Eyes, Nose, Mouth, and Temporomandibular Joint

A thorough examination of the face, head, and neck structures is needed to detect organic disease. Examine the ears for signs of infection.

Anisocoria is when right and left pupils are not equal. It can be benign but is associated with eye infection or injury or increased intracranial pressure. Ipsilateral lacrimation, ptosis, and pupillary constriction are seen with cluster headache. Test extraocular movement (EOM) in all fields of gaze. If a patient cannot look completely to the right or the left (lateral gaze), suspect a CN VI palsy, possibly the result of increased ICP. If EOMs are painful, consider optic neuritis.

Observe nasal mucosa for redness and swelling. Rhinorrhea and congestion are seen with sinus headaches. Observe teeth and oral mucosa because upper molar disease and poor dentition can cause headache. Tapping on the teeth or biting down on a tongue blade can elicit pain from sinusitis.

Temporomandibular joint instability can cause headache pain. See Chapter 15 for a discussion of examination techniques.

Enlarged pupils seen during a headache indicate migraine; however, if they outlast a headache, then organic disease should be suspected.

Upper motor neuron facial weakness may be present in hemiplegic migraine.

Perform Ophthalmoscopy

On ophthalmoscopic examination, note contour of the optic disc and clarity of margins. Note the disc for papilledema and inspect vasculature for hemorrhage or exudate, venous pulsations, and arterial spasm.

Papilledema is often caused by an expanding intracranial mass and increased ICP. Optic disc atrophy suggests a chronically increased ICP or a lesion in the optic chiasm.

Meningitis does not produce fundus changes. Retinal hemorrhage in children may indicate abuse.

Assess Cranial Nerve Function

A complete assessment of CN function may provide evidence for more serious causes of headaches secondary to inflammation, traction, or metabolic imbalance.

- *CN I:* Assess for smell. The sense of smell may be lost when the olfactory nerve is damaged by head injury or by a tumor in the vicinity of the olfactory groove. Herpes simplex encephalitis can lead to a destruction of the olfactory cortex or olfactory nerve.

- *CN II:* Check visual acuity. Rarely does poor vision contribute to a headache. Poor vision may contribute to eye pain, but children equate this with headache. Double vision may be the presenting ocular symptom of increased ICP caused by a unilateral CN VI palsy or a posterior fossa lesion.
- *CNs III, IV, and VI:* Check visual fields. Headaches as a result of pituitary tumors are usually associated with defects in the peripheral vision. Unilateral or homonymous hemianopsia (a loss of the same half of the visual field of both eyes) can occur with migraines or brain tumor headaches when the tumor is in the occipital lobes or adjacent to the visual pathways. A half-field defect is seen with parietal lobe tumor. CN III palsy can cause an enlargement of the pupil from compression of the nerve by an expanding lesion. The dilated pupil is always on the side of the expanding lesion. CN VI palsy (inability to move eyes in a lateral direction) may be found with acute hydrocephalus or cerebral edema. Nystagmus suggests a brainstem or cerebellar lesion and is usually ipsilateral. Lateral gaze nystagmus is also present with an elevated blood alcohol level. Vertical and rotatory nystagmus suggests central posterior fossa abnormality.
- *CN V:* Test jaw strength, pain, and touch sensation to face. Trigeminal neuralgia pain can be triggered by stimulation of the affected nerve.
- *CN VII:* Ask the patient to frown, raise eyebrows, show teeth, close eyes against resistance, and puff out cheeks. Test taste on the anterior two thirds of the tongue for sweet and salt discrimination. Salivary and lacrimal glands are innervated by CN VII.
- *CN VIII:* Test hearing acuity. Unilateral deafness should be investigated to rule out acoustic neuroma.
- *CNs IX and X:* Observe swallowing and uvula rise.
- *CN XI:* Test trapezius strength and sternocleidomastoid strength against resistance.
- *CN XII:* Test tongue strength. An intracranial vascular event may cause a hemiplegia or hemiparesis that can be assessed by observing the protruded tongue drift laterally or by the inability to hold position against resistance.

Examine the Neck

Ask the patient to perform full range of motion (ROM) of the neck to observe for stiffness or difficulty with movement, which may indicate muscle tension or meningismus. If there is a history of trauma involved, the patient should only perform an active ROM examination. A passive ROM may worsen the acute injury, and the patient's neurologic function in the presence of a neck injury and should be avoided.

Test for Meningismus

Normally, the chin can be flexed passively to touch the chest. If neck stiffness (nuchal rigidity) is present, this maneuver is not possible. With the patient supine, attempts to flex the neck cause involuntary hip flexion, and the hips rise (Brudzinski sign). Attempts to extend the knee joint when the hip joint is flexed may cause the other limb to flex at the hip (Kernig sign).

Assess Motor Strength and Coordination of Extremities

Asymmetrical increase in muscle tone on the affected side, contralateral to the hemisphere lesion, suggests a cerebral lesion.

Patients who exhibit forearm drift with arms extended and eyes closed may have a motor neuron or cerebellar disturbance with an expanding intracranial lesion.

Test Balance and Gait

Midline cerebellar abnormalities cause marked ataxia. The patient has difficulty standing on the ipsilateral leg and has a tendency to fall or stumble toward the side of the lesion. The gait is also wide-based and halting, and the patient turns with jerky movements. Minimal disturbance is observed when the patient hops on either foot or stands tandem (one foot behind the other).

Assess Deep Tendon Reflexes

Note asymmetry, absence of reflexes, or hyperactive responses. Increase in, or asymmetry of, reflexes is seen with cerebral lesions. The plantar or Babinski response is often present with cerebral lesions.

Have Children Draw Pictures of Their Headaches

Having a child draw a headache is an inexpensive and accurate way to help diagnosis headaches. The child is given a plain piece of paper and asked to draw a picture of how his or her headache felt before any history of the headache is taken. These drawings help to diagnose migraine headaches. Drawings for migraines include visual images such as flashing. Showing the lights being turned off, a dark room, or a blanket over the head depicts photophobia. The need to lie down is also associated with migraine headache. Images for nonmigraine headaches show pictures of pounding or tight headbands. Even very young children (age 4 years) are able to draw stick figures with significant detail.

LABORATORY AND DIAGNOSTIC STUDIES

Complete Blood Count

A complete blood count with differential is obtained to detect major blood dyscrasias. Hypoxia secondary to severe anemia can cause headache. In bacterial meningitis the polymorphonuclear leukocytes will be high with a left shift.

Blood Cultures

Blood cultures should be drawn in a patient who has a fever, headache, nuchal rigidity, and altered mental status.

Computed Tomography Scan

Computed tomography scanning is a noninvasive diagnostic tool used to detect intracranial disease and should be done with sudden-onset severe headaches that occur every day or headache associated with abnormal neurologic signs.

Magnetic Resonance Imaging

A magnetic resonance image changes over time as red blood cells lyse and hemoglobin degrades. It is the first imaging choice for a brain abscess.

Lumbar Puncture

Lumbar puncture can measure CSF pressure directly and can be analyzed for normal values of components that are altered by disease such as lymphocytes, glucose, protein, and the presence of bacteria. An LP is performed when a central nervous system (CNS) infection is suspected but is contraindicated if there is suspicion of increased ICP.

Erythrocyte Sedimentation Rate

Erythrocyte sedimentation rate (ESR) is a nonspecific test that is elevated in the presence of inflammation. An ESR should be performed when temporal arteritis is suspected.

Skull Radiograph

A radiograph of the skull is useful in posttraumatic headache. Specific views must be obtained to better observe intracranial structures such as the pituitary gland or paranasal sinuses.

DIFFERENTIAL DIAGNOSIS

Primary Headaches

Tension-type headache (muscle)

Tension-type headache is the most common type of headache in adults and occurs most often in women. The exact mechanism of tension headache is uncertain but is related to sustained muscle contraction. Tension headache produces a bilateral pain, general or localized, often described as a frontotemporal bandlike distribution. The discomfort is described as a mild to moderate, nonthrobbing pain, tightness, or pressure with a gradual onset. It may last for hours or days, and recurrences may extend over weeks or months. It is associated with hunger, depression, or stress.

Migraine without aura (common)

About 20% of adults experience migraines, and episodes are not uncommon in children as young as 5 years old. The headache is unilateral and throbbing and most often accompanied by nausea, photophobia, and exacerbation from physical activity. The headache is usually frontal or periorbital. The onset is rapid, and crescendo is within hours. Migraines may recur daily, weekly, or less often. Migraine headaches are most commonly found in adults 25 to 34 years of age and are rare during pregnancy. Chronic migraine is present when attacks occur more than 15 days in a month.

Migraine with aura (classic)

Neurologic signs that indicate cortical or brainstem involvement precede classic migraine headaches. Bright lights, noise, or tension may precipitate headaches. Auras may include visual disturbances (e.g., scintillating scotoma: a pattern of twinkling colored lights), ascending paresthesias or numbness, weakness, and aphasia. The pain may be associated with photophobia, phonophobia (noise sensitivity), nausea, and vomiting. Aura usually precedes but may accompany a headache or occur without headache.

Mixed headache

Mixed headaches are a combination of muscular contraction and vascular dysfunction. The headache is experienced as a throbbing, constant pain during waking hours with symptoms of tightness, pressure, and muscle contraction. A family history of migraine is common.

Cluster headache

Cluster headaches are of vascular origin and are less common than migraines. The onset is abrupt, often during the night, and the severity increases steadily. The pain is unilateral, ocular, or periocular, and described as burning, piercing, or neuralgic. Cluster headaches occur more often in men and last 15 minutes to 2 hours. The episodic recurrences are "clustered" in cycles of days or weeks with remission lasting months to years. Associated symptoms include ipsilateral rhinorrhea, conjunctival injections, facial sweating, ptosis, and eyelid edema. Alcohol ingestion, stress, or vasodilation secondary to wind or heat exposure may precipitate the pain.

Benign exertional headache

These headaches occur suddenly and are related to coughing, sneezing, straining, running, or orgasm. Headache is the result of stretching the pain-sensitive structures in the posterior fossa. They are more common in men. The onset is sudden and "splitting" and pain may last from seconds up to 30 minutes. They should be distinguished from headache of SAH or arterial dissection.

Secondary Headaches

Infectious origin

Sinusitis

Sinusitis is frequently associated with a sore throat irritated by postnasal discharge, facial or tooth pain, or a headache over the affected sinus that increases in intensity with coughing or bending forward. There frequently are a cough that worsens in a lying position, morning periorbital swelling, fever, malaise, and recent upper respiratory tract infection. The maxillary sinuses are the most often affected. Whereas pain in the temporal and periorbital area suggests frontal sinusitis, maxillary sinusitis produces pain below the eye, in the upper teeth, or both. Ethmoid sinusitis produces medial orbit pain.

Dental Disorders

Patients with dental abscess, nerve root dysfunction, or infection may have headache and facial pain located near the site of the lesion. Tenderness elicited by tapping on the maxillary teeth with a tongue blade may indicate dental root infection or maxillary sinusitis. Inspection of the mouth may reveal ulceration or infection of pain-sensitive structures in the oral mucosa and gingiva.

Pharyngitis

Bacterial infection may irritate pain-sensitive structures in the oropharynx, leading to headache.

Otitis Media

Recurrent otitis media with sequelae of mastoiditis or chronic infection may result in headache. Signs of otitis will be seen on examination of the tympanic membrane.

Meningitis

Bacterial meningitis begins as bacteria colonize in the nasopharynx and enter the CNS through the dural venous sinuses or choroid plexus into the subarachnoid space. Common causal organisms in adults are *Staphylococcus pneumoniae* and *meningitidis*. In children, common organisms are *S. pneumoniae* and *Haemophilus influenzae*; in neonates, common organisms group B *Streptococcus* spp. and *Escherichia coli*. Bacterial meningitis is usually accompanied by severe systemic toxicity and mental status changes (encephalitis). In contrast, aseptic meningitis caused by enteroviruses or mumps virus produces a mild illness sometimes without fever. Photophobia and stiff neck are present in varying degrees. The person usually appears ill with a severe headache, fever, chills, myalgias, photophobia, and stiff neck. The Brudzinski and Kernig signs may be positive. A petechial skin rash may suggest meningeal disease. Patients may progress to coma and have seizures.

Neurogenic origin

Trigeminal Neuralgia

The pain associated with malfunction of the trigeminal nerve (CN V) is characterized by episodes of a series of bursts or jabs of sharp electrical, stabbing pain lasting seconds that occur repeatedly over minutes or hours with a minute or so of relief between episodes. The pain is limited to the distribution of the three branches of CN V. Headaches caused by trigeminal neuralgia are stimulated by sensory stimuli to the involved nerves, produced by rubbing or touching the face or swallowing. Trigeminal neuralgia usually occurs in women and individuals older than age 55 years. In younger patients, episodes may indicate multiple sclerosis.

Optic Neuritis

Optic neuritis refers to a variety of conditions that affect the optic nerve and reduce visual function. Disorders include demyelinating disease (e.g., multiple sclerosis), inflammation, viral illness, metabolic disorders, and toxin exposure. The patient has an acute onset of blurred vision with extraocular motion pain that precedes the visual changes by several days. Ophthalmoscopic examination reveals a slightly elevated (hyperemic) disc and a blurred disc margin. Treatment is focused on the underlying disease.

Cervical Spine Disorders

The three upper cervical nerves are sensory pathways for pain sensation felt in the posterior head and ipsilateral temporal and eye areas (see Fig. 19.2). Disturbances in the neck may cause muscle spasms and pressure on other neck structures. Patients with neck-related headache have pain associated with motion of the neck. Downward pressure on the head makes the pain worse and may cause it to travel down the arms.

Temporal Arteritis (Giant Cell Arteritis)

Temporal arteritis is a vasculitis of the ophthalmic and posterior ciliary branches of the internal carotid artery. It almost always affects people older than age 50 years. It produces a sharp, localized pain over a tender, nodular temporal artery. Other symptoms include fever, malaise, anorexia, weight loss, or polymyalgia rheumatica. Ischemic jaw pain and face pain are rare but highly suggestive. Headaches precede the major danger of temporal arteritis (blindness) by weeks. Unilateral blindness may occur suddenly and is not reversible. Left untreated, blindness may occur in the other eye. An ESR greater than 50 mm/hr is almost always present. Suspected temporal arteritis is an emergency, and the patient needs referral to an emergency center for immediate evaluation and treatment.

Metabolic origin

Carbon Monoxide Poisoning

Carbon monoxide is a colorless, odorless gas with an affinity for binding with hemoglobin to produce carboxyhemoglobin (COHb), which impairs oxygen transport. Symptoms are nonspecific and are dose related. Low

COHb levels may produce mild dyspnea and tightness across the head; however, as COHb concentration increases, the headache becomes more severe and is associated with dizziness, nausea, fatigue, and dimmed vision. As COHb levels rise, symptoms increase in severity and lead to loss of consciousness and seizures. Blood gases and COHb blood levels are diagnostic. History may suggest recent smoke inhalation or similar symptoms in multiple family members.

Severe Hypoglycemia

Hypoglycemia is more likely to occur in individuals with type 1 diabetes but can occur in anyone taking oral hypoglycemic agents, in younger people who experience reactive hypoglycemia, or in people who have ingested excessive amounts of alcohol. A dietary and medication history may lead to a specific causative factor. Headache is generalized and bilateral and is associated with dizziness and a sense of not feeling well. Some people with diabetes may have nocturnal hypoglycemia and report nightmares and vivid dreams, night sweats, and a headache on awakening. Blood glucose levels can confirm the presence of hypoglycemia.

Drug Withdrawal

Withdrawal from prolonged use of steroids may cause migraine headaches. Nitrites may precipitate headache. Other drugs causing cranial dilation and an aftereffect of rebound vasoconstriction include hydralazine, alcohol, histamine, nicotinic acid, and caffeine.

Dietary Ingestion

A mild to moderately severe generalized headache may occur after ingestion of tyramines (e.g., aged cheese, red wine), monosodium glutamate, and nitrites in smoked meats. A headache diary will help identify the pattern of headache related to specific foods.

Cerebrovascular origin

Intracranial Tumor

Primary intracranial tumors are more common in children than adults. Brain metastases from primary sites in the lung, breast, or kidney are more common in adults. Pain is constant and progressive, is felt in a discrete location, changes with head position, and awakens the person from sleep. Objective neurologic signs are present in 98% of all children with brain tumors.

Hydrocephalus

Hydrocephalus is an excessive collection of CSF in the ventricles of the brain and can be caused by tumors or cysts. If fontanels are still open, hydrocephalus will cause an enlargement of the head on measurement. Headache will be progressive and may be associated with neurologic findings and mental status changes similar to those observed with dementia. Radiographic techniques are diagnostic, and LP may detect increased CSF pressure.

Subdural Hematoma

Acute subdural hematoma produces a sudden, severe headache and may be associated with a history of head trauma, exertional physical activity, or pharmacologic anticoagulation. There is transient loss of consciousness, stiff neck, nausea, vomiting, photophobia, pupillary dilation, and pain over the eye. It is essential to obtain a thorough history of trauma. Posttrauma headache can occur hours or a day after injury.

Pseudotumor Cerebri

Teenagers being treated with topical acne preparations, menopausal women, and individuals ingesting large amounts of vitamin A are at increased risk for pain from pseudotumor cerebri. Papilledema will be present in many cases, but without it, the headache may be diagnosed as mixed type. A neurology referral is indicated to ensure that no local obstruction is present before an LP is done to assess for increased ICP. An LP sometimes leads to herniation of the brainstem.

Brain Abscess

Onset of pain can be gradual or severe, deep, and aching in nature, often worse in morning and aggravated by coughing or straining. Pain is usually localized to the side of the abscess. Other signs of increased ICP may be present, such as papilledema and widening pulse pressure. There may be a recent history of head injury, infections (e.g., dental abscess, otitis media, or sinusitis), or assault to the CNS.

Intracerebral Hemorrhage

Intracerebral hemorrhage may result in a stroke or sudden coma and is associated with neurologic findings defined by the site of bleeding. A person may present with a sudden-onset, severe headache, with or without a history of trauma. The severity of symptoms from bleeding intracranial aneurysms is correlated to the rate of hemorrhage and graded from I (asymptomatic to minimal headache with nuchal rigidity) to V (deep coma, decerebrate rigidity). Geriatric patients with AIDS and patients prescribed anticoagulation therapy are at increased risk for ICH. CT scan is diagnostic.

▶ DIFFERENTIAL DIAGNOSIS OF *Common Causes of Headache*

CONDITION	HISTORY	PHYSICAL FINDINGS	DIAGNOSTIC STUDIES
PRIMARY HEADACHES WITHOUT STRUCTURAL OR SYSTEMIC PATHOLOGY			
Tension-type headache (muscle)	Common in adults; bilateral pain, general or localized in bandlike distribution; history of anxiety, stress, or depression	Normal physical examination; neck muscle tightness or fasciculations may be palpated	None
Migraine without aura (common)	More common in children; unilateral, throbbing pain; nausea	Photophobia and phonophobia	None
Migraine with aura (classic)	Pain precipitated by environmental stimuli; visual disturbances (scintillating scotoma) precede pain	Nausea and vomiting, photophobia and phonophobia	None
Mixed headache	Throbbing, constant pain during waking hours; muscle tightness; family history of migraine	Mix of findings related to tension and migraine headache pain	None
Cluster headache	Rare in children; abrupt, nighttime onset; unilateral periorbital pain that is severe	Ipsilateral rhinorrhea, nasal stuffiness, conjunctival injection, sweating, ptosis	None
Benign exertional headache	Sudden onset related to physical exertion, Valsalva maneuver, or coitus	Normal physical examination	May need to distinguish from subarachnoid hemorrhage with CT scan
SECONDARY HEADACHES WITH STRUCTURAL OR SYSTEMIC PATHOLOGY			
INFECTIOUS ORIGIN			
Sinusitis	Frontal, upper molar, or periorbital pain; cough, rhinorrhea	Low to no fever; pain on palpation of frontal, maxillary sinuses; purulent nasal or postnasal discharge	Radiographs (Waters view)
Dental disorders	Localized pain in jaw and top of head	Malocclusion, caries, abscesses of teeth present, gum disease	Dental referral

DIFFERENTIAL DIAGNOSIS OF *Common Causes of Headache—cont'd*

CONDITION	HISTORY	PHYSICAL FINDINGS	DIAGNOSTIC STUDIES
Pharyngitis	Sore throat	Fever; infection of posterior pharynx	Throat culture
Otitis media	Ear pain, pain with swallowing	Fever; red, bulging tympanic membrane	None
Meningitis	Severe headache, chills, myalgias, stiff neck; toxic child or adult	Positive Kernig and Brudzinski signs; fever, photophobia, petechial rash may be present; mental status changes	Lumbar puncture
NEUROGENIC ORIGIN			
Trigeminal neuralgia	People older than 55 yr; bursts of sharp pain over face innervated by affected nerve; triggered by stimulus to affected nerve	Normal physical examination; stimulation of triggers may provoke pain	None
Optic neuritis	Acute onset of pain with OM followed by blurred vision	Diminished visual acuity, decreased papillary reflex, hyperemia of optic disc; pain with EOM	Ophthalmology referral
Cervical spine disorders	May have history of trauma; occipital pain, muscle stiffness	Normal physical examination findings or pain associated with neck motion	Cervical spine radiographs
Temporal arteritis	Age older than 50 yr; sharp, localized temporal pain; malaise, anorexia; history of polymyalgia rheumatica	Fever, weight loss; tender over a nodular temporal artery	Elevated ESR (>50); immediate referral for treatment
METABOLIC ORIGIN			
Carbon monoxide poisoning	History of exposure; throbbing headache, mild dyspnea	Nausea, vomiting, change in mental status, lethargy, loss of consciousness	Blood gases and carboxyhemoglobin level
Severe hypoglycemia	History of diabetes or medication, alcohol, and food ingestion; generalized headache, dizziness, sense of not feeling well	Normal physical examination findings or pallor, sweating, and weakness	Blood glucose level; may need self-monitoring of blood glucose to establish pattern
Drug withdrawal	Pattern of headache associated with stopping medication or substance use	Normal physical examination findings	Blood chemistry
Dietary ingestion	Mild to moderately severe headache after ingestion of foods or medication	Normal physical examination findings	Blood chemistry

Continued

▶ **DIFFERENTIAL DIAGNOSIS OF** *Common Causes of Headache—cont'd*

CONDITION	HISTORY	PHYSICAL FINDINGS	DIAGNOSTIC STUDIES
CEREBROVASCULAR ORIGIN			
Intracranial tumor	Sudden-onset headache that is progressive, exacerbated by coughing or exercise; worse in morning; history of trauma increases risk	Papilledema, vomiting, asymmetrical reflexes, weakness, sensory deficit, or other neurologic deficit	CT scan for adults, MRI for children preferred
Hydrocephalus	Progressive headache, vomiting, irritability	Rapid enlargement of head, bulging fontanels	CT scan and referral
Subdural hematoma	History of head trauma, bleeding disorders, child abuse; adult older than 35 yr; sudden onset of "worst headache ever," often over eye; transient loss of consciousness	Unequal pupils, photophobia, neurologic changes, seizure	CT scan and neurosurgical referral
Pseudotumor cerebri	Teens, menopausal women; history of vitamin A or tetracycline ingestion; progressive headache	Papilledema may be present	CT scan, neurology referral to assess risk related to lumbar puncture
Brain abscess	History of chronic ear infection or cyanotic heart disease	Fever, seizures, focal neurologic deficits	MRI
Intracerebral hemorrhage	Risk factors: people older than 50 yr, with AIDS, taking anticoagulation therapy, hypertension	If conscious, abnormal neurologic findings correlated with extent of lesion	Emergency transport for immediate evaluation (CT, MRI, and possible surgical treatment)

AIDS, acquired immune deficiency syndrome; *CT,* computed tomography; *EOM,* extraocular movement; *ESR,* erythrocyte sedimentation rate; *MRI,* magnetic resonance imaging.

Heartburn and Indigestion

Heartburn is a sensation of burning, warmth, or heat in the retrosternal area between the xiphoid and manubrium. In contrast, indigestion refers to pain or discomfort in the upper abdomen without radiation that occurs with eating or soon after a meal.

Patients describe heartburn using a variety of terms, including *indigestion, acid regurgitation, sour stomach,* and *bitter belching.* The burning sensation often begins inferiorly and radiates up the entire retrosternal area to the neck, occasionally to the back, and rarely into the arms. Heartburn can be a result of gastroesophageal acid reflux that occurs as a consequence of lower esophageal sphincter relaxation. Acid reflux may or may not cause tissue damage and erosions. In erosive reflux disease (erosive esophagitis or Barrett esophagus), mucosal breakdown allows refluxed acid to irritate local nociceptors. Not all reflux results in heartburn, and not all heartburn is caused by reflux. For example, heartburn can be a symptom of angina or myocardial infarction (MI). Heartburn is different from localized gastric or epigastric burning, which most likely represents dyspepsia.

Indigestion is commonly triggered by overeating; eating too fast; stress; excess alcohol; caffeine intake; and fatty, greasy, or spicy foods. Patients may report associated symptoms of postprandial fullness, upper abdominal bloating, early satiation, epigastric burning, belching, nausea, and vomiting. Indigestion that is chronic or recurrent is typically associated with dyspepsia. Indigestion that occurs with other symptoms such as chest pain and shortness of breath that suggest a cardiac origin; painful or difficult swallowing, unintentional weight loss, persistent vomiting, or gastrointestinal (GI) bleeding suggests serious upper GI conditions. Although heartburn and indigestion can be symptoms of distinct entities, they often co-occur in conditions such as gastroesophageal reflux disease (GERD), peptic ulcer disease (PUD), gastritis, and gastric cancer.

The immediate concern when patients present with heartburn or indigestion is to assess for symptoms that require immediate endoscopy.

DIAGNOSTIC REASONING: FOCUSED HISTORY

Is immediate endoscopy necessary?

Key Questions
- Do you have trouble swallowing? If yes, is it solids or liquids?
- Do you have pain with swallowing?
- Have you had unintentional weight loss?
- Do you have persistent vomiting?
- Have you had rectal bleeding, blood in your stool, or been told that you have anemia?

Alarm Symptoms

The symptoms of most concern are dysphagia, odynophagia, unintentional weight loss, persistent vomiting, GI bleeding, and unexplained anemia. These are symptoms for a serious condition and require immediate evaluation. These symptoms suggest either the presence of upper GI cancer, PUD, or the development of a GERD-related complication. Dysphagia suggests erosive or Barrett esophagus or gastric or esophageal cancer. Pain with swallowing suggests esophageal ulcer. Unintentional weight loss in the presence of dysphagia or odynophagia is suggestive of cancer. GI bleeding and anemia are suggestive of cancer or ulcer disease. Unexplained iron deficiency anemia indicates esophageal ulcer.

Mechanical obstruction of solid foods is suggestive of peptic stricture. Liquid obstruction suggests a neuromuscular disorder, neoplasm, or esophageal diverticulum.

Could this be cardiac in origin?

Key Questions
- Are the symptoms provoked by exertion or activity?
- Are the symptoms relieved by rest?
- Does the sensation radiate (e.g., to the left shoulder, down the arm, or to the neck or jaw)?
- Is there shortness of breath, nausea, vomiting, or diaphoresis?
- How long do the symptoms last?
- Does the patient have risk factors for cardiac disease (older age, smoker, hyperlipidemia, hypertension, diabetes, obesity, history of coronary artery disease [CAD], family history of CAD)?

Symptom Characteristics

Heartburn and indigestion can be symptoms of angina or MI. Pain arising from the GI and cardiac systems transmits to the same spinal cord segments, T1 through T5, and makes identification of the specific origin of discomfort difficult. Therefore, it is essential to determine if the symptoms are cardiac or GI in origin. The typical onset of angina occurs during exercise or exertion. Symptoms typically last 2 to 10 minutes and are relieved by rest or nitroglycerin. Symptoms from acute coronary insufficiency last no longer than 30 minutes. Anginal pain typically radiates to the left shoulder and down the left arm and can extend to the neck and lower jaw. Heartburn from noncardiac conditions rarely radiates down the arms.

Myocardial infarction can occur at any time and is not relieved by rest or nitroglycerin. The onset is acute. Pain can radiate to the throat or neck, across both sides of the chest to the shoulder, or down the medial aspects of either or both arms. The chest symptoms are often associated with shortness of breath, nausea, vomiting, and diaphoresis.

See Chapter 8 for additional assessment of chest pain.

Cardiac Risk Factors

A quick review of risk factors for cardiac disease helps provide context for the presenting symptom(s) (https://www.cdc.gov/heart disease/risk_factors.htm).

What symptom characteristics will help me narrow the differential diagnosis?

Key Questions
- Describe the sensation.
- Do you regurgitate gastric contents into the mouth?
- Do you have fullness after eating or satisfy your appetite easily?
- What are the aggravating or precipitating factors?
- What relieves the heartburn?
- Do you have nighttime symptoms?
- Do you have hoarseness, wheezing, or cough?

Description of the Sensation

Heartburn that is burning and stinging is a classic symptom of GERD. The burning sensation or unpleasant subjective sensation of heat often begins inferiorly and radiates up the entire retrosternal area to the neck, occasionally to the back, and rarely into the arms. Burning epigastric pain is a symptom of dyspepsia and is not considered to be heartburn unless the pain radiates retrosternally.

Patients with dyspepsia (both ulcer and functional) report epigastric pain or burning. Epigastric pain is located in the region between the umbilicus and lower end of the sternum, within the midclavicular lines. Epigastric pain may or may not have a burning quality.

Regurgitation

The regurgitation of gastric contents into the mouth (water brash or pyrosis) is a cardinal symptom of GERD. Infants 6 months of age or younger often have the return of small amounts of swallowed food or liquid shortly after feeding. This is referred to as spitting up.

Postprandial Fullness or Early Satiation

Dyspepsia commonly presents with postprandial fullness or early satiation. Postprandial fullness is described as an unpleasant sensation of prolonged persistence of food in the stomach. Early satiation is the loss of appetite during a meal and is described as a feeling that the stomach is full soon after starting to eat so that the meal cannot be finished.

Aggravating or Precipitating Factors

Symptoms from reflux occur postprandially, particularly after large meals, or after ingesting spicy foods, citrus products, fats, chocolates, and alcohol.

The supine position and bending over may exacerbate heartburn from GERD. Symptoms from hiatal hernia may worsen on reclining. In gas entrapment, pain is intensified by bending over or wearing tight garments.

Relieving Factors

Heartburn caused by GERD may be relieved by the ingestion of antacids, baking soda, or milk. Heartburn that is relieved by reducing the meal size, avoiding high-fat meals, and eating slowly suggests GERD. Ingesting food may relieve symptoms from ulcer disease. Symptoms from gas or gas entrapment are relieved by passage of flatus.

Nocturnal Symptoms

Many patients with GERD report nocturnal symptoms that interrupt sleep and health-related quality of life. Patients with PUD also report nocturnal symptoms.

Extraesophageal Symptoms

Additional symptoms of hoarseness, wheezing, and cough support a diagnosis of GERD. The causal relationship between asthma and GERD is difficult to establish because either condition can aggravate the other. Asthma can cause increased reflux by creating negative intrathoracic pressure and overcoming the lower esophageal sphincter barrier.

Is this patient at risk for a serious underlying condition?

Key Questions

- If the patient is older than 45 years old, is this a new-onset symptom?
- How long have you been having symptoms?
- Do you have a family history of gastric cancer or PUD?

At-Risk Patients

Patients at high risk for a serious underlying condition such as esophageal or gastric cancer or PUD include patients older than 45 years with new onset of symptoms, patients with longstanding symptoms, and those with a family history of gastric cancer. The prevalence of erosive esophagitis and Barrett esophagus increases with age.

 EVIDENCE-BASED PRACTICE *Can Gastroesophageal Reflux Disease Be Diagnosed by Symptoms Alone?*

The symptoms of heartburn and regurgitation are used for making a presumptive diagnosis of gastroesophageal reflux disease. Included in a larger systematic review was a review of seven studies to assess the accuracy of clinical opinion in diagnosing esophagitis. A total of 5134 patients were included; 894 (17%) had esophagitis on endoscopy. The sensitivities of heartburn and regurgitation for determining the presence of erosive esophagitis were 30% to 76%, with specificities ranging from 62% to 96%. The authors concluded that symptoms alone do not have high diagnostic accuracy. However, the clinical history is important in distinguishing upper gastrointestinal disorders from other disorders such as angina.

Reference: Moayyedi et al, 2006.

Key Questions

- Is the patient a child?
- Have you had recent GI surgery?
- What medications are you taking?
- How much alcohol do you drink?

Child

In infants, gastroesophageal reflux (GER) is the most common esophageal disorder. Symptoms often peak at 4 months of age and resolve by 12 to 24 months. Infants with GER may present with postprandial regurgitation, irritability, arching, choking, gagging, feeding aversion, failure to thrive, obstructive apnea, or stridor. Cow's milk protein is a common cause of GER in infants, and a trial of elimination should be considered. Older children with GER experience abdominal pain, chest pain, asthma, hoarseness, and sinusitis.

Allergic eosinophilic esophagitis (AEE) occurs primarily in young children and adolescents and presents with dyspepsia symptoms of reflux or vomiting, irritability, food refusal, and early satiation.

Recent Gastrointestinal Surgery

Reflux of bile can occur after partial gastrectomy, truncal vagotomy, and pyloroplasty for peptic ulcer reflux or cholecystectomy. Bile reflux can cause severe epigastric abdominal pain accompanied by bilious vomiting and weight loss.

Medications

The ingestion of aspirin, nonsteroidal antiinflammatory drugs (NSAIDs), or corticosteroids can cause mucosal irritation of the esophagus and stomach. This acute injury is produced by contact with a damaging agent. Other medications that cause esophagitis or gastritis include tetracycline, potassium chloride, ferrous sulfate, and alendronate. ACE inhibitors and angiotensin receptor inhibitors can cause angioedema and swelling of the larynx producing hoarseness.

Medications that may decrease lower esophageal sphincter pressure and are associated with GERD include calcium channel blockers, alpha adrenergic antagonists, anticholinergic drugs, theophylline, nitrates, sildenafil, albuterol sedatives, and prostaglandins.

Alcohol

Chronic or excessive alcohol intake is associated with GERD, esophagitis, gastritis, and dyspepsia.

DIAGNOSTIC REASONING: FOCUSED PHYSICAL EXAMINATION

Note General Appearance

Physical examination often has no specific findings. Look for pallor, diaphoresis, distress, and anxiety that would suggest MI. Pallor may also suggest anemia or allergic disorder as a cause of the symptoms. Cachexia points to advanced cancer or compromised nutrition.

Assess Vital Signs

Vital signs will generally be within normal range. Variation in pulse, blood pressure, or presence of fever should alert you to infection or a serious underlying condition.

Assess Weight

Compare previously recorded weights. Unintentional, unexplained weight loss suggests the presence of cancer (see Chapter 39). Weight loss in an adult is clinically significant when it exceeds 5% of usual body weight over a 6- to 12-month period. In infants, a decrease in weight of more than 8% necessitates follow-up within 48 hours. A loss of more than 10% of birth weight warrants careful assessment and consideration for hospital admission.

Obesity is associated with the development of GERD, esophagitis, hiatal hernia, and upper GI cancers. Obesity results in an increase in intragastric pressure, which increases the gastroesophageal pressure gradient and the frequency of transient lower esophageal sphincter relaxation, thereby predisposing gastric contents to migrate into the esophagus. In addition, obesity enhances the spatial separation of the crural diaphragm and the lower esophageal sphincter, thereby predisposing to a hiatal hernia.

Inspect the Eyes, Nose, and Mouth

Evidence of allergic rhinitis, such as pale boggy nasal mucosa, clear rhinorrhea, and cobblestone conjunctivae suggest AEE. Ill-fitting dentures may be a cause of aerophagia and gas.

The presence of ipsilateral Horner syndrome (miosis, ptosis, absence of sweating on ipsilateral face and neck) points to advanced esophageal cancer.

Palpate Supraclavicular Lymph Nodes

Supraclavicular lymphadenopathy points to esophageal, breast, or gastric cancer.

Examine the Skin

Evidence of atopic dermatitis suggests AEE and may include acute and chronic eczematous lesions. Acute lesions may be erythematous papules that are inflamed or crusty and oozing if they have been scratched. Chronic lesions may be discolored, thickened, or scaly. The symptoms of atopic dermatitis vary with the age of the patient. In infants, the condition usually causes red, scaly, oozy, and crusty cheeks, and the symptoms may also appear on the neck and extensor surfaces of the legs and arms. Adolescents are more likely to develop thick, leathery, and dull-looking lesions on the face and neck and in the flexural folds of the extremities.

Auscultate the Lungs and Percuss the Chest

Absent breath sounds, the ability to hear peristalsis in the chest, or dullness of the left lung base suggests a large hiatal hernia.

Wheezing may be present if the patient has asthma.

Auscultate Heart Sounds

Abnormal sounds, such as paradoxical second heart sound (S_2) during pain, are a sign of coronary ischemia. A transient S_3 (ventricular gallop) or mitral regurgitation murmur at the apex can occur occasionally with myocardial ischemia. An S_4 (atrial gallop) typically indicates a stressed heart, which can be the result of hypertension, MI, or CAD. Abnormal rhythms and heart rates are often heard during MI assessment. Electrocardiograms (ECGs) are necessary to identify the specific rhythm.

Percuss and Palpate the Abdomen

Some patients with gastritis have midepigastric tenderness on percussion and palpation. A palpable epigastric or abdominal mass suggests cancer. A palpable hard lymph node in the umbilicus points to gastric cancer.

LABORATORY AND DIAGNOSTIC STUDIES

Complete Blood Count

The initial evaluation should include a complete blood count (CBC) to rule out anemia.

Blood Chemistries

Patients with nausea, vomiting, and epigastric fullness may also have generalized electrolyte imbalances. If the history and physical examination suggest the presence of a hepatobiliary condition, liver function tests should be ordered.

> **EVIDENCE-BASED PRACTICE** *Can a Trial of Proton Pump Inhibitor Confirm the Diagnosis of Gastroesophageal Reflux Disease?*
>
> This meta-analysis included 15 studies that compared clinical response to a short course of a proton pump inhibitor (PPI) with an objective measure of gastroesophageal reflux disease (GERD) such as 24-hour pH monitoring. Sensitivity of the trial response in detecting GERD was 78% (95% confidence interval [CI], 0.66–0.86), and specificity was 54% (95% CI, 0.44–0.65). This analysis concluded that a PPI trial in patients suspected of having GERD does not confidently establish or exclude the diagnosis of GERD. The authors suggest that despite diagnostic uncertainty, a PPI trial might be reasonable in patients without alarm symptoms or other suspected complications of GERD.
>
> Reference: Numans et al, 2004.

Response to Antacids

A diagnosis of acid-induced heartburn can be indirectly established through response to antacids; however, lack of response does not exclude reflux.

Trial of Proton Pump Inhibitors

A trial of proton pump inhibitors (PPIs) for 4 to 6 weeks may be useful in patients with classic symptoms of reflux without alarm symptoms. A negative result does not rule out GERD.

Sublingual Nitroglycerin

Both angina and reflux may respond to the administration of nitroglycerin.

Helicobacter pylori Testing

Screening for *Helicobacter pylori* infection is not recommended in patients suspected of having GERD. *H. pylori* testing may be useful in high-prevalence areas or in patients with dyspepsia symptoms that suggest PUD or gastritis. Laboratory methods for testing include antibody or antigen testing with serology, urine, or stool, or urea breath test.

Endoscopy

Upper endoscopy is the gold standard to determine abnormal esophageal mucosal pathology. It is indicated to evaluate for alarm symptoms: esophageal or gastric malignancy, eosinophilic esophagitis, and screening of high-risk patients (family history of gastric cancer, emigrated from a country with a high rate of gastric cancer, or had a prior partial gastrectomy) and in patients unresponsive to PPIs. Endoscopy is the procedure of choice in cases in which mucosal lesions or growths are suspected. It is not useful for identifying hiatal hernia. Upper endoscopy is not required in the presence of typical GERD symptoms without alarm features.

Esophageal pH Monitoring

Esophageal pH monitoring provides direct physiologic measurement of acid in the esophagus through use of a probe or endoscopically placed capsule. Twenty-four-hour esophageal pH monitoring is useful in patients with atypical manifestations of GERD such as chest pain or chronic cough. Esophageal pH monitoring with symptom recording may identify a relationship between heartburn and acid reflux with a pH lower than 4.

Esophageal Manometry

Esophageal manometry is indicated in patients with refractory reflux in whom surgical therapy is planned to determine the functional capacity of the lower esophageal sphincter (LES). It is not recommended for GERD diagnosis.

Upper Gastrointestinal Series

An upper GI series (barium swallow) is useful in patients unwilling to have endoscopy or with medical contraindications to the procedure. It is useful in diagnosing hiatal hernia. It can identify ulcerations and strictures; however, it

---

> **EVIDENCE-BASED PRACTICE** *Screening with Endoscopy*
>
> Based on review of the available evidence, the American College of Gastroenterology does not recommend endoscopy to screen for Barrett esophagitis (BE) in the general population. Screening for BE may be considered for those at high risk. Risk factors include men with chronic (>5 years) or frequent (weekly or more) symptoms of GER (heartburn or acid regurgitation) and 2 or more risk factors for BE or esophageal adenocarcinoma (EAC). These risk factors include age older than 50 years, white race, presence of central obesity (waist circumference >102 cm or waist–hip ratio >0.9), current or past history of smoking, and a confirmed family history of BE or EAC in a first-degree relative. Women with chronic gastroesophageal symptoms are at lower risk of EAC compared with men, and routine screening is not recommended. However, screening could be considered in individual cases as determined by the presence of multiple risk factors for BE or EAC.
>
> Reference: Shaheen et al, 2013.

may miss mucosal abnormalities and is not used to diagnose GERD.

Electrocardiography and Cardiac Enzymes

If the clinical history is suggestive of a cardiac origin, coronary artery disease or MI should be excluded through ECG or cardiac enzyme testing. The preferred biomarker is a cardiac troponin (T or I; cTnT, or cTnI); creatinine kinase MB isoenzyme (CK-MB) is less sensitive (see Chapter 8).

DIFFERENTIAL DIAGNOSIS

Gastroesophageal Reflux

Gastroesophageal reflux is seen in all age groups but is most common in newborns and infants (younger than 6 months of age). In infants, GER occurs three to four times a day because of transient relaxation of an immature esophageal sphincter. This can be a functional diagnosis and does not necessarily indicate pathology. This is sometimes referred to as the "happy spitter"; the condition improves with age and simple feeding techniques. In adults, GER generally occurs after a meal, lasts for a few minutes, and has no other symptoms.

Gastroesophageal Reflux Disease or Reflux Esophagitis

Gastroesophageal reflux disease is defined as symptoms and complications resulting from the reflux of gastric contents into the esophagus into the oral cavity (including larynx) or into the lung. GERD can be either erosive or nonerosive. The severity of esophageal damage does not correlate with the severity of symptoms.

Classic symptoms include heartburn that is caustic and stinging, typically without radiation to the back. Regurgitation of gastric contents into the mouth (acid regurgitation, water brash, or pyrosis) suggests progressing GERD. Lying supine or leaning forward provoke both heartburn and regurgitation.

Additional symptoms may include chronic cough and bronchospasm, chest pain, hoarseness, early satiety, abdominal fullness, bloating with belching, and dental erosion in children.

Causes of GERD include transient relaxation of the LES, medications that lower LES pressure (calcium channel blockers, alpha-adrenergic antagonists, anticholinergic drugs, theophylline, nitrates, sildenafil, albuterol sedatives, and prostaglandins); foods that lower LES pressure (chocolate, yellow onions, peppermint), tobacco abuse, alcohol, coffee, pregnancy, and gastric acid hypersecretion. Hiatal hernia may or may not be a causative factor. Obesity is associated with a significant increase in the risk for reflux.

Complications of reflux esophagitis include esophageal ulceration, hematemesis, melena, stricture development, and Barrett esophagus.

The presence of frequent and typical reflux symptoms should lead to a provisional diagnosis of GERD rather than dyspepsia. In the absence of alarm features, the diagnosis is typically made by careful history and physical examination and a trial of medication with antacids or PPI. Generally, when symptoms of GER are typical, and the patient responds to therapy, there is no need for further diagnostic tests to verify a diagnosis of GERD. However, overlap of GERD with dyspepsia is probably frequent and needs to be considered when symptoms do not respond to appropriate management of GERD.

Upper endoscopy or 24-hour pH monitoring is indicated for complicated or refractory cases.

Other Causes of Esophagitis

Esophagitis can cause pain with swallowing and weight loss. Other causes of esophagitis include infective esophagitis, AEE, and so-called pill esophagitis.

Infective esophagitis

Infective esophagitis is caused by fungal agents, such as *Candida* spp. and *Torulopsis glabrata*; viral agents, such as herpes simplex, cytomegalovirus, HIV, and varicella zoster; and, rarely, bacterial infections including diphtheria and tuberculosis. The typical presenting signs and symptoms are odynophagia, dysphagia, and retrosternal pain. Patients may also experience fever, nausea, and vomiting. Diagnosis of infectious esophagitis is made by endoscopy (ulcerations, exudates) and histopathology examination; adding polymerase chain reaction, tissue viral culture, and immunocytochemistry enhances the diagnostic sensitivity and precision.

Allergic eosinophilic esophagitis

Allergic eosinophilic esophagitis occurs primarily in young children and adolescents with dyspepsia symptoms of reflux such as vomiting, irritability, food refusal, and early satiation. Adults report reflux, epigastric or chest pain, and dysphagia. The failure of high-dose PPI treatment and the absence of acid reflux are necessary for diagnosis. Patients often have a personal or family history of other allergic disorders. Most patients with AEE have atopic dermatitis, allergic rhinitis, asthma, or modest peripheral eosinophilia. The diagnosis is made by classic findings on endoscopy, such as linear furrowing, and multiple rings accompanied by biopsies that show eosinophilic infiltration.

Pill esophagitis

Oral medications of any type can cause esophageal injury by producing a caustic acid solution (e.g., ferrous sulfate), producing a caustic alkaline solution (e.g., alendronate), placing a hyperosmolar solution in contact with the esophageal mucosa (e.g., potassium chloride), or causing direct injury to the esophageal mucosa (e.g., tetracycline). Medications that can cause esophagitis include tetracycline, potassium chloride, ferrous sulfate, NSAIDs, and bisphosphonates. The patient may report taking the medication at bedtime with insufficient water or lying down directly after taking the medication. The patient may also report acute discomfort followed by progressive retrosternal pain. Ulcer formation can cause odynophagia, dysphagia, and weight loss. Physical examination is normal. Endoscopy shows a focal lesion.

Functional Heartburn

Functional heartburn is a GI disorder characterized by symptoms of heartburn not related

---

Box 20.1   **Diagnostic Criteria for Functional GI Disorders**

The Rome criteria is a system developed to classify functional gastrointestinal (GI) disorders. The most recent version of the criteria—Rome IV—created a new term for functional disorders: disorders of gut–brain interaction (DGBIs). These disorders are defined as a group of disorders classified by GI symptoms related to any combination of motility disturbances, visceral hypersensitivity, altered mucosal and immune function, gut microbiota, or central nervous system processing. Criteria for the specific disorders are available at http://theromefoundation.org.

Drossman and Hasler, 2016.

---

to GER or other organic causes. Findings include normal endoscopy findings and normal esophageal acid exposure during esophageal pH monitoring.

The patient reports vague nonspecific symptoms and obtains no consistent relief with medication. The patient may report anxiety. Physical examination is normal with no evidence of systemic disease or weight loss. Box 20.1 describes a source for diagnostic criteria for functional GI disorders.

Hiatal Hernia

Hiatal hernia is stomach herniation via esophageal hiatus of the diaphragm. It causes pain in the epigastrium or lower chest that worsens on reclining and is relieved on standing. The pain may be retrosternal with radiation down the left arm. Physical examination findings are generally normal. A large hernia may create dullness on percussion over the left lung base, absent breath sounds, or bowel sounds present in the chest. The causal association of hiatal hernia with GERD is unclear. Hiatal hernia is diagnosed by barium swallow. Upper endoscopy is poor at identifying hiatal hernia.

Peptic Ulcer Disease

Peptic ulcer disease includes gastric and duodenal ulcer disease. Uncomplicated PUD may have no symptoms. PUD is characterized by episodic gnawing or epigastric pain usually

2 to 5 hours after meals or on empty stomach; nighttime awakening as a result of pain; and symptom relief with food intake, antacids, or antisecretory agents. Other symptoms include fullness, bloating, early satiation, vomiting, indigestion, loss of appetite, heartburn, hematemesis, back pain, and unexplained weight loss. Children may present with generalized abdominal pain. Older adults are more likely to be asymptomatic but may also have nonspecific complaints including confusion, restlessness, abdominal distention, and falls.

Most peptic ulcers are caused by *H. pylori* infection or NSAIDs, including aspirin. Other high-risk medications include corticosteroids (in high doses or when combined with NSAIDs), bisphosphonates, mycophenolate, potassium chloride, and fluorouracil.

Diagnosis is made by endoscopy. In patients with isolated dyspepsia who do not exhibit alarm symptoms, testing for and treating for *H. pylori* infection is effective and less expensive than initial endoscopy.

Also see Chapter 3 on abdominal pain for assessment of acute upper abdominal pain.

Esophageal Cancer

Carcinomas of the esophagus include both squamous cell and adenocarcinoma. Patients are usually asymptomatic until advanced stage III or stage IV. They typically present with alarm symptoms of dysphagia (initially occurs with solid foods and gradually progresses to include semisolids and liquids), odynophagia, anorexia, and unintentional weight loss. Esophageal cancer is likely caused by repeated exposure to irritants such as smoking, alcohol, or chronic GERD in combination with genetic predisposition. There is a strong association between Barrett esophagus and development of esophageal adenocarcinoma.

Physical examination findings that suggest advanced disease include cachexia, ipsilateral Horner syndrome (miosis, ptosis, absence of sweating on ipsilateral face and neck), supraclavicular adenopathy, hoarseness, and halitosis. Epigastric swelling or a mass may be present on palpation. Patients may have anemia. Diagnosis is made with endoscopy.

Gastric Cancer

The most common gastric cancer is adenocarcinoma. The presenting symptoms are dyspepsia unrelieved by antacids, epigastric discomfort (usually lessened by fasting and exacerbated by food intake), and early satiation. Alarm symptoms include dysphagia, anorexia, and weight loss. Symptoms occur late in the disease.

Physical examination findings indicative of advanced disease include a palpable left supraclavicular (Virchow) node and a palpable hard lymph node in the umbilicus. An epigastric or abdominal mass may be palpable. A hard, nodular liver generally indicates metastatic disease. The patient may be pale from anemia. Ascites, lymphadenopathy, or pleural effusion may indicate metastasis. Stools may be positive on fecal occult blood testing.

Diagnosis is made with endoscopy.

Gastritis

Gastritis is caused by inflammation of the lining of the stomach that can be acute or chronic. Acute gastritis is caused by irritation caused by excessive alcohol use, chronic vomiting, stress, or the ingestion of aspirin, NSAIDs, or steroids. The most common cause of chronic gastritis is *H. pylori* infection. Other causes include other bacterial, viral, fungal, or parasitic infection; bile reflux; or pernicious anemia. Bile gastritis can occur after a partial gastrectomy, truncal vagotomy and pyloroplasty for peptic ulcer reflux, or cholecystectomy. Bile reflux can cause severe epigastric abdominal pain accompanied by bilious vomiting and weight loss.

The most common gastritis symptoms are those of dyspepsia. They include abdominal pain, indigestion, heartburn, epigastric discomfort that is worse after eating, loss of appetite, sense of fullness, nausea, occasional vomiting, and a burning or gnawing feeling in the stomach between meals or at night.

On physical examination, epigastric tenderness may be present on palpation.

Endoscopy is indicated in patients with alarm features or persistent symptoms. Upper endoscopy demonstrates friable, beefy red mucosa. Additional workup may include testing for *H. pylori* infection, a CBC to assess for anemia, and fecal occult blood testing.

Dyspepsia

Dyspepsia refers to recurrent or chronic pain or discomfort in the upper abdomen without radiation that occurs with eating or soon after a meal. Burning pain confined to the epigastrium is a cardinal symptom of dyspepsia. Other symptoms may include postprandial fullness, upper abdominal bloating, early satiation, belching, nausea, and vomiting. Heartburn may occur as part of the symptom constellation, but when heartburn is the predominant symptom, the patient should be considered to have gastroesophageal reflux disease and not dyspepsia.

Dyspepsia can be caused by structural disease such as gastroesophageal reflux, PUD, gastritis, and gastric cancer. American Gastroenterological Association Guidelines recommend endoscopy for patients older than age 55 years with new-onset dyspepsia symptoms and for younger high-risk patients (those with weight loss, progressive dysphagia, recurrent vomiting, evidence of GI bleeding, or a family history of cancer). Biopsy specimens should be obtained during endoscopy for *H. pylori*.

Functional Dyspepsia (Nonulcer Dyspepsia)

In some patients with dyspepsia, diagnostic testing shows no evidence of structural disease. Box 20.1 lists diagnostic criteria for functional dyspepsia.

The etiology and pathophysiology of nonulcer dyspepsia include abnormalities of gastric motor function (e.g., delayed gastric emptying and antral hypomotility), visceral hypersensitivity, *H. pylori* infection, and psychosocial factors associated with anxiety and depression. Risk factors include excessive amounts of caffeine, alcohol, and smoking; taking steroids, NSAIDs, or other medications; and living in a high *H. pylori* prevalence area.

Gas and Gas Entrapment

Excessive abdominal gas can produce abdominal discomfort, vague feelings of indigestion, abdominal bloating, belching, and chest pain. Excessive gas comes from bacterial degradation of large intestine contents as a result of ingestion of flatulogenic foods, GI stasis, constipation, malabsorption, gas in the stomach from air swallowing (aerophagia), hurried eating or drinking, smoking, chewing gum, poorly fitting dentures, and dry mouth from anxiety or anticholinergics. Gas can become trapped in the hepatic or splenic flexures (hepatic or splenic flexure syndrome). Bending over or wearing tight garments intensifies pain, and pain is relieved by the passage of flatus.

Physical examination findings may include visible abdominal distention on inspection. The abdomen may be distended with hyperresonance on percussion and diffuse tenderness on palpation.

Cardiac Causes of Heartburn and Indigestion (see Chapter 8)

Acute coronary insufficiency

Acute coronary insufficiency refers to those situations in which chest pain is caused by a lack of oxygen to the myocardium but there is no evidence of infarct. The patient reports severe, oppressive, constricting, retrosternal discomfort lasting longer than 30 minutes. The patient may report a prior history of MI or angina.

On physical examination, abnormal sounds, such as paradoxical second heart sound (S_2) during pain, are a sign of coronary ischemia. A transient S_3 (ventricular gallop) or mitral regurgitation murmur at the apex can occur occasionally with myocardial ischemia. An S_4 (atrial gallop) typically indicates a stressed heart, which can be the result of hypertension, MI, or CAD.

The ECG may show intermittent ischemic changes or may be normal. Cardiac isozyme test results are normal.

Stable angina

Stable angina refers to chest pain typically described as substernal chest pressure or heaviness, radiating to the left shoulder and arm, neck, or jaw. The pain onset is usually gradual, brought on and exacerbated by exercise and stress; it is associated with nausea, diaphoresis, and shortness of breath and is alleviated with rest or nitroglycerin. Pain typically lasts 2 to 10 minutes. Physical examination findings are usually normal with no tenderness on palpation of the abdomen. An S_4 gallop can be transiently present during an episode of pain. Tests for angina include performing an ECG during an episode of pain, which can show ST-segment depression and T-wave inversions, or the findings may be normal. Administration of sublingual nitroglycerin during an episode of pain relieves the pain.

Myocardial infarction

The patient with an acute MI generally describes a sudden onset of pain at rest. It is a persistent, often severe, deep, central chest pain and can radiate, as does angina, to the throat or neck, across both sides of the chest to the shoulder, or down the medial aspect of

either or both arms. Rest or nitroglycerin does not relieve the pain. The chest pain is often associated with shortness of breath, nausea, vomiting, and diaphoresis.

Patients can also express a sense of impending doom. A review of risk factors includes men 45 years and older, women 55 years and older, cigarette smoking, hyperlipidemia, hypertension, diabetes, obesity, history of CAD, and family history of CAD. Objective evidence of an MI can include skin pallor, cool diaphoretic skin, and transient paradoxical S_2. The patient can be hypertensive or hypotensive. Abnormal rhythms include tachycardia and bradycardia.

The patient with a suspected MI should be placed on a cardiac monitor as soon as possible. Observe for premature ventricular contractions and classic ECG changes that indicate MI, including ST-segment elevations, T-wave inversions, and Q waves. Performing a 12-lead ECG and determining levels of cardiac isozymes will help confirm a diagnosis.

> **DIFFERENTIAL DIAGNOSIS OF** *Common Causes of Heartburn and Dyspepsia*

CONDITION	HISTORY	PHYSICAL FINDINGS	DIAGNOSTIC STUDIES
GER	*Infants:* Spitting up three to five times a day *Adults:* Pain occurs after a meal and lasts a few minutes No other symptoms	None	None
GERD	Heartburn, pyrosis Possible extraesophageal symptoms, laryngitis, wheezing, cough *Infants:* weight loss, arching of back, vomiting, irritability	None Possible wheezing with asthma Obesity Growth chart change	Trial of antacids Trial of PPI pH monitoring Endoscopy for refractory symptoms to rule out erosions
Infective esophagitis	Odynophagia, dysphagia, retrosternal pain; possible fever, nausea, and vomiting	None Possible fever	Endoscopy: ulcerations, exudates
AEE	*Young children and adolescents:* dyspepsia, heartburn, vomiting, irritability, food refusal, early satiation *Adults:* heartburn, epigastric or chest pain, dysphagia, and food impaction Personal or family history of allergic disorders	None Possible allergic rhinitis, atopic dermatitis	Endoscopy: linear furrowing and multiple rings

Continued

> **DIFFERENTIAL DIAGNOSIS OF** *Common Causes of Heartburn and Dyspepsia—cont'd*

CONDITION	HISTORY	PHYSICAL FINDINGS	DIAGNOSTIC STUDIES
Pill esophagitis	Medication history: tetracycline, potassium chloride, ferrous sulfate, NSAIDs, and bisphosphonates Takes medication at bedtime with insufficient water or lying down directly after taking Acute discomfort followed by progressive retrosternal pain	None	Endoscopy: focal lesion
Functional heartburn	Burning retrosternal discomfort or pain Symptoms present for the past 3 mo	None	Endoscopy
Hiatal hernia	Pain in epigastrium or lower chest that worsens on reclining; relieved on standing Pain may be retrosternal with radiation down left arm	None Large hernia may create dullness on percussion over the left lung base, absent breath sounds, or bowel sounds resent in the chest	Barium swallow
PUD	Episodic gnawing or epigastric pain usually 2–5 hr after meals or on empty stomach Nighttime awakening because of pain; symptom relief with food intake, antacids, or antisecretory agents Fullness, bloating, early satiation, vomiting, indigestion, loss of appetite, heartburn, hematemesis, back pain, and unexplained weight loss Medication history: NSAIDs, aspirin, high-dose corticosteroids, bisphosphonates, mycophenolate, potassium chloride, and fluorouracil Children may present with generalized abdominal pain Older patients may be asymptomatic, but may also present with nonspecific complaints, including confusion, restlessness, abdominal distention, and falls	None	Endoscopy: ulcers; *Helicobacter pylori* testing CBC if suspect anemia FOBT for bleeding

DIFFERENTIAL DIAGNOSIS OF *Common Causes of Heartburn and Dyspepsia—cont'd*

CONDITION	HISTORY	PHYSICAL FINDINGS	DIAGNOSTIC STUDIES
Esophageal cancer	Alarm symptoms: dysphagia (solids or liquids), odynophagia, anorexia, and unintentional weight loss Repeated exposure to irritants such as smoking, alcohol History of Barrett esophagus	Advanced disease: cachexia, ipsilateral Horner syndrome (miosis, ptosis, absence of sweating on ipsilateral face and neck), supraclavicular adenopathy, hoarseness, halitosis Epigastric swelling or mass may be present on palpation	Endoscopy
Gastric cancer	Dyspepsia unrelieved by antacids, epigastric discomfort, usually lessened by fasting, and exacerbated by food intake and early satiation Alarm symptoms of dysphagia, anorexia, and weight loss	Advanced disease: cachexia, palpable left supraclavicular (Virchow) node, palpable hard lymph node in umbilicus A hard, nodular liver indicates metastatic disease May be pale from anemia Ascites, pleural effusions may indicate metastasis	Endoscopy and FOBT
Gastritis	Dyspepsia with abdominal pain, indigestion, heartburn, and epigastric discomfort that is worse after eating, loss of appetite, sense of fullness, nausea, occasional vomiting, burning or gnawing feeling in the stomach between meals or at night Excessive alcohol use, chronic vomiting, stress, or the ingestion of aspirin, NSAIDs, or steroid Bile gastritis can occur after partial gastrectomy, truncal vagotomy and pyloroplasty for peptic ulcer reflux, or cholecystectomy Bile reflux can cause severe epigastric abdominal pain, accompanied by bilious vomiting and weight loss	Possible epigastric tenderness	Endoscopy for patients with alarm features or persistent symptoms Additional workup may include testing for *H. pylori* CBC if anemia suspected FOBT for bleeding

Continued

> **DIFFERENTIAL DIAGNOSIS OF** *Common Causes of Heartburn and Dyspepsia—cont'd*

CONDITION	HISTORY	PHYSICAL FINDINGS	DIAGNOSTIC STUDIES
Dyspepsia	Epigastric pain or burning with postprandial fullness, early satiation Symptoms for 3–6 mo	May have epigastric tenderness	Endoscopy: for patients 55 yr and older, those with weight loss, progressive dysphagia, recurrent vomiting, evidence of GI bleeding, or family history of cancer, new-onset dyspepsia *H. pylori* testing: patients 55 yr and younger without alarm features
Functional dyspepsia (nonulcer dyspepsia)	Risk factors: excessive amounts of caffeine or alcohol, smoking, steroids, NSAIDs, living in an area with a high prevalence of *H. pylori*	None	*H. pylori* testing Testing for structural disease, negative findings
Gas or gas entrapment	Abdominal discomfort, vague feelings of indigestion; abdominal bloating, belching, chest pain Ingestion of flatulogenic foods, GI stasis, constipation, malabsorption, air swallowing (aerophagia), hurried eating or drinking, smoking or chewing gum, poorly fitting dentures, or dry mouth from anxiety or anticholinergics Pain worsens by bending over or wearing tight garments and is relieved by passage of flatus	Possible distended abdomen with hyperresonance on percussion	None
Acute coronary insufficiency	Severe, oppressive, constricting, retrosternal discomfort lasting >30 min Possible prior history of MI or angina	Possible abnormal heart sounds such as paradoxical S_2 during pain; transient S_3 (ventricular gallop) or mitral regurgitation murmur at the apex; S_4 (atrial gallop)	ECG: intermittent ischemic changes or normal Cardiac isoenzymes normal

> ## DIFFERENTIAL DIAGNOSIS OF *Common Causes of Heartburn and Dyspepsia—cont'd*

CONDITION	HISTORY	PHYSICAL FINDINGS	DIAGNOSTIC STUDIES
Stable angina	Chest pain typically described as substernal chest pressure or heaviness, radiating to the left shoulder and arm, neck, or jaw Onset brought on and exacerbated by exercise and stress; typically lasts 2–10 min Alleviated with rest or nitroglycerin	Possible diaphoresis and shortness of breath Transient S_4 gallop during an episode of pain	ECG during an episode of pain: ST-segment depression and T wave inversions, or the findings can be normal
MI	Sudden onset of pain at rest Persistent, often severe, deep, central chest pain; and may radiate to the throat or neck, across both sides of the chest to the shoulder, or down the medial aspect of either or both arms Nitroglycerin does not relieve the pain Possible sense of impending doom Risk factors: men 45 yr and older; women 55 yr and older; cigarette smoker; hyperlipidemia; hypertension; diabetes; obesity; history of CAD; family history of CAD	Skin pallor, cool diaphoretic skin Hypertensive or hypotensive Possible transient paradoxical S_2 or abnormal rhythms including tachycardia and bradycardia	ECG: ST-segment elevations, T-wave inversions, and Q waves Cardiac enzymes elevated

AEE, allergic eosinophilic esophagitis; *CAD,* coronary artery disease; *CBC,* complete blood count; *ECG,* electrocardiogram; *FOBT,* fecal occult blood testing; *GER,* gastroesophageal reflux; *GERD,* gastroesophageal reflux disease; *GI,* gastrointestinal; *MI,* myocardial infarction; *NSAID,* nonsteroidal antiinflammatory drugs; *PPI,* proton pump inhibitors; *PUD,* peptic ulcer disease.

Hoarseness is a disturbance of the normal voice pitch by an abnormal vibration of the vocal cords. It is a term used to describe an unnaturally rough, harsh, or deep voice. Voice is the sound produced when the vocal folds are approximated and expired airflow between the cords causes them to vibrate. The sound produced by the larynx is amplified by the pharynx, oral cavity, sinuses, and nasal cavity and is modified by movements of the tongue, uvula, and soft palate. Hoarseness may be an early sign of local disease or a manifestation of a systemic illness. Hoarseness is a cardinal symptom of laryngeal disease.

The larynx is a musculocartilaginous structure lined with a mucous membrane connected superiorly to the pharynx (below the tongue and hyoid) and inferiorly to the trachea. It is the sphincter that guards the entrance into the trachea and functions secondarily as the organ of voice. Nine cartilages connected by ligaments and eight muscles form the larynx. The lower portion of the thyroarytenoid muscle forms the true vocal fold, or folds, which are highly elastic and account for the extraordinary versatility of the voice and the wide range of pitch, volume, and quality. The glottis is the triangular opening between the true vocal cords. The supraglottic area includes the ventricular folds (false vocal cords), the aryepiglottic folds, and the epiglottis (Fig. 21.1). The epiglottis is the lidlike cartilaginous structure that overhangs the entrance to the larynx and serves to prevent food from entering the larynx and trachea while swallowing.

Many benign conditions cause hoarseness such as functional disorders from voice overuse and upper respiratory infections (URIs). Acute laryngitis is the most common cause of hoarseness. Functional causes are unrelated to organic disease and may have a psychosocial component, such as restraint in expressing anger, crying, or a history of psychological trauma.

However, persistent hoarseness for more than 2 weeks in an adult and 1 week in a child may indicate secondary changes to the vocal cords. These changes may be caused by structural changes resulting from palsies, polyps, or cysts; laryngeal neoplasm; or congenital disorders of the larynx. Hoarseness may also be a symptom of systemic disease, such as hypothyroidism, or a symptom of inflammation caused by a variety of processes. Many forms of laryngitis that appear alike on physical examination have very different causes. Critical clues to the specific etiology of laryngitis depend on taking a careful history.

DIAGNOSTIC REASONING: FOCUSED HISTORY

Is the hoarseness acute or chronic?

Key Questions

- How long has the symptom been present?
- Has this happened before? Is it recurrent?
- Is it getting better or worse?
- Have you noticed other symptoms?

Duration

Symptoms of less than 2 weeks' duration are considered to be acute; the most likely cause is a viral upper respiratory tract infection. Inflammations secondary to acute viral infection or voice overuse are the most common causes of acute laryngitis. Chronic symptoms suggest structural change in the larynx or hoarseness secondary to disorders, such as gastroesophageal reflux disease (GERD), or

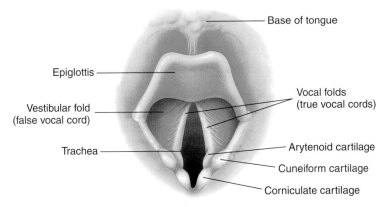

FIGURE 21.1 View of the interior of the larynx. (From Christensen B, Kockrow E: *Foundations and adult health nursing,* ed. 6, St. Louis, 2011, Mosby.)

systemic disease such as hypothyroidism. If the duration of hoarseness is longer than 2 weeks, referral to an ear, nose, and throat specialist is indicated to evaluate for possible neoplasm, most often squamous cell carcinoma because chronic laryngitis rarely has an infectious cause.

Recurrence

Recurrent episodes of hoarseness may indicate allergies or sinusitis with postnasal drip, laryngeal reflux, or systemic disease.

Progression

Progressive hoarseness usually indicates a lesion such as a laryngeal or hypopharyngeal cyst.

> *What does the onset of hoarseness tell me?*

Key Questions
- How did the hoarseness develop?
- Is there any history of trauma to the throat?
- Have you had any recent surgery around the throat or neck?

Onset

Acute onset of hoarseness is usually the result of infection or trauma. The trauma can be from direct injury (foreign body, accidents) or overuse from screaming. The overuse can be gradual, resulting in progressive hoarseness and vocal cord changes.

This hoarseness is worse in the afternoon or evening.

Hoarseness from birth may indicate a congenital problem, such as laryngeal web, cyst, palsy, or angioma. Newborns with aphonia, or a hoarse cry that does not resolve, may have a congenital anomaly, papilloma, or vocal cord paralysis.

Trauma

External trauma to the throat is rarely a cause of hoarseness, but it can result in hematoma formation in the laryngeal soft tissues. There can also be mucosal lacerations, arytenoid cartilage dislocation, or fracture of the laryngeal cartilage. Internal trauma can occur with endotracheal intubation associated with surgery when an endotracheal tube catches on laryngeal structures and is pushed against resistance.

Surgical History

Hoarseness or voice change is a sign of the vagus nerve (cranial nerve [CN] X). Surgery such as tonsillectomy, thyroidectomy, or rhinoplasty can alter the quality of the voice secondary to structural change and scarring. Damage to CN X can also be the result of hormone imbalance, bacterial infection, or tumor. Voice surgery undertaken by transgender persons to alter the pitch of their voice can injure the delicate tissue of the vocal fold and negatively alter normal vocal quality.

Key Questions

- Have you had a recent cold or upper respiratory tract infection?
- Do you have allergies or asthma?
- Do you smoke? How long have you been a smoker?
- How much alcohol do you drink?
- Can you describe your voice habits, such as singing, talking, and shouting?
- Are you frequently exposed to dust, fumes, or loud noise?
- Are your immunizations up to date?

Upper Respiratory Infection

Acute laryngitis, epiglottitis, and acute laryngotracheobronchitis (croup) are sequelae from a viral URI that can result in vocal cord inflammation. Postnasal discharge that is thick and purulent may pool around the larynx and cause chronic secondary edema. Nasal congestion that leads to mouth breathing produces laryngeal dryness, with resultant hoarseness on arising in the morning.

Children who have epiglottitis are not hoarse, but as the epiglottis swells, the voice becomes muffled and drooling is observed.

Allergies and Asthma

Poorly controlled or undiagnosed asthma can result in a chronic cough with subsequent hoarseness. Allergies can cause chronic or recurrent irritation and swelling of both the upper and lower airways. Children who have a history of asthma or allergies can develop vocal cord edema, inflammation, and hoarseness.

Smoking

Cigarette smoking is the most significant risk factor for laryngeal cancer. Smoking is also a risk factor for acute or chronic laryngitis because smoke irritates all mucous membranes and impairs ciliary function, causing pooling of secretions around the larynx.

Alcohol Consumption

Chronic consumption of hard liquor is a direct irritant to the throat and is associated with laryngeal cancer.

Voice Habits

Voice misuse occurs when the true vocal cords are forced to vibrate under undue stress and tension. Voice abuse is exuberant overuse and can lead to inflammation and edema of the larynx, hemorrhage, or vocal cord polyps. A gradual progression of hoarseness may go unnoticed by the patient. In an attempt to elevate pitch, transgender persons may voluntarily increase the tension in the vocal folds, which requires continuous muscular effort and may produce increased vocal effort and fatigue. Often a precipitating incident (e.g., shouting, excessive speaking, or singing) produces acute laryngitis. Specific questions may need to be asked to make the patient aware of conditions that lead to voice abuse, such as the following:

- Have others noticed a change in the quality of your voice?
- Do you talk frequently to people who are hard of hearing?
- Do you yell at children?
- Do you work in an environment that is noisy or contains dust and fumes?
- Have you recently attended a sporting event?

Exposures

Patients who are chronically exposed to work environments that contain dust, fumes, or a high noise level that leads to chronic voice abuse are at increased risk for laryngeal cancer.

Children exposed to poor indoor air quality may be at risk for hoarseness.

Immunizations

Laryngeal diphtheria should be considered in patients who have failed to update their diphtheria immunizations. For adults, the tetanus, diphtheria, and acellular pertussis (Td/Tdap) vaccination is recommended once and then tetanus and diphtheria (Td) boosters every 10 years; pregnant women are advised to have a Tdap during each pregnancy (http://www.cdc.gov/vaccines/schedules/hcp/adult.html). Laryngeal diphtheria usually develops as a downward progression of the tonsillar pharyngeal membrane.

What other clues will help narrow the diagnostic possibilities?

Key Questions
• Does the hoarseness change during the day?
• Is it painful?
• What other symptoms are present?
• Do you have a neurological disorder?

Timing

Hoarseness that is altered by a position change suggests a mobile lesion, such as a pedunculated polyp. Patients with myasthenia gravis have a normal voice in the morning with progressive hoarseness throughout the day.

Pain

Pain may be associated with an inflammatory process, such as a viral URI or GERD. Pain occurs late in laryngeal cancer. Neurologic and hormonal causes do not usually produce pain.

Associated Symptoms

The presence of cough, shortness of breath, weight loss, dysphagia, ear pain, or throat pain should raise concerns about neoplasm, systemic disease, or neurologic causes. Hormonal disorders, such as hypothyroidism, also produce signs and symptoms that vary in severity according to the duration and degree of hormone deficiency. Early symptoms of hypothyroidism include cold intolerance, heavy menses, weight gain, dry skin, fatigue, and constipation. Later signs and symptoms include hoarseness, very dry skin, hair loss of lateral eyebrows, and neurological symptoms, such as delayed deep tendon reflex recovery, depression, and mental confusion.

Neurologic Disease

Patients with parkinsonism, myasthenia gravis, or amyotrophic lateral sclerosis have progressive dysarthria and dysphagia. As neurologic disease progresses, patients develop a chronic cough and throat clearing caused by microaspiration of pooled secretions.

Gastroesophageal Reflux Disease

Reflux of gastric contents causes inflammation of the posterior larynx, especially the arytenoid mucosa. The patient may also report a habit of frequent throat clearing and a sensation of a lump in the throat. Chronic cough or throat clearing further damages already irritated vocal folds. Generally patients have hoarseness in the morning and coughing at night. In children, GERD presents with dysphagia, hoarseness, vomiting, and chronic cough.

DIAGNOSTIC REASONING: FOCUSED PHYSICAL EXAMINATION

Listen to the Quality of the Voice

Acoustic evaluation criteria for voice include range (monotonic to extremely variable), loudness (soft to loud), pitch (low-pitched voice requires more effort to produce adequate volume; sudden changes in pitch), register (temporary loss of voice because of abductor spasm), and quality (roughness, breathiness, and hoarseness). Table 21.1 lists common criteria used in evaluating the voice.

Table 21.1	Diagnostics Used in Evaluating Voice	
ACOUSTIC QUALITY	**MEASUREMENT**	**DISORDER**
Range	Monotonal to extremely variable	Monotonal: Parkinson disease, depression
Loudness	Soft to loud	Environmental, psychological, systemic disease
Pitch	Low to high; glottal, raspy to falsetto	Variable: puberty Low: male gender, overuse
Register	Presence of voice	Vocal fatigue, overuse
Quality	Breathy to resonant	Vocal cord mass, paresis, bowing, atrophy

Examine the Respiratory System

Assess the airway. Stridor, a high-pitched inspiratory sound caused by turbulent air passing through a narrowed glottis secondary to inflammation or tumor, indicates an immediate referral to a specialist. If the patient is able to cough and laugh but cannot speak, this indicates a functional problem because coughing and laughing require total adduction of the vocal cords. Auscultate the lungs for quality of breath sounds, asthmatic wheezing, and signs of consolidation.

Note any associated stridor in children. Inspiratory stridor may indicate an extrathoracic problem, such as supraglottic collapse or vocal fold paralysis. An intrathoracic lesion may cause an expiratory stridor.

Perform a General Inspection

Note hair distribution, especially signs of hair loss over lateral eyebrows and hair loss on the scalp, to assess thyroid function. Look for the placement of the trachea and thyroid gland. Bulges or asymmetry of the neck suggest a tumor. A head and neck hemangioma or lymphangioma increases the possibility of a similar laryngeal lesion as the source of hoarseness.

Examine the Head and Neck

Examine the oral, pharyngeal, and nasal mucosa for signs of excessive dryness, inflammation, or infection. Excessive mucosal dryness, including the conjunctiva, may be secondary to use of medications such as decongestants and antidepressants or may be a symptom of an autoimmune disorder such as Sjögren syndrome.

Otoscopy may indicate otitis media with effusion contributing to hearing loss, a factor to be considered in voice abuse. Inspect the nasal mucosa for color, edema, and purulent discharge and examine the nasal septa for deviation that may cause obstruction. Hypertrophic tonsils and severe dental abnormalities (malocclusion, cleft palate) can contribute to hoarseness.

Any indication of airway obstruction associated with hoarseness is a potentially life-threatening situation. Do not perform a physical examination of the pharynx if you suspect acute epiglottitis. Examination may trigger laryngospasms and airway obstruction. Refer immediately for emergency treatment and airway support.

Examine the larynx indirectly using a laryngeal mirror. Patient cooperation is critical.

EVIDENCE-BASED PRACTICE *Are Specialists More Accurate Than Primary Care Providers in Diagnosing Voice Disorders?*

Accurate diagnosis of a voice disorder is an essential first step in choosing appropriate treatment. The objective of this study was to examine differences in laryngeal diagnosis over time in outpatients evaluated by primary care physicians (PCPs), otolaryngologists, or both. The study retrospectively analyzed data from a large, national, administrative US claims database. Participants were patients with a laryngeal disorder diagnosis from 2004 to 2008, with at least two outpatient visits by a PCP, otolaryngologist, or both and continuously enrolled for 12 months; 29,501 individuals met the inclusion criteria. The initial and final laryngeal diagnoses were tabulated. Results showed that more than half the patients in the PCP-to-otolaryngology group (referred), and one-third of the otolaryngology-to-otolaryngology group had different laryngeal diagnoses over time. Three-fourths of patients with an initial acute laryngitis diagnosis in the PCP–to-otolaryngology group and half of patients in the otolaryngology-to-otolaryngology group had a different final laryngeal diagnosis. Of patients with a final diagnosis of laryngeal cancer, one-fourth of the otolaryngology-to-otolaryngology group had an initial diagnosis of nonspecific dysphonia, and one-fifth of the PCP-to-otolaryngology group had an initial diagnosis of acute laryngitis.

Conclusion: Differential diagnosis of voice disorders often evolves over time, and the impacts on treatment and health care use are important areas of future study.

Reference: Cohen et al, 2014.

Ask the patient to open the mouth wide and extend the neck while protruding the tongue. The mirror is advanced to contact and lift the uvula while the patient breathes through the mouth. Focus the light on the mirror after the mirror is angled to visualize the larynx. Ask the patient to say "e" or "a" to observe movement. Sometimes the epiglottis obscures visualization. Direct examination of the larynx with a laryngoscope requires the skill and experience of a specialist.

Observe the larynx for the presence of secretions and evidence of ulcers, polyps, masses, edema, or redness. Observe for vocal cord motion, especially adduction and abduction of vocal cords, and the presence of spasm or tremor.

Assess Cranial Nerve Function

Most of the CNs play a part in speech and voice production, and any disease process that affects neurological function, especially vocal cord paralysis, may affect the voice. Specifically examine CNs V, VII, VIII, IX, X, XI, and XII.

Assess Hearing (Cranial Nerve VIII)

Voice or whisper testing for hearing acuity is the first level of hearing screening. An audible whisper is approximately 20 decibels (dB), and normal speech is about 50 dB. Patients with neurosensory hearing loss may speak at an abnormally loud volume.

Palpate Lymph Nodes

Palpate the cervicofacial lymph nodes. Tender nodes indicate inflammation; nontender nodes may indicate neoplasm. Enlarged nodes in the deep cervical chain in the absence of other symptoms may indicate laryngeal cancer.

Palpate Thyroid

Palpate the thyroid for size, tenderness, and crepitus by moving the thyroid cartilage across the cervical spine.

LABORATORY AND DIAGNOSTIC STUDIES

Flexible Fiberoptic Laryngoscopy

Laryngoscopy allows direct examination of the hypopharynx and larynx. A local anesthetic is applied to the oral or nasal mucosa, and the instrument is passed through the nose or oral cavity for excellent visualization of laryngeal structures. Laryngoscopy is also performed using a general anesthetic.

Radiography

Lateral view radiographs of soft tissues of the neck are used to evaluate structures for abnormalities.

Barium Esophagram

This contrast radiographic technique can be used to differentiate between mechanical lesions and motility disorders, providing important information about the latter in particular. For patients with esophageal dysphagia and a suspected motility disorder, barium esophagraphy should be performed first.

DIFFERENTIAL DIAGNOSIS

Acute Laryngitis

Acute laryngitis is a self-limiting condition caused by a viral infection, environmental irritants, postnasal drainage secondary to poorly controlled allergic rhinitis, or voice overuse. The loudness and quality of voice are affected, and the patient may report a sore throat. Hoarseness often progresses throughout the course of the day. Indirect examination of the larynx reveals redness and edema of the vocal cords. Physical pathology may be absent in mild cases.

Acute Epiglottitis

Adults will report severe and rapidly progressing symptoms of sore throat, dyspnea, and hoarseness. In children, there is no cough or hoarseness, but drooling with a forward leaning posture is observed. This condition is most commonly associated with *Haemophilus influenzae* infection. Voice quality is froglike. The patient will also have a high temperature and will be anxious, fearful, and restless with respiratory distress.

Trauma

Any swelling in response to trauma, directly to the larynx or indirectly to the throat, will cause hoarseness. Swelling might be secondary to head and neck surgery such as dental surgery, tonsillectomy, or thyroidectomy. Postintubation trauma may be acute if secondary to inflammation, or chronic if neurological or structural damage is irreversible. Mucosal abrasion or ulcer may be caused by direct trauma to the larynx and is associated with painful phonation and a breathy voice.

Acute Laryngeal Edema

Laryngeal edema may be one symptom in a generalized allergic response that involves the lips, tongue, and other hypopharyngeal structures. Drug reactions and food allergies, especially to seafood and nuts, often precipitate this response. This condition is a medical emergency because of the high risk of airway obstruction.

Laryngotracheobronchitis (Croup)

Subglottic edema is caused by a viral infection, most often parainfluenza virus 1 that can obstruct the airway. This condition is most common in children ages 3 months to 3 years and is more prevalent in the fall and winter. It is associated with a barking cough, dyspnea, wheezing, low-grade fever, and hoarseness. Inspiratory stridor occurs abruptly because of narrowing of the passage, causing negative pressures generated on inspiration. Physical examination can determine the degree of respiratory distress such as color, stridor, nasal flaring, and level of consciousness.

Chronic Laryngitis

This condition is associated with a combination of chronic exposure to working conditions with high levels of dust, fumes, or noise; hard liquor consumption; cigarette smoking; and a history of frequent and persistent cough. Physical examination reveals edema or nodules of the vocal cords.

Polyps

Vocal cord polyps develop as a result of chronic inflammation from voice abuse, allergies, or GERD. The voice quality is breathy. With dependent polyps, the patient may report that symptoms of hoarseness change with position.

Neoplasm

Laryngeal cancer usually occurs in patients who have a long history of cigarette smoking and alcohol consumption. Hoarseness is characterized by a raspy or harsh voice. Physical examination may reveal leukoplakia or a white scaly appearance of the vocal cords. Patients do not usually report pain until carcinoma is advanced. Pain secondary to ulceration is late and is often perceived as ear pain, especially when swallowing.

Gastroesophageal Reflux Disease

Patients with GERD will report retrosternal burning (heartburn) that radiates upward. The regurgitation of gastric acid is exacerbated by consuming large meals, lying in a supine position, or bending over. Patients may describe a sour taste, experience salivary hypersecretion, have painful swallowing, or have a chronic cough or habit of throat clearing. Physical examination will be normal or epigastric tenderness may be elicited by abdominal examination. Inflammation or ulceration may be visible on the vocal cords.

Hypothyroidism

One symptom of hypothyroidism is a low, gravelly voice. The degree of hoarseness depends on the severity of thyroid deficiency. Usually hypothyroidism is suspected when other symptoms are present such as cold intolerance; rough, scaly skin texture; weight gain; and signs such as bradycardia and prolonged deep tendon reflex recovery. Risk factors for hypothyroidism include increased age, postpartum status, and a family history of thyroid disease. The thyroid gland may be nonpalpable or enlarged. Examination of the larynx may reveal edema or polyps. An elevated serum thyroid-stimulating hormone level will confirm the diagnosis.

Vocal Cord Paralysis

Paralysis is usually unilateral and produces a weak, breathy voice. Unilateral abductor paralysis on the left side is caused by pressure on the vagus or recurrent laryngeal nerve by a mass of malignant glands in the superior mediastinum or carcinoma of the thyroid or esophagus.

Psychogenic Hoarseness

Patients with psychogenic hoarseness will have a low, breathy voice caused by voluntarily abducting the vocal cords during phonation. Physical examination will reveal no abnormalities. Psychogenic hoarseness may follow a traumatic event.

Laryngeal Papillomas

These are the most common laryngeal lesions that occur during childhood. Most patients are between the ages of 2 and 7 years and present with hoarseness. Occasionally papillomas, caused by the human papillomavirus, are seen in newborns.

▶ **DIFFERENTIAL DIAGNOSIS OF** *Common Causes of Hoarseness*

CONDITION	HISTORY	PHYSICAL FINDINGS	DIAGNOSTIC STUDIES
Acute laryngitis	Voice overuse, exposure to environmental irritants, recent URI	Voice quality: aphonia, cervical lymphadenopathy; pharyngitis; edema and redness of vocal cords	None, if duration of hoarseness is <3 wk
Acute epiglottitis	*Adults:* rapid onset of sore throat, dyspnea, hoarseness *Children:* drooling, forward-leaning posture	Voice quality froglike; fever, signs of respiratory distress; drooling	Possible airway support; lateral and AP radiographic views of neck
Trauma	Hoarseness after intubation; direct throat trauma or foreign body	Subluxation of cricoarytenoid joint	Lateral and AP radiographic views of neck; laryngoscopy
Acute laryngeal edema	History of food or drug allergy	Edema of lips, tongue, and hypopharynx; observe for respiratory distress; voice quality breathy	Possible airway support
Laryngotracheobronchitis (croup)	Children 3 mo–3 yr; recent URI	Barking cough, low-grade fever, wheezing, hoarseness; edema of vocal cords; observe for signs of respiratory distress	None initially, airway support may be necessary
Chronic laryngitis	Chronic history of smoking and alcohol use; exposure to environmental irritants; chronic cough; duration of hoarseness >3 wk	Edema of vocal cords; nodules may be present	Lateral and AP radiographic views of neck; laryngoscopy
Polyps	History of allergy; voice abuse, GERD, smoker; duration of symptoms >3 wk; progressive hoarseness, worse at end of day, but near normal in morning; hoarseness may change with position	Polyps visible on vocal cords	ENT referral for biopsy

Continued

▶ DIFFERENTIAL DIAGNOSIS OF *Common Causes of Hoarseness—cont'd*

CONDITION	HISTORY	PHYSICAL FINDINGS	DIAGNOSTIC STUDIES
Neoplasm	Smoking, airborne exposure, chronic alcohol use, history of chronic cough, hoarseness for >3 wk	Tracheal deviation; pain with advanced tumor; hoarseness may be only sign	ENT referral for biopsy
GERD	History of upper GI burning; cough especially at night; chronic use of alcohol, NSAIDs, or aspirin; history of ulcer disease, smoker, age younger than 45 yr; frequent throat clearing	May have epigastric tenderness on palpation; vocal cord inflammation or ulcers	Referral for endoscopy if symptoms not relieved with medication or dietary alterations
Hypothyroidism	Presence of systemic symptoms, such as cold intolerance, weight gain, fatigue; age older than 65 yr; postpartum; family history of thyroid disease	Normal or enlarged thyroid gland, coarse hair, very dry skin, prolonged DTR recovery	TSH, free T_4 index
Vocal cord paralysis	Chronic cough; inspiratory or expiratory stridor with exertion	Breathy, weak, soft voice; abnormal movement (usually unilateral) of vocal cords; examination may suggest specific CN involvement	Refer for ENT evaluation
Psychogenic hoarseness	History of psychiatric illness, or psychological trauma	Breathy, low voice; larynx will appear normal	As indicated to rule out other causes (i.e., lateral and AP radiographic views of neck); laryngoscopy
Laryngeal papillomas	Children 2–12 yr and may occur in infants; history of maternal human papillomavirus; may be recurrent, progressive	Faint cry, severe stridor, voice change, or complete aphonia	Refer for ENT evaluation

AP, anteroposterior; *CN,* cranial nerve; *DTR,* deep tendon reflex; *ENT,* ear, nose, and throat; *GERD,* gastroesophageal reflux disease; *GI,* gastrointestinal; *NSAIDs,* nonsteroidal antiinflammatory drugs; *T₄,* thyroxine; *TSH,* thyroid-stimulating hormone; *URI,* upper respiratory tract infection.

Lower Extremity Limb Pain

A useful framework for differentiating limb pain involves determining whether symptoms are caused by musculoskeletal injury, musculoskeletal or joint disease, systemic disease, or a combination of factors. Pain can result from direct reaction in tissues, secondary reaction in adjacent tissues, or referral from a proximal or distal lesion or from organs such as the heart or kidney. For example, lower extremity pain is often referred from the low back and emanates from irritated nerve roots, or pain is secondary to myofascial syndromes of the low back, pelvic, and hip musculature. In children, aches and pains in limbs are common. However, the presence, location, and intensity of the pain are often difficult to assess.

DIAGNOSTIC REASONING: FOCUSED HISTORY

Is the pain related to an urgent problem that needs immediate treatment to avoid disability or death?

Key Questions
- Have you had a recent injury?
- Can you describe exactly how the injury occurred?
- Do you have any other symptoms such as fatigue, fever, or swollen joints?
- What is the severity of the pain? Does it occur with exercise or rest?

Injury
Injuries to the musculoskeletal system can range from simple muscle strain to a significant fracture associated with nerve or vascular injury. Therefore, when a patient has a history of trauma, the priority is to assess the vascular integrity of the limb. Neurologic integrity is next. Symptoms of coldness,

severe pain, or paresthesia are signals the that physical examination should immediately assess the extent of injury and the need for emergency treatment. Acute pain and swelling that follow trauma usually indicate injury to a previously normal structure. Compartment syndrome is an injury that involves both vascular integrity and neurologic functioning. This condition develops when trauma to an extremity causes swelling and pressure that compromises blood flow to the affected muscles and nerves. Surgical decompression is needed, and prompt diagnosis is crucial to avoid amputation and other complications.

If the injury does not warrant urgent attention, obtain further history. Ask questions that specify the mechanism of injury, such as a direct blow or impact, landing position after a fall, twisting, jumping, running, overstretching, or overuse. A severe crush injury puts the patient at high risk for developing compartment syndrome—among other complications—in the crushed limb. When discussing the precipitating event, ask the patient to describe any noise, such as snapping, popping, or breaking that may have occurred with the injury.

Constitutional Symptoms
The presence of generalized symptoms, such as fever, weight loss, general malaise, or hot swollen joints, suggests the presence of a systemic disorder such as infection or rheumatic disease. Infection in a child causes systemic illness and the child appears ill.

Fever related to joint problems can be the result of hematogenous seeding by an organism, direct invasion as a result of trauma or puncture, or migration from an adjacent area of infection. In rheumatic fever, a β-hemolytic streptococcal infection precedes the initial joint pain by 1 to 3 weeks. Often the hip joint may be the first of many joints affected before polyarticular migratory involvement occurs. The fever is sustained, not intermittent. Fever spikes are seen with chronic forms of arthritis in children.

Severity of Pain

Unrelenting diffuse pain, often occurring at night, is an indication of bone involvement either through bone cancer or an infection such as osteomyelitis, arthritis, or septic hip. Claudication and neurogenic pain increase with activity and decrease with rest; more immediately for vascular causes and more slowly for neurogenic causes.

Severe nontraumatic pain that occurs with pallor, paresthesia, or paralysis in a cold limb may be the result of acute limb ischemia, which requires emergent treatment to avoid amputation. Acute limb ischemia is often the result of worsening atherosclerotic peripheral vascular disease, in which a narrowed artery becomes occluded secondary to thrombosis or embolism. On examination, the affected limb will have diminished or absent peripheral pulses. Acute limb ischemia requires urgent consultation with a vascular surgeon for possible revascularization.

In young children, failure to voluntarily move an arm or leg can be a sign of pain and is called pseudoparalysis.

Radiating leg pain associated with saddle anesthesia and loss of bladder or bowel control may indicate cauda equine syndrome and requires immediate surgical intervention (see Chapter 24).

What does the location of the pain tell me?

Key Questions
- Where does it hurt?
- Is the pain local or generalized?

Location

Location of pain provides a clue for identifying the site where the pain originates. Local pain receptors signal the site of irritation, and an increase in sensitivity (hyperesthesia) results. Referred pain generally involves the muscle chains, nerve pathways, and vessels. Unilateral, circumscribed limb or quadrant pain involves autonomic nerve fibers.

Bilateral pain is more likely to originate from systemic involvement. Diffuse pain with inconsistent distribution may be the result of psychosomatic conditions such as depression and anxiety. Diffuse pain over trigger points is indicative of fibromyalgia. Collagen diseases and connective tissue diseases can affect one or more joints. The more vaguely defined the boundaries of the pain, the deeper or more central is the location of the somatic irritation. The obturator nerve has sensory branches that innervate the hip and skin on the medial aspect of the thigh, causing pain that originates in the hip but is referred to the knee.

Could this be caused by a sprain or strain?

Key Questions
- Describe how the injury occurred.
- Did you hear a noise with the injury, such as a ripping or cracking sound?
- Were you able to use the limb after the injury?

Strain

Whereas strains involve injury to muscles and tendons, sprains involve injury to ligamentous structures. Both types of injuries can produce a ripping or tearing sound and range in severity from minor damage to a complete tear. Injuries are generally classified as mild, moderate, or severe. A moderate to severe strain or sprain may involve some loss of joint or ligament stability. Strains may be acute or chronic. Ankle injury commonly occurs when lateral stress is applied while the joint is plantar flexed. This position is the least stable position of the ankle, and the overstretched ligaments are more susceptible to eversion or inversion forces.

Sprain

Sprains cause minimal to moderate pain, increasing 1 to 2 days after the trauma when the inflammatory process begins. A complete disruption that severs the sensory nerve fibers within the structure will cause little pain, whereas a partial injury irritates sensory fibers, and may produce intense pain.

In children, ligaments and joint capsules are two to five times stronger than the epiphysis; therefore, growth plate injuries are more common than sprains.

Fracture

A fracture produces diffuse swelling around the injured bone soon after injury. Deformity will be present if the fracture is displaced. A patient may report hearing a crack and being disabled by the increased severity of pain with weight bearing or movement of the limb. With a stress fracture, there may be mild swelling and tenderness and pain with weight bearing.

If there is no history of trauma or a precipitating event, what else is causing the pain?

Key Questions

- Can you describe your usual daily activities at home, at work, and with hobbies?
- How does the pain affect your activities?
- Do you have other illnesses?

Activities

A person may adapt to chronic musculoskeletal problems by using an assistive device, such as a cane, or by limiting activities. Rheumatic disorders produce symmetrical discomfort and pain with inactivity. Noninflammatory conditions are often associated with asymmetrical pain after extended use. Children will often avoid walking on a limb that causes pain. Infants will have lack of movement of the limb with irritability and fussiness when the limb is moved passively.

Other Illnesses

The presence of coronary artery disease increases the risk of arterial insufficiency and associated claudication pain. Peripheral neuropathy associated with diabetes can produce numbness and burning pain or "pins and needles" sensation, especially in the lower extremities. Pain may be sequelae of a prior cerebrovascular accident or Gillian-Barre syndrome.

History of Injury

In joint pain with injury, what do I need to know about the specific joints involved?

Key Questions

- Is the pain affected by weight bearing or activity?
- Did you feel a sense of "giving way"?
- Did you hear a pop, tear, or other sound?
- In what position was your leg when the injury occurred?

Continuing with an activity means the injury did not totally disrupt any ligamentous structures. An inability to straighten or bend the knee suggests a mechanical disruption such as a patellar dislocation or meniscus tear. In chondromalacia, the patient can bend the knee, but the movement is usually painful.

A loud pop is virtually diagnostic of an anterior cruciate ligament (ACL) tear. A ripping sound suggests a meniscus injury. A cracking sound may signify a bony injury or dislocation of the patella.

A quick change in direction, or a sudden stop, may put more force on the ligaments than they can dissipate, resulting in an acute rupture. A sudden twisting injury is likely to represent a meniscus tear and a serious ligament disruption. Running or jumping activities are commonly associated with knee and ankle injuries.

In children, 10% to 20% of knee symptoms are the result of a problem in the hip joint.

Could this be musculoskeletal or joint disease?

Key Questions

- Can you describe the pain?

In general, sharp, piercing, stabbing, cutting, pinching, and gnawing pain is most common with lesions of the nerves and skin. Dull, tearing, boring, burning, and cramping are common terms used to describe pain arising from deeper structures such as muscles and joints. Pulsating, pounding, throbbing, and hammering are common descriptions of vascular pain. Gradually increasing sensations of pressure, tension, heaviness, and calf pain indicate venous obstruction. Severe pain that develops over 1 to 4 days is typical of osteomyelitis or septic arthritis and is an emergency condition.

Muscle pain is caused by receptors located in bursa, muscle fibers, ligaments, and tendon attachments. It is a diffuse, dull, gnawing, boring, or tearing pain that increases with use and decreases with rest.

Intraarticular pain arises from receptors of the synovial membrane, joint capsule, or the fibrochondral layers of the articular surfaces. Joint pain is either inflammatory or degenerative. Inflammatory joint pain radiates diffusely to surrounding tissues. It is intense, sharp, burning, boring, or pulsating (effusion) pain. It persists during rest and is evident especially at night, worsening in the morning with stiffness that lasts more than 45 minutes and improving throughout the day.

Degenerative joint pain radiates to the soft tissue structures around the joint (i.e., muscles, ligaments, tendons). It is a dull, gnawing sensation associated with muscle pain, or it can be a sharp, acute pain that increases with overuse.

Bone lesions cause a dull ache; periosteal pain is sharp, not well localized, and increases in intensity with dependency of the extremity.

Neuralgic pain occurs in the distribution of a peripheral nerve or nerve root. The pain is stabbing, burning or cutting.

What does the history of swelling tell me?

Key Questions
- Is there any swelling?
- When did the swelling begin?

Swelling

Swelling around a joint is always abnormal. Children do not always recognize swelling; they often report that they cannot squat down or flex their knee fully because it feels "full or tight." Generally, swelling secondary to trauma develops immediately or within 2 hours after an injury; swelling 6 to 24 hours after an injury is usually of synovial origin such as a meniscal tear, subluxation, dislocation, or ligamentous damage. Swelling after 24 hours suggests an inflammatory response.

Is this an acute or a chronic problem?

Key Questions
- When did the pain first occur?
- When did you first notice a problem?

Pain experienced hours after an injury or physical activity is usually caused by acute extensor injury or overuse. Severe ligament sprain is manifested as an immediately disabling pain at the moment of the injury.

Determining if the complaint is acute or chronic helps differentiate the cause. Whereas chronic joint problems compound each other, intermittent or episodic pain is characteristic of diseases of the musculoskeletal system. In children, limping or not using the extremity may be a signal that the child is experiencing pain. Parents will often note the loss of motion in an extremity or an awkward gait; they often report that the child is unable to perform routine activities.

How is activity affected?

Key Questions
- What are your usual activities?
- What activity makes the pain worse?
- What movements make the pain worse?

Repetitive microtrauma in the lower extremities from inappropriate rate and intensity of training, poorly fitting shoes, or unsuitable playing surfaces can cause stress fractures of the weight-bearing bones of the lower limbs. Pain is worse over the site of the fracture.

In children, pain in the groin or referred to the knee and anterior thigh that is intermittent after activity and gradually becomes constant may indicate Legg-Calvé-Perthes disease (LCPD).

Intraarticular lesions usually worsen with joint motion and sports activities. Intraosseous tumors are less sensitive to joint motion.

In children with a septic hip, pain increases with movement.

What does joint stiffness or locking tell me?

Key Questions
- Have you had any joint stiffness?
- Does activity make the stiffness worse or better?
- Do you have locking of the knee?

Joint Locking

Locking of the knee is an abrupt occurrence in which the patient complains that something "gets in the way" and is unable to fully extend the knee. Manipulation of the leg often results in an equally abrupt unlocking. This is usually a sign of a chronic unstable meniscus tear. Stiffness is a common feature of any inflammatory arthropathy. Whereas arthritic stiffness and pain are alleviated by activity, mechanical problems are aggravated by activity.

What does the history of a limp tell me?

Key Questions
• Is there pain with the limp?
• Did the limp develop suddenly?
• Is the limp constant or intermittent?
• What is the effect of running or climbing stairs?

Limp

Limping is a pathological alteration of a smooth, regular gait pattern and is never normal. Gait can be divided into two phases: stance and swing. The stance phase starts with the foot in contact with the ground and ends with the toe being lifted off the ground; the limb supports all the body weight. The swing phase begins with the toe elevated from the ground and ends with the heel strike. During the swing phase, the foot is not touching the ground; the pelvis rotates forward and tilts slightly while the trunk maintains a neutral position. Limp after strenuous running may indicate a stress fracture.

Quadriceps weakness causes difficulty in climbing stairs. During ambulation, this weakness causes the knee to be unstable on heel strike, and assistance is needed to push the knee manually into an extended position. A knee flexion contracture of just 5 degrees increases risk for fall.

Neuromuscular diseases can result in progressive and painless muscle weakness or spasticity that affects ambulation in a variety of ways.

Symptoms of pain and limping in children may be incorrectly attributed to trauma instead of a more serious problem such as neoplastic tumors or bone infections.

Could this be caused by systemic disease?

Key Questions
• Have you been treated with antibiotics recently?
• Have you had any recent immunizations?
• Does the pain awaken you at night?
• Is the pain worse at night?

Medications

Certain antibiotics can cause serum sickness in children, producing joint pain and fever. In adults, fluoroquinolone antibiotics can produce tendinitis or tendon rupture.

Night Pain

Intense pain may occur at rest and during the night. At first, the pain may occur only when the patient changes position while sleeping. However, sleep becomes disrupted as the pain increases. Report by an adolescent of night pain is a red flag for the intraosseous pain of a bone tumor. Pain in the lower limbs in children 6 to 12 years of age who are in a rapid linear growth period may cause the child to awaken at night. The cause of these "growing pains" is unknown, but they are thought to result from muscle structures that have to catch up with bone growth. The pains are usually bilateral with no objective findings.

Could Lyme disease be the cause of pain?

Key Questions
• Have you been camping or spending time in wooded areas?
• Have you noticed any skin rashes?

Lyme Disease

Lyme disease is an infection caused by the tick-borne spirochete *Borrelia burgdorferi*. Early symptoms include diffuse arthralgias, myalgias, fever, chills, and a characteristic targetlike rash. The arthralgia may involve multiple joints, but the knee is most often affected. Joint manifestations occur 1 week to 2 years after the initial illness. Patients may or may not recall the antecedent tick bite or exposure.

Key Questions

- Have you had anything like this before?
- Do you have a chronic disease?
- Could you have been exposed to any sexually transmitted infection?
- Have you been treated with cortisone?

Chronic Conditions

Chronic diseases, such as sickle cell anemia, inflammatory bowel disease, Crohn disease, hypothyroidism, hyperthyroidism, and collagen vascular diseases, are frequently associated with skin rashes, psoriasis, and limb and joint pain.

Gonorrhea disseminates to the musculoskeletal system in 1% to 3% of individuals with the disease. Of these, more than 80% develop arthritis. *C. trachomatis infection can produce a triad of symptoms that include arthritis, uveitis, and urethritis.*

Patients with chronic illness that requires long-term administration of corticosteroids are at risk for cortisone-induced necrosis of the hip. Sickle cell anemia can cause hip pain during a sickle cell crisis. Viral infections may cause diffuse myalgia.

Is this a mixed condition?

Consider the possibility that a patient may have a condition that is a mix of factors such as a systemic disorder that has resulted in an acute injury. Clues to mixed etiology might include an injury that seems out of proportion to the extent of the precipitating activity or the presence of a chronic condition and other symptoms that might point to an undetected chronic condition. It is important to evaluate the limb pain in the context of the whole person.

DIAGNOSTIC REASONING: FOCUSED PHYSICAL EXAMINATION

Evaluation of musculoskeletal injuries should include examination of joint stability, deformity, and function. Examination should be done as soon as possible after an injury for an accurate diagnosis. Observe for symmetry, and then functionally assess limbs and joints bilaterally beginning with the unaffected side. Order the examination so that the most painful tests will be done last. Figures 22.1 and 22.2 illustrate anatomical landmarks of the knee and ankle. Table 22.2 describes selected tests used to assess for lower extremity musculoskeletal disorders.

Observe the Patient

Subtle clues of physical abuse must be considered when the patient history is not consistent with the type or extent of injury. Abuse should always be considered in an infant when symptoms and history suggest a fracture, multiple injuries, rotational injuries, or multiple bruises in different stages of healing. Radiographs may show previous fractures.

People who have septic joints appear ill, and movement of the joint will increase the pain. Inspect the patient with minimal clothing obstructing your view of movements. A child with a septic hip lies with the thigh in a position of flexion, abduction, and external rotation and cries when the lower limb is moved.

In adults, an internally rotated abducted leg is the posture assumed with a posterior hip dislocation. An externally rotated hip and shortened lower extremity are signs of hip fracture.

General stiffness or limitation of motion of a joint causes the surrounding joints to accommodate by moving with greater excursion or range of movement than usual. This makes the gait appear irregular or jerky.

Look for Limp

Pain, weakness, and deformity cause limping. Limping will be accentuated if the patient is asked to walk on the heels or tiptoes.

Common abnormal gaits related to limping are Trendelenburg gait, antalgic gait, and circumduction gait. Trendelenburg gait is a ducklike gait that reflects unilateral weakness of the gluteus medius muscle. The pelvis drops on the unaffected side during weight bearing on the affected side. In antalgic gait, there is an acute one-sided limp because the patient takes quick soft steps to shorten the

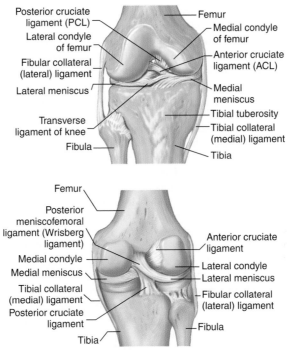

FIGURE 22.1 Basic anatomy of the right knee. (From Patton K, Thibodeau G: *Anatomy and physiology,* ed. 9, St. Louis, 2016, Elsevier.)

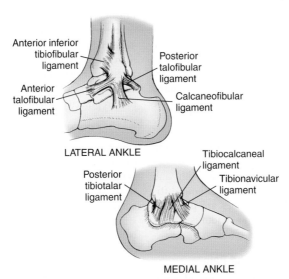

FIGURE 22.2 The lateral ankle ligaments—anterior and posterior talofibular (ATF and PTF, respectively) and calcaneofibular (CF). Also shown are the anterior inferior tibiofibular (AITF) ligament and the beginning of the interosseous membrane (IM). (From Auerbach P: *Wilderness medicine,* St. Louis, 2007, Mosby.)

period of weight bearing on the involved extremity. Stance time on the affected limb is decreased while stride length of the opposite side is shortened, allowing a quicker return of weight bearing to the unaffected limb. This is a reflex response to weight bearing on a painful limb.

Circumduction gait is seen with pathology of the foot or ankle and reduces discomfort by limiting movement of the ankle. The gait is characterized by a circular outward swing of the leg and external rotation of the foot that requires less ankle movement. External rotation of the entire extremity is seen with slipped capital femoral epiphysis. A video of abnormal gaits can be viewed at https://www.youtube.com/watch?v=Q98WKpwIpkE.

Have the patient stand on one foot and then the other. When standing on one leg, the gluteus medius on that side maintains the opposite side of the pelvis level, balancing the trunk over the weight-bearing hip. If the hip abductors are weak or painful, the opposite side of the pelvis dips down during the stance phase. With each step, the trunk shifts toward the side of a painful or weak extremity to decrease the force transmitted through the extremity to the hip.

Assessment of gait is best done either before or after examination, when patients are less aware that they are being observed.

Ankle plantar flexion and dorsiflexion are necessary for normal gait. If plantar flexion is restricted, there is no push-off, and the forefoot and heel come off the floor at the same time. The result is a higher knee lift, and the forefoot may slap against the floor. This condition is seen with weakness from peroneal nerve injury or with the painful dorsiflexion associated with shin splints.

Observe the patient walking with and without shoes. If a child walks without difficulty with shoes off, the shoes are probably the problem. Inadequate shoe width is a common source of foot pain in children.

Have the Patient Locate the Pain

Have the patient point to the area of pain. Location of pain and the actual area of pathology may not be consistent. Hip pain often is referred to the knee area because the anterior branch of the obturator nerve passes close to the hip joint and, if irritated, provides a painful sensation to the medial side of the knee. True hip joint pain arises in the trochanteric bursa and is perceived in the groin area.

Pain in the groin, lateral hip, or knee in a child may indicate LCPD.

Pain in the groin, buttocks, or lateral hip in a child may indicate slipped femoral capital epiphysis.

Vague, nebulous discomfort in the front of the thighs, in the calves, and behind the knees located outside of the joints in a child may indicate growing pains.

Note Any Deformities

Fractures generally produce unilateral deformities or swelling in the extremities. Inflammatory and degenerative joint diseases produce observable joint swelling and deformity that usually occurs bilaterally.

Assess Vital Signs

Elevated temperatures are seen with neoplastic, systemic, and infectious processes such as osteomyelitis, septic arthritis and septic hip in children, and rheumatic disease. Neonates may not exhibit a fever with a septic hip but may refuse to feed and will exhibit other symptoms of septicemia such as lethargy and subnormal temperature. Palpate for the quality and presence of pulses in any injured limb and compare with the opposite side. Assess peripheral pulses for presence, rate, regularity, strength, and equality.

Inspect the Skin and Nails

Chronic venous obstruction in the lower extremities causes a brownish coloring of the skin, and arterial insufficiency causes thin, shiny skin with an absence of hair and brittle nails.

Lyme disease usually presents with a rash before joint involvement; however, rash may occur concurrently. The rash, characteristically found on the trunk, begins as an erythematous papule that develops into an annular lesion with a clear center. Concentric rings may develop, giving it a bull's-eye appearance (erythema migrans).

Inspect the skin for redness and inflammation. Look for a puncture or an abscess that could be the source of infection and seeding if a septic joint or osteomyelitis is suspected. Swelling and redness in a joint or in the midshaft of the tibia may be caused by osteomyelitis.

Look for an ingrown toenail that may alter gait. When the nails are trimmed by rounding off the edges, the hypertrophied and inflamed soft tissue fold can overlap the nail, and ingrowth at the distal margin will occur. Ingrown toenail pain is enhanced when tight-fitting shoes compress the soft tissues around the nail.

Look for ecchymosis and bruising. These indicate trauma as a source for pain and raise the suspicion of abuse. Ecchymosis indicates underlying bleeding and disruption of soft tissue or bone. Ecchymosis changes color over a period of days. Initially, the color is dark red or violet, and in 1 to 3 days, the bruise is blue-brown; in 1 week, it is yellow-green; and after 1 week, it is light brown. Ecchymosis resolves within 2 to 4 weeks.

Ecchymosis in the popliteal fossa after dislocation of the knee may be a sign of arterial disruption. Hemarthrosis, or bleeding into a joint, usually occurs within 1 to 2 hours after an injury and can occur secondary to hemophilia or other bleeding disorders, or it can be associated with visible ecchymoses caused by blood leaking into soft tissues.

Swelling and redness of a joint indicate underlying infection or inflammation. Edema will present as an asymmetrical area of swelling. Effusion, or fluid in the joint capsule, distends the joint in a smooth, symmetrical manner.

Observe the muscles around the painful limb area. Decreased muscle tone or atrophy from disuse begins immediately after injury, although it will not be clinically apparent for approximately 1 week. Neurologic injury may also be a cause of atrophy.

Asymmetrical gluteal folds may indicate a congenital dislocated hip (Fig. 22.3).

Measure Limb Circumference and Length

Use a tape measure to locate points at which to measure and compare limb circumference. Differences may be the result of muscle atrophy or edema. Measure the circumference of both calves in a patient who has unilateral lower limb edema. Measurements are taken 10 cm inferior to the anterior tibial tuberosity and compared bilaterally. A difference of 2 to 3 cm is considered a significant discrepancy and may indicate deep vein thrombosis (DVT) in a swollen leg.

To measure leg length, have the patient lie supine with legs in comparable positions and measure the distance from the anterior iliac spine to the medial malleoli of the ankles. If a discrepancy is found, ask the patient to lie supine with knees flexed 90 degrees and

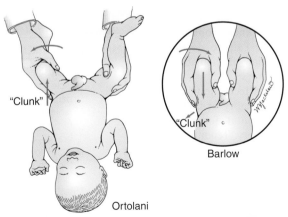

FIGURE 22.3 Ortolani sign for congenital dislocation of the hip. A "click" is palpable or audible as the hip is reduced by abduction. If the test result is negative, the examination should always be repeated in 2 to 4 months. (Swartz MH: *Textbook of physical diagnosis: history and examination*, ed. 7, Philadelphia, 2014, Saunders.)

feet flat on the table. If one knee is higher, the tibia of that extremity is longer. If one knee projects further anteriorly, the femur of that extremity is longer.

Palpate Extremities and Joints

Always palpate those areas that are suspected to be painless first and then compare with the affected limb.

Determine if there is edema (e.g., presence of interstitial fluid). Induration is interstitial swelling that has progressed and is now firm. An effusion is a collection of fluid in the joint capsule, which can be the result of rupture of a vascular structure or a synovial secretory response to an inflammatory process. The consistency of the fluid is noteworthy. Pus has a thick consistency and is less fluctuant than synovial fluid. Hematoma has a more gel-like consistency. Swelling in an ankle sprain is diffuse and nonfluctuant. Knee ligament sprain is much more fluctuant. To assess for fluid in the knee joint, press above the knee and watch the concave or shallow areas of the joint become distended and bulge on either side of the kneecap. Note that swelling can extend above and below the point of pathology.

In severe knee trauma, rupture of the capsule allows fluid to escape into surrounding tissues, and less distention may be more apparent than with lesser injuries.

Palpate for fluid bulge if the knee is painful. Milk up the fluid into the suprapatellar pouch and then bring the hand down the lateral aspect of the knee, looking for a medial fluid bulge. Palpate deeply to detect muscle fibrillation, fasciculation, or tumors.

Feel for heat in the affected joint, which can indicate an inflammatory or infectious process. Evaluate the joint for crepitus, both palpable and auditory. Tendinitis may produce a grating sensation on palpation of the ligament or a grating sound with movement.

Perform Passive and Active Range of Motion of the Hips, Knees, and Ankles

Range of motion (ROM) may be limited because of pain, weakness, or deformity.

If there is joint pathology, pain will be the same with active and passive motion. If the disease is outside the joint or extraarticular, passive motion may be painless, but active motion produces pain. During passive tests, move the joint until an end point or end range is felt to help determine the affected structure.

There are six end points to note when assessing joint movement: (1) bone-to-bone sensation, felt with an osteophyte or abnormal bone development; (2) spasm, which can indicate severe ligamentous injury; (3) capsular feel or a firm arrested movement with some give to it, which can indicate chronic joint effusion, arthritis, or capsular scarring; (4) spring block or joint rebound at the end of range of movement, caused by an articular derangement or an intraarticular body; (5) tissue approximation, a normal end feel caused by tissue limiting further movement, such as the biceps muscle limiting elbow flexion; and (6) empty end feel, present when there is no tissue resistance, but the patient stops the movement because of pain. This last condition indicates bursitis, extraarticular abscess, or tumor.

Test for Muscle Strength

Test for lower extremity flexor and extensor strength against resistance of both the proximal and distal muscle groups (Table 22.1). Proximal muscle weakness is seen in myopathic

Table 22.1	**Muscle Strength Test**	
GRADE	MUSCLE STRENGTH	TERM
0	No palpable contraction	Zero
1	Muscle contracts but part does not move	Trace
2	Muscle moves part but not against gravity	Poor
3	Muscle moves part through range against gravity	Fair
4	Muscle moves part even with resistance	Good
5	Normal strength against resistance present	Excellent

disorders. Distal muscle weakness is seen secondary to a neuropathic process. Generally, if the opposite side is normal, strength should be compared with it.

In the presence of significant pain, muscle strength may be unreliable. If the contraction is strong and painful, the pathology is caused by mild musculotendinous damage. If the contraction is weak and painful, the pathology is the result of severe musculotendinous damage. If the contraction is weak and painless, the pathology results from a neurologic lesion (paresis).

Perform a Neurologic Examination

A complete assessment of sensory and motor function and deep tendon reflexes should be done on the affected and contralateral limbs. If systemic illness is suspected, perform a complete neurologic examination. A referral is indicated if initial treatment does not adequately control pain, if function loss is present, or if the patient is immunocompromised.

LABORATORY AND DIAGNOSTIC STUDIES

Complete Blood Count

A complete blood count is obtained to evaluate for anemia associated with chronic disease, infection, or neoplasm. An altered white blood cell (WBC) count may indicate infection or leukemia.

Erythrocyte Sedimentation Rate

An erythrocyte sedimentation rate (ESR) is elevated when inflammation is present. It is a nonspecific test.

Joint Aspiration

Joint aspiration is performed to assess synovial fluid for elevated WBC count, Gram stain, culture and sensitivity, crystal analysis, presence of glucose, and consistency or "string test." This procedure is performed using local anesthesia under sterile technique. Synovial fluid will flow easily when the joint capsule is penetrated.

Radiography

Obtain at least two radiographic views, anteroposterior and lateral, because injuries are not always apparent on a single view. Any evidence of fracture or dislocation will require orthopedic attention. Sometimes radiographic comparisons with the opposite limb may be useful. Traumatic knee injuries should include four radiographic views: anteroposterior, lateral, tunnel (intracondylar notch), and a 30-degree sunrise (patella). Magnetic resonance imaging (MRI), computed tomography (CT), or bone scanning is usually ordered by a specialist. MRI is usually used in spine, joint, and soft tissue imaging. CT scans are usually performed for bone visualization.

Antinuclear Antibodies

Antinuclear antibody (ANA) tests are positive with high titers in rheumatoid arthritis (RA) and systemic lupus erythematosus (SLE). However, other conditions, such as advanced age, medications, and other connective tissue disease, can produce positive antibody titers.

Rheumatoid Factor

Rheumatoid factor (RF) is the single most useful test to confirm a diagnosis of RA and is positive in 80% of patients with this disease. RF can be positive years before clinical symptoms appear.

C4 Complement

C4 complement determines serum hemolytic complement activity, a protein that binds antigen–antibody complexes for the purpose of lysis. Complement is increased in active inflammatory disease and in autoimmune disorders such as juvenile rheumatoid arthritis.

C-Reactive Protein

C-reactive protein (CRP) indicates the presence of abnormal plasma protein or a nonspecific response to inflammation caused by both infectious and noninfectious processes. CRP is elevated in RA and infection.

Lyme Titer Enzyme-Linked Immunosorbent Assay Serology

Enzyme-linked immunosorbent assay (ELISA) detects antibodies against *B. burgdorferi*, which causes Lyme disease. However, it may not detect antibodies for several weeks after the onset of infection.

DIFFERENTIAL DIAGNOSIS

Causes of emergent lower extremity pain

Compartment syndrome

Acute compartment syndrome is an injury that involves both vascular integrity and neurological functioning. This condition develops when trauma to an extremity, often fractures to long bones, causes swelling and pressure that compromises blood flow to the affected muscles and nerves. Surgical decompression is needed, and prompt diagnosis is crucial to avoid amputation and other complications.

Cauda equine syndrome

Compression of the S1 nerve root produces back pain, bladder and bowel dysfunction, and motor weakness of the lower extremities with radiculopathy (see Chapter 24). This syndrome is a surgical emergency.

Causes of non-emergent lower extremity pain
Musculoskeletal Inflammation

Tenosynovitis (tendinitis)

Soft tissue disorders of tendinitis, bursitis, and fibrositis tend to co-occur. *Tenosynovitis* is a term that refers to inflammation of the tendon and tendon sheath.

The patient's chief concern will be pain that is worse with movement and swelling around the affected area. Occupational and recreational history will provide vital clues to a traumatic or overuse cause of pain. People with arthritis may have tendinitis secondary to joint disease. Crepitus may be felt on palpation of the tendon.

Bursitis

Bursitis is inflammation of a sac lined with synovial fluid, most often secondary to traumatic tenosynovitis of the hips and knees. Bursitis is caused by overuse and trauma and may be associated with RA. If isometric contraction of a group of muscles causes pain, the muscles, tendons, or both may be involved. Bursitis causes an aching pain that radiates to points of tendon insertion or further along the limb. Muscle weakness may also be present. Palpation reveals local tenderness and swelling without full range of joint motion.

Osteomyelitis

Osteomyelitis, a pyogenic infection of bone, presents differently depending on the age of the patient as well as the bone involved. It should be suspected in any patient who reports pain in long or flat bones and walks with an antalgic limp. Pressure ulcers caused by immobility or neuropathy are a major cause of osteomyelitis. Fever, chills, and vomiting are present in acute osteomyelitis but may not occur in the neonate or young infant. Chronic osteomyelitis is characterized by relapse of pain, erythema, swelling, or purulent discharge. The hallmark symptom is a constant local pain that progressively worsens. The slightest motion of the limb aggravates the pain. The child keeps the limb motionless. Laboratory findings show increased WBC count, ESR, and CRP. Radiographs may show bone destruction or deep soft tissue swelling at the site of infection.

Joint Inflammation

Osteoarthritis

Osteoarthritis (OA) is a degenerative disease of joint cartilage that results in osteophyte (spur) development and synovial inflammation. It is the most common form of arthritis and is present to some extent in all older adults. Patients report joint stiffness, pain, and limited movement, most often of the spine (cervical and lumbar) and large proximal joints (e.g., knee, hip). Symptoms may be asymmetrical. Heberden nodes develop on the distal interphalangeal joints. Patients at increased risk have a history of joint trauma, are obese, or have diabetes mellitus. Acute arthritis is associated with an increased ESR, and radiographs will show spurs, joint deformity, and erosive changes.

Rheumatoid arthritis

Symptoms of RA include morning stiffness of symmetrical small joints in the hands and feet, swelling, and progressive fatigue. Other symptoms include fever, weight loss, anorexia, and diaphoresis. Pericarditis, pleuritis, and vasculitis are associated conditions. Laboratory data may disclose a normochromic, normocytic anemia, an elevated ESR, and a positive rheumatoid factor in 75% to 90% of patients. Radiographs may show bony erosion at the joint margins and joint deformities. Box 22.1 lists criteria for the diagnosis of RA.

Juvenile rheumatoid arthritis

Juvenile rheumatoid arthritis is the most common connective tissue disease in children. The patient presents with fatigue, low-grade fever, weight loss, and failure to grow. Night pain and morning stiffness that improve with activity are common symptoms. Younger children may present with irritability, refusal to walk, or guarding of a joint. The disease may be systemic, affect fewer than four joints (pauciarticular), or affect more than four joints (polyarticular). Laboratory findings show anemia, leukocytosis, and thrombocytosis. Rheumatoid factor and ANA may be negative. ESR is elevated.

Box 22.1	**Diagnostic Criteria for Rheumatoid Arthritis (Four Criteria Must Be Present)**

- Morning stiffness ≤1 hour before improvement for >6 weeks
- Arthritis of three or more joints for >6 weeks
- Arthritis of hand joints for >6 weeks
- Symmetrical arthritis of same joint
- Rheumatoid nodules
- Positive serum rheumatoid factor
- Radiographic changes showing erosions or bony decalcification

Modified from Arnett FC, Edworthy SM, Bloch DA, et al: The American Rheumatism Association 1987 revised criteria for the classification of rheumatoid arthritis, *Arthritis Rheum* 31:315, 1988.

Septic arthritis

Septic arthritis is sudden pain and inflammation of a single joint, sometimes associated with systemic signs such as fever, malaise, and diaphoresis. The hip is a common site of blood-borne joint infection in neonates, infants, and young children. The presentation depends on the age of the child. A neonate may be afebrile but irritable, refusing to feed and failing to gain weight. In an older child, the onset of pain and fever is acute, and the child refuses to bear weight. ROM of the hip is markedly restricted and very painful.

In adults, migratory joint pain and tenosynovitis may follow 2 to 4 weeks after a mucosal site infection with *Neisseria gonorrhoeae.* Knee, wrist, ankle, and hand joints are most commonly affected. Joint aspiration shows increased WBC count, and culture of fluid or pus may reveal bacterial, tubercular, fungal, syphilitic, and viral organisms. The ESR and CRP are also elevated. Exposure to *Chlamydia trachomatis* (sexually transmitted) and *Chlamydia pneumonia* (respiratory tract) can trigger an autoimmune response when these organisms migrate through the blood to joint tissue; this is called reactive arthritis.

With hip involvement, ultrasound shows marked distention of the hip joint with varying degrees of femoral hip displacement. Septic arthritis is an emergency situation, and treatment must be initiated immediately.

Gout

Gout is a joint inflammation caused by deposits of urate crystals and is associated with an inborn error of uric acid secretion or with metabolic disorders (e.g., hemolytic anemia, renal insufficiency, sarcoidosis). Men older than 30 years and those with a family history of gout are most often affected. The patient reports a recurrent, sudden onset of pain early in the morning that subsides over several days, especially of the first metatarsophalangeal joint. The joint is warm, tender, and red; tophi (chalky subcutaneous deposits of sodium urate) may be present on extensor surfaces. Gout can be differentiated from pseudogout by the presence of calcium pyrophosphate crystals, involvement of large joints, and secondary osteoarthritis. Laboratory findings during an acute attack show elevated serum uric acid level, ESR, and WBC count. The joint may be aspirated for fluid to observe uric acid crystals and cultured to exclude septic arthritis.

Musculoskeletal Pain Related to Trauma or Overuse

Hip and leg

Slipped Capital Femoral Epiphysis

In children undergoing a rapid growth spurt, the onset of knee pain, an antalgic limp, and leg weakness may indicate a slipped capital femoral epiphysis (SCFE). Pain may be of several weeks' or months' duration and is exaggerated by strenuous physical activity. Examine the child in a prone position and assess the symmetry of medial rotation of the hip. A reduction of medial rotation may indicate an SCFE. A widening of the epiphyseal plate can be visualized in a lateral view radiograph.

Transient Synovitis of the Hip

A nonspecific inflammatory condition of the hip, transient synovitis is the most common cause of a painful hip in children younger than 10 years. History may reveal a recent upper respiratory tract infection or minor injury. The child complains of pain in the anteromedial aspect of the thigh and knee and walks with an antalgic limp; there is tenderness on palpation over the anterior aspect of the hip joint. Hip movement is limited and painful. There may be a low-grade fever. Ultrasound should be used for diagnosis, and both hips should be compared. WBC count is usually normal, although the ESR may be elevated.

Legg-Calvé-Perthes Disease

This disease occurs as osteochondritis of the femoral head epiphysis. It is characterized by a period of avascular necrosis of the femoral head, followed by revascularization and bone healing. It occurs most commonly in boys between the ages of 3 and 11 years. The child has groin or medial thigh pain and a limp. The pain may be recurring, and the child may have been limping for several months. The loss of medial hip motion is an early sign. There is a high incidence of hernia, undescended testicles, and kidney abnormalities in children with this condition. Radiographs show the ossific nucleus of the femoral head combined with the widened articular cartilage space compared with the opposite hip.

Iliopsoas Tendinitis

This tendinitis is caused by frequent repetitive flexion of the hip joint and is common in weight lifters, rowers, and football players. The patient complains of mildly intense groin pain on the anterior hip, which worsens with movement. An acute injury involves forced extension of a flexed leg. In younger age groups, radiographic evaluation is done if evulsion of the epiphysis is suspected. Test for iliopsoas tendinitis by having the seated patient place the heel of the affected leg on the knee of the other leg. This movement will create pain and a tense iliopsoas muscle (Table 22.2).

Proximal Fibula Fracture

Most proximal fibula fractures are caused by direct trauma to the lateral leg. However, some fractures can be the result of forces transferred from a lateral malleolar injury of the ankle, especially when the force is a combination of compressive and rotational trauma. The peroneal nerve and anterior tibial artery pass near the fibular head, thus injury to either of these structures can be a complication of a proximal fibular fracture. If foot drop is present or a diminished dorsalis pedal pulse is noted, the patient needs immediate referral to an orthopedic surgeon (Fig. 22.4).

Stress Fracture

Stress fractures occur most often in the weight-bearing bones of the lower leg and foot. They occur in adolescents whose bodies are not able to accommodate an increase in intensity of training and in adults who engage in high-intensity exercise. Patients will note pain with activity several weeks after beginning a sport. Injury progresses from

Table 22.2	Selected Tests Used to Assess for Lower Extremity Musculoskeletal Disorders	

TEST	DESCRIPTION	FINDINGS
LEG OR HIP		
Iliopsoas	Have seated patient place heel of affected leg on knee of other leg.	Pain with this movement indicates muscle iliopsoas tendinitis.
KNEE		
Foucher sign	Look for change in consistency of a mass in popliteal fossa that hardens with extension and softens with flexion.	A positive sign indicates a popliteal tumor or aneurysm; a negative sign indicates a Baker cyst.
Bulge sign	Apply lateral pressure to area adjacent to patella.	Medial bulge will appear if fluid is in knee joint.
Drawer sign	With patient supine, flex knee 90 degrees and hip 45 degrees with foot on table; apply slow, steady anterior pull, and in same position, gently push tibia back.	Tests for cruciate ligament stability; abnormal anterior or posterior movement of tibia on femur is a positive drawer sign and indicates ligamentous instability.
McMurray maneuver	With patient supine, maximally flex knee and hip; externally and internally rotate tibia with one hand on distal end of tibia; with other hand, palpate joint. Extend knee with slight lateral pressure with tibia internally rotated. Extend knee with slight internal pressure on tibia externally rotated.	Pain and a palpable or audible click are positive findings and indicate a meniscus injury. Positive finding in this position indicates a lateral meniscus injury. Positive finding in this position indicates a medial meniscus injury.
Collateral ligament test	Apply medial or lateral pressure when knee is flexed 30 degrees and when it is extended.	Medial or lateral collateral ligament sprain will show laxity in movement and no solid end points, depending on degree of sprain.
Lachman test (cruciate ligaments)	With knee flexed 30 degrees, pull tibia forward with one hand while other hand stabilizes femur.	Positive test result is a mushy or soft end feel when tibia is moved forward, indicating damage to anterior cruciate ligament.

trabecular microfractures in the bone to the osteoclastic action exceeding the rate of osteoblastic bone formation, resulting in the bone breaking. Plain radiographs may not demonstrate injury, so MRI is used to identify location of injury and CT is used for follow-up.

Knee

Chondromalacia Patellae
Chondromalacia of the patella is a change in the patellofemoral joint cartilage that is most common in female adolescents. The condition can be caused by trauma, anatomic anomalies, and misalignment of the patella. Softening of

joint cartilage, tufts of patellar cartilage, fissures, or ulcers occur. Patients present with anterior knee pain that is worse while climbing stairs or biking. Radiographic studies of the knee, including tangential and sunrise views, show irregularities of the patellofemoral joint.

Patellar Tendinitis (Jumper's Knee)
This overuse syndrome is characterized by inflammation in the distal extensors of the knee joint. Patellar tendinitis is more common in athletes who habitually place excessive strain on their knees from jumping or running. Determine the quadriceps angle by measuring the angle between the center of the patella

partial or complete (rupture) tear. It is often an injury in recreational sports. Patients will report a jumping, falling, or stepping injury and hearing a pop followed by sharp pain in the ankle and difficulty ambulating. The patient will not be able to stand on the toes with the affected limb. Ankle swelling may be present.

Plantar Fasciitis

Plantar fasciitis is a condition caused by chronic weight-bearing stress when laxity of foot structures allows the talus to slide forward and medially and plantar ligaments and fascia that connect the heel to the toes to stretch. Tendons and joints become inflamed, and muscles spasm because of the misalignment of structures. People who are obese or who engage in excessive standing are at greatest risk. Pain in the heel is worse on awakening and is relieved with non–weight-bearing activity.

Muscle Pain (Myalgia)

Viral infections

Viral infections can produce diffuse myalgias that are usually associated with fever, chills, upper respiratory tract symptoms, and malaise. A patient with influenza will have intense myalgia and a high fever and appear quite ill. Because viral illnesses are highly contagious, epidemics in both children and adults in a community may be a useful clue to diagnosis. A paraviral immunoglobulin M (IgM) titer is diagnostic of an acute parvovirus B19 infection.

Night leg cramps

Leg cramps occur at night, mostly in the calf, and are relieved with flexion of the ankle, can be caused by muscle fatigue and nerve problems, although often there is no specific cause identified. Risk factors include middle-aged adults, pregnancy, diuretics, and diabetes.

Psychogenic

Pain that is diffuse, varies in pattern, and is unaffected by activity or rest may be psychogenic in origin. A careful history may reveal any secondary gain the patient may derive from the pain and suggest the presence of an anxiety or depression disorder. On examination, the patient may display facial expressions and descriptions of discomfort to palpation and movement that are inconsistent. This diagnosis involves excluding other causes.

Fibromyalgia

Fibromyalgia is a syndrome characterized by chronic fatigue, generalized musculoskeletal pain, and multiple trigger points of pain on physical examination. It primarily affects women between 20 and 50 years of age, and the symptoms are worse in the morning. Other symptoms associated with this syndrome include stage IV sleep disturbance, anxiety or depression, obsessive-compulsive behavior, and irritable bowel syndrome. Symptoms are exacerbated by stress. Physical examination shows focal tenderness without signs of synovitis. Diagnostic criteria for fibromyalgia include diffuse pain present for 3 months and tenderness at 11 or more of 18 trigger points.

Systemic Disorders

Acute leukemia

Leukemia is the most common cancer in children, and bone and joint pain is the most common presenting complaint. The bone pain is diffuse and nonspecific and may extend to adjacent joints. Laboratory findings may show the WBC count as elevated, depressed, or normal. Severe anemia is common, as is a depressed platelet count. Radiographs of the limb at the distal end of the femur and the proximal end of the tibia show abnormal areas of radiolucency.

Sickle cell disease

Sickle cell disease is a genetic disorder characterized by production of hemoglobin S, an anemia secondary to short erythrocyte survival, and sickle-shaped erythrocytes. It affects mainly African American, Mediterranean, and Southeast Asian population groups. Sickle cell disease manifests itself after the first 6 months of life. The child presents with painful or vaso-occlusive crises characterized by symmetrical, painful swelling of the hands and feet. Older people report pain in long bones and joints, abdominal pain, decreased appetite, fever, and malaise. The laboratory findings reveal a hemoglobin S genotype and anemia, but findings can vary depending on the hemoglobin genotype, age, gender, and presence of other organ involvement. Sickle cell disease is associated with osteonecrosis of the hip.

Systemic lupus erythematosus

Systemic lupus erythematosus is a systemic inflammatory condition that occurs most often in women. It is characterized by arthritis that commonly involves the small joints of the hands, wrists, ankles, knees, and hips as well as malar rash, oral ulcers, glomerulonephritis, hematologic disorders, and psychological symptoms. The pain is transient but severe. Laboratory findings show leukopenia with neutrophils predominating the peripheral count, and the ANA is positive.

Lyme arthritis

The bite of the deer tick may transmit the spirochete *B. burgdorferi*. Patients may not recall a tick bite but will have been in an endemic area. The presenting complaints in Lyme disease are diffuse joint pain and swelling, a target like skin rash (erythema migrans), fever, and chills. These symptoms may be present for weeks before the spirochete spreads via blood and lymph tissue to the myocardium and central nervous system. A chronic arthritis may appear months after the initial infection. The arthritis is asymmetrical and occurs in the large joints. The knee is a commonly affected joint. The patient has an antalgic limp with diffuse swelling and warmth of the knee joint anteriorly, as well as local synovial thickening. Laboratory diagnosis reveals elevation of IgM titers and immunoglobulin G (IgG) antibodies against the spirochete. The ESR is elevated.

Neuroblastoma

Neuroblastoma is a malignant tumor that usually occurs in children younger than 5 years of age. It originates from cells in the sympathetic ganglia and adrenal medulla but can arise from any part of the sympathetic nervous system and metastasize to the bone. The presenting complaint may be varied, but bone pain, limp, pallor, and fatigue may be present. CT or MRI is used to identify the primary location of the tumor. In the urine, 3-methoxy-4-hydroxymandelic acid and homovanillic acid levels are elevated.

Osteogenic sarcoma

Osteogenic sarcoma occurs in people 10 to 25 years old, with the most common site being the distal femur or the proximal tibia. The patient initially complains of local intermittent pain that quickly progresses to a constant and severe pain, and an antalgic limp may develop. Palpation reveals tenderness over the area affected. Laboratory findings show an increase in serum alkaline phosphatase level; radiograph shows a "sunburst" image.

Nerve Entrapment Syndromes

Peroneal nerve compression

Peroneal nerve compression can be caused by a cast, sports injury, or trauma. Pain is felt across the head of the fibula and can result in footdrop.

Tarsal tunnel syndrome

Tarsal tunnel syndrome is occasionally associated with motor weakness of the proximal toe flexors. The posterior tibial nerve is involved, and the pain is felt across the ankle and proximal foot. Patients may not remember a specific onset but report pain and weakness of the foot muscles. Tapping the posterior tibial nerve posterior and inferior to the medial malleolus elicits pain. Ask the patient about shoe fit and use of any orthotic devices.

Neuritis

Vascular metabolism affected by systemic disorders, such as diabetes mellitus, can cause a nerve to become ischemic, producing toxins that can directly damage the nerve. Inflammation can be of the nerve axon, myelin sheath, or both. Soft tissue inflammation contributing to neuropathy can be caused by collagen disorders (e.g., SLE, scleroderma).

Diabetes mellitus is commonly associated with sensory peripheral neuropathy and results in pain and sensory loss that is more intense in the lower extremities.

Alcoholism is associated with distal, demyelinating neuropathy that may resolve with cessation of alcohol ingestion.

> ## DIFFERENTIAL DIAGNOSIS OF *Common Causes of Lower Extremity Limb Pain*

CONDITION	HISTORY	PHYSICAL FINDINGS	DIAGNOSTIC STUDIES
MUSCULOSKELETAL INFLAMMATION			
Tenosynovitis (tendinitis)	Repetitive trauma activities; pain with movement	Swelling over tendon, crepitus	None
Bursitis	History of overuse; aching pain over affected bursae that radiates along limb	Local tenderness, swelling; limited joint motion; muscle weakness	None
Osteomyelitis	Presentation depends on age, location of infection; history of infection, trauma, penetration, invasive procedure; refusal to bear weight (hip); constant pain	Fever, chills, vomiting; pain localized over affected area but progressively worsens; soft tissue injury or abscess	Increased WBC count, ESR, CRP; radiographs
JOINT INFLAMMATION			
Osteoarthritis	Older adults; asymmetrical joint pain and stiffness that improves throughout day; history of repetitive joint trauma; obesity	DIP, PIP joints enlarged; Heberden nodes; limited cervical spine ROM	ESR; radiograph may reveal osteophytes, loss of joint space
Rheumatoid arthritis	Morning stiffness of small joints; symmetrical involvement; anorexia, weight loss	Fever, rheumatoid nodules, ulnar deviation of wrists	Increased ESR, positive rheumatoid factor, anemia on CBC; radiograph shows bony erosion
Juvenile rheumatoid arthritis	Fatigue, weight loss, failure to thrive, refusal to walk, joint pain and stiffness	Fever, rash, guarding of joints, limited ROM; joint swelling, nodules	Elevated WBC count, ESR; positive rheumatoid factor and antinuclear antibody
Septic arthritis	History of systemic infection, malaise, diaphoresis, refusal to bear weight (hip), acute joint pain	Fever; red, swollen joint; limited range of motion	WBC count, culture of joint aspirate, ESR, CRP, ultrasound of joint

> **DIFFERENTIAL DIAGNOSIS OF *Common Causes of Lower Extremity Limb Pain—cont'd***

CONDITION	HISTORY	PHYSICAL FINDINGS	DIAGNOSTIC STUDIES
Gout	Acute pain of large joint, asymmetrical; men older than 30 yr of age, history of gout	Inflamed, swollen joint; tophi; sodium urate crystals	Increased serum uric acid level, ESR, WBC count
MUSCULOSKELETAL PAIN RELATED TO TRAUMA OR OVERUSE			
Slipped capital femoral epiphysis	*Children:* During rapid growth spurts; knee pain worse with activity	Limitation of medial hip rotation, limp	Radiograph of epiphyseal plate
Transient synovitis of hip	Children younger than 10 yr; history of upper respiratory tract infection; limp, pain in anteromedial thigh and knee	Tenderness on palpation over anterior hip; hip movement increases pain and is limited; low-grade fever	Ultrasound, ESR
Legg-Calvé-Perthes disease (LCPD)	Boys age 3–11 yr; groin or medial thigh pain, limp	Decreased hip ROM	AP and frog lateral radiographs of hip; LCPD may show increased density of femoral head
Iliopsoas tendinitis	History of repetitive flexion of hip; pain worse with movement	With patient sitting, place heel of affected leg on knee of other; test is positive if pain is elicited	None
Proximal fibular fracture	History of direct trauma to the fibula or ankle	Pain on weight bearing, edema and tenderness to palpation over fracture	Radiography, CT if soft tissue injury is suspected
Stress fracture	Younger age, history of overuse of lower extremities	Pain with activity	Radiography, MRI
Chondromalacia patellae	Female adolescents; history of knee trauma or misalignment, knee pain worse with activity	Tenderness to palpation over knee	Four-view radiographs of knees to rule out arthritis
Patellar tendinitis	History of overuse, especially running or jumping; dull, achy knee pain; click	Q angle >10 degrees in males, 15 degrees in females; clicking or popping with knee movement	None
Medial collateral ligament sprain	History of valgus stress to knee; limp; pain	Effusion and point tenderness over knee; valgus and varus pressure to assess instability	AP and lateral radiographs may reveal a ligament avulsion of femoral origin

Continued

> **DIFFERENTIAL DIAGNOSIS OF** *Common Causes of Lower Extremity Limb Pain—cont'd*

CONDITION	HISTORY	PHYSICAL FINDINGS	DIAGNOSTIC STUDIES
Medial meniscus tear	History of twisting injury to the knee, pain, difficulty flexing, bearing weight, clicking or catching of knee with movement	Positive McMurray test, Thessaly test, clicking or locking during joint movement, joint tenderness	Four-knee view radiographs to rule out bony abnormality; MRI
Anterior cruciate ligament tear	History of twisting or extension knee injury; audible "pop"	Swelling; positive Lachman test	Radiograph to rule out fracture; MRI
Osgood-Schlatter disease	Adolescent males; knee pain and swelling aggravated by activity, limp	Tenderness, warmth, swelling over anterior tibial tubercle	Radiograph with knee rotated inward may show soft tissue swelling
Baker cyst	Fullness or swelling of posterior knee, aggravated by walking	Negative Foucher sign; normal joint examination; positive Homans sign in ruptured cyst	None
Ankle sprain	History of inversion stress with audible "pop," immediate swelling	Swelling, soft tissue trauma, able to perform active ROM with ligament sprain	Radiograph needed only with tenderness over the lateral malleolus to rule out fracture
Shin splints	Ache or pain over medial tibia that is worse with exercise, history of running	Tenderness over medial tibia	AP and lateral radiographs may show a stress fracture; a bone scan will be positive with increased uptake along the medial tibia
Achilles tendinitis	Pain and tightness over Achilles tendon, especially with walking or running	Tenderness over Achilles tendon; pain worse with dorsiflexion ankle; calf weakness	Lateral ankle radiograph reveals enlarged posterosuperior tuberosity of the calcaneus
Achilles tendon rupture	History of a jumping, falling, or stepping injury; hearing a pop; ankle pain	Inability to stand on toes; difficulty with ambulation; ankle swelling	None
Plantar fasciitis	History of chronic weight bearing; aching feet, muscle spasms, obesity	Misalignment of foot structures, especially talus, calcaneus, and plantar ligaments	None
MUSCLE PAIN (MYALGIA)			
Viral infections	History of upper respiratory tract infection; malaise, chills, cold symptoms, general muscle aches	Fever, ill-appearing adult or child	Viral serum titer

▶ **DIFFERENTIAL DIAGNOSIS OF** *Common Causes of Lower Extremity Limb Pain—cont'd*

CONDITION	HISTORY	PHYSICAL FINDINGS	DIAGNOSTIC STUDIES
Night leg cramps	History of night calf pain or spasms relieved with foot flexion	Normal examination	None
Psychogenic	Pain is diffuse; varies in pattern of activity, setting; history of depression or anxiety	Normal examination or patient response to examination maneuvers disproportionate to physical findings or subjective complaints	None
Fibromyalgia	Adult 20–50 yr; history of depression, sleep disturbance, chronic fatigue, general muscle and joint aches	Palpation of trigger points will produce pain; normal physical examination	None
SYSTEMIC DISORDERS			
Acute leukemia	Hip pain in children, refusal to walk	Fever, hepatosplenomegaly, bruising	CBC
Sickle cell disease	African American, family history; appears after 6 mo of age; acute pain with swelling of hands and feet, abdominal pain, decreased appetite, malaise	Normal examination	Hemoglobin S genotype
Systemic lupus erythematosus	Transient arthritis of small joints, malar rash	Joint tenderness on palpation	Kidney function tests, antinuclear antibody, CBC
Lyme arthritis	History of exposure to endemic areas of deer tick; chills, diffuse joint pain and swelling; often knee is affected	Asymmetrical swelling, warmth of joint; erythema migrans; may have myocardial involvement	Serum IgM and IgG antibodies, ESR
Neuroblastoma	Younger than age 5 yr; pain in bones	Unexplained fever	Urine for vanillylmandelic or homovanillic acid; CT scan
Osteogenic sarcoma	Age 10–25 yr; intermittent pain of lower femur, upper tibia; limp	Tenderness over affected area	Radiograph, serum alkaline phosphatase
NERVE ENTRAPMENT SYNDROMES			
Peroneal compression	History of pressure to knee from a cast, sports injury, or trauma; pain over head of fibula; clumsy gait	Unilateral footdrop	None

Continued

> **DIFFERENTIAL DIAGNOSIS OF** *Common Causes of Lower Extremity Limb Pain—cont'd*

CONDITION	HISTORY	PHYSICAL FINDINGS	DIAGNOSTIC STUDIES
Tarsal tunnel syndrome	Pain in ankle and proximal foot; weakness of toe flexors; ill-fitting shoes	Tapping posterior tibial nerve elicits pain	None
Neuritis	Pain and sensory loss, usually of lower extremities; history of alcohol ingestion, diabetes mellitus	Decreased sensory and pain sensation	Liver function tests, hemoglobin A_{1c} to rule out diabetes mellitus

AP, anteroposterior; *CBC,* complete blood cell count; *CRP,* C-reactive protein; *CT,* computed tomography; *DIP,* distal interphalangeal; *ESR,* erythrocyte sedimentation rate; *MRI,* magnetic resonance imaging; *PA,* posteroanterior; *PIP,* proximal interphalangeal; *ROM,* range of motion; *WBC,* white blood cell.

Upper Extremity Limb Pain

Reports of pain in a limb present a diagnostic challenge because of the many possible pathophysiological causes. It is helpful to distinguish among limb pain that affects the bones, muscles, and tendons. Injury or inflammation of a joint can affect surrounding musculature, nerves, and blood vessels. Pain may also be the result of upper extremity peripheral vascular disease, cardiovascular etiology or cervical spine pathology

A useful mnemonic to assist clinicians in assessing the symptom of pain in any body location is PQRST: Provoke (or alleviate), Quality, Radiation, Severity, and Timing.

DIAGNOSTIC REASONING: FOCUSED HISTORY

Is the pain related to a problem that needs immediate treatment to avoid disability or death?

Key Questions
- Have you had a recent injury? Is this an emergent condition?
- Can you describe exactly how the injury occurred?
- Do you have any other symptoms, such as fatigue, fever, neck or chest pain or swollen joints?
- What is the severity of the pain? On a scale from 0 with no pain to 10 as the worst pain you've had, how do you rate this pain?

Injury
Acute compartment syndrome (ACS) is a condition that causes severe pain, burning or numbness when pressure increases within a compartment or group of muscles surrounded by fascia, usually after an injury. In the upper extremity it often involves the forearm. ACS is a surgical emergency.

The majority of patients with a cervical spine injury due to a fall or trauma are adults. The causative mechanisms of cervical spine injury for children and adolescents are related to motor vehicle trauma, diving, and sports injuries. The patient needs to be immobilized and immediately transported for emergency care. A less severe traumatic injury or degenerative processes can produce neck pain with upper extremity radiculopathy. Presence of neurologic signs and symptoms warrant prompt radiologic evaluation.

If the injury does not warrant urgent attention, obtain further history related to it (see Chapter 22).

Constitutional Symptoms
The presence of generalized symptoms, such as fever, weight loss, general malaise, or hot, swollen joints, suggests a systemic disorder such as infection or rheumatic disease.

Other systemic infections associated with polyarthritis include bacterial endocarditis, Lyme disease, syphilis, and such viruses as hepatitis B, rubella, cytomegalovirus, human immunodeficiency virus, Epstein-Barr virus, and varicella zoster.

Severity of Pain
Unrelenting diffuse pain, often occurring at night, is an indication of bone involvement, either through bone cancer or an infection such as osteomyelitis. Pain or sensation related to myocardial ischemia warrants immediate referral for evaluation.

What does the location of the pain tell me?

Key Questions
- Where does it hurt?
- Is pain associated with discomfort in your chest or neck?
- Is the pain local or generalized?

319

Location

Pain localized at the top of the shoulder suggests arthritis or acromioclavicular joint separation. Pain from an inflamed bursa or torn rotator cuff begins in the deltoid region and radiates to the lateral upper arm. Pain at the base of the thumb that occurs with grip or pinching moving suggests arthritis. Bilateral pain is more suggestive of a generalized condition, such as arthritis, or systemic causes. Pain in the chest or neck may indicate cervical spine or cardiac involvement.

Could this be caused by a sprain or strain?

Key Questions
- Describe how the injury occurred.
- Did you hear a noise with the injury, such as a ripping or cracking sound?
- Were you able to use the limb after the injury?

Strain

A strain is an injury to a muscle or tendon (fibrous cords that connect muscles to bone) and usually involves repetitive trauma. The most common wrist or hand complaint is pain caused by inflammation of any of the tendons that cross the wrist (tendonitis). Treatment usually consists of rest, splinting, ice, and nonsteroidal antiinflammatory medicines. Golfers often have wrist and elbow strain.

Sprain

A sprain is a stretch or tear of a ligament (i.e., fibrous bands that connect bone to bone across a joint). Sprains of the fingers are common. Patients almost always report a history of trauma.

Fracture

A Bennett fracture of the first metacarpal is an oblique fracture at the base of the thumb often after a blow to the thumb and commonly caused by direct trauma as a result of sports, accidents and punching an object. It occurs most often in young males. Fractures to the phalanges are more common in children. Humeral fracture is fairly common after a blow to the arm.

Scaphoid fractures frequently occur as a result of a fall on an outstretched hand.

A Colles fracture involves the distal radius and is most common in adolescents engaged in sports and in older adults with osteoporotic bones. A fracture of the metacarpal, known as Boxer's fracture, is sustained by a punching motion or direct blunt force to the dorsum of the hand. A displaced fracture is characterized by severe arm pain, swelling, and deformity.

If there is no history of trauma or a precipitating event, what else is causing the pain?

Key Questions
- Can you describe your usual daily activities at home and at work and your hobbies?
- How does the pain affect your activities?

Overuse

Cumulative injury or overuse is a problem caused by repetitive microtrauma, which most often affects the fingers, wrists, and upper extremities. People who work on keyboards for long periods of time may complain of paresthesia of the fingers and pain and soreness of the wrists and fingers. Weekend hobbies or participation in sports may result in overuse of certain muscle groups associated with those activities. Some overuse conditions include carpal tunnel syndrome, ulnar nerve entrapment and tennis elbow.

Activities

A person may adapt to chronic musculoskeletal problems by limiting activities. Inflammatory disorders produce symmetrical discomfort and pain with inactivity while noninflammatory conditions are often associated with asymmetrical pain.

In upper extremity (shoulder, wrist, elbow) joint pain with injury, what do I need to know about the specific joints involved?

Key Questions
- Is the pain in your dominant limb?
- Did you fall on an outstretched hand or arm?

- Did you engage in any activities that required overuse of one or more joints?

Pain in the dominant hand may indicate repetitive microtrauma caused by overuse. Breaking a fall with an outstretched arm is a common mechanism of injury for a fracture or dislocation of the hand or wrist. Patients who participate in sports using racquets, clubs, or bats are particularly at risk for injury.

Could this be musculoskeletal or joint disease?

Key Question
- Can you describe the pain?

Pain associated with fracture is often severe. Older adults often report chronic joint pain. Bursitis pain is often associated with swelling and limited joint motion (see Chapter 22).

 EVIDENCE-BASED PRACTICE *Is Childhood Obesity a Risk Factor for the Type and Severity of Humeral Fracture?*

Obese children have an increased risk of sustaining musculoskeletal injuries compared with normal-weight peers and are at greater risk of sustaining forearm fractures, particularly from low-energy mechanisms. This study explored whether children who sustain lateral condyle (LC) fractures have a higher body mass index (BMI) than those with supracondyle (SC) humerus fractures and if children with higher BMI sustain more severe fractures. Results showed that the LC group had a higher mean BMI than the SC group as well as more obese patients (37% versus 19%). Among patients with SC fractures, there was no difference in the BMI or percentage of obese children when analyzed by fracture subtype. The authors conclude that obesity places a child at greater risk for sustaining an LC fracture and that these fractures are often more severe compared with those in nonobese children.

Reference: Fornari, et al, 2013.

What does the history of swelling tell me?

Key Questions
- Is there any swelling?
- When did the swelling begin?

Swelling

Generally, swelling secondary to trauma such as a strain develops immediately or within 2 hours after an injury. Swelling 6 to 24 hours after an injury is usually of synovial origin, such as a subluxation, dislocation, or ligamentous damage (sprain). Swelling after 24 hours suggests an inflammatory response.

Is this an acute or a chronic problem?

Key Questions
- When did the pain first occur?
- When did you first notice a problem?

Severe ligament sprain is manifested as an immediately disabling pain at the moment of the injury. Pain experienced hours after an injury or physical activity is usually caused by acute extensor injury or overuse. Chronic pain that occurs over months and years suggests a structural cause or a systemic condition.

How is activity affected?

Key Questions
- What are your usual activities?
- What activity makes the pain worse?
- What movements make the pain worse?

Patients may report noticing pain, weakness, or difficulty in activities of daily living, such as using a hair dryer, opening jars, holding a pen, or handling eating utensils.

A large percentage of musculoskeletal injuries are caused by repetitive motion that leads to microtrauma and eventually cumulative damage.

What does joint stiffness tell me?

Key Questions
- Have you had any joint stiffness?
- Does activity make the stiffness worse or better?

Joint Stiffness

Stiffness is a common feature of any inflammatory arthropathy. It is important to know whether it is localized or generalized. The length of time the stiffness lasts in the morning is a useful index of active synovitis in disease states such as rheumatoid arthritis (RA) or systemic lupus erythematosus (SLE). With most inflammatory arthropathies, stiffness and pain are alleviated by activity; in contrast, mechanical problems are aggravated by activity. Musculoskeletal tumors commonly present with mild joint stiffness because of muscle involvement but rarely demonstrate instability.

Could this be caused by systemic disease?

Key Questions

- Have you been treated with antibiotics recently?
- Have you had any recent immunizations?
- Does the pain awaken you at night?
- Is the pain worse at night?

Medications

Transient arthralgia may occur 6 to 8 weeks after receiving immunizations, especially in women. Myalgia can begin hours after the injection and last up to 3 weeks.

Night Pain

Rotator cuff tears can cause shoulder pain and upper extremity numbness when sleeping on one's affected side.

What does the health history tell me?

Key Questions

- Do you have a chronic disease?
- Could you have been exposed to any sexually transmitted infection?
- Have you recently been treated with a cortisone injection?

Chronic Disease

Chronic diseases, such as sickle cell anemia, inflammatory bowel disease, Crohn disease, hypothyroidism and hyperthyroidism, and collagen vascular diseases, are frequently associated with skin rashes, psoriasis, and limb and joint pain.

Sexually Transmitted Infection

Gonorrhea disseminates to the musculoskeletal system in 1% to 3% of infected individuals. One form involves skin rashes and many joints, usually large joints such as the knee, wrist, and ankle. Exposure to other infectious agents, such as *Chlamydia trachomatis* (sexually transmitted) and *Chlamydia pneumonia* (respiratory tract), can trigger an autoimmune response when these organisms migrate through the blood to joint tissue; this is called reactive arthritis. Untreated syphilis, caused by the spirochete *Treponema pallidum*, occurs in stages over time and secondary infection can be manifested as a diffuse truncal and extremity rash.

Cortisone Treatment

About 50% of patients experience increased pain after a corticosteroid injection to the hand or elbow, and the symptom lasts for a couple of days before pain relief is achieved. The pain is primarily due to the increased volume in the enclosed space.

DIAGNOSTIC REASONING: FOCUSED PHYSICAL EXAMINATION

Figures 23.1 to 23.3 depict anatomic landmarks of the shoulder, elbow, hand, and wrist. Table 23.1 describes selected tests used to assess for upper extremity musculoskeletal disorders.

Observe the Patient Walking and Removing a Coat or Jacket

People who have septic joints appear ill, and movement of the joint will increase pain. Inspect the patient with minimal clothing obstructing your view of movements.

Have the Patient Locate the Pain

Have the patient point to the area of pain. Location of pain and actual area of pathology may not be the same because of referred pain. Shoulder pain from rotator cuff tendinitis is felt over the lateral aspect

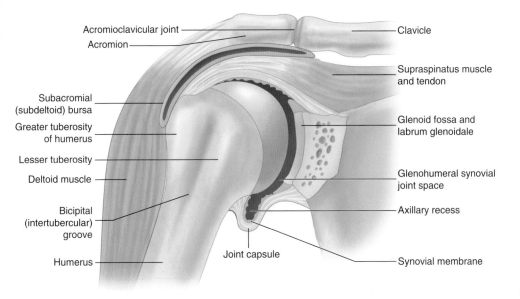

Acromioclavicular joint

Acromion

Clavicle

Supraspinatus muscle
and tendon

Subacromial
(subdeltoid) bursa

Greater tuberosity
of humerus

Lesser tuberosity

Deltoid muscle

Bicipital
(intertubercular)
groove

Humerus

Glenoid fossa and
labrum glenoidale

Glenohumeral synovial
joint space

Axillary recess

Joint capsule

Synovial membrane

FIGURE 23.1 Anterior view of bones and ligaments of the right shoulder. (From Fam A, Lawry G, Kreder H: *Musculoskeletal examination and joint injection techniques,* Philadelphia, 2005, Mosby.)

of the deltoid. Swelling of the elbow may compress the ulnar nerve, producing a tingling sensation in the fourth and fifth fingers and numbness, pain or burning in sensory areas supplied by the ulnar nerve.

Note Any Deformities

Fractures generally produce unilateral deformities or swelling in the extremities. Inflammatory and degenerative joint diseases produce observable joint swelling and deformity that usually occurs bilaterally. Examine the cervical spine for deformity, tenderness, and range of joint motion.

Osteoarthritis typically involves the distal interphalangeal (DIP) and proximal interphalangeal (PIP) joints, spine, hips, knees, and first metatarsophalangeal (MTP) joints. Joints are enlarged with Heberden (DIP joints) and Bouchard (PIP joints) nodes (Fig. 23.4).

Joints affected by RA include PIPs, metacarpophalangeal (MCP) joints, wrists, knees, elbows, cervical spine, and MTPs. Joints are swollen with a fusiform-shaped swelling of the PIP joints. Subluxation, ankylosis, and ulnar deviation may be observed as a result of joint destruction from chronic inflammation.

Assess Vital Signs

Elevated temperatures are seen with neoplastic, systemic, and infectious processes such as osteomyelitis, septic arthritis and septic hip in children, and rheumatic disease. Palpate for quality and presence of pulses in any injured limb and compare with the opposite side. Assess peripheral pulses for presence, rate, regularity, strength, and symmetry.

Inspect the Skin and Nails

Inspect the skin for redness and inflammation.

Look for a puncture or an abscess that could be the source of infection and seeding if a septic joint or osteomyelitis is suspected. Look for ecchymosis and bruising. These indicate trauma as a source for pain as well as raise a suspicion of abuse. Swelling and redness of a joint indicate underlying infection or inflammation. Effusion, or fluid in the joint capsule, always distends the joint in a smooth, symmetrical manner.

Observe the muscles around the painful limb area. Decreased muscle tone or atrophy

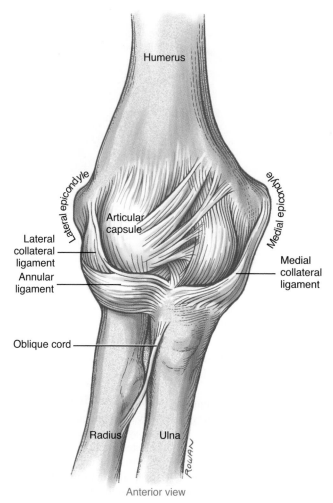

FIGURE 23.2 Bony and ligamentous anatomy of the elbow. (From Neumann D: *Kinesiology of the musculoskeletal system,* St. Louis, 2010, Mosby.)

from disuse begins immediately after injury; however, it will not be clinically apparent for approximately 1 week.

Measure Limb Circumference and Length

Use a tape measure to locate points at which to measure and compare limb circumference. Differences may be the result of muscle atrophy or edema.

Palpate Extremities and Joints

Palpate those areas that are painful last and then compare with the unaffected limb.

Determine if there is edema (e.g., presence of interstitial fluid). Induration is interstitial swelling that has progressed and is now firm. An effusion is a collection of fluid in the joint capsule, which can be the result of rupture of a vascular structure or a synovial secretory response to an inflammatory process. The consistency of the fluid is noteworthy. Pus has a thick consistency and is less fluctuant than synovial fluid. Hematoma has a more gelatinous consistency.

Heat over the affected joint can indicate inflammation or infection. Evaluate the joint for crepitus, both palpable and auditory.

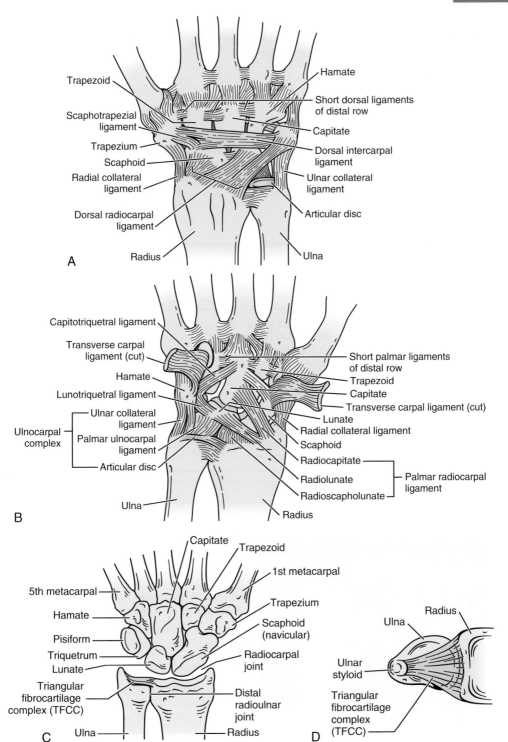

FIGURE 23.3 Bones and ligaments of the wrist. **A,** Ligaments, dorsal view. **B,** Ligaments, palmar view. **C,** Bones, dorsal view. **D,** Close-up view of triangular fibrocartilage complex. (From Magee D: *Orthopedic physical assessment,* St. Louis, 2008, Mosby.)

Table 23.1	**Selected Tests Used to Assess for Upper Extremity Musculoskeletal Disorders**	
TEST	**DESCRIPTION**	**FINDINGS**
Shoulder		
Yergason test	Have patient supinate forearm against resistance.	A positive test produces pain in bicipital groove and is suggestive of bicipital tendinitis.
Rotator cuff tear	Ask patient to externally rotate and abduct shoulder.	In a partial tear, patient can raise arm but cannot maintain position against resistance; in a complete tear, attempts to abduct arm will produce a shoulder shrug.
Elbow		
Tennis elbow	Have patient resist forearm supination with elbow flexed 90 degrees.	Pain with this movement indicates lateral humeral epicondylitis.
Wrist		
Finkelstein test	Have patient flex fingers over a clenched thumb; then passively deviate wrist ulnarly.	Movement produces pain in De Quervain disease (first dorsal compartment tenosynovitis).
Tinel sign	Tap over median nerve (palmar surface of wrist) to assess for compression neuropathy.	In a positive test result, patient reports a tingling or prickling sensation distal to site tapped along first three digits, wrist pain, and weak grip.
Phalen test	Ask patient to maintain palmar flexion for 1 min with dorsal surfaces of each hand pressed together.	Test result is positive if maneuver produces numbness and paresthesia in fingers innervated by median nerve.

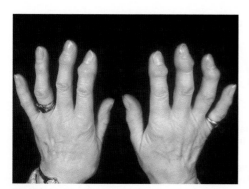

FIGURE 23.4 Osteoarthritis of the hand. Heberden nodes are shown at the distal interphalangeal joints. (From Waldman S: *Pain management,* Philadelphia, 2007, Saunders.)

Tendonitis can produce a grating sensation on palpation of the ligament or a grating sound with movement.

Perform Passive and Active Range of Motion of All Limbs and the spine

Range of motion (ROM) may be limited because of pain, weakness, or deformity.

Test for Muscle Strength

Test for upper extremity flexor and extensor strength against resistance of both the proximal and distal muscle groups. Proximal muscle weakness is seen in myopathic disorders. Distal muscle weakness is seen secondary to a neuropathic process. Generally, if the

Table 23.2	**Muscle Strength Test**	
GRADE	MUSCLE STRENGTH	TERM
0	No palpable contraction	Zero
1	Muscle contracts but part does not move	Trace
2	Muscle moves part but not against gravity	Poor
3	Muscle moves part through range against gravity	Fair
4	Muscle moves part even with resistance	Good
5	Normal strength against resistance present	Excellent

opposite side is normal, strength should be compared with it. A scale of 0 to 5 is used to rate muscle strength (Table 23.2).

Perform a Neurologic Examination

Assessment of sensory and motor function and deep tendon reflexes should be done on the affected and contralateral limbs and cervical spine. If systemic illness is suspected, perform a neurologic examination.

LABORATORY AND DIAGNOSTIC STUDIES

Complete Blood Count

A complete blood count is obtained to evaluate for anemia associated with chronic disease, infection, or neoplasm. An altered white blood cell (WBC) count may indicate infection or leukemia.

Erythrocyte Sedimentation Rate

An erythrocyte sedimentation rate (ESR) is elevated when inflammation is present. It is a nonspecific test.

Joint Aspiration

Joint aspiration is performed to assess synovial fluid for elevated WBC count, Gram stain, culture and sensitivity, crystal analysis, presence of glucose, and consistency or "string test." This procedure is performed using local anesthesia under sterile technique. Synovial fluid will flow easily when the joint capsule is penetrated.

Radiography

Obtain at least two radiographic views, anteroposterior and lateral, because injuries are not always apparent on a single view. Any evidence of fracture or dislocation will require orthopedic attention. Sometimes radiographic comparisons with the opposite limb may be useful. Magnetic resonance imaging (MRI) is usually used in spine, joint, and soft tissue imaging. Computed tomography (CT) scans are usually performed for bone visualization. An MRI can confirm a chronic or acute rotator cuff tear in tendons and bone swelling after an acute injury.

Antinuclear Antibodies

Antinuclear antibody (ANA) test results are positive with high titers in RA and SLE; however, other factors such as advanced age, medications, and other connective tissue disease can produce positive antibody titers.

Rheumatoid Factor

Rheumatoid factor (RF) is the single most useful test to confirm a diagnosis of RA and is positive in 80% of patients with this disease.

C4 Complement

C4 complement determines serum hemolytic complement activity, a protein that binds antigen–antibody complexes for the purpose of lysis. Complement is increased in active inflammatory disease and in autoimmune disorders such as juvenile RA.

C-Reactive Protein

C-reactive protein (CRP) indicates the presence of abnormal plasma protein or a nonspecific response to inflammation caused by both infectious and noninfectious processes. CRP is elevated in RA and infection.

DIFFERENTIAL DIAGNOSIS

Emergent Causes of Upper Extremity Pain

Acute compartment syndrome

Acute compartment syndrome (ACS) causes severe pain, burning or numbness when pressure increases within a muscle compartment, usually after an injury. In the upper extremity it often involves the forearm. A patient with symptoms suggestive of ACS need immediate referral for surgical intervention.

Cervical spine injury

Most cervical spine injuries occur as a result of a fall or trauma to the head and neck related to motor vehicle trauma, diving, and sports injuries. The patient needs to be immobilized and immediately transported for emergency care. Presence of neurologic signs and symptoms warrant prompt radiologic evaluation.

NONEMERGENT CAUSES OF UPPER EXTREMITY PAIN

Musculoskeletal Inflammation

Tenosynovitis (tendinitis)

Soft tissue disorders of tendinitis, bursitis, and fibrositis tend to occur together. Tenosynovitis is inflammation of the tendon and tendon sheath. In an acute inflammation, usually caused by trauma related to recreational or occupational activities, effusion may accumulate and result in swelling. With chronic inflammation, ROM will be limited by fibrosis of the tendon sheath.

Pain is worse with movement. Occupational and recreational history will provide vital clues to differentiate between overuse and trauma as the cause of pain. People with arthritis may have tendinitis secondary to joint disease. Crepitus may be felt on palpation of the tendon.

Bursitis

Bursitis is inflammation of a sac lined with synovial fluid, most often secondary to traumatic tenosynovitis of the shoulder and elbow. Numerous bursae lie over bony prominences and reduce friction from motion of fascial planes. Bursitis is caused by overuse and trauma and may be associated with RA. If isometric contraction of a group of muscles causes pain, the muscles or tendons, or both, may be involved. Bursitis causes an aching pain that radiates to points of tendon insertion or further along the limb. Muscle weakness may also be present. Palpation reveals local tenderness and swelling without full range of joint motion.

Myositis (myofascitis, fibromyositis)

Myositis is an inflammatory response that leads to immune mediated muscle injury. The exact process of how inflammation produces muscle injury are is well understood. Conditions, such as polymyalgia rheumatica, RA, ankylosing spondylitis, hypothyroidism, neuritis, and viral infection, generate major muscle tension around a large, weight-bearing proximal joint. Fatty and fibrous nodules may be palpable, and painful trigger sites can be located throughout the shoulder and pelvic girdle or lower extremities. Patients complain of stress and anxiety, sleep disturbance, painful trigger points, and joint stiffness. Creatine kinase levels will be elevated.

Osteomyelitis

The presentation of osteomyelitis, a pyogenic infection of bone, depends on the patient's age as well as the bone involved. The hallmark is a constant, local pain that progressively worsens. The slightest motion of the limb aggravates the pain. Laboratory findings show increased WBC counts, ESR, and CRP. Radiographs may show bone destruction or deep soft tissue swelling at the site of infection.

Joint Inflammation

Osteoarthritis

Osteoarthritis (OA) is the most common form of arthritis and is present to some extent in all elderly people. Patients report joint stiffness, pain, and limited movement. Symptoms may be asymmetric. Patients at increased risk have a history of performing repetitive weight-lifting tasks, have sustained some form of joint trauma, are obese, or have been diagnosed with diabetes mellitus. Acute arthritis is associated with an increased ESR, and radiographs will show spurs, joint deformity, and erosive changes.

Rheumatoid arthritis

Rheumatoid arthritis is a chronic inflammatory disease characterized by joint swelling and tenderness and destruction of synovial joints, leading to severe disability and premature mortality. There is a wide clinical presentation of RA, and symptoms include morning stiffness of symmetrical small joints in the hands and feet, swelling, and progressive fatigue. Rheumatoid nodules are soft and spongy and appear on the elbows, forearms, and hands. Pericarditis, pleuritis, and vasculitis are associated conditions. Laboratory data may disclose a normochromic/normocytic anemia, an elevated ESR, and a positive rheumatoid factor (RF) in 75% to 90% of patients. A positive RF test result may precede symptoms by many years. Radiographs may show bony erosion at the joint margins and joint deformities.

Musculoskeletal Pain Related to Trauma or Overuse

Shoulder

Dislocation (Glenohumeral Joint Instability)

A patient with shoulder dislocation presents with anterior or posterior joint pain (or both anterior and posterior), periarticular muscle spasm, anxiety, and limited movement. An anterior dislocation causes inability to internally rotate and abduct the humerus. Posterior dislocation causes limitation of external rotation, arm abduction, and hand supination with the shoulder flexed forward. Radiographs of the shoulder (anteroposterior, lateral, and axillary views) will exclude fracture of surrounding bones.

Acromioclavicular Joint Injury

Acromioclavicular joint injuries usually result from sports injuries or motor vehicle accidents. Injury occurs when the acromion, scapula, and upper extremity are driven inferiorly, and the supporting ligamentous structures are sprained or torn. There are three grades of severity: (1) partial tear (dislocation) of the acromioclavicular ligament, (2) partial tear of the acromioclavicular and coracoclavicular ligaments, and (3) complete rupture of the acromioclavicular and coracoclavicular ligaments and joint separation. History will reveal the nature of the injury. The patient will have pain and limited shoulder movement and may present with obvious deformity if there is a severe injury.

Bicipital Tendinitis

Bicipital tendinitis is an overuse syndrome of the biceps brachii muscle that ends in two tendons, one attached to the radial tuberosity (arm adduction) and one to the forearm fascia (arm abduction and internal rotation). The syndrome may be associated with other shoulder disorders, such as impingement syndrome. Children may have anomalies of the intertubercular groove when presenting with repeated trauma from swimming, volleyball, baseball, or golf. Pain is localized to the intertubercular groove, is aggravated by the offending movement, and subsides with rest. A Yergason test can indicate bicipital tendinitis. A positive test result is characterized by pain in the intertubercular groove with resistance to supination of the forearm while the elbow is flexed 90 degrees. A Fisk radiographic view enables the examiner to determine the size of the intertubercular groove.

Rotator Cuff Tear

Rotator cuff tears are acute injuries in children and young adults but occur as chronic injuries in older adults. In acute tears, the shoulder pain is severe, and the patient is unable to raise the arm sideways because of pain. In a complete tear, attempts to raise the arm laterally will produce a shoulder shrug. In a partial tear, the patient can raise the arm but cannot maintain the position with any resistance. Inflammation secondary to injury can cause rotator cuff tendinitis that produces shoulder and upper arm pain, weakness, and a grating sound with movement.

Chronic rotator cuff tears are most common in people older than 50 years; they result from cumulative and repeated impingement processes. The onset of pain is insidious and is made worse with the arm in an overhead position. Patients experience shoulder pain with sleep and tenderness over the acromioclavicular joint. Examination may reveal minimal restriction in movement, crepitus, and weakness in external rotation of the shoulder. Radiographs will show any bony abnormality, such as an acromial spur.

Elbow

Olecranon Bursitis

Olecranon bursitis is commonly seen in people who engage in contact sports, repetitive motion, rubbing or placing pressure on the elbow, or overuse. Pain is localized over the bursae, and swelling may be the result of hemorrhage in a traumatic injury. The joint's ROM is usually normal. The joint may be warm and red. When these signs are present, carefully examine the skin over the elbow to ensure intactness because a penetrating injury may cause septic bursitis. Radiography will exclude underlying bone infection and show the plane of soft tissue swelling.

Lateral Humeral Epicondylitis (Tennis Elbow)

Epicondylitis is an aseptic inflammation of the bone–tendon junction, resulting from repetitive concentric contractions that transmit force via the muscles to the origin on the lateral epicondyle. People most at risk for tennis elbow are nonathletes who have occupations that require repeated contractions of extensor and supinator muscles. Athletes at risk are tennis players, bowlers, and hockey players. Patients present with gradual onset of pain and tenderness over the lateral epicondyle that progresses in intensity. Palpation over the lateral epicondyle produces point tenderness, although elbow movement is not limited. Resisted forearm supination with the elbow flexed at 90 degrees will intensify symptoms.

Subluxation of the Radial Head

A rapid upward pulling of a child's hand or wrist causes subluxation of the radial head. The radial head is pulled out of the annular ligament. This ligament then becomes caught between the radial head and the joint, causing the elbow to be flexed and pronated. The child cries at the event and then refuses to move the arm and may complain of pain in the elbow. Radiographs may not reveal a fracture but dislocation of the radial head.

Wrist and hand

Wrist Fracture

Wrist fractures usually result from falling on an outstretched hand and may involve a number of types of fracture. Patients present with a painful, swollen distal forearm and wrist and may report numbness if the median nerve is involved. Gently palpate to locate the site of maximal pain, particularly the navicular ("snuffbox") area located between the extensor pollicis longus and the extensor pollicis brevis tendons when the mechanism of injury is hyperextension of the wrist. Pain localized here indicates a scaphoid (navicular) fracture that may be missed on radiograph. Assess pulses, pain sensation, and motor function (range and strength). Radiographic views (posteroanterior, lateral, and oblique) will reveal the bone involved. In a Colles fracture, the distal radius is displaced dorsally and shows up as a "silver fork" deformity on lateral view radiographs.

Finger Fracture

Fractures of the phalanges (fingers) and metacarpals (hand) are common sports injuries. Older people usually sustain fractures as a result of falls. Correct diagnosis of a fractured finger is important in preventing long-term functional disability. Patients present with a history of trauma or injury. Physical examination includes assessment of vascular and neurologic function, tenderness and swelling, ROM of each joint, and signs of joint instability or deformity. Three radiographic views (posteroanterior, lateral, and oblique) are needed for a complete evaluation.

Ganglion

Ganglions are cysts that contain a gelatinous fluid formed by an "outpouching" of a joint capsule or tendon sheath. They most often occur on the dorsum of the wrist. A ganglion can be distinguished from a tumor by its soft consistency and transillumination.

De Quervain Tendonitis

This is a painful condition affecting the tendons on the thumb side of the wrist caused by overuse or joint inflammation secondary to arthritis. Pain and sometimes swelling are located at the base of the thumb. The patient has difficulty moving the thumb and wrist with grasping or pinching movements. A "sticking" sensation can be felt with thumb movement. The Finkelstein test (see Table 23.1) will produce pain on the thumb side of the wrist.

Muscle Pain (Myalgia)

Viral infections

Viral infections can produce diffuse myalgias that are usually associated with fever, chills, upper respiratory tract symptoms, and malaise. A patient with influenza will have intense myalgia and high fever and appear quite ill. A paraviral immunoglobulin M (IgM) titer is diagnostic of an acute parvovirus B19 infection.

Psychogenic

Pain that is diffuse, variable in pattern, and unaffected by activity or rest may be psychogenic in origin. A careful history may reveal any secondary gain the patient may derive from the pain and suggest the presence of an anxiety or depression disorder. On examination, the patient may display facial expressions and descriptions of discomfort to palpation and movement that are inconsistent. This diagnosis involves excluding other causes.

Fibromyalgia

Fibromyalgia is a syndrome characterized by chronic fatigue, generalized musculoskeletal pain, and multiple trigger points of pain on physical examination (see Chapter 22).

Systemic Disorders

Dupuytren contracture

Dupuytren contracture is a condition that mainly involves the ring and pinky finger and most often occurs on one side. A thick patch of skin can be felt on the palm. The patient will not be able to press the hand flat against a surface. The contracture grows slowly and restricts finger movement and the ability to open up the hand. The cause is not known, but Northern Europeans and adults older than 50 years of age are at greater risk.

Sickle cell disease

Sickle cell disease is a genetic disorder characterized by production of hemoglobin S, an anemia secondary to short erythrocyte survival, and sickle-shaped erythrocytes. It affects mainly African American, Mediterranean, and Southeast Asian population groups. Sickle cell disease manifests itself after the first 6 months of life. The child presents with painful or vaso-occlusive crises characterized by symmetrical, painful swelling of the hands and feet. Older people report pain in long bones and joints, abdominal pain, decreased appetite, fever, and malaise. The laboratory findings reveal a hemoglobin S genotype and anemia, but findings can vary depending on the hemoglobin genotype, age, gender, and presence of other organ involvement.

Systemic lupus erythematosus

Systemic lupus erythematosus is a systemic inflammatory condition that occurs most often in women. It is characterized by arthritis that commonly involves the small joints of the hands, wrists, ankles, knees, and hips as well as malar rash, oral ulcers, glomerulonephritis, hematological disorders, and psychological symptoms. The pain is transient but severe. Laboratory findings show leukopenia with neutrophils predominating the peripheral count, and the antinuclear antibody test result is positive.

Nerve Entrapment Syndromes

Thoracic outlet syndrome

Thoracic outlet syndrome is the result of compression of nerve and vascular structures in the neck area. Arterial compression creates pallor and decreased pulses and weakness, with eventual skin and nail atrophy in the affected extremity. Nerve compression creates paresthesias, dysesthesias, and pain. History may disclose that the patient sleeps with the arm extended against the head, causing morning symptoms of pain and paresthesias. Reaching, working with the arm raised, and lifting exacerbate pain. Other risk factors include a rounded, sagging shoulder posture and shoulder muscle deformities. A common compression occurs with the cervical rib compressing the subclavian artery. A bruit may be heard over the supraclavicular fossa. Electromyographic studies help to delineate the specific nerve involvement, although they may not identify the vascular involvement.

Carpal tunnel syndrome

Carpal tunnel syndrome involves entrapment of the median nerve in the dominant hand, resulting from repeated strain that causes thickening of the flexor tendon sheath. A dull, achy pain is felt across the wrist and forearm with paresthesia, weakness, or clumsiness of the hand; atrophy; dry skin; and skin color changes of the hand secondary to impaired nerve innervation. Symptoms are often worse at night. History reveals repetitive activity of the upper extremity. Carpal tunnel syndrome most often occurs in women and in people older than 30 years. Examination discloses dry skin on the thumb, index finger, and middle finger (median nerve distribution). Thenar atrophy may be present. Tinel sign and Phalen test results are often positive (Table 23-2). EMG and nerve conduction testing can confirm the diagnosis and determine the extent of damage.

Cubital tunnel syndrome

Ulnar nerve entrapment occurs when the ulnar nerve, one of the three main nerves in the arm, becomes compressed or irritated. Numbness and tingling in the ring and small fingers, pain in the forearm, and weakness in the hand are common symptoms. A positive Tinel sign is when percussing over the ulnar nerve at the wrist produces a tingling sensation. The major risk factors for cubital tunnel syndrome are diabetes, obesity, holding a tool in a constant position, especially with a bent elbow, and performing a repetitive task. Symptoms may subside and recur over time. The diagnosis can be confirmed with nerve conduction studies.

Neuritis

Vascular metabolism affected by systemic disorders such as diabetes mellitus can cause a nerve to become ischemic, producing toxins that can directly damage the nerve. The nerve axon, myelin sheath, or both, can be inflamed. Soft tissue inflammation contributing to neuropathy can be caused by collagen disorders (e.g., SLE, scleroderma).

> ▶ **DIFFERENTIAL DIAGNOSIS OF** *Common Nonemergent Causes of Upper Extremity Limb Pain*

CONDITION	HISTORY	PHYSICAL FINDINGS	DIAGNOSTIC STUDIES
Musculoskeletal Inflammation			
Tenosynovitis (tendinitis)	Repetitive trauma activities; pain with movement	Swelling over tendon, crepitus	None
Bursitis	History of overuse; aching pain over affected bursae that radiates along limb	Local tenderness, swelling; limited joint motion; muscle weakness	None
Myositis	Pain in trigger sites throughout body, joint stiffness, disturbed sleep	Fatty, fibrous nodules in muscles; palpation of trigger points elicits pain	Elevated creatine kinase

> **DIFFERENTIAL DIAGNOSIS OF** *Common Nonemergent Causes of Upper Extremity Limb Pain—cont'd*

CONDITION	HISTORY	PHYSICAL FINDINGS	DIAGNOSTIC STUDIES
Osteomyelitis	Presentation depends on age, location of infection; history of infection, trauma, penetration, invasive procedure; refusal to bear weight (hip); constant pain	Fever, chills, vomiting; pain localized over affected area but progressively worsens; soft tissue injury or abscess	Increased WBC count, ESR, CRP; radiographs
Joint Inflammation			
Osteoarthritis	Older adults; asymmetrical joint pain and stiffness that improves throughout day; history of repetitive joint trauma; obesity	DIP, PIP joints enlarged; Heberden nodes; limited cervical spine ROM	ESR; radiograph may reveal osteophytes, loss of joint space
Rheumatoid arthritis	Morning stiffness of small joints; symmetrical involvement; anorexia, weight loss	Fever, rheumatoid nodules, ulnar deviation of wrists	Increased ESR, positive rheumatoid factor, anemia on CBC count; radiograph shows bony erosion
Septic arthritis	History of systemic infection, malaise, diaphoresis, refusal to bear weight (hip), acute joint pain	Fever; red, swollen joint; limited range of motion	WBC count, culture of joint aspirate, ESR, CRP, ultrasound of joint
Musculoskeletal Pain Related to Trauma or Overuse			
Shoulder dislocation	History of trauma, pain	Limited rotation, arm abduction, and hand supination	Radiograph of shoulder with AP view and internal/external rotation
Acromioclavicular joint injury	History of trauma, pain	Limited shoulder movement; obvious deformity	Radiograph of shoulder with AP view and internal/external rotation
Bicipital tendinitis	History of overuse of biceps; pain worse with movement	Positive Yergason test; pain localized over intertubercular groove	Radiograph (Fisk view)
Rotator cuff tear	Acute: younger people, history of trauma, severe pain; chronic: older, pain worse with overhead movement, sleep disturbance	Acute: inability to raise arm laterally, shrug shoulders; chronic: tenderness over AC joint, crepitus, weakness in external shoulder rotation	Radiograph may reveal humeral displacement or spurs; MRI

Continued

> **DIFFERENTIAL DIAGNOSIS OF** *Common Nonemergent Causes of Upper Extremity Limb Pain—cont'd*

CONDITION	HISTORY	PHYSICAL FINDINGS	DIAGNOSTIC STUDIES
Olecranon bursitis	Repetitive motion of or pressure to elbow; localized pain	Warmth, redness, and swelling over joint; full ROM	Radiograph to rule out fracture of olecranon process
Lateral humeral epicondylitis	History of repetitive contraction of extensor and supinator muscles; pain over lateral epicondyle that progresses	Tenderness over lateral epicondyle; palpation produces pain, motion does not; supination against resistance worsens pain	None
Subluxation of radial head	Occurs in children; pain in elbow or arm	Affected arm is flexed; child cries when attempts are made to move joint	Radiograph of elbow
Wrist fracture	History of fall on an outstretched hand; pain and swelling of forearm and wrist	Palpation of snuffbox increases pain; observe for joint deformity	Three-view radiographs to determine scaphoid or Colles fracture
Bennett fracture (first metacarpal)	History of fall or direct impact to the thumb; pain, swelling and limited thumb movement	Palpate base of thumb for tenderness or deformity	Radiograph shows fracture or subluxation of the first metacarpal
Finger fracture	History of trauma or fall, joint tenderness	Joint swelling, instability	Three-view radiographs (PA, lateral, and oblique)
Ganglion	Noticeable lump on dorsal surface of wrist	Gelatinous filled nodule, soft, transilluminates	None
De Quervain tendinitis	History of pain with thumb movement	Positive Finkelstein test	none
Muscle Pain (Myalgia)			
Viral infections	History of upper respiratory tract infection; malaise, chills, cold symptoms, general muscle aches	Fever, ill-appearing adult or child	Viral serum titer
Psychogenic	Diffuse pain; varies in pattern of activity, setting; history of depression or anxiety	Normal examination or patient response to examination maneuvers disproportionate to physical findings or subjective complaints	None
Fibromyalgia	Women 20–50 yr old; history of depression, sleep disturbance, chronic fatigue, general muscle and joint aches	Palpation of trigger points will produce pain; normal physical examination	None

Continued

> ▶ **DIFFERENTIAL DIAGNOSIS OF** *Common Nonemergent Causes of Upper Extremity Limb Pain—cont'd*

CONDITION	HISTORY	PHYSICAL FINDINGS	DIAGNOSTIC STUDIES
Systemic Disorders			
Dupuytren contracture	Gradual thickening of tissue of ring and pinky fingers	Contracture of ring or pinky finger, usually unilateral	Surgical referral if severe
Sickle cell disease	African American, family history; appears after age 6 mo; acute pain with swelling of hands and feet, abdominal pain, decreased appetite, malaise	Normal examination	Hemoglobin S genotype
Systemic lupus erythematosus	Female; transient arthritis of small joints, malar rash	Normal examination may have joint tenderness on palpation	Kidney function tests, antinuclear antibody, CBC
Nerve Entrapment Syndromes			
Thoracic outlet syndrome	History of sleeping with arm against head; morning shoulder pain; pain worse with lifting; paresthesia, weakness, or clumsiness of hand; symptoms worse at night	Bruit over supraclavicular fossa; pallor, decreased pulses of upper extremity, weakness, skin and nail atrophy	None
Carpal tunnel syndrome	History of repetitive upper extremity motion; paresthesia, weakness, or clumsiness of hand; symptoms worse at night	Positive Phalen test result and Tinel sign; weakness of hand; dry skin over distribution of median nerve	None
Cubital tunnel syndrome	History of diabetes, repetitive movement, especially with elbow, pain and tingling of fingers	Clumsy hand movement; positive Tinel sign	Nerve conduction studies if symptoms are severe

AC, acromioclavicular joint capsule; *AP,* anteroposterior; *CBC,* complete blood cell count; *CRP,* C-reactive protein; *CT,* computed tomography; *DIP,* distal interphalangeal; *ESR,* erythrocyte sedimentation rate; *MRI,* magnetic resonance imaging; *PA,* posteroanterior; *PIP,* proximal interphalangeal; *ROM,* range of motion; *WBC,* white blood cell.

Low Back Pain (Acute)

A report of acute low back pain (ALBP), although quite common, requires a thorough evaluation. The underlying pathophysiology of back pain is frequently multifactorial and includes both physiological and psychological components. The most common causes of ALBP relate to musculoligamentous injuries and age-related degenerative processes. About 90% of ALBP episodes in adults are related to mechanical causes that resolve within 4 weeks without serious sequelae. A smaller percentage of patients will continue to have chronic symptoms without organic pathology or have underlying disease.

In children, the prevalence of back pain increases with age and with involvement in sports. Anthropometric variations in children place them at risk for excess strain on the spine, producing back pain. These variations include reduced hip mobility, decreased lumbar extension and increased lumbar flexion, poor abdominal muscle strength, tight hamstring muscles, and lumbar hyperlordosis.

Acute low back pain is defined as activity intolerance producing lower back or back-related leg symptoms of less than 3 months' duration. The Agency for Healthcare Research and Quality (AHRQ) guidelines provide the following framework for causes of ALBP:

- Potentially serious conditions (e.g., spinal fracture, tumor, infection, or cauda equina syndrome)
- Sciatica, or leg pain and numbness of the lateral thigh, leg, and foot, suggesting nerve root compression (Fig. 24.1)
- Nonspecific back problems such as musculoskeletal strain, diskogenic pain, or bony deformity secondary to inflammatory disease
- Nonspinal causes secondary to abdominal involvement (e.g., gallbladder, liver, renal,

pelvic inflammatory disease, prostate tumor, ovarian cyst, uterine fibroids, aortic aneurysm, or thoracic disease)
- Psychological causes such as stress related to work environment (e.g., disability, workers' compensation, secondary gains).

When evaluating ALBP, the goal of the clinician is to first identify signs and symptoms of potentially serious conditions through a careful history and physical examination. A holistic approach to the patient is needed to appreciate the extent to which pain affects the patient's daily routine or work-related activities. Because ALBP is a common occupation-related complaint and a cause of disability and lost productivity, the clinician must gain insight into the patient's psychosocial and economic situation to help arrive at a correct diagnosis.

DIAGNOSTIC REASONING: FOCUSED HISTORY

Is this a potentially serious cause of ALBP?

Key Questions
- Do you have a fever?
- Have you experienced any trauma to the spine or back?
- Do you have any other health problems?
- Have you been treated for cancer?
- What is your age?
- Have you had loss of control of your bowels or bladder?
- Are you taking any medications?

Fever

The presence of a fever indicates an inflammatory condition such as spondyloarthropathy or systemic infection. Infection is a likely diagnosis when there are chills and fever, weight loss, a recent history of bacterial infection,

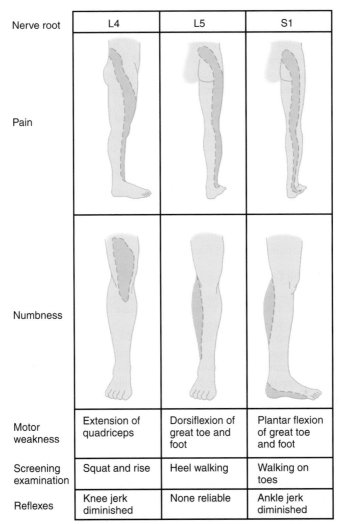

Nerve root	L4	L5	S1
Pain			
Numbness			
Motor weakness	Extension of quadriceps	Dorsiflexion of great toe and foot	Plantar flexion of great toe and foot
Screening examination	Squat and rise	Heel walking	Walking on toes
Reflexes	Knee jerk diminished	None reliable	Ankle jerk diminished

FIGURE 24.1 Testing for lumbar nerve root compromise. (From Bigos S, Bowyer OR, Braen GR, et al: *Acute low back problems in adults, clinical practice guidelines,* Quick Reference Guide Number 14, Rockville, Md., 1994, Department of Health and Human Services, U.S. Public Health Service, Agency for Health Care Policy and Research, AHCPR Publication No. 95-0643.)

intravenous drug use, or immunosuppression. Ewing sarcoma is a malignant tumor and can mimic spinal infection, occurring as back pain that can be accompanied by fever. Children with discitis will have a fever and refuse to walk because of back pain. In adults, vertebral osteomyelitis or discitis occurs most often as a result of hematogenous seeding of *S. aureus,* introduced through invasive procedures or surgery. Pain localizes over the infected disc area and is made worse with physical activity. Pain may radiate to the abdomen, leg, scrotum, groin, or perineum.

Trauma

Acute trauma to the spinal cord can result in fracture, dislocation, or damage to muscles, ligaments, and intervertebral disks. Trauma may be caused by blunt impact, repetitive injury, or sudden stress caused by lifting or pulling. Low back pain is the most common occupational injury reported, so knowing a patient's occupation helps assess specific risk factors. Injury to the back usually results in contusions and abrasions but can also cause spinal fracture if the force is major, such as that sustained in a motor vehicle accident or fall. Adults can have an acute compression spinal fracture as a result of strenuous lifting when osteoporosis is present. Most cases of ALBP in adolescents who are athletically active are caused by injury to the posterior structures of the spine.

Injury to the spinal column should be suspected in anyone whose level of consciousness is impaired after an accident. Cervical, thoracic and lumbar spine fractures are sustained during flexion, extension, compression, rotation, or a combination of forces.

Systemic Disease and Cancer

Metabolic disease, inflammatory disorders, and fibromyalgia can lead to back pain. Patients with a history of cancer may have increased risk of a metastatic spinal tumor. Neuroblastoma is common in young children, and although it occurs in the abdomen, metastases to the spine may produce back pain. People younger than 20 years and older than 50 years are at increased risk for tumor, as are those with a history of cancer.

Age

In the absence of trauma, the sudden onset of severe low or middle back pain in people older than 30 years might suggest a dissecting aortic aneurysm; the pain is not alleviated by rest. Patients older than 50 years are at increased risk for compression fracture as well as cancer.

Bowel and Bladder Symptoms

Loss of urinary or stool continence are early signs of conus medularis syndrome (vertebral involvement at L2) and late signs of cauda equina syndrome which involves nerve root compromise in the lower lumbar and sacral nerve roots secondary to a herniated disk, nerve root entrapment, spinal stenosis, infection, or tumor. Cauda equine is considered a surgical emergency. Other symptoms include constant lumbar pain with saddle anesthesia, urinary retention or overflow incontinence, and fecal incontinence due to an atonic anal sphincter.

Cauda equina

Children are embarrassed to talk about urinary or bowel habits and changes. Hidden spinal cord tumors might have a relationship to developmental delays in bladder and bowel control. Children younger than 4 years of age who have back pain should be evaluated for serious diseases, such as intraspinal tumors, dermoid cysts, and malignant astrocytomas.

Medications

Long-term use of corticosteroids can lead to compression fractures of the vertebrae. Use of intravenous drugs may suggest infection as a cause.

What does the location of pain tell me?

Key Question
• Where does it hurt?

Location of Pain

In general, children are less specific than adults when describing location of pain. Traumatic lesions are more likely to occur in the cervical and lumbar portions of the spine, where there is more motion and less protection. Generalized pain or pain over a fairly wide anatomical area is frequently seen with overuse problems and inflammatory conditions.

Sciatica pain is a sharp, burning pain that radiates down the posterior and lateral leg to the foot or ankle. Rheumatoid arthritis produces pain in the upper back and neck. Localized pain is seen with spondylolysis and tumors. Flank pain in adults may indicate a kidney infection. Pain from gallbladder disease radiates to the subscapular areas. Compression fractures of vertebrae associated with osteoporosis or malignancy may produce pain over the area where the fracture has occurred.

Children with traumatic low back derangement will have pain and muscle spasm in the lumbar area from the shock of an impact injury.

What does the pattern of pain tell me?

Key Questions
• When did the pain start?
• How long have you had this pain?

- What does the pain feel like?
- Does it interfere with sleep?
- Have you had this pain before?

Onset

The onset of ALBP is sudden, and more than half of patients do not associate it with a specific precipitating event or injury. The vast majority of cases of ALBP resolve with conservative treatment in 4 weeks, and radiographic or further diagnostic studies are not recommended unless it associated with trauma or symptoms such as radiating pain to an extremity, extremity weakness or bladder or bowel dysfunction.

Children are frequently poor historians, and parents may have a difficult time remembering when the pain started. Association with events such as birthdays, holidays, and activities is helpful in establishing the onset of a child's pain. Mild pain of short duration (1–2 weeks) is rarely serious.

Back pain lasting longer than 4 weeks needs to be reevaluated for further diagnostic studies.

Duration

Subacute back pain is of 6 to 12 weeks' duration. Chronic back pain is pain lasting for more than 3 months. In people younger than 40 years of age, the cause may be postural, related to weak abdominal or back muscles, or may indicate congenital spinal deformity, such as scoliosis or ankylosing spondylitis. In older people, chronic back pain is more likely to indicate degenerative disease, such as spinal stenosis or disk herniation. In children, back pain present for more than 3 weeks is often caused by organic and serious causes.

Pain Characteristics

In children, expression of pain depends on the child's ability to put feelings of pain into behavior; observing for these behaviors is important. Ask children to rate the pain using a 10-point pain scale with happy to sad faces (see Chapter 3). Ask adults to rate pain from 0 (no pain) to 10 (worst pain ever) and assess how much the pain interferes with daily activities. Intractable back pain, especially night pain with constitutional findings, is likely to indicate neoplastic disease. Hyperalgesia is increased sensitivity to pain in damaged tissue; this can develop after long-term use of opioids for chronic pain.

Night Pain

Nighttime back pain is a worrisome symptom that often signals a serious problem, such as tumor, infection, or inflammation. Generally, muscle strains, overuse injuries, spondylolysis, spondylolisthesis, and Scheuermann disease (an exaggeration of the normal posterior convex curvature of the thoracic spine) produce less pain at night. Morning stiffness that improves as the day progresses suggests osteoarthritis or ankylosing spondylitis.

Nighttime back pain is unusual and indicates the need for a complete and thorough workup.

Recurring Pain

Back pain in young children who have had previous injuries or fractures may be a symptom of child abuse. In older adults, it may be an indication of compression fractures of the spine. As with young children, it may also signal abuse by a caregiver.

What does the pain in relation to activity tell me?

Key Questions
- What makes the pain worse?
- What makes the pain better?
- School children: do you carry a backpack?

Aggravating Factors

Pain in the lumbar area after strenuous sporting activities is usually the result of trauma to the muscles and tendons, causing contusions and sprain. It occurs when the patient pushes the muscles and ligaments past the normal level of tolerance. Repeated injury can cause soft tissue scarring and shortening.

Stress and fatigue fractures of the pars interarticularis, the region between the superior and inferior articulating facets of the vertebra, occur when lumbar lordosis places more stress on the pars, such as in gymnastics and tennis.

Pain that is aggravated by activity is usually musculoskeletal in origin. Pain of ankylosing spondylitis is relieved with exercise. Spinal stenosis is associated with increased pain with standing, sneezing, or coughing. In an active adult, poor preparation before exercise can lead to back injury and pain. Severe low back pain is often the first symptom reported with spinal cord compression. When pain is not improved with lying down it suggests cancer or infection. Pain with movement suggests vertebral instability.

Any child who has voluntarily given up a pleasurable activity because of back pain has a severe symptom.

Alleviating Factors

Back pain not associated with any activity and not relieved by rest may indicate tumor. In children, back pain relieved with aspirin or nonsteroidal antiinflammatory drugs may indicate an inflammatory cause. Pain that is alleviated by rest and heat indicates a musculoskeletal cause. Pain of spinal stenosis is relieved by flexion of the spine.

Suspect spondylolisthesis, or forward slippage of one vertebra over another, if the onset of pain is during hyperextension, which can occur with a back handspring, butterfly stroke in swimming, or a tennis serve. The defect can be the result of degenerative processes in older patients or arise from a stress fracture or stress reaction of the isthmus of the pars interarticularis in the area of L5 to S1. The pain localizes to the low back and occurs during a growth spurt and after engaging in sporting events. The pain improves with rest and is worse with standing.

Backpack

School children often carry heavy backpacks, increasing the risk of back pain and injury.

What does radiation of pain tell me?

Key Questions
- Does the pain travel?
- Can you show me where the pain travels?

Radiation of Pain

Referred pain is of two types: (1) pain referred from the spine into areas lying within the lumbar and upper sacral dermatomes and (2) pain referred from the pelvic and abdominal viscera to the spine. Pain from the upper lumbar spine usually radiates to the anterior aspects of the thighs and legs, and pain from the lower lumbar spine radiates to the gluteal regions, posterior thighs, and calves (see Figure 24.4).

Pain from visceral disease is usually felt within the abdomen or flanks. Gallbladder pain radiates around the trunk to the right scapula. Position does not affect the pain.

In children and adolescent athletes, spondylolysis typically represents a fracture of the posterior arch in the lower lumbar spine due to overuse and is a relatively common cause of low back pain. Spondylolisthesis, an anterior displacement of a vertebra, is less common. Patients often develop pain that spreads across their lumbar region and radiates into their buttocks or posterior legs.

Pain that is sharp and burning and radiates down the lateral or posterior aspect of the leg to the lateral ankle or foot is called sciatica and is a classic symptom of nerve root irritation most often caused by disk herniation.

Are there signs of neurological damage?

Key Questions
- Have you been stumbling?
- Have you noticed any change in your balance or coordination?
- Does the child frequently stumble or fall?
- Do you have numbness or tingling in your extremities?

Stumbling

Spinal cord tumors, such as astrocytoma or ependymoma, may present as a disturbance of movement, posture, or strength in the spine or extremities. Impairment of proprioception or sensation from an upper motor neuron lesion, exhibited by foot drop or ataxia, may produce stumbling.

Numbness and Tingling

Radiculopathy (nerve root pain) is sharp pain felt in a dermatomal pattern and is sometimes associated with numbness and tingling.

Is there a family history of back pain?

Key Question
- Does anyone in your family have scoliosis or a crooked spine?

EVIDENCE-BASED PRACTICE *Does Low Back Pain in Adolescents Indicate a Serious Problem?*

A study of more than 200,000 adolescents who presented to a health care provider with low back pain were followed for 1 year. At 1 year, more than 80% of the adolescents had no identifiable diagnosis. The most common diagnoses found at 1 year were lumbar sprain-strain, less than 8%; scoliosis, less than 4%; and lumbar degenerative disk disease, less than 1%. Spondylolysis, spondylolisthesis, infection, tumor, and fracture had a less than 1% association with LBP.

Reference: Yang et al, 2017.

Family History

Spondylolysis and scoliosis are often seen in families, with a 40% familial occurrence in Native Alaskans.

Could this pain be caused by systemic disease?

Key Question
• Have you been ill?

Illness

Pharyngitis or upper respiratory tract infections, such as pneumonia, can be the precursor to diskitis, inflammation of the vertebral disk space, in children. The intervertebral disk in children receives its blood supply from the surface of the adjacent vertebral bodies, providing the mechanism necessary for infection. Uveitis and iritis may be associated with juvenile rheumatoid arthritis or juvenile ankylosing spondylitis.

A female patient with pelvic inflammatory disease (PID) may have mild to moderate dull, aching, lower abdominal, pelvic, or possibly back pain. With pyelonephritis, the patient may report fever, nausea and vomiting, headache, and back or flank pain. A urinary tract infection may present as back pain.

DIAGNOSTIC REASONING: FOCUSED PHYSICAL EXAMINATION

Observe the Patient's General Appearance and Behavior

Any person appearing ill with a fever, limp, or unwillingness to walk is highly suspect for having an infectious cause of back pain; however, a number of these symptoms may have a psychological component that should be explored.

Observe for symmetry of posture and movement from direct anterior, posterior, and lateral views of the patient. Note the amount of thoracic kyphosis (anteroposterior curve) and lumbar lordosis (anterior convexity) and the alignment of the head and neck above the center of gravity. Children with diskitis often protect their backs by sitting in a hyperextended position, using the arms as support, and may lie down and cry if they are made to sit.

Observe Gait

Shifting or leaning to one side (listing) and atypical scoliosis may indicate a tumor. Listing is caused by asymmetric sustained muscle contraction. The spinal curvature serves to relieve the discomfort and reduce pressure on a nerve root.

Severely affected gait in spondylosis is caused by hamstring tightness and results in uneven stride length with a persistently fixed knee to prevent hip flexion, which would stretch the tight hamstring muscles and increase pain.

Assess Vital Signs

Fever may indicate systemic infection as well as diskitis. Unexplained weight loss may suggest neoplasm, infection, or depression.

Examine Skin

Dermal cysts or a hairy patch over the spine may indicate spinal anomaly or tumor.

A doughy, fatty mass in the midline of the back (sometimes covered with hair [a Faun beard]) is evidence of a lipoma, which may extend into the spinal cord and produce neurologic symptoms.

Examine Eyes, Ears, Nose, and Mouth

Uveitis iritis is seen in juvenile rheumatoid arthritis and ankylosing spondylitis. Pharyngitis, otitis media, or infection of hematogenous origin may be the cause of diskitis in children.

Inspect the Back and Extremities

Observe for spinal alignment and symmetry of the tips of the scapula, iliac crests, and gluteal crease. If indicated, measure and compare leg lengths from the anterosuperior iliac crest to the medial malleolus. Measurements can be performed with the patient standing or supine. Legs should be of equal length or have less than 1 cm difference in length. Leg length differences are associated with pathologic conditions of the sacroiliac, facet joint, and disk.

From posterior and lateral viewpoints, observe the patient bending forward with feet together to detect scoliosis, kyphosis, or stiffness and guarding.

Percuss and Palpate Back and Spine

Painful scoliosis and stiffness are common in osteoid osteoma. Idiopathic scoliosis is usually painless without functional limitation. Point tenderness over the affected area is a finding associated with a compression fracture of the vertebrae or an infection of the spine.

Palpate and percuss the back to determine if tenderness is in the paravertebral muscular or midline spinous processes, which may indicate diskitis or osteomyelitis. To rule out the sacroiliac joint as the site of origin of ALBP, conduct a FABER test (Fig. 24.2). Place the patient in the supine position. Flex the leg and put the foot of the tested leg on the opposite knee. The motion is that of **fl**exion, **ab**duction, **e**xternal **r**otation at the hip. Slowly press down on the superior aspect of the tested knee joint lowering the leg into further abduction. The test result is positive if there is pain at the hip or sacral joint or if the leg cannot lower to the point of being parallel to the opposite leg.

Use fist percussion over the costovertebral angles to discriminate flank pain caused by renal disease from spinal pathology. Apply fist percussion over the costovertebral angles and over the spine to localize tenderness.

Perform Range of Motion of the Spine

Ask the patient to flex, extend, rotate, and bend the spine laterally. Decreased mobility and back pain along the spine may indicate muscle spasm, neoplasm, or bony deformity. Pain with forward flexion usually indicates a mechanical cause. Back extension pain increases with spinal stenosis.

Look for compensating effects of hip motion on the spine. The absence of lumbar flexion may be totally masked by a normal range of hip flexion when the patient bends forward. Test lumbar flexion by placing a mark

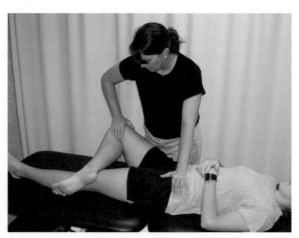

FIGURE 24.2 The FABER maneuver (**fl**exion, **ab**duction, **e**xternal **r**otation at the hip). (From Cummings N, Stanley-Green S, Huggs P: *Perspectives in athletic training,* St. Louis, 2009, Mosby.)

over the fourth lumbar vertebra and another over the sacrum. Lumbar flexion is demonstrated by an increased distance between these two marks when the patient bends forward.

A modified Schober test can be used to assess lumbar mobility. With the patient standing erect and heels together, draw a mark on the skin 5 cm below an imaginary line between the buttock dimples overlying the posterior superior iliac spine. A second mark is made 15 cm above this line. Then have the patient bend forward touching their toes. An increase in distance between these lines of 6 cm or more is normal; less than 6 cm indicates decreased lumbar spine mobility (Fig. 24.3).

Observe for limitation of motion on forward bending caused by hip flexion contracture. Lumbar lordosis does not flatten with forward bending and is an organic cause for back pain. In children, Scheuermann disease, an exaggeration of the normal posterior convex curvature of the thoracic spine, produces pain with forward flexion, and spondylolysis produces pain with hyperextension.

Perform Straight Leg Raising

The straight leg raising (SLR) test can assess sciatic (L5 and S1) nerve root tension. With the patient supine, place one hand above the knee,

the other cupping the heel, and slowly raise the limb. Instruct the patient to say when to stop because of pain. Observe for pelvic movement and the degree of leg elevation when the patient tells you to stop. Ask the patient to tell you the most distal point of pain sensation, such as the back, hip, thigh, or knee. While holding the leg at the limit of elevation, dorsiflexing the ankle and internally rotating will add tension to the neural structures and increase the pain if nerve root tension is present.

Pain below the knee at less than 70 degrees of elevation that is aggravated by dorsiflexing the ankle or hip rotation is a sign of L5 or S1 nerve root tension, suggestive of a herniated disk. This test can also be performed with the patient sitting. In a positive test result, the patient will resist extension or will compensate with hyperextension of the spine.

Lift each leg in succession to detect contralateral pain in patients with nerve root compression.

Results of the SLR test in children with a tumor can be unremarkable.

Check Hip Mobility

With the patient prone and supine, check active hip flexion, extension, internal and external

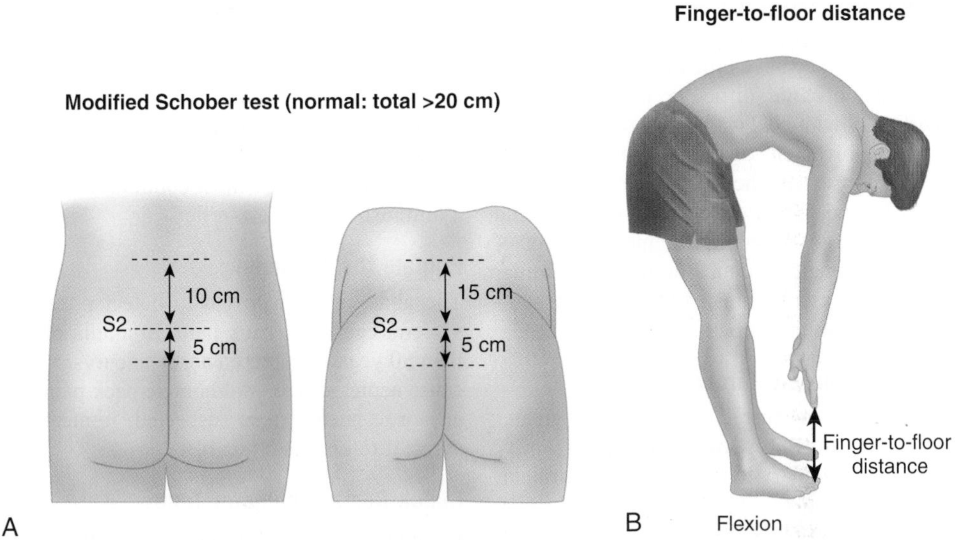

FIGURE 24.3 Performing the modified Schober test for spinal flexibility. (From Lawry G, Kreder H, Hawker G, Jerome D: *Fam's musculoskeletal examination and joint injection techniques,* ed. 2, Philadelphia, 2011, Mosby.)

rotation, and strength against resistance. Weakness of the gluteus maximus is associated with lumbar or referred pain from L5 nerve roots or gluteal nerve injury. In small children, check for congenital hip dysplasia with the child supine and abducting the hips (see Chapter 22). The knees should appear of equal height and should rotate externally by equal degrees. The presence of a hip click, joint instability, uneven hip-to-knee length with hips and knees flexed, and uneven gluteal skinfolds suggests congenital hip dislocation.

Examine Feet

Perform active range of motion of the ankle, feet, and toes against resistance. Weakness, pain, or limitation of dorsiflexion movement indicates an L4 nerve root injury. Similar symptoms produced by plantar flexion indicate S1 involvement, while symptoms produced by dorsiflexion of the big toe indicate L5 involvement. Deformities of the foot, such as talipes equinovarus (clubfoot) or hallux malleus (claw toes), may aggravate misalignment of back structures because of asymmetry.

Evaluate Muscle Strength

Evaluate strength against resistance of the lower extremity muscle groups. Test the patient's ability to stand on the toes and heels and to squat. A person with S1 nerve root involvement may have little motor weakness but may demonstrate difficulty in toe walking. Difficulty with heel walking or squatting indicates involvement of L5 and L4 nerve roots. Leg extension at the knee against resistance tests L4 root function. In young children who are unable to cooperate for measurement of muscle strength, use measurements of similar limb girths as an estimate of the bilateral symmetry of muscle strength.

Measure Muscle Circumference

Differences in muscle circumference greater than 2 cm in two opposite limbs may signify atrophy secondary to neurologic impairment.

Test Sensory Function

Neurologic test results are evaluated by comparing the symmetry of responses or perceptions. Bilateral comparison is the simplest, most efficient way to determine the presence, location, and extent of any abnormality. A sensory examination is a general guide in determining the level of spinal cord involvement. Test for light touch and pain sensation in the sensory areas of L3 to S1 dermatomes (see Fig. 24.4). Dermatomes overlap and vary greatly in individuals; thus, only gross changes can be detected by pinprick. Test 5 to 10 pinpricks in each dermatomal area if the patient reports numbness and tingling. Disk lesions rarely produce bilateral symptoms. It is sometimes difficult to distinguish numbness from a cutaneous nerve versus a dermatomal origin. Numbness from cutaneous nerve lesions does not occur in a dermatomal pattern. Numbness and tingling are uncommon symptoms in most children with back pain. When these symptoms are present, it suggests a serious problem.

Assess Deep Tendon Reflexes

Normal deep tendon reflexes (DTRs) are symmetrical. DTRs are increased when an upper motor neuron lesion is present and decreased with a lower motor neuron lesion. A positive Babinski sign indicates a disorder of upper motor neurons affecting the motor area of the brain or corticospinal tracts caused by spinal tumors or demyelinating disease. DTRs are decreased if a tumor is pressing on a peripheral nerve. Asymmetric abdominal reflexes are seen in tumors of the spine.

An absent or a decreased ankle-jerk reflex suggests an S1 nerve root lesion. An L3 to L4 disk herniation is the most common cause of a diminished knee-jerk reflex.

Palpate the Abdomen

The abdomen is palpated to detect possible visceral causes of back pain. In adults older than 50 years, a ruptured aortic aneurysm can cause acute, severe, midthoracic back pain. If an aortic aneurysm is suspected, immediate surgical referral is critical.

Check Rectal Sphincter Tone

In cauda equina syndrome, the compression of S1 to S2 nerve roots results in decreased sphincter tone and decreased sensation in the

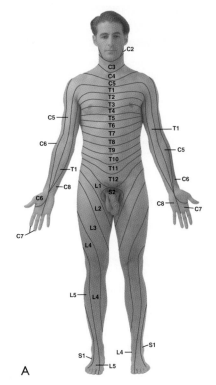
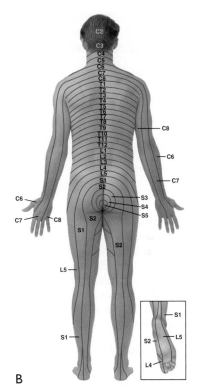

A   B

FIGURE 24.4 Dermatomes of the body, the area of body surface innervated by particular spinal nerves; C1 has no cutaneous distribution. **A**, anterior view. **B**, posterior view. (From A: Rudy, EB: *Advanced neurological and neurosurgical nursing.* 1984, Mosby, St Louis. B: Thibodeau, GA, Patton, KT: *Anatomy and physiology.* ed 5, 2003, Mosby, St Louis)

perianal area. This syndrome is a surgical emergency.

LABORATORY AND DIAGNOSTIC STUDIES

According to national practice guidelines, no diagnostic tests are warranted within the first 4 weeks for onset of ALBP without neurological signs or symptoms.

Spinal Radiographs

A flat lumbosacral spinal radiograph is obtained when there is a history of trauma or in people older than 50 years who have ALBP with signs of neurologic deficit a history of straining or lifting. Anterior and posterior view radiographs are useful in ruling out fracture, tumor, osteophytes (bone spurs), or vertebral infection.

Oblique and flexion views increase the sensitivity for determining instability.

Bone Mineral Density

Bone mineral density (BMD) uses radiography to assess the amount of calcium in bone. The distal wrist and lumbosacral spine can be scanned to assess BMD and the risk of osteoporosis. Density is measured as a T-score, reported as the number of standard deviations that a patient's BMD value is above or below the reference value for a healthy 30-year-old adult. A T-score cutoff value for osteoporosis is −2.5.

Bone Scan

Bone scanning uses a radioisotope to assess blood flow and bone formation or destruction. It can reveal inflammatory and infiltrative processes and occult fractures.

> **EVIDENCE-BASED PRACTICE** *How Important Is Obtaining Radiographic Imaging When Managing Acute Low Back Pain?*

A systematic review and meta-analysis was conducted to compare care with and without immediate routine lumbar imaging for ALBP without indications of serious underlying conditions. Outcomes examined included pain, function, mental health, quality of life, patient satisfaction, and overall patient improvement.

Results showed no differences in short-term or long-term follow-up between the group that underwent imaging and the group that did not. In addition to no clinical benefit from immediate imaging with ALBP, routine lumbar imaging is associated with radiation exposure and increased cost related to unnecessary procedures.

Reference: Andersen JC: 2011.

Electromyography

Electromyography (EMG) with nerve conduction study is a diagnostic procedure to assess the health of muscles and the nerve cells (motor neurons) that control them. In nerve conduction electrodes are placed on the skin to measure speed and strength of signals traveling between two points.

Diagnostic Imaging

Magnetic resonance imaging (MRI) is useful in evaluating soft tissue detail, such as disk herniations, tumors, and spinal cord pathologies, especially in vertebral osteomyelitis. Computed tomography is usually used for bone visualization.

Urinalysis

Urinalysis is performed to assess kidney and metabolic function, including infectious processes, to rule out a visceral cause of back pain, such as the pain of pyelonephritis.

Erythrocyte Sedimentation Rate

The erythrocyte sedimentation rate (ESR) will be elevated in about 90% of patients with a serious musculoskeletal infection; however, there is no direct relationship between ESR and severity of infection. The test is nonspecific.

Complete Blood Count

The complete blood count will detect anemia as well as other conditions that might manifest as back pain, such as tumor or infection. The anemia of chronic disease is usually hypochromic or normochromic with low iron indices.

DIFFERENTIAL DIAGNOSIS

Potentially Serious Causes of Acute Low Back Pain

Spinal fracture

The patient may relate a history of major trauma to the back from an impact or fall or, if the patient is an older adult, a history of strenuous lifting or a minor fall. Pain is felt near the site of injury. Any suspicion of spinal fracture should be treated as an emergency. The patient is immobilized to prevent further damage and transported by emergency personnel to obtain radiographs of the suspected area of fracture.

Tumor (osteoblastoma, spinal metastasis, osteoid osteoma)

Whereas primary tumors are a more common cause of back pain in children, metastases are a more common cause in adults. The lower thoracic and upper lumbar vertebrae are the most common sites of bony metastatic disease from marrow tumors. A health history and diagnostic tests may reveal other signs of poor general health, such as weight loss, fatigue, weakness, and anemia.

Infection (osteomyelitis, diskitis, epidural abcess)

The spine is the most common site of osteomyelitis in adults, secondary to adjacent infection or following invasive instrumentation that results in bacterial seeding of the bone via arterial blood. *Staphylococcus aureus* is the most frequently identified organism. Vertebral osteomyelitis causes stiffness and pain, usually localized over the site of infection. A tender spinous process, positive SLR test result, and paravertebral muscle spasm may be seen in vertebral osteomyelitis or septic diskitis. Patients may have hip pain secondary to involvement of L2 to S1.

Diskitis is usually a benign disorder in children that results in intervertebral disk inflammation. Children will be reluctant to walk, sit, or stand. Pain will be aggravated by motion and relieved by rest. History will reveal a recent bacterial infection, often secondary to pharyngitis or otitis media, intravenous drug use, diabetes mellitus, or immunosuppression. A small percentage of adults will report an acute onset of fever, weight loss, and general malaise; however, the majority will only have the symptom of back pain, present from 2 weeks to years.

Epidural abscess is a rare and serious infection of the central nervous system (CNS). Abscesses that occur within the bony confines of the skull or spinal column can expand to compress the brain or spinal cord and cause severe symptoms, permanent complications, or even death. Prompt diagnosis and treatment is critical and treatment often includes aspiration guided by magnetic resonance imaging or surgical drainage of the abscess.

Herniated disk

Disk herniation causes nerve root irritation and produces ALBP that radiates down the buttock to below the knee. Pain is the prominent symptom, with numbness and weakness less common. Physical examination will reveal a positive SLR test result. If the pain persists longer than 1 month consider MRI. Urgent neuroimaging is indicated if neurologic deficits, urinary retention, saddle anesthesia are present, or if neoplasm or epidural abcess are suspected.

Cauda equina syndrome

Compression of the S1 nerve root produces constant back pain with saddle distribution anesthesia (buttock and medial and posterior thighs), fecal incontinence, bladder dysfunction, motor weakness of the lower limbs, and radiculopathy. The patient may limp and guard lumbar spine movement, will not be able to heel walk or toe walk, and will have abnormal or asymmetrical knee and ankle DTRs. The SLR test result will be positive. This syndrome is a surgical emergency.

Nonspecific Back Problems

Sciatica

The most common cause of sciatica radiculopathy, or pain related to spinal nerve root involvement, is herniated vertebral disk. History may disclose repetitive motion strain or strenuous lifting, twisting, and bending. ALBP is associated with pain and burning that radiates along the lateral thigh, leg, and foot, sometimes associated with numbness along the dermatomal areas. SLR and sitting knee extension produce radicular pain below the knee at less than 60 degrees of limb elevation, and pain may be felt in the buttocks or posterior thigh. Bowel and bladder functions are normal.

Musculoskeletal strain (postural, overuse)

Back structures such as muscles and ligaments can become inflamed from overuse or strain. History often reveals no precipitating event for the onset of pain. Patients may report that pain is alleviated by rest, especially in the supine position with hips and knees flexed, and by the application of heat or cold. Pain is aggravated by sitting, walking, standing, and with certain motions. On physical examination, palpation will localize the pain, and muscle spasms may be felt. Range of motion of the spine will increase the pain, especially with forward flexion. Neurologic examination shows no abnormalities.

Spondylolisthesis

Pain can be the result of disruption of the vertebral spinous process, where the disruption results in subluxation of the vertebral body onto adjacent structures. This usually occurs between L5 and S1. Pain is usually chronic. Examination of the spine may disclose a palpable, prominent spinous process. Forward flexion may be limited.

Ankylosing spondylitis

Ankylosing spondylitis is a systemic inflammatory condition of the vertebral column and sacroiliac joints. Peak incidence is in people 20 to 30 years old; males are most often affected. Patients report chronic LBP, which is worse on morning rising and lessens as the day progresses. Examination shows an excessive thoracic kyphosis and rounding of the posterior thoracic spine with forward flexion of the head, neck, and lower back. About 30% of patients will have arthritis of other joints. Radiographs may reveal fusion of vertebrae, and ESR is elevated.

Spinal stenosis

Spinal stenosis is a bony encroachment on the nerve roots of the lumbar spine and is the most common cause of ALBP in adults older than 50 years. Patients report ALBP associated with lumbosacral radiculopathy, pain with walking or standing, and pain relief with sitting or forward flexion of the spine. Neurogenic (pseudo) claudication pain of the lower extremities is made worse with prolonged standing, walking, bending, or hyperextending the back.

Scheuermann disease

Adolescents develop this disease as a result of anterior disk protrusion, causing wedging of the thoracic vertebrae and exaggeration of the normal posterior convex curvature of the thoracic spine. The cause is unknown but may develop from excessive lifting or spinal flexion. The patient reports mild to moderate pain, worsening toward the end of the day or after physical activity but relieved by rest. Physical examination demonstrates an increase in thoracic kyphosis on lateral view, made sharper by forward bending.

Osteoporosis

Osteoporosis is loss of mineralized bone mass that can result in a compression fracture of the vertebral body, usually occurring in the thoracic area. Back pain is often chronic and poorly localized. Multiple compression fractures may produce dorsal kyphosis and cervical lordosis. Estrogen deficiency, through menopause or medications, is a risk factor. It is also common in people older than 70 years who have age-related reduction in vitamin D synthesis. Osteoporosis can also be secondary to endocrine imbalance (e.g., hyperthyroidism), organ disease, drugs (e.g., corticosteroids), or excessive intake of alcohol. The Fracture Risk Assessment Tool (FRAX[R]) is a web-based algorithm used to calculate the 10-year probability of hip and femur fracture based on clinical risk factors and BMD results.

Vertebral compression fracture

Causes of vertebral compression fractures are trauma, osteoporosis, and systemic disease. In older adults, compression fractures secondary to osteoporosis may be without symptoms. Patients may report pain, loss of sensation, or loss of continence after a trauma. A history of cancer may indicate metastasis. Radiograph will detect a fracture.

Nonspinal Causes

Aortic aneurysm (dissecting)

Sudden onset of severe low or middle back pain that is not alleviated by rest in people older than 30 years might suggest a dissecting aortic aneurysm. The patient may exhibit pallor, diaphoresis, and confusion. Pulses and blood pressure measured on each upper extremity will be asymmetric. Emergency surgery is indicated.

Gallstones

Gallbladder problems increase with age. A gallbladder attack often follows a fatty meal. Crampy right upper quadrant (RUQ) pain following a fatty meal is produced by spasms of the cystic duct that is obstructed with a stone. Gallbladder pain radiates around the trunk to the right scapula. Position does not affect the pain. Patients report belching and bloating. Attacks may increase in frequency and severity and cause nighttime wakening. During an attack, palpation will show RUQ tenderness. Physical findings between attacks may be normal, or there may be tenderness to palpation of the RUQ on inspiration (Murphy sign) if the gallbladder is inflamed. An RUQ mass may be felt if the gallbladder is obstructed. Obstruction is an emergency surgical situation.

Pyelonephritis

With pyelonephritis, the patient will appear ill and diaphoretic and may report nausea and vomiting, headache, and back or flank pain. The patient may have a fever. Severe lumbar tenderness will be found on fist percussion for costovertebral angle tenderness. Urinalysis will show cloudy, malodorous urine, and microscopy will show casts and cells (i.e., red blood cells, white blood cells, and epithelial cells).

Pleuritis

Inflammation of the pleural lining of the lungs often follows an upper respiratory tract infection. Pleuritic pain is sharp, worsens on inspiration or with coughing, and is lessened by lying on the affected side. Physical examination of the lungs may be normal, or crackles and bronchial breath sounds will be heard on auscultation. A chest radiograph will provide information on the condition of the lungs.

Pelvic inflammatory disease

The symptoms of PID depend on the extent of infection. Infection usually begins in the lower urinary tract or cervix and spreads to the endometrium, Fallopian tubes, and peritoneum. The sexually active patient may have mild to moderate dull, aching, lower abdominal, pelvic, or possibly back pain. The patient will report tenderness during cervical motion, uterine motion, or palpation of the adnexa. History may be positive for sexually transmitted infections (usually *Neisseria gonorrhoeae* or *Chlamydia trachomatis*), vaginal symptoms, or use of an intrauterine device for contraception.

Psychogenic Causes

Psychologic back pain

A careful history is needed to gain insight into the psychosocial and economic issues surrounding report of back pain. The patient may have a history of recent life stressors, be involved in a legal injury or workers' compensation action, or have a history of depression or alcohol abuse. The clinician should be aware of exaggerated signs of pain, such as moaning, grimacing, or overreacting. A malingerer pretends to suffer but, when distracted, will show inconsistent and variable results on examination such as SLR, or will describe radiation of pain inconsistent with dermatome distribution.

▶ DIFFERENTIAL DIAGNOSIS OF *Common Causes of Acute Low Back Pain*

CONDITION	HISTORY	PHYSICAL FINDINGS	DIAGNOSTIC STUDIES
POTENTIALLY SERIOUS CAUSES			
Spinal fracture	Trauma to spine or back; pain is felt near site of injury	Palpable tenderness over site of fracture	Considered an emergency; immobilize patient and transport for radiographs
Tumor	History of cancer; progressive pain is unremitting; occurs at night and at rest	Weight loss, fever, tenderness near tumor	ESR; bone scan; MRI

Continued

> **DIFFERENTIAL DIAGNOSIS OF** *Common Causes of Acute Low Back Pain—cont'd*

CONDITION	HISTORY	PHYSICAL FINDINGS	DIAGNOSTIC STUDIES
Osteoblastoma	Neck or back pain not relieved by aspirin; occurs in older adolescents and young adults	Localized tenderness; may have scoliosis with muscle pain	Plain film shows an expansive osteolytic lesion surrounded by thin peripheral rim of bone; bone scan; CT scan
Osteoid osteoma	Occurs primarily in adolescents; rare in patients older than age 40 yr; well-localized pain that may be more severe at night and relieved by aspirin or other prostaglandin inhibitors	Painful, well-localized scoliosis may be present	Bone scan
Infection (vertebral osteomyelitis)	History of infection, invasive procedure; continuous, dull back pain; chronic back pain	Acute onset with fever, diaphoresis; tenderness over affected disk; positive SLR	ESR; blood culture; bone biopsy; CT scan; MRI
Diskitis	Pain aggravated by movement; more common in children	Tenderness over affected disk	ESR; CT
Herniated disk	LBP radiating down the buttock to below the knee, symptoms present <1 mo	Positive SLR	MRI
Cauda equina syndrome	Constant pain in a saddle distribution; urinary retention, fecal incontinence, radiculopathy	Positive SLR, abnormal DTRs, motor weakness	MRI, surgical emergency
NONSPECIFIC BACK PROBLEMS			
Sciatica	Acute back pain with radiculopathy; history of strain or trauma, relief with sitting	Paravertebral tenderness and spasm; positive SLR; sitting knee extension, sensory findings	MRI
Musculoskeletal strain	Pain in back, buttocks; history of new activity or exertion; relief of pain with sitting	Paravertebral tenderness, scoliosis, or loss of lumbar lordosis; no neurological signs	None

▶ DIFFERENTIAL DIAGNOSIS OF *Common Causes of Acute Low Back Pain—cont'd*

CONDITION	HISTORY	PHYSICAL FINDINGS	DIAGNOSTIC STUDIES
Spondylolisthesis	Young person in a sport that demands rapid movement between hyperflexion and hyperextension or requires excess loading in hyperextension	No neurological signs; pain localized to low back, just below level of iliac crest; tight hamstrings	Lumbar spine radiographs
Ankylosing spondylitis	Younger than age 40 yr: insidious onset; progressive morning back pain relieved with exercise	Painful sacroiliac joints, reduced spine mobility; may have uveitis	ESR; spinal radiographs
Spinal stenosis	Pain worse throughout day; aggravated by standing, relieved by rest; pseudoclaudication	Signs of osteoarthritis of joints; may have neurological signs	MRI
Scheuermann disease	Affects mostly adolescent males; mild to moderately severe pain, worse at end of day, relieved by rest	Normal examination; may show an exaggerated thoracic kyphosis that is fixed in attempted hyperextension	Thoracic spine radiographs
Osteoporosis	Chronic, poorly localized back pain; postmenopausal; slight build; history of inactivity or endocrine disorder	Palpable tenderness over area of compression fracture; kyphosis or lordosis; loss of height	Bone densitometry; FRAX^R score; spinal radiograph to assess fracture
Vertebral compression fracture	Pain, loss of sensation, incontinence; trauma to the spine; history of cancer, osteoporosis	Palpable tenderness over fracture, observation of spine deformity	Radiograph to detect fracture
NONSPINAL CAUSES			
Aortic aneurysm	Severe, acute-onset pain not related to activity or movement; increased risk older than age 30 yr; pallor, diaphoresis, anxiety, confusion	Intact aneurysm will be a visible pulsatile midline upper quadrant abdominal mass; in a dissected aneurysm, upper extremity pulse and pulse pressures are asymmetric; posterior thoracic pain may be felt	Emergency surgical referral

Continued

DIFFERENTIAL DIAGNOSIS OF *Common Causes of Acute Low Back Pain—cont'd*

CONDITION	HISTORY	PHYSICAL FINDINGS	DIAGNOSTIC STUDIES
Gallstones	Increased incidence with age; steady, intense pain in RUQ with radiation to right scapula or shoulder; belching, bloating, fatty food intolerance	Normal physical examination or positive Murphy sign on palpation of abdomen	Surgical referral
Pyelonephritis	Ill-appearing; sweating, nausea, back or flank pain, headache	Fever; cloudy, malodorous urine; CVA tenderness on percussion	Urinalysis; urine culture
Pleuritis	History of recent URI; pleuritic pain	Normal examination or crackles and bronchial breath sounds	PPD; chest radiograph
Pelvic inflammatory disease	Sexually active female; low back and abdominal pain; history of urinary or vaginal symptoms, sexually transmitted disease, IUD, multiple sex partners	Cervical and uterine motion tenderness, adnexal tenderness; cervicitis, fever	Gonorrhea, Chlamydia cultures; ESR
PSYCHOGENIC CAUSES			
Psychological back pain	History of psychosocial stressors, depression, exaggerated expressions of pain	Exaggerated or inconsistent reactions to testing; normal examination	None

CT, computed tomography; *CVA*, costovertebral angle; *DTRs*, deep tendon reflexes; *EMG*, electromyography; *ESR*, erythrocyte sedimentation rate; *IUD*, intrauterine device; *LBP*, lower back pain; *MRI*, magnetic resonance imaging; *PPD*, purified protein derivative; *RUQ*, right upper quadrant; *SLR*, straight leg raising; *URI*, upper respiratory tract infection.

CHAPTER
25

Nasal Symptoms and Sinus Congestion

Concern about symptoms of the "common cold" accounts for a significant proportion of primary care visits by both children and adults, especially in the winter months. Viral infections and self-limiting causes of symptoms require the clinician to provide primarily symptom relief and to avoid overuse of antibiotic treatment. Symptoms include nasal congestion, rhinorrhea, postnasal drip, sneezing, itchy nose, watery and itchy eyes, and frontal headache. Severe symptoms are associated with ageusia (loss of taste) and anosmia (loss of smell).

The nose humidifies, warms, and filters inspired air. The nasal turbinates located in the nasal cavity promote turbulent airflow that causes particulate matter to fall on the mucosa, where it is swept away by ciliated pseudostratified columnar cells to the nasopharynx (Fig. 25.1). Rhinitis, or inflammation of the mucous membranes, is a frequent nasal symptom that is caused by bacterial or viral infection, a response to allergens, a response to medication, or a reaction to extremes in environmental temperature.

Nasal polyps, septal deviation, or congenital anomaly can cause nasal obstruction. In children, nasal obstruction is frequently unilateral and may be secondary to a foreign body inserted into the nose.

Epistaxis is a common symptom in both adults and children, with most cases occurring before the age of 10 or between 45 and 65 years of age. Causes are trauma to the nose, mucosal changes related to fluctuations in temperature and humidity, and anticoagulation therapy. Blood or structural alterations can lead to nasal obstruction.

Respiratory epithelium lines the paranasal sinuses and creates drainage into the nasal cavity via the superior meatus and middle meatus. The maxillary sinus is the most frequently involved paranasal sinus because its ciliated cells carry maxillary sinus drainage against gravity. When drainage systems become impaired as a result of mucosal edema, mechanical obstruction, or impaired ciliary activity, viruses and bacteria proliferate.

The paranasal sinuses include the frontal, ethmoid, maxillary, and sphenoid (Fig. 25.2). Most sinus infections are caused by bacteria common to the nasopharynx that proliferate when local or systemic defenses are impaired. The most common causative organisms producing bacterial sinusitis in both adults and children are *Streptococcus pneumoniae* and *Haemophilus influenzae*. Sinusitis may also be associated with allergies and asthmatic exacerbations or with contiguous infection of the mouth or face.

DIAGNOSTIC REASONING: FOCUSED HISTORY

What symptoms will help me narrow the possibilities?

Key Questions
- Can you describe your symptoms?
- Do you have pain? If so, where is the pain located?
- How long have symptoms been present?
- Do the symptoms occur at any particular time of the year? Do you have a history of nasal problems?
- Is there a family history of allergies or asthma?

Acute Symptoms

Acute sinusitis is an abrupt onset of infection of one or more of the paranasal sinuses, and it occurs when the sinus ostia become obstructed, usually after an upper respiratory tract infection. Sinusitis is frequently associated with a sore throat, often irritated by postnasal discharge, facial or tooth pain, or

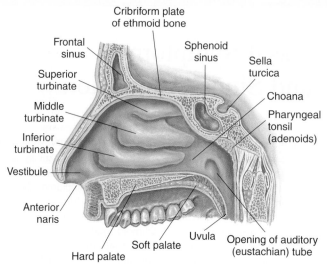

Cribriform plate
of ethmoid bone

Frontal
sinus

Sphenoid
sinus

Sella
turcica

Superior
turbinate

Choana

Middle
turbinate

Pharyngeal
tonsil
(adenoids)

Inferior
turbinate

Vestibule

Anterior
naris

Uvula   Opening of auditory
Soft palate   (eustachian) tube
Hard palate

FIGURE 25.1 Lateral view of the left nasal cavity. (From Ball JW, Dains JE, Flynn J, et al: *Seidel's guide to physical examination*, ed. 8, St. Louis, 2015, Elsevier.)

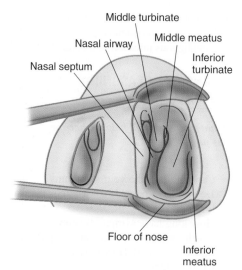

Middle turbinate

Nasal airway

Middle meatus

Inferior
turbinate

Nasal septum

Floor of nose

Inferior
meatus

FIGURE 25.2 Anterior and lateral views of the paranasal sinuses. (From Ball JW, Dains JE, Flynn J, et al: *Seidel's guide to physical examination*, ed. 8, St. Louis, 2015, Elsevier.)

Acute symptoms of rhinitis or sinus congestion, usually lasting 48 to 72 hours, are caused by edematous mucosa obstructing the sinus ostia. Systemic symptoms such as fever, myalgias, chills, and acute infectious rhinitis are often caused by rhinoviruses or parainfluenza virus.

Acute symptoms of epistaxis may be related to trauma to the nose, exposure to changes in air temperature or humidity level, or symptoms associated with a rhinosinusitis infection.

Chronic Symptoms

Chronic symptoms can be caused by prolonged obstruction of the osteomeatal complex, which leads to dysfunction of ciliary motility and movement of mucus within the sinuses. Local factors that cause mechanical obstruction include adenoid hypertrophy, conchae bullosa, nasal polyps, foreign bodies, and nasal deviations. Adults with symptoms that last more than 3 weeks experience upper molar pain or headache, postnasal drip, and nausea. Chronic rhinitis lasting weeks to years is rarely infectious; rather, it is often associated with anatomical abnormalities that impair the sinus drainage system, although the mucociliary clearance mechanisms are normal.

In children, chronic sinusitis is defined as the presence of symptoms for longer than 30 days.

headache over the affected sinus, as well as morning periorbital swelling, fever, and malaise. Other less common causes include anatomical abnormality, adenoid hypertrophy, and contiguous infection, such as a dental abscess or periorbital cellulitis.

Chronic epistaxis can be related to nose picking, foreign body (especially in children), platelet disorders, and anticoagulation therapy

Location of Pain

An adult with sinusitis most often reports prolonged symptoms of nasal congestion and facial pain. Children rarely complain of headache or facial pain. The location of pain may indicate which sinus is involved. Pain of maxillary sinusitis occurs over the sinuses and is sometimes perceived as a maxillary toothache. Frontal sinusitis produces a frontal headache that is worse on morning wakening. Whereas ethmoid sinusitis causes pain that refers to the vertex, forehead, or occipital or temporal region, the pain of sphenoid sinusitis is perceived on the top of the head.

Seasonal Occurrence of Symptoms

Suspect allergic rhinitis if a person describes seasonal occurrence of nasal symptoms associated with sneezing and itchy or burning eyes. A distinguishing feature of the allergic individual is the propensity to develop sustained immunoglobulin E (IgE) response after antigenic stimulation. IgE is an antibody capable of interacting with target cells that release mediators on contact with specific antigens. This reaction is the manifestation of an allergy.

People with perennial allergies have an allergen present in the environment on a year-round basis from such sources as animal dander, house dust, mold, feathers, and cockroaches. Seasonal allergies usually occur in early spring (tree pollens), early summer (grass pollens), and early fall (weed pollens).

Family History

Family history of asthma or allergies is frequently associated with allergic rhinitis. Other symptoms may include a sensation of head stuffiness, ear discomfort, fatigue, and a scratchy or mild sore throat.

If I suspect sinus problems, what do I need to know?

Key Questions
- Do your symptoms change with position changes?
- Do you have a history of sinus problems?

Position Change

Maxillary sinusitis produces pain that worsens with bending or leaning forward. The postnasal discharge associated with sinusitis produces a cough that worsens while lying down.

History of Sinus Problems

Chronic sinusitis can be attributed to infection, growths in the sinuses (nasal polyps) or a deviated nasal septum. The condition most commonly affects young and middle-aged adults, but it also can affect children.

Does the presence of other symptoms provide any clues?

Key Questions
- Do you have other acute symptoms, such as cough, fever, or muscle aches?
- Do you have other chronic symptoms, such as eye pain, bad breath, or fatigue?

Other Acute Symptoms

Seropurulent nasal discharge is often present with acute bacterial infection of the nasal and sinus mucosa. Acute rhinitis caused by a bacterial or viral infection produces systemic symptoms such as fever, myalgia, and chills. Allergic rhinitis is associated with sneezing, nasal congestion, clear and profuse rhinorrhea, as well as pruritus of the nose, palate, pharynx, and middle ear. Eye symptoms include conjunctival irritation, itching, erythema, and tearing. Ear symptoms involve a feeling of fullness in the ears with popping. Sinus symptoms are pressure or pain of the cheeks, forehead, or behind the eyes.

Acute sinusitis in children involves the presence of symptoms for less than 30 days, a persistent cough, fever with a temperature greater than 39°C (102.2°F) for more than 3 days, and malodorous breath. The maxillary and ethmoid sinuses are most commonly affected, the frontal sinus is occasionally affected, and the sphenoid sinus is rarely affected.

Other Chronic Symptoms

Chronic sinusitis involves long episodes of inflammation or repeated infections that lead to anatomical destruction. The recurrent symptoms interfere with daily activities and are not relieved with nonpharmacological measures or over-the-counter medications. Patients often report a cold that does not go away, eye pain, halitosis, chronic cough, fatigue, anorexia, and malaise.

Is the cause viral, bacterial, or allergic?

Key Question
• What color is your nasal drainage?
Acute rhinitis is caused by a bacterial or viral infection that produces a watery, profuse nasal discharge early in the onset, and later becomes more mucoid and purulent. Purulent discharge may be the result of a primary viral infection or a secondary bacterial infection. The color of the nasal discharge is not diagnostic. Watery or clear discharge occurs with allergic reactions and is usually persistent or seasonal.

Are there factors that will narrow the diagnosis?

Key Questions
• Are symptoms on one side or both sides?
• Do you smoke?
• Are you exposed to others who smoke?
• Have you had a recent history of head or facial trauma?
• Have you been diving or swimming?
• Have you been exposed to infections in day care, school, or work settings?
• Are you pregnant?

Unilateral or Bilateral Symptoms

Infectious rhinitis and allergic rhinitis are usually bilateral. Unilateral symptoms are more indicative of an anatomical cause such as nasal polyps, septal deviation, unilateral choanal atresia, or a foreign body (typically occurs in children).

Smoking History

Smokers have an increased risk of sinusitis. Smoking can lead to the production of more tenacious mucus and to temporary paralysis of the nasal cilia. Exposure to passive smoke causes an increased risk of upper and lower respiratory tract infections.

Trauma History

Nasal trauma or fracture may lead to nasal congestion. A rare but serious posttrauma cerebrospinal fluid rhinorrhea can be present. Up to 80% of head injuries involve the paranasal sinuses.

Diving and Swimming

Sinusitis from diving or swimming is secondary to barotrauma, infection from contaminated water, or an allergic response to chlorine. Chlorine exposure can cause inflammation of the sinus mucosa, restricting nasal discharge.

Exposure

Exposure to viral infections increases when children are exposed to other children. The spread of a virus occurs by direct secretion of droplets or contact with contaminated objects.

 EVIDENCE-BASED PRACTICE *Do Symptoms Distinguish Between Viral and Bacterial Acute Sinusitis?*

This systematic literature search was done to assess the diagnostic value of fever and facial and dental pain in adults suspected of acute bacterial rhinosinusitis (ABRS). The prevalence of positive predictive values and negative predictive values were extracted from 3171 records where the diagnosis was confirmed by culture from either sinus puncture or endoscopically obtained antral aspirate. Only one study was deemed to be of good quality. The study reported an odds ratio for fever of 1.02 (0.52–2.00) and 1.65 (0.83–3.28) for facial and dental pain. The authors concluded that evidence is inadequate to support the value of fever and facial and dental pain to differentiate viral or bacterial causes of ABRS in adults. These symptoms should not be used in clinical practice for decision making about prescribing antibiotic treatment.

Reference: Hauer et al, 2014.

Pregnancy

The hormonal changes of pregnancy can cause nasal congestion.

Is the patient using any drugs that would cause nasal congestion?

Key Questions

- Are you using nasal sprays or drops?
- Do you use cocaine or other recreational drugs?
- What other medications are you taking?

Nasal Spray

The use of topical sympathomimetic sprays or drops for more than 1 week can lead to rebound nasal congestion or vasodilation after short periods of vasoconstriction. The use of decongestants and antihistamines with low ambient humidity leads to excessive dryness and impaired ciliary function.

Recreational Drug Use

Chronic or acute cocaine use can cause rebound nasal congestion. Nasal congestion associated with conjunctivitis and irritation of the eyes may be seen in people who abuse drugs by inhalation.

Medications

Oral contraceptives, phenothiazines, angiotensin-converting enzyme inhibitors, and β-blockers may cause nasal congestion.

Is there systemic disease present?

Key Questions

- Have you noticed any other body symptoms?
- Do you have any chronic health problems?

Systemic Disorders and Chronic Health Problems

Systemic causes of decreased mucociliary clearance include cystic fibrosis, ciliary dyskinesia syndrome, and immunoglobulin deficiency. Individuals with congenital or acquired immune deficiencies, such as diabetes mellitus, leukemia, acquired immunodeficiency syndrome, and cystic fibrosis, have an increased risk of developing acute

and chronic sinusitis. Hypothyroidism, acromegaly, Horner syndrome, neoplasm, and granulomatosis disorder can cause nasal symptoms.

DIAGNOSTIC REASONING: FOCUSED PHYSICAL EXAMINATION

Perform a General Inspection

Note the patient's general appearance. Observe for signs of impaired mental status. A severe, unremitting, or new-onset headache, vomiting, or alteration in consciousness requires consideration for immediate referral.

Take Vital Signs

Patients with acute viral rhinitis or acute sinusitis may be afebrile or have a low-grade fever. Patients with allergic rhinitis are afebrile. The presence of mouth breathing suggests chronic nasal obstruction caused by hypertrophied pharyngeal lymphoid tissues.

Inspect the Face

Children with chronic allergic conditions have an allergic "salute"; this is a crease on the nose from continued wiping up of nasal drainage. Allergic "shiners" are dark circles under the eyes suggestive of venous congestion and stasis. Observe for allergic facies from chronic mouth breathing: open mouth, receding chin, overbite, elongated face, and arched hard palate. Observe for facial symmetry and signs of periorbital edema. Periorbital cellulitis is the most common serious complication of severe bacterial sinusitis.

Perform a Regional Examination of the Head and Neck

Examine the eyes (including visual acuity), ears, and cervicofacial lymph nodes. Complications of severe fulminant sinusitis are rare and are caused by the direct spread of infection, secondary to destruction of the wall between the sinuses and the orbit. Symptoms can include a sudden increase in pain, acute edema of the eyelids, periorbital edema and erythema, decreased visual acuity, diplopia, and displacement of the eye laterally. The patient may experience pain on testing of extraocular muscles. These symptoms mandate immediate referral.

Observe for symptoms of coryza (acute rhinitis) as well as ear and eye drainage. Erythematous tympanic membranes are seen in acute viral rhinitis.

Examine the Mouth and Teeth

Examine the teeth for the presence of abscesses, especially the first and secondary maxillary molars and the alveolar margin of the teeth. Tenderness elicited by tapping on the maxillary teeth with a tongue blade may indicate dental root infection or maxillary sinusitis. Lymphoid hyperplasia, "cobblestoning," may be seen on the posterior pharynx with chronic allergies. Mouth breathing is associated with hypertrophied gingival mucosa and halitosis. Halitosis can also be a sign of dental abscess or sinusitis.

Children with acute viral rhinitis have mild erythema of the tonsils and posterior pharynx. If there is vasomotor rhinitis, mucus is present in the posterior pharynx.

Test for Smell

Test for smell by asking the patient to close their eyes and identify simple odors (e.g., coffee, vinegar, chocolate) presented to each naris separately. Severe nasal congestion or ethmoid sinusitis causes anosmia, as do neurodegenerative diseases such as Alzheimer and Parkinson diseases.

Inspect Condition of Nasal Mucosa and Turbinates

Use a nasal speculum and pen light or head mirror to optimally visualize the condition of the nasal mucosa and turbinates. A topical vasoconstrictive agent may be needed to shrink the swollen mucosa to visualize the middle meatus.

In infants and young children, the nares tend to open forward, and tilting the tip of the nose up with the thumb and directing the light into the nares will allow inspection of the nasal cavities.

Pale, swollen, and wet turbinates are seen with allergic rhinitis. Inflamed mucous membranes are seen with acute coryza or hay fever. Allergic rhinitis may also produce a violet-colored mucous membrane. Ulceration of the nasal mucosa may be found in individuals who abuse drugs by inhalation.

Inspect for Masses

Observe for the presence of nasal polyps, which look like skinned grapes and are usually bilateral and hang from the middle turbinate into the lumen of the nose. Septal deviation or anatomical anomalies may predispose to infection. Nasal septum deviation can also lead to nasal obstruction. Squamous cell carcinoma usually occurs unilaterally. Masses that increase in size and pulsate on Valsalva maneuver may indicate a meningocele.

Note the Presence and Color of Any Discharge

Pus in the ostium of the middle turbinate suggests a bacterial sinusitis. Cerebrospinal fluid (CSF) drainage will increase in a forward position. Identify CSF by testing nasal drainage for glucose and protein levels comparable to those of CSF. Foul-smelling nasal discharge is a characteristic feature of sinusitis of dental origin. Foul-smelling unilateral purulent discharge may indicate a foreign body in the nasal cavity.

Transilluminate the Sinuses

Frontal sinuses can be transilluminated by placing a light source below the supraorbital rim. Transillumination of maxillary sinuses can be done in two ways. Place a transilluminator over the infraorbital rim, blocking light from the examiner's vision with the free hand, and judge the amount of light transmission (opaque, dull, normal) through the hard palate. This should be performed in a completely darkened room. Dentures must be removed. A second method is to place the transilluminator in the patient's mouth, sealing the lips, and observe the amount of light transmitted through the maxillary sinuses.

Light will pass through air-filled sinuses. Transillumination is used to assess the presence of fluid in the frontal and maxillary sinuses and cannot be used to examine the ethmoid or sphenoid sinuses. Normal transillumination of the frontal sinus rules out frontal sinusitis in 90% of cases. Complete opacity of sinuses suggests infection. However, the results of transillumination are often nonspecific, and reduced illumination does not lead to a diagnosis.

Palpate and Percuss Frontal and Maxillary Sinuses for Tenderness

Percuss and palpate the cheeks for tenderness and swelling, indicating maxillary sinusitis of dental origin. To assess for tenderness in the frontal sinuses, exert pressure over the eyebrow or slightly upward pressure under the brow. Direct percussion may elicit tenderness over the affected sinus.

Test for Facial Fullness and Pressure

Bending forward from the waist (with head dropping downward) or performing a Valsalva maneuver will worsen the symptoms if a partial or complete sinus obstruction is present.

Examine the Lungs

Auscultate the lungs for signs of wheezing, rales, and loudness of breath sounds. Peak flow volume or PO_2 saturation as measured using a pulse oximeter will detect the presence of reactive upper airway disease that may be associated with nasal symptoms.

Perform Neurologic Testing if Indicated

To detect any complications from sinusitis, assess neurologic and cranial nerve function if the patient appears severely ill. A rare but severe complication of sinusitis is cavernous sinus thrombosis. Cavernous sinuses are trabeculated sinuses located at the base of the skull that drain venous blood from facial veins. Cranial nerves III, IV, V, and VI are commonly affected because they are adjacent to the cavernous sinuses.

LABORATORY AND DIAGNOSTIC STUDIES

C-Reactive Protein

C-reactive protein is a glucoprotein produced by the liver in response to inflammation caused by infectious or noninfectious processes.

Nasal Smear

A nasal smear performed to look for eosinophils confirms the diagnosis of allergic rhinitis. Nasal scraping of the surface epithelium and a sample of secretions are more reliable in detecting the presence of eosinophils than is the sampling of secretions alone. Either method can be used to detect the presence of neutrophils. Specimens are graded using a scale of 0 to 4+, based on the concentration of cells.

Sinus Radiographs

Radiographs are not routinely indicated but may be obtained in patients who have severe symptoms and fail to respond to treatment. Severe symptoms may indicate complications of sinusitis such as orbital cellulitis, brain abscess, osteomyelitis, or cavernous sinus thrombosis. A sinus radiographic series consists of four views: an anteroposterior (Caldwell) view of the ethmoid sinus, a view (Chamberlain) of the frontal sinus, a lateral view of the sphenoid and frontal sinuses, and an occipitomental (Waters) view of the maxillary sinuses.

Computed Tomography Scan

A computed tomography (CT) scan shows air, bone, and soft tissue and optimally facilitates definition of regional anatomy and the extent of disease. A CT scan is done when sinusitis becomes chronic and does not respond to symptomatic or antibiotic treatment. A CT scan may also show causes for chronic sinusitis by visualizing disorders not detected by plain films such as facial fractures, nasal polyps, cysts, chronic mucosal thickening, temporomandibular joint disorders, foreign bodies, and tumors.

Magnetic Resonance Imaging

Magnetic resonance imaging (MRI) is used to image soft tissue pathology of the face and neck, especially neoplastic conditions. CT does not delineate soft tissue pathology as well as MRI.

Sinus Aspiration

Sinus aspiration is the only way to confirm the diagnosis of bacterial sinusitis and is performed by an otolaryngologist. A trocar is introduced into the maxillary sinus through the upper gingival recess.

Nasal Endoscopy

Nasal endoscopy allows direct observation of the nasal passages, larynx, pharynx, and surrounding tissue and aids in the diagnosis of nasal polyps, chronic sinusitis, or laryngeal trauma. Before a flexible fiberoptic scope is threaded through the nasal passages, an anesthetic spray is applied to the nasal tissue while the patient is in a sitting position. This procedure is generally performed by an otolaryngologist.

Allergy Skin Testing

Results of skin testing can confirm immunological disease and identify specific antigens responsible for allergic rhinitis, which may come from exposure to irritants in the patient's environment. The presence of serum IgE antibody suggests an allergic response.

DIFFERENTIAL DIAGNOSIS

Infectious Rhinitis

Infectious rhinitis is an acute condition frequently associated with a history of recent upper respiratory tract infection. A definitive sign of this condition is the presence of yellow or green purulent discharge and red nasal mucosa.

Allergic Rhinitis

Allergic rhinitis is distinguished by a recurrent rhinorrhea with clear watery mucus, sneezing, and pruritus. Nasal turbinates are pale and swollen. There is often a family history of allergies. About 25% of the population has some type of allergy. Diagnosis of IgE-mediated reactions to aeroallergens is based on a combination of history, physical examination, and skin tests. Nasal smears can be tested for the presence of eosinophils to confirm an allergenic response.

Seasonal allergies are associated with short bursts of intense exposure to an allergen that creates symptoms consistent with a histamine-mediated response such as pruritus, swelling, sneezing, and rhinorrhea. Perennial allergies are caused by continuous exposure to allergens associated with chronic congestion. Common indoor allergens are animal dander, dust mites, and cockroaches. Outdoor allergens include grasses, trees, pollens, and weeds. A history or pattern of symptoms and exposure is critical in diagnosis.

Nonallergic Rhinitis

Nonallergic rhinitis may be associated with eosinophilia on a nasal smear. Nonallergic rhinitis with eosinophilia syndrome (NARES) is a diagnosis based on nasal cytology and involves symptoms similar to allergic rhinitis without an identifiable allergen cause. A history will reveal aspirin or nonsteroidal antiinflammatory drug intolerance and rhinorrhea. Noneosinophilia is associated with any other nonallergic cause of rhinitis.

Rhinitis Medicamentosa

Drug-induced rebound congestion can follow the long-term use of topical nasal decongestants. Rhinitis medicamentosa is also used to describe nasal symptoms secondary to other medications, such as nasal congestion associated with hormone changes of pregnancy. Other drugs that have vasodilative effects include antihypertensives that interfere with adrenergic neuronal function and hormones in oral contraceptives. Nasal vasoconstriction response is completely abolished after the administration of reserpine.

Acute Sinusitis

Acute sinusitis is characterized by purulent nasal discharge, postnasal drip, and localized facial pain over the sinus involved. It often follows a viral upper respiratory tract infection. However, symptoms such as halitosis, reduced sense of smell, and morning cough have been reported in children in the absence of facial pain. Physical examination will elicit localized tenderness to palpation or percussion over the affected sinus. Pressure and pain will increase in a forward-bending position. Purulent discharge may be visible in the posterior pharynx or may be seen emerging from the ostia of the middle turbinate. Transillumination will indicate unilateral or bilateral obstruction. Ciliary function is impaired with infection and may not be completely restored for 2 to 6 weeks. The diagnosis of sinusitis in children requires two of three major criteria (cough, purulent nasal discharge, purulent pharyngeal drainage), or one major and two minor criteria (sore throat, wheezing, foul breath, facial pain, periorbital edema, headache, earache, fever, toothache).

Chronic Sinusitis

An incompletely treated acute sinusitis can lead to a chronic condition. The patient has persistent symptoms of low-grade infection and intermittent acute exacerbations typical of acute sinusitis. Symptoms are recurrent and not controlled with over-the-counter or nonpharmacologic remedies. Multiple pathogens may be causative organisms, with the most common being *Moraxella catarrhalis, H. influenzae,* and *S. pneumoniae.* A diagnosis of chronic sinusitis requires sinus radiographs or a CT scan that reveals mucosal thickening of 5 mm or greater. Allergy testing may reveal a perennial allergy that creates chronic inflammation.

Nasal or Sinus Obstruction

A history of aspirin intolerance or asthma with polyps is associated with obstruction.

Acute obstruction suggests edema secondary to infection, allergic response, exposure to irritants, or foreign body (in children). Chronic obstruction may be secondary to congenital deformity, nasal polyps, or septal deviation. In infants, congenital choanal atresia can cause obstruction.

Nasal Polyposis

This syndrome has multiple causative factors, including a history of asthma and aspirin intolerance. The polyps are translucent, grapelike growths that are mobile, rarely bleed, and prolapse into the nasal cavity. The resulting obstruction can be associated with chronic sinusitis. Any suspicious polyps should be biopsied.

Osteomyelitis of the Frontal Bone

Osteomyelitis can occur as a complication of sinusitis. Osteomyelitis occurs in children and young adults and may follow head trauma or scuba diving. *Staphylococcus pyogenes* or anaerobic streptococci are the causative organisms. Patients appear severely ill and may have edema of the upper eyelid and puffy swelling over the frontal bone. Diagnosis is by radiography and blood culture.

▶ **DIFFERENTIAL DIAGNOSIS OF** *Common Causes of Nasal Symptoms and Sinus Congestion*

CONDITION	HISTORY	PHYSICAL FINDINGS	DIAGNOSTIC STUDIES
Infectious rhinitis	Perennial, but more common in winter months; recent URI	Red, swollen mucosa; purulent discharge	Nasal smear for neutrophils, intracellular bacteria, CRP
Allergic rhinitis	Family history of allergies; sneezing; recurrent pattern; more common in children and young adults	Pale, boggy mucosa; rhinorrhea with clear, watery mucus	Nasal smear for eosinophils; allergy testing
Nonallergic rhinitis	No allergenic cause identified	Similar to allergic rhinitis	Absence of eosinophilia on nasal cytology
Rhinitis medicamentosa	History of medication use: oral contraceptives, nasal sprays, antihypertensives; nasal congestion	Swollen mucosa; clear mucus or dry mucosa	None

Continued

> **DIFFERENTIAL DIAGNOSIS OF** *Common Causes of Nasal Symptoms and Sinus Congestion—cont'd*

CONDITION	HISTORY	PHYSICAL FINDINGS	DIAGNOSTIC STUDIES
Acute sinusitis	Smoker; recent URI; winter months; frontal headaches made worse with forward bending; sensation of fullness or pressure In children nasal discharge, cough, for >10 days, fever >38°C with purulent rhinorrhea for 3 days	Purulent discharge; maxillary toothache on percussion; postnasal drainage; decreased transillumination; fever	None
Chronic sinusitis	History of previous sinus infections; dull ache or no pain; persistent symptoms	Same as in acute sinusitis; decreased or no transillumination; obstruction such as deviated septum, polyps	CT scan; nasal endoscopy; allergy testing
Obstruction	History of asthma, aspirin intolerance; foreign body in children; tumor in adults; infants with choanal atresia: difficulty feeding; cyanosis if bilateral	Increased pain with forward motion or Valsalva; pain with percussion and palpation of sinuses; no transillumination; septal deviation	Sinus radiographs; CT scan
Nasal polyposis	History of asthma, aspirin intolerance	Presence of polyps	Nasal endoscopy; may require biopsy
Osteomyelitis of frontal bone	History of head trauma, diving	Appears severely ill; periorbital and frontal edema	Sinus and skull radiographs; blood culture

CRP, C-reactive protein; *CT,* computed tomography; *URI,* upper respiratory infection.

CHAPTER

26 Palpitations

Palpitations are defined as an unpleasant awareness of the forceful, rapid, or irregular beating of the heart. It is a common presenting symptom that is usually benign; however, occasionally palpitations can indicate a life-threatening arrhythmia.

Palpitations are described by patients as a thumping, pounding, or fluttering sensation in the chest. This sensation can be either intermittent or sustained, and either regular or irregular. Patients often note palpitations when quietly resting, a time when other stimuli are minimal.

Causes of palpitations can be of cardiac or noncardiac origin. Cardiac causes include arrhythmias; structural abnormalities such as mitral valve prolapse, valvular disease, cardiomyopathy; and congenital heart lesions. Noncardiac causes include psychological conditions such as anxiety; systemic conditions, including thyroid disorders, anemia, and hyperdynamic cardiovascular states; and drugs, medications, and stimulants. Any condition that can cause sinus tachycardia (anxiety, pain, fever, caffeine, hypovolemia, pulmonary embolism, hyperventilation) can result in the reported symptom of palpitations. During menopause, women often report experiencing palpitations. Pheochromocytoma is a rare but serious cause of palpitations. Fever, anxiety, exercise, and anemia are common causes of palpitations.

The principal goals in assessing patients with palpitations is to distinguish cardiac from noncardiac causes and determine if the symptom is caused by a life-threatening arrhythmia.

DIAGNOSTIC REASONING: FOCUSED HISTORY

Could this patient have a life-threatening arrhythmia?

Key Questions
- Do you have a history of coronary artery disease (CAD)?
- Are you lightheaded or have you had episodes of passing out?
- Are you having chest pain?
- Have you had difficulty breathing?
- Do you have a family history of sudden cardiac death (SCD)?
- Have you had heart surgery?

Coronary Artery Disease

Patients with risk factors for or preexisting CAD are at greater risk for ventricular arrhythmias as a cause for palpitations. Risk factors include smoking, hypertension, diabetes, a history of myocardial infarction (MI), and a family history of heart attack or stroke before age 60 years.

Lightheadedness and Syncope

Palpitations associated with other symptoms suggestive of hemodynamic compromise, including lightheadedness or syncope, may signify a life-threatening cardiac arrhythmia.

Chest Pain and Dyspnea

Palpitations caused by sustained tachyarrhythmias in patients with CAD can be accompanied by angina pectoris or dyspnea (shortness of breath). Palpitations associated with chest pain suggest ischemic heart disease; if the chest pain is relieved by leaning forward, pericardial disease is suspected. Exertional palpitations associated with chest pain, lightheadedness, or both in the athlete may indicate an underlying cardiovascular disorder.

Sudden Cardiac Death

A family history of SCD may indicate an inherited cardiac problem.

Cardiac Surgery

Children and adults who have had cardiac surgery are at risk for arrhythmias and palpitations.

What else do I need to know about the palpitation?

Key Questions

• How would you describe the palpitation or sensation?
• When do the palpitations occur? Are they associated with rest or activity?
• How long do the palpitations last?
• Do the palpitations start or stop abruptly?

Description of Palpitations

Flip flopping

Single skipped beats or a sensation of the heart stopping and then starting with a pounding, flipping, or jumping sensation, especially while sitting quietly or lying in bed and lasting only for brief periods, are typically attributed to premature contraction of the atria or ventricles. The sensation that the heart has stopped results from the pause following the premature contraction, and the pounding or flipping sensation results from the forceful contraction following the pause.

Rapid fluttering in the chest

A feeling of rapid fluttering in the chest may result from atrial or ventricular arrhythmias, including sinus tachycardia.

Pounding in the neck

A pounding feeling in the neck is caused by the dissociation of atrial and ventricular

contractions so that the atria contract against closed tricuspid and mitral valves, producing cannon A waves, which are large pressure waves seen in the neck as a result of the simultaneous contraction of the atria and ventricles. The sensation of rapid and regular pounding in the neck is typical of reentrant supraventricular arrhythmias, particularly atrioventricular (AV) nodal tachycardia.

Occurrence of Palpitations

Palpitations that start during sleep or states of increased vagal tone (e.g., at termination of exercise) may be associated with vagal-mediated atrial fibrillation or certain subtypes of long QT syndromes. Palpitations that are worse at night may be caused by benign ectopy or atrial fibrillation.

Palpitations that start and stop abruptly suggest supraventricular or ventricular tachycardias. Palpitations that can be stopped using patient-initiated vagal maneuvers, such as the Valsalva maneuver, suggest supraventricular tachycardia.

Rapid palpitations during catecholamine excess, such as during exercise, suggest ventricular tachycardia, sinus tachycardia, or atrial fibrillation. Palpitations that occur regularly with exertion suggest hypertrophic cardiomyopathy or CAD. Palpitations at rest that are exacerbated by exercise suggest anemia. Persistent palpitations at rest may indicate a systemic condition.

Positional palpitations may reflect AV nodal tachycardia, pericarditis, or a structural process within the heart (e.g., atrial myxoma) or adjacent to the heart (e.g., mediastinal mass).

Could this be related to stress or a psychological condition?

Key Questions

• Have you experienced panic attacks (brief periods [seconds or minutes] of an overwhelming panic or terror accompanied by racing heartbeats, shortness of breath, or dizziness)?
• Can you describe your stress level and how you cope with stress in your life?
• Do you or anyone in your family have a problem with panic attacks, anxiety, or depression?
• What other symptoms are you having?

Panic Disorder, Stress, and Anxiety

The most common psychological causes of palpitations are anxiety and panic disorder. The release of catecholamines during a panic attack or significant stress can trigger an arrhythmia. Patients with psychological causes more commonly report a longer duration of the sensation (>15 minutes) and accompanying symptoms than patients with other causes. It is essential to rule out clinically significant arrhythmias before attributing palpitations to psychological causes. Panic attacks, however, may also indicate pheochromocytoma, a rare tumor of the adrenal tissue, resulting in the release of too much epinephrine and norepinephrine.

EVIDENCE-BASED PRACTICE *Can Patient History Predict Arrhythmias?*

This systematic review included 23 studies. Seven studies examined the utility of the patient history in diagnosing an arrhythmia as the cause of palpitations. A slightly increased likelihood of a cardiac arrhythmia was associated with a history of cardiac disease and palpitations affected by sleeping or while at work. A history of panic disorder or having palpitations lasting less than 5 minutes made the presence of cardiac arrhythmia slightly less likely. A regular rapid-pounding sensation in the neck that occurred with the palpitations increased the likelihood that the palpitations were due to a specific arrhythmia (i.e., atrioventricular node [AV] reentry tachycardia). Likewise, the absence of that symptom made the likelihood of AV tachycardia unlikely. The authors concluded that patient history cannot exclude clinically significant arrhythmias in most patients, and electrocardiographic monitoring is required.

Reference: Thavendiranathan et al, 2009.

Other Symptoms

Palpitations associated with hyperventilation, hand tingling, nervousness, shortness of breath, or dizziness are common when anxiety or panic disorder is the underlying cause. Children with serious arrhythmias may not report palpitations. Young infants may exhibit poor feeding or be irritable when palpitations are present.

Could this be secondary to a systemic condition?

Key Questions
- What other symptoms are you having?
- Have you been ill?
- Are you pregnant?

Symptoms or Illness

Noncardiac symptoms should be elicited because the palpitations may be caused by a normal heart responding to a metabolic or inflammatory condition. Palpitations can be precipitated by vomiting or diarrhea that lead to electrolyte disorders and hypovolemia. Other systemic causes of palpitations include exercise, fever, dehydration, hypoglycemia, anemia, anorexia, hyperthyroidism, hyperventilation, caffeine, menopause, and pheochromocytoma.

A complete blood count (CBC) may identify anemia, infection, or hypovolemia as possible underlying causes. Evaluation of electrolytes can identify an imbalance.

Fatigue and shortness of breath can suggest anemia. Weight loss and heat intolerance may indicate hyperthyroidism. Patients with hyperthyroidism also report nervousness, emotional lability, fatigue, muscle weakness, increased sweating, menstrual changes (oligomenorrhea), increased appetite, insomnia, thinning hair, tremors, and anxiety. A fever with hypotension may indicate myocarditis.

A pheochromocytoma, although rare, can lead to palpitations. Patients typically report headache (usually severe, pounding, and paroxysmal), sweating, nausea and vomiting, visual problems, episodic flushing, weight loss, diarrhea, nervousness, abdominal or chest pain, panic attacks, flank pain, pallor, tremor, fatigue, anxiety, weakness, dyspnea, warmth, fever, dizziness, constipation, paresthesias, hematuria, and anorexia.

Pregnancy

Pregnancy produces a hyperdynamic cardiovascular state that may cause palpitations.

Are drugs, medications, or other stimulants implicated?

Key Questions

- What prescription and over-the-counter (OTC) medications are you taking?
- What recreational drugs do you use?
- Are the palpitations associated with caffeine or tobacco use?

Medications

Palpitations can result from OTC and prescription medications. Medications that prolong the QT interval and predispose patients to arrhythmias include antidysrhythmics, antimicrobials, antihistamines, psychotropic drugs, and other medications, such as motility medications, electrolyte-depleting diuretics, and protease inhibitors for human immunodeficiency virus. Palpitations may occur with the use of sympathomimetic agents, vasodilators, anticholinergic drugs, or β-agonists. Acetylcholinesterase inhibitors cause arrhythmia in about 25% of people who take them.

In children, cold medicines may cause palpitations.

Stimulants

Stimulants such as caffeine, cocaine, amphetamines, and nicotine enhance the strength of myocardial contraction and may cause palpitations. Energy drinks and workout supplements marketed to increase endurance, concentration, and performance also have a high caffeine content and may therefore lead to the occurrence of palpitations.

DIAGNOSTIC REASONING: FOCUSED PHYSICAL EXAMINATION

Most patients with episodic palpitations are asymptomatic on physical examination. Typically, the purpose of the physical examination is to identify structural heart abnormalities to help confirm or rule out the presence of an arrhythmia.

Note General Appearance

Observe the patient entering the room. Note signs of stress or anxiety. Tremors may indicate hyperthyroidism or pheochromocytoma. Flushing or sweating may occur with pheochromocytoma. Pallor suggests anemia.

Take Vital Signs

Vital signs can provide information on cardiac function. Blood pressure and pulse should be taken in the supine, sitting, and standing positions. Atrial fibrillation is suggested by an irregular pulse that has no repeating pattern (irregularly irregular). The presence of a pulse deficit (obtaining a lower pulse rate at the wrist than at the apex) or the auscultation of a variable intensity of the first heart sound suggests atrial fibrillation. These findings are attributable to beat-to-beat variation in stroke volume that occurs during atrial fibrillation. Hypertension may indicate underlying CAD or pheochromocytoma. Weight loss from anorexia nervosa or bulimia nervosa may cause palpitations as a result of dehydration. In addition, the possible use of appetite suppressants, diuretics, or vomiting may result in an electrolyte imbalance. A fever with hypotension and the presence of a murmur may indicate myocarditis or pericarditis.

Assess Jugular Venous Pressure

The presence of cannon A waves on the jugular venous pressure (JVP) examination of the jugular veins suggests an arrhythmia that is associated with AV dissociation, such as complete heart block or ventricular tachycardia. Cannon A waves are prominent waves in the JVP that occur with the contraction of the right atrium against a closed tricuspid valve. Cannon A waves are perceived as neck pulsations and when rapid and regular may be seen as a bulging in the neck, sometimes termed a "frog sign."

Auscultate the Heart

A displaced and enlarged cardiac point-of-maximal impulse suggests the presence of left ventricular hypertrophy or cardiomyopathy. Hypertrophic and dilated cardiomyopathies can increase the likelihood of ventricular tachycardia and atrial fibrillation.

An irregular heartbeat, in both rhythm and strength, that begins and terminates abruptly suggests atrial fibrillation.

Listen for murmurs. A midsystolic click suggests mitral valve prolapse. Mitral valve prolapse has an association with supraventricular arrhythmias. The harsh holosystolic murmur of hypertrophic cardiomyopathy, which occurs along the left sternal border and increases with the Valsalva maneuver, can be associated with atrial fibrillation or ventricular tachycardia.

Assess Mental Status

Assess general behavior. Irritability may occur in patients with anxiety. Note body posture, movement, and facial expressions. Assess thought content for delusions that may occur with substance abuse or psychoses. Young infants may exhibit poor feeding or be irritable when palpitations are present.

Inspect the Head and Neck

Intranasal substance users may have chronic rhinorrhea, frequent nosebleeds, or lesions in the nose and around the nostrils. Pupils may be dilated secondary to substance use. The patient may have dry lips, halitosis, and an odor of alcohol or tobacco. Patients with hyperthyroidism may display exophthalmos and thinning hair. Patients with anemia may have pale mucous membranes.

Examine the Thyroid

In patients with thyroid disease, the thyroid may be enlarged, and a bruit may be present in hyperthyroidism.

Examine the Extremities

Look for onycholysis (detachment of the nail from the nail bed) and localized myxedema (edematous skin thickening) of the legs (pretibial) or dorsa of the feet if you suspect hyperthyroidism. The nail beds should be examined for cyanosis and clubbing.

Check Reflexes

Hyperthyroidism can produce overly brisk reflexes.

LABORATORY AND DIAGNOSTIC STUDIES

Twelve-Lead Electrocardiogram

A standard 12-lead electrocardiogram (ECG) is the initial test in patients with palpitations and may identify the arrhythmia or provide insight into underlying structural and electrical abnormalities that may be causing the arrhythmia. Patients with electrical or structural abnormalities on a 12-lead ECG require further evaluation.

Electrocardiogram exercise stress testing is appropriate in patients who have palpitations with physical exertion and patients with suspected CAD or myocardial ischemia (see Chapter 8).

Cardiac Monitoring: Event or Continuous Loop

These measures are used in patients with suspected cardiac arrhythmias as the cause of the palpitations. Holter monitoring or long-term (weeks, months) event monitoring is used to document ECG recordings. Holter monitoring is a continuous 24- or 48-hour ECG recording to evaluate the type and amount of irregular heartbeats during regular activities, exercise, and sleep. The patient keeps a diary to record daily activities and any symptoms experienced. At the end of the monitoring period, the data are analyzed for arrhythmias and are correlated with symptoms recorded by the patient. Cardiac event monitoring is a continuous-loop, digital memory recorder worn for extended periods of time (up to 30 days or longer) that saves and records transient events felt by the patient. These monitors are patient-activated as symptoms occur or can be automatically triggered by a predefined high or low heart rate. Implantable loop monitors save information for a predetermined period before the patient trigger and can help identify the initiation sequence for arrhythmias. These stored events can be transmitted for review.

Echocardiogram

An echocardiogram is a noninvasive ultrasound test for examining the heart that provides information about the ventricular function and position, size, and movements of the valves and chambers, and velocity of blood flow through the heart. This test is used to determine, detect, or rule out structural abnormalities or hypertrophy; to evaluate velocity and direction of blood flow; and to provide direction for further diagnostic evaluation.

Complete Blood Count

A CBC with differential can be done to establish the presence of a systemic infection. An increase in white blood cells and bands is seen with systemic infection. Hemoglobin and hematocrit levels are useful if anemia is suspected as an underlying cause of palpitations.

Electrolytes

Evaluation of electrolytes is useful when the palpitation is from a suspected electrolyte imbalance.

Thyroid-Stimulating Hormone and Free Thyroxine

Thyroid-stimulating hormone (TSH) and free thyroxine (fT$_4$) levels are used to detect thyroid disease. An abnormal level requires further testing. An undetectable TSH level is diagnostic of hyperthyroidism.

Catecholamines and Metanephrines

Catecholamines and metanephrines are measured in a 24-hour urine collection to rule out pheochromocytoma. Metanephrines may also be measured in the blood. If levels are greater than two times the reference range, imaging studies are usually performed to evaluate the adrenal glands.

DIFFERENTIAL DIAGNOSIS

Cardiac Causes

Cardiac arrhythmias

Cardiac arrhythmias that result in palpitations include atrial fibrillation or flutter, supraventricular and ventricular tachycardia, premature ventricular and atrial contractions, sick sinus syndrome, and advanced AV block. The causes are primary electrical abnormalities or electrical abnormalities secondary to structural cardiac disease or

---

Box 26.1	**Arrhythmias That Can Cause Palpitations**

- Atrial fibrillation or flutter
- Bradycardia caused by advanced arteriovenous block or sinus node dysfunction
- Bradycardia-tachycardia syndrome (sick sinus syndrome)
- Multifocal atrial tachycardia
- Premature supraventricular complexes
- Premature ventricular complexes
- Sinus tachycardia or arrhythmia
- Supraventricular tachycardia
- Ventricular tachycardia
- Wolff-Parkinson-White syndrome (atrioventricular nodal reentrant tachycardia)

From Abbott AV: Diagnostic approach to palpitations, *Am Fam Physician* 71:743, 2005.

---

comorbid conditions. The association of palpitations with other symptoms that indicate hemodynamic compromise, including syncope or lightheadedness, may signify a life-threatening cardiac arrhythmia, and referral to a cardiologist is warranted. Chest pain and dyspnea may be the result of sustained tachyarrhythmias.

Physical findings such as a pulse deficit, irregular heartbeat, or cannon A waves on JVP measurement indicate a cardiac arrhythmia as the cause of the palpitations. ECG and cardiac monitoring may reveal the arrhythmia. Box 26.1 lists arrhythmias that can cause palpitations.

Structural abnormalities

Structural cardiac causes of palpitations include valvular heart diseases such as aortic insufficiency or stenosis, atrial or ventricular septal defect, cardiomyopathy, congenital heart disease, and pericarditis. Positional palpitations may reflect a structural process within the heart (e.g., atrial myxoma) or adjacent to the heart (e.g., mediastinal mass), AV nodal tachycardia, or pericarditis. An echocardiogram can be useful in detecting structural cardiac causes of palpitations. Box 26.2 lists some structural cardiac causes of palpitations.

EVIDENCE-BASED PRACTICE *What Diagnostic Device Is Best to Use?*

This systematic review included 28 studies, both descriptive and experimental, that compared the yield of two or more devices or diagnostic strategies in detecting cardiac arrhythmias. With the continuous event recorder (CER), a diagnosis was established in 21% to 62% of the studied patients, compared with a maximum of 30% diagnosed with Holter monitoring. The CER was better at excluding arrhythmias during symptoms than the Holter monitor (34% and 2%, respectively). Automatically triggered recorders detected more arrhythmias (72%–80%) than patient-triggered devices (17%–75%). Implantable devices are used for prolonged monitoring periods in patients with infrequent symptoms or unexplained syncope. The authors concluded that the choice of the device depends on the characteristics of the symptoms and the patient. As a result of methodological shortcomings of the included studies, no evidence-based diagnostic strategy was proposed.

Reference: Hoefman et al, 2010.

Box 26.2 Structural Cardiac Causes of Palpitations

- Atrial or ventricular septal defect
- Cardiomyopathy
- Congenital heart disease
- Congestive heart failure
- Mitral valve prolapse
- Pacemaker-mediated tachycardia
- Pericarditis
- Valvular disease (e.g., aortic insufficiency, stenosis)

From Abbott AV: Diagnostic approach to palpitations, *Am Fam Physician* 71:743, 2005.

Noncardiac Causes

Psychological causes

Panic Disorder

Panic disorder is manifested by sudden attacks of fear accompanied by symptoms that may resemble a heart attack (e.g., palpitations, chest pain, dizziness). Often the symptoms develop rapidly and without an identifiable stressor. The individual may have had periods of high anxiety in the past or may have been involved in a recent stressful situation; however, the underlying cause is typically subtle. Panic attacks subside as abruptly as they begin, typically lasting a few minutes, although they can last several hours. Asking a single question, "Have you experienced brief periods, for seconds or minutes, of an overwhelming panic or terror that was accompanied by racing heartbeats, shortness of breath, or dizziness?" can help identify patients with panic disorder.

Generalized Anxiety Disorder

Chronic anxiety, also referred to as generalized anxiety disorder (GAD), manifests as persistent worries, fears, and negative thoughts lasting at least 6 months. Excessive worry over daily activities and a tendency to have symptoms of headache and nausea are seen. Typically, GAD develops over a period of time and may not be noticed until it is significant enough to cause problems with functioning. Anxiety is persistent, pervasive, and occurs in many different settings.

Systemic causes

Anemia

Fatigue and pallor may indicate anemia. Hemoglobin and hematocrit levels will be low.

Hyperthyroidism

Patients with hyperthyroidism may report nervousness, emotional lability, fatigue, muscle weakness, weight loss with good appetite, hyperdefecation, heat intolerance, menstrual changes (oligomenorrhea), increased appetite, insomnia, and tremors. On physical examination, exophthalmos, warm skin, onycholysis, increased sweating, and thinning hair may be evident. Patients may have localized myxedema (edematous skin thickening) of the legs (pretibial) or dorsa of the feet. The thyroid may be enlarged and a bruit may be present. Deep tendon reflexes may be brisk. High fever, congestive heart failure, and mental status changes suggest thyroid storm. TSH level will be low or undetectable. Older adult patients have less obvious signs and symptoms than younger patients and a higher prevalence of cardiac manifestations such as atrial fibrillation.

Pheochromocytoma

Pheochromocytomas are rare catecholamine-producing tumors of the adrenal glands. In addition to palpitations, patients with pheochromocytoma often report severe, pounding, and paroxysmal headaches, sweating, nausea and vomiting, visual problems, flushing, weight loss, diarrhea, nervousness, abdominal or chest pain, panic attacks, flank pain, pallor,

tremor, fatigue, anxiety, weakness, dyspnea, warmth, fever, dizziness, constipation, paresthesias, painless hematuria, and anorexia. On physical examination, patients may exhibit hypertension, tremors, postural (orthostatic) hypotension, and pallor. The heart may be enlarged.

Drugs and Stimulants

Palpitations that coincide with the use of a drug suggest them as a probable cause. Drugs and stimulants that commonly cause palpitations include alcohol, caffeine, tobacco, digitalis, phenothiazine, theophylline, β-agonists, acetylcholinesterase inhibitors and cocaine.

On physical examination, look for telltale signs of stimulant use: chronic rhinorrhea, frequent nosebleeds, and lesions in the nose or around the nostrils. Pupils may be dilated secondary to substance use. Notice if the patient has an odor of alcohol or tobacco.

▶ DIFFERENTIAL DIAGNOSIS OF *Common Causes of Palpitations*

CONDITION	HISTORY	PHYSICAL FINDINGS	DIAGNOSTIC STUDIES
CARDIAC CAUSES			
Cardiac arrhythmias	CAD, lightheadedness, syncope, chest pain, dyspnea	Pulse deficit, irregular heartbeat, cannon A waves on JVP	ECG, continuous event or loop monitoring, CAD evaluation (stress test)
Structural causes	May have positional palpitations	Murmur may be present	ECG, continuous event or loop monitoring; echocardiogram
NONCARDIAC CAUSES			
Psychological Causes			
Panic disorder	Panic attacks, terror	None	ECG, continuous event or loop monitoring
Stress or anxiety	Persistent worries, fears, and negative thoughts	None	ECG, continuous event or loop monitoring
Systemic Causes			
Anemia	Fatigue	Pallor; pale mucous membranes	ECG, continuous event or loop monitoring; Hct or Hgb

► DIFFERENTIAL DIAGNOSIS OF *Common Causes of Palpitations—cont'd*

CONDITION	HISTORY	PHYSICAL FINDINGS	DIAGNOSTIC STUDIES
Hyperthyroidism	Nervousness, emotional lability, fatigue, muscle weakness, weight loss with good appetite, hyperdefecation, heat intolerance, menstrual changes (oligomenorrhea), increased appetite, insomnia, and tremors	Exophthalmos, warm skin, onycholysis, increased sweating and thinning hair, localized myxedema of legs (pretibial) or dorsa of feet; enlarged thyroid, bruit may be present; brisk DTRs	ECG, continuous event or loop monitoring; TSH, free T_4
Pheochromocytoma	Severe pounding and paroxysmal headaches, sweating, nausea, visual problems, flushing, weight loss, diarrhea, nervousness, abdominal or chest pain, panic attacks	Sweating, tremors hypertension, postural hypotension, heart may be enlarged	ECG, continuous event or loop monitoring; 24-hr urine; catecholamines and metanephrines; plasma metanephrines; abdominal imaging
Drugs and Stimulants			
	Use of alcohol, caffeine, tobacco, digitalis, phenothiazine, theophylline, β-agonists, acetylcholinesterase inhibitors, and recreational drugs such as cocaine and amphetamines	Nasal substance users may have chronic rhinorrhea, frequent nosebleeds, and lesions in the nose or around the nostrils; pupils may be dilated secondary to substance use; dry lips, halitosis; odor of alcohol, or tobacco	ECG, continuous event or loop monitoring; toxicology screen

CAD, coronary artery disease; *DTR,* deep tendon reflex; *ECG,* electrocardiogram; *Hct,* hematocrit; *Hgb,* hemoglobin; *JVP,* jugular venous pressure; *TSH,* thyroid-stimulating hormone.

Penile Discharge

Penile discharge results from an infectious or inflammatory process secondary to exposure and contact with organisms that enter and ascend the urethra. Patients infected with *Chlamydia trachomatis* may be asymptomatic 25% of the time, and symptoms may be absent with gonorrhea infections as well. Coinfection with both *Neisseria gonorrhoeae* and *Chlamydia* organisms may be present in up to 25% of heterosexual patients.

Urethritis related to a sexually transmitted infection (STI) is classified as either gonococcal urethritis or nongonococcal urethritis (NGU). It is not possible to determine the causative organism based on symptoms or physical examination alone. Although patients may be tentatively classified clinically, laboratory tests are necessary to direct diagnosis and treatment. The most frequently identified organism (40%) in nongonococcal infection is *C. trachomatis*. Other organisms identified in NGU include *Ureaplasma urealyticum,* and less frequently, *Trichomonas* species. STIs remain prevalent in older adults.

DIAGNOSTIC REASONING: FOCUSED HISTORY

Is this likely a sexually transmitted infection?

Key Questions
- Are you sexually active? How many sexual partners do you have?
- Do you have any new partners?
- When was the last time you had unprotected sex?
- When did you first notice the symptoms?

Sexual History

A history of multiple sexual partners signifies a risk of exposure to STIs. You cannot assume that a married patient or the spouse is monogamous and exclude a STI. A new partner is also a risk factor, as is a sexual partner who has other sexual partners. Sexually active adolescents are at risk for STIs because of impetuous sexual activities, lack of barrier protection use, and use of alcohol or drugs. STIs are a serious health problem, occurring in about 25% of sexually active adolescents.

Unprotected Sex

Unprotected sexual intercourse, whether vaginal, oral, or anal, increases the chances of STIs.

Number of Days Between Exposure and Symptom Onset

For patients with a single exposure, a shorter incubation period (2 to 6 days) is characteristic for *N. gonorrhoeae* and a longer period (2–3 weeks) for *C. trachomatis*. For patients with multiple or unknown exposures, the time interval may not be useful.

Are there any risk factors that point me in the right direction?

Key Question
- Have you used street or other drugs?

History of Drug or Substance Abuse

Substance or drug abuse is a risk factor for unprotected and indiscriminate sexual activity.

What do the characteristics of the discharge tell me?

Key Questions
- What color is the discharge?
- How much discharge are you having?
- What is the consistency of the discharge?

Color, Consistency, and Amount of Discharge

The presence of copious amounts of spontaneous yellow-greenish drainage is indicative of a gonococcal infection. A scant mucoid discharge is characteristic of a nongonococcal infection. Substance or drug abuse may produce a scant, whitish penile discharge.

Is this a local infection or process?

Key Questions
- Is the tip of your penis red and inflamed?
- Can you describe how you clean yourself?

Red, Inflamed Glans Penis

A beefy-red, inflamed glans penis is indicative of a yeast infection or a fixed drug reaction often caused by tetracycline. Lubricated condoms or spermicidal gel can cause contact dermatitis.

Hygienic Practices

Poor hygiene or aggressive hygiene with inappropriate and harsh cleansers can cause local irritation and result in inflammation.

Is this complicated urethritis?

Key Questions
- Do you have frequency, urgency, or nocturia?
- Do you have rectal, testicular, or low back pain?
- Do you have pain in any joints or muscles?
- Do you have any skin sores or lesions?

Symptoms of Complicated Urethritis

Symptoms of urinary frequency, urgency, and nocturia may indicate complications of a urethral infection caused by spreading of the infection to other urinary tract structures such as the prostate (see Chapter 18). Symptoms of perirectal, testicular, or low back pain indicate involvement of the vas deferens and the epididymis, which can lead to acute epididymitis or the involvement of the testicles and the development of orchitis.

Symptoms That May Indicate Reiter Syndrome

Reiter syndrome is a complication of NGU that follows urogenital infection and classically includes arthritis, conjunctivitis, oral mucosal ulcers, and dermatitis. More common is the joint and tendon involvement after *C. trachomatis* infection. This complication has also been reported in HIV-positive patients. It is less common in nonwhite populations, and the incubation period is usually 1 to 4 weeks after the onset of urethritis.

Symptoms That May Indicate Disseminated Systemic Urethral Infection

A disseminated gonococcal infection can produce papules or petechiae that progress to pustules on the skin surfaces of the hands, arms, and legs.

Is this an upper urinary tract problem?

Key Questions
- Have you had a fever or chills?
- Have you noticed any blood in your urine?
- Are you having any acute pain?
- Where is the pain?

Fever

The presence of fever indicates an ascending infection of the upper urinary tract (e.g., pyelonephritis) or a descending infection of the lower urinary tract (e.g., prostatitis, epididymitis). A fever with a temperature of greater than 101°F (39°C) should be cause for concern and requires aggressive treatment.

Hematuria

Blood in the urine signifies renal involvement—specifically, pyelonephritis or lithiasis. Painless hematuria in older adults is characteristic of a bladder tumor or is a late symptom of carcinoma of the kidney.

Acute Pain

Abdominal pain, flank pain, and costovertebral angle (CVA) pain are characteristic of bladder, ureter, and kidney involvement.

Urinary tract pain is usually perceived locally in the area where sensory fibers of nerves are located. However, pain can be referred to a site distant from the area that is affected because sensory nerves of the lower body are concentrated in the same segments of the spinal cord. A dull ache may be felt at the CVA or flank. Pain may be elicited by applying tension to the renal capsule, pelvis, or ureter. Ureter pain may be perceived in the bladder, penis, scrotum, or perineum. Testicular pain may be a result of renal calculi. Pain may vary in intensity from a dull ache to a sharp, stabbing, colicky pain that is unbearable.

What else could this be?

Key Questions
- Do you have scrotal pain or fever?
- Have you had recent urinary tract surgery or a urinary catheter?
- Have you been treated recently for an STI?
- Are you or your partner international or have you recently engaged in international travel?

Scrotal Pain or Fever

Epididymitis usually presents with scrotal pain that developed over a period of several hours. The patient often is also febrile.

Recent Surgery or Instrumentation

Recent surgery or instrumentation in the urethra results in a risk of infection. Older patients are especially at risk because they often undergo urinary tract surgery or procedures using instrumentation secondary to benign prostatic hypertrophy.

Recent Treatment for a Sexually Transmitted Infection

Recent treatment for an STI may indicate treatment failure, a coinfection that was not sensitive to the prescribed drug, or recent exposure. The appropriate laboratory test may not have been done or might not have been available, or treatment may have been empirically based on presenting symptoms. Infection with more than one organism indicates coinfection. Urethritis can also develop from a nongonococcal organism that has a longer incubation period and was not sensitive to the drug prescribed. The urethritis episode may also indicate a recent exposure after treatment. Another possibility could be a lack of patient compliance with treatment. The patient might not take the medication as directed or stop taking the medication when the symptoms disappear but before the causative organism is eliminated from the urethra.

International Patient or Partner or Recent International Travel

Patients who are international, have partner(s) from another country, or have a history of international travel may have exposure to STIs that are not seen frequently in the United States but have a higher incidence and prevalence in other countries. Resistant strains of common organisms are also prevalent in other countries. Referral or consultation with urologists, infectious disease departments, or public health departments may be necessary to identify and treat patients with unusual STIs.

DIAGNOSTIC REASONING: FOCUSED PHYSICAL EXAMINATION

Note General Appearance

If the patient appears systemically ill, a more aggressive and immediate approach should be taken and an expanded examination becomes appropriate. An ascending infection is usually limited to the anterior portion of the male urethra and is most likely to cause local signs and symptoms in the patient. The patient who appears to be in acute pain from sites other than the urethra warrants more than a focused physical examination.

Examine all skin surfaces including exposed orifices, eyes, mucous membranes, and bordering areas around sites that may have been exposed during sexual activity.

Note eyes for discharge or infection. Check around nares and lips for signs of infection or lesions. Inspect the chest, back, palms, and bottoms of the feet for rashes or lesions. Secondary syphilis produces typical rashes and lesions in these areas, as does

Reiter syndrome. Spontaneous greenish-yellow discharge from the eyes may indicate gonococcal infections.

Inspect the skin of the abdomen, inguinal areas, and thighs for lesions or rashes. Disseminated gonococcal infections may produce papules, petechiae, and pustules on the hands, arms, and feet. *Chlamydia* may produce hyperkeratotic lesions on skin surfaces and a rash on the penis in the uncircumcised patient.

Palpate Lymph Nodes

Palpate the cervical, axillary, inguinal, and femoral lymph nodes for adenopathy. Although a nonspecific indicator of infection, lymph nodes may enlarge in response to exposure from a variety of organisms. Virus exposure may cause lymph node enlargement, or there may be an extension of bacterial organisms into adjacent lymph chains, indicating regional infections. It is important to ascertain how long the nodes have been enlarged and what symptoms have appeared during the course of enlargement. Assess the state of the nodes such as any redness, swelling, heat, or pain, and note if they are firm, mobile, or boggy. Sexually active patients may have some inguinal lymph node enlargement, and the patient may or may not be aware of the enlargement. Lymph node enlargement should be documented and described.

Examine Body Hair

Examine hair on the head and in the pubic area, and inspect underlying skin areas. Hair shafts can be infected with lice and nits. Hair follicles can be irritated from scratching and from secondary infection by other organisms.

Examine the Penis and Urethral Meatus

Inspect penile skin surfaces for lesions, especially the underside of the head of the penis around the area of the frenulum, where viral lesions may be found. Palpate the shaft of the penis for tenderness or for strictures of the urethra. Retract the foreskin, if present, and inspect the glans penis, corona, and frenulum for lesions. Inspect the meatus for redness, discharge, patency, or growths. If there is discharge, note if it is spontaneous or produced by milking or stripping the penis. Document a tender urethra and describe the character of any discharge. Note whether the discharge is profuse and yellow-green, which indicates gonococcal infection, or scant and mucoid-like, which is characteristic of *C. trachomatis* and nongonococcal infections. Collect a specimen for testing.

Examine the Scrotum and Testicles

Inspect and palpate the scrotum for lesions. Palpate the testicles and epididymis for tenderness and any signs of inflammation. Elevating a tender testicle may alleviate pain and reduce discomfort in epididymitis. The testicle may not be defined when there is an acute infection present because of examiner-produced pain with palpation. The borders of the testicle may also be obliterated by swelling and edema.

Inspect and Examine Other Sites for Lesions and Discharge

Inspect other sites such as the mouth and pharynx using a tongue depressor to visualize buccal skinfolds for any lesions. The pharyngeal area may be asymptomatic. Depending on the patient's sexual practices and preferences, other sites exposed to sexual contact, such as the rectum, need to be examined. Rectal bleeding, pus, and mucus may indicate proctitis and require further anoscopic examination with special cultural and laboratory consideration (see Chapter 29). Examine any joints or tendons that are inflamed or tender or have limited range of motion.

LABORATORY AND DIAGNOSTIC STUDIES

To improve the probability of identifying the causative organism, the patient should be examined and specimens obtained at least 1 hour after the last voiding and ideally up to 4 hours after voiding. Manufacturer's directions should be followed for all materials used to collect specimens, and policies and procedures should be followed to obtain valid and reliable results from laboratory and diagnostic tests.

Urine Dipstick

Urine dipstick is used as a screening test for urethritis. A positive leukocyte esterase (LE) result is indicative of urethritis (75%–90% sensitivity, 95% specificity). A positive nitrite signifies bacterial infection. Urine that tests positive for leukocyte esterase and nitrites should be cultured for bacteria. However, note that some organisms that cause urinary tract infections do not convert nitrate to nitrites (e.g., staphylococci and streptococci).

Urinalysis with Microscopic Examination

Look for proteinuria and glycosuria, which suggest kidney involvement. Casts indicate hemorrhage or pathological conditions of the nephrons. RBCs indicate acute inflammatory or vascular disorders of the glomerulus. More than 1 or 2 RBCs/high-power field (HPF) is abnormal and may indicate renal or systemic disease or kidney trauma. Microscopic examination of the urine resulting in 20 or more organisms/HPF indicates UTI. Fewer than 20 organisms/HPF merits further study such as culture and sensitivity.

Segmented Urine Collection for Culture and Sensitivity

Obtaining segmented urine specimens is a procedure used to identify the site along the urinary tract where the colonization of organisms occurs and is useful in diagnosing prostatitis (see Chapter 18).

Gram Stain of Specimens

The Gram stain has 95% specificity in gonococcal urethritis. Sensitivity in urethritis is nearly 100%. A Gram stain of urethral discharge should be performed to determine inflammation (WBCs) and the presence of either gram-negative or gram-positive bacteria.

If the stain is positive for polymorphonuclear neutrophils, then the smear is examined for gram-negative intracellular diplococci (GNICDCs). If diplococci are found, the smear is considered positive for gonococcal urethritis. Lack of GNICDCs, indicate an NGU.

Culture and Sensitivity

Culture and sensitivity should be performed on specimens to confirm the identity of the causative organism and its sensitivity to antibiotics. This is especially important in populations with resistant organisms. A urethral swab and cultures are necessary in cases of suspected rectal or pharyngeal infection.

Molecular Testing for Infectious Organisms

Molecular testing using a first-void sample or a sample taken from the urethra or rectum provides rapid, sensitive, and specific results. Tests include DNA probes, nucleic acid amplification tests, and polymerase chain reaction assays. Tests are available for *C. trachomatis*, *N. gonorrhoeae*, *U. urealyticum*, and other organisms.

Doppler Blood Flow

Doppler blood flow studies can be performed to support the diagnoses of testicular torsion and epididymitis. Testicular torsion results in a lack of blood flow to the testicle, but in epididymitis, the blood flow is intact. Color-flow Doppler studies also provide information concerning blood flow to the testicles and identify hot areas of infection.

Complete Blood Count

A complete blood count with differential can be performed to indicate a systemic response to infection.

Syphilis Testing

Serologic tests are used for screening and diagnosing syphilis and are recommended if other STIs are found, if high risk, or exposure suspected. The screening tests are nontreponemal and include Venereal Disease Research Laboratory, rapid plasma reagin, and enzyme immunoassay tests. Diagnostic tests are *Treponema pallidum*–specific IgM hemagglutination test, fluorescent treponemal antibody absorption test, and the *Treponema pallidum* particle agglutination assay. Detection of *T. pallidum* can also be done using DNA testing.

DIFFERENTIAL DIAGNOSIS

Urethritis

Urethritis presents with itching, burning, or pain around the urethral opening. Symptoms vary in severity. Discharge may range from copious amounts of greenish-yellow discharge to scant mucoid-like discharge that may only be visible before the first voiding of the day. The patient may report symptoms such as urinary frequency, urgency, or burning with urination, as well as penile discharge. Patients may also report a known sexual partner or indicate that the public health department has informed them to get checked for an STI. If you are unable to make a diagnosis based on history and physical findings, diagnostic testing is necessary for specific organism identification.

N. gonorrhoeae and NGU caused by C. trachomatis are the two most common infectious causes of urethritis. A coinfection with both organisms is found in up to 25% of cases. Therefore, regardless of the timing of infection or appearance of the discharge, clinicians should always consider and test for both gonorrhea and chlamydia in any patient with urethritis.

Gonococcal Urethritis

Gonococcal STIs are usually the easiest to diagnose because the patient often presents with complaints of a yellow-green discharge and burning on urination. Unprotected sexual relations increase the risk for contracting this STI. Gonococcal infection often becomes symptomatic 2 to 6 days after exposure and produces the classic yellow-green, profuse, spontaneous drainage. On examination, the penis will be normal in appearance except for the copious discharge. Diagnosis is established by DNA testing and is confirmed by Gram staining and urethral culture.

Nongonococcal Urethritis

Nongonococcal urethritis can produce penile discharge, although on examination, discharge may not be present. NGU typically develops over a longer incubation period of 8 to 21 days, and 75% of patients have a clear or mucoid discharge.

Chlamydia is the most common nongonococcal causative organism. The resulting urethritis is characterized by a scant mucoid discharge visible before the first urination of the day. The patient may complain of irritation around the meatus of the urethra and have vague symptoms. On examination, stripping the penis may produce scant mucoid discharge. Molecular testing is used to diagnose Chlamydia. Gram staining is used to rule out or confirm nongonococcal disease, which is usually a chlamydial infection. Urine screening tests can be used to identify DNA chlamydial particles. It is important to test for both gonococcal infection and chlamydial infection in patients suspected of a STI.

Complicated Urethritis

Periurethritis may progress to urethral stricture in untreated cases, causing banding of the penile urethra in the shaft of the penis.

 EVIDENCE-BASED PRACTICE *Partner Notification for Sexually Transmitted Infections*

Partner notification is a process in which sexual partners of patients with an STI are informed of their exposure and the need to receive treatment. This systematic review covers four partner notification strategies: (1) patient referral (the patient tells his sexual partners that they need to be treated, either with [enhanced] or without [simple] additional support), (2) expedited partner therapy (the patient delivers medication or a prescription for medication to his partner[s] without the need for a medical examination of the partner), (3) provider referral (health service personnel notify the partners); or (4) contract referral (the patient is encouraged to notify partners, but health service personnel will contact them if they do not visit the health service by a certain date). In this review, expedited partner therapy was more successful than simple patient referral in reducing repeat infection in patients with gonorrhea, chlamydia, or nongonococcal urethritis (six trials). Expedited partner therapy and enhanced patient referral resulted in similar levels of repeat infection (three trials). There were too few trials to allow consistent conclusions about the relative effects of provider, contract, or other patient referral methods for different sexually transmitted infections (STIs). The authors concluded that the evidence assessed in this review does not identify a single optimal strategy for partner referral for any particular STI.

Reference: Ferreira et al, 2013.

Prostatitis can develop and progress to a systemic inflammatory response, causing chills and fever. Extension of inflammation to other structures of the urinary tract may result in acute infection of the epididymis and testicles. Orchitis, a testicular inflammation, presents with a swollen and tender testicle. Disseminated systemic urethral infection produces small tender papules or petechiae on the skin surfaces of the hands, arms, and legs. They may further develop into pustules and become hemorrhagic or necrotic. Joints may become involved, with tenosynovitis and arthritis with synovial effusion indicating reactive arthritis (Reiter syndrome). Monarticular joint or tendon involvement should be investigated further.

Prostatitis

Patients with acute bacterial prostatitis are typically febrile and look and feel ill. They usually complain of dysuria, burning, frequency, and nocturia (see Chapter 18). Prostatic massage is contraindicated in acute bacterial prostatitis.

Patients with chronic prostatitis do not appear acutely ill but have a history of prostate problems. A causative organism may not be identified (see Chapter 18).

Epididymitis and Orchitis

The patient with epididymitis or orchitis is usually a sexually active young male patient, and pain is likely the presenting symptom. The patient may also have a urethral discharge and be febrile. The history usually indicates a slower onset of discomfort over hours or days compared with testicular torsion, which has a rapid onset of symptoms. Elevation of the affected testicle may reduce the discomfort. Swelling of the scrotum and testicle may be present. Doppler flow studies with color can locate hot spots and identify intact blood flow (see Chapter 18). Urethral Gram staining, urinalysis and culture, and DNA testing for *C. trachomatis* and *N. gonorrhoeae* may be indicated.

Balanitis

Balanitis is inflammation of the glans penis. Balanitis involving the foreskin or prepuce is called balanoposthitis. Uncircumcised patients with poor personal hygiene are most affected by balanitis. Lack of aeration and irritation from smegma and discharge surrounding the glans penis cause inflammation and edema. The most common complication of balanitis is phimosis or inability to retract the foreskin from the glans penis.

▶ **DIFFERENTIAL DIAGNOSIS OF** *Common Causes of Penile Discharge*

CONDITION	HISTORY	PHYSICAL FINDINGS	DIAGNOSTIC STUDIES
Balanitis	Not circumcised; poor hygiene practices	Localized erythema and edema; presence of smegma	None; history and physical examination
URETHRITIS Gonococcal urethritis	Unprotected sexual activity; abrupt onset of symptoms 3–5 days after exposure; yellow-green discharge; classic symptoms reported: frequency, urgency, dysuria; dysuria may be worse at beginning of urine flow	Yellow-green discharge; spontaneous or copious amounts with stripping of penis	Collect specimens at least 1 hr, preferably 4 hr, after last voiding; Gram stain, culture; urine molecular testing for gonococcus

> **DIFFERENTIAL DIAGNOSIS OF** *Common Causes of Penile Discharge—cont'd*

CONDITION	HISTORY	PHYSICAL FINDINGS	DIAGNOSTIC STUDIES
Nongonococcal urethritis	Unprotected sexual activity; longer incubation period (8–21 days); meatal itching or irritation; scant mucoid-like discharge, if present, before first voiding of day; symptoms vary and range in severity for urgency, frequency, and dysuria	Thin mucoid discharge may be absent or minimal with penile milking or stripping	Gram stain; culture; urine molecular testing for Chlamydia
COMPLICATED URETHRITIS			
Acute bacterial prostatitis	Chills, fever; 30–50 yr of age; onset of symptoms over days; pain in rectal, perianal area, low back, and abdomen	May have fever; painful prostate; do not massage	Segmental urine specimens; culture and sensitivity
Epididymitis or orchitis	Abrupt onset over several hours; febrile, pain in scrotum, testicles, or both	Tender, swollen epididymis, testicles, or both; elevation of affected testicle may lessen discomfort; may have fever	Doppler flow studies with color; urethral Gram stain, urinalysis and culture, and molecular testing for *Chlamydia trachomatis* and *Neisseria gonorrhoeae*

28 Rashes and Skin Lesions

Dermatologic problems result from a number of mechanisms, including inflammatory, infectious, immunologic, and environmental (traumatic and exposure induced). At times, the mechanism may be readily identified, such as the infectious bacterial etiology in impetigo. However, some dermatologic lesions may be classified in more than one way. Most insect bites, for example, involve both environmental (the bite) and inflammatory (the response) mechanisms. Awareness of the potential mechanism of any skin disorder is most helpful in identifying the risk a person may have for other illnesses. For example, people with eczema are also frequently at risk for other atopic conditions, notably asthma and allergic rhinitis. Thousands of skin disorders have been described, but only a small number account for the majority of patient visits.

Evaluation of rashes and skin lesions depends on a carefully focused history and physical examination. The provider needs to be familiar with the characteristics of various skin lesions; anatomy, physiology, and pathophysiology of the skin; clinical appearance of the basic lesion; arrangement and distribution of the lesion; and associated pathological conditions. It is also important to know common symptoms associated with specific lesions such as itching or fever. It is necessary to quickly identify life-threatening diseases and those that are highly contagious. Ultimately, competence in dermatologic assessment involves recognition through repetition.

DIAGNOSTIC REASONING: INITIAL FOCUSED PHYSICAL EXAMINATION

Initial Inspection

Dermatologic assessment is similar to the assessment of most other body systems in that it depends on patient history and physical assessment. However, sometimes a brief physical assessment preceding the history can assist in the development of the initial differential diagnoses followed by a focused history and further physical examination.

Morphologic Criteria

Examination involves the classification of the lesion based on a number of morphologic features (examples are listed in Tables 28.1 and 28.2 and illustrated in Figs. 28.1 and 28.2). Evaluation should be systematic. Generally, morphologic features should be analyzed as follows:

- Identify the location of the lesion(s).
- Identify the distribution of the lesions as localized, regional, or generalized.
- Identify whether the lesion is primary (appearing initially) or secondary (resulting from a change in a primary lesion).
- Identify the shape of the lesion and any arrangement if numerous lesions are present.
- Assess the margins (borders).
- Assess the pigmentation, including variations.
- Palpate to assess texture and consistency.
- Measure the size of an individual lesion or estimate the size if lesions are numerous or widespread.

Perform a systematic physical examination before obtaining the majority of the history to provide greater relevance to the information given by the patient. Use gloves when palpating rashes and lesions.

DIAGNOSTIC REASONING: FOCUSED HISTORY

Is the rash associated with an immediate life-threatening condition?

Key Questions
- Do you have a fever?
- Are you short of breath?

Table 28.1   **Morphologic Criteria of Rashes and Skin Lesions**

NATURE OF LESION	DESCRIPTION	EXAMPLES
PRIMARY LESIONS (DEVELOP INITIALLY IN RESPONSE TO CHANGE IN INTERNAL OR EXTERNAL ENVIRONMENT OF SKIN)		
Macule	Discrete flat change in color of skin; usually <1.5-cm diameter	Freckle, lentigo, purpura
Patch	Discrete flat lesion (large macule); usually >1.5-cm diameter	Pityriasis rosea, melasma, lentigo
Papule	Discrete palpable elevation of skin; <1-cm diameter; origin may be epidermal, dermal, or both	Nevi, seborrheic keratosis, dermatofibroma
Nodule	Discrete palpable elevation of skin; may evolve from papule; may involve any level of skin from epidermis to subcutis	Nevi, basal cell carcinoma, keratoacanthoma
Plaque	Slightly raised lesion, typically with flat surface; >1-cm diameter; scaling frequently present	Psoriasis, mycosis fungoides
Wheal	Transient pink/red swelling of skin; often displaying central clearing; various shapes and sizes; usually pruritic and lasts <24 hr	Urticaria
Tumor	Large papule or nodule; usually >1-cm diameter	Basal cell carcinoma, squamous cell carcinoma, malignant melanoma
Pustule	Raised lesion <0.5-cm diameter containing yellow cloudy fluid (usually infected)	Folliculitis, acne (closed comedones)
Vesicle	Raised lesion <0.5-cm diameter containing clear fluid	Herpes simplex, herpes zoster, contact (irritant) dermatitis
Bulla	Vesicle >0.5-cm diameter	Bullous pemphigoid, contact (irritant) dermatitis, blisters of second-degree sunburn
Cyst	Semisolid lesion; varies in size from several mm to several cm; may become infected	Sebaceous cyst
SECONDARY LESIONS (APPEAR AS RESULT OF CHANGES IN PRIMARY LESIONS)		
Crust	Dried exudate that may have been serous, purulent, or hemorrhagic	Impetigo, herpes zoster (late phase)
Scale	Thin plates of desquamated stratum corneum that flake off rather easily	Xerosis, ichthyosis, psoriasis
Excoriation	Shallow hemorrhagic excavation; linear or punctate; results from scratching	Contact (irritant) dermatitis
Lichenification	Thickening of skin with exaggeration of skin creases; hallmark of chronic eczematous dermatitis	Chronic eczema
Erosion	Partial break in epidermis	Herpes simplex or zoster, pemphigus vulgaris
Fissure	Linear crack in epidermis	Xerosis, angular cheilitis, severe eczema

Continued

Table 28.1	**Morphologic Criteria of Rashes and Skin Lesions—cont'd**	
NATURE OF LESION	**DESCRIPTION**	**EXAMPLES**
DISTRIBUTION OF LESIONS		
Localized	Lesion appears in one small area	Impetigo, herpes simplex (e.g., labialis), tinea corporis ("ringworm")
Regional	Lesions involve specific region of body	Acne vulgaris (pilosebaceous gland distribution), psoriasis (extensor surfaces and skinfolds)
Generalized	Lesions appear widely distributed or in numerous areas simultaneously	Urticaria, disseminated drug eruptions
SHAPE AND ARRANGEMENT		
Round or discoid	Coin or ring shaped (no central clearing)	Nummular eczema
Oval	Ovoid shape	Pityriasis rosea
Annular	Round, active margins with central clearing	Tinea corporis, sarcoidosis
Zosteriform (dermatomal)	Following nerve or segment of body	Herpes zoster
Polycyclic	Interlocking or coalesced circles (formed by enlargement of annular lesions)	Psoriasis, urticaria
Linear	In a line	Contact dermatitis
Iris/target lesion	Pink macules with purple central papules	Erythema multiforme
Stellate	Star shaped	Meningococcal septicemia
Serpiginous	Snakelike or wavy line track	Cutanea larva migrans
Reticulate	Netlike or lacy	Polyarteritis nodosa, lichen planus lesions of erythema infectiosum
Morbilliform	Confluent and salmon colored	Rubeola
BORDER OR MARGIN		
Discrete	Well demarcated or defined; able to draw a line around it with confidence	Psoriasis
Indistinct	Poorly defined; having borders that merge into normal skin or outlying ill-defined papules	Nummular eczema
Active	Margin of lesion shows greater activity than center	Tinea species eruptions
Irregular	Nonsmooth or notched margin	Malignant melanoma
Border raised above center	Center of lesion depressed compared to edge	Basal cell carcinoma
Advancing	Expanding at margins	Cellulitis
ASSOCIATED CHANGES WITHIN LESIONS		
Central clearing	Erythematous border surrounds lighter skin	Tinea eruptions
Desquamation	Peeling or sloughing of skin	Rash of toxic shock syndrome
Keratotic	Hypertrophic stratum corneum	Calluses, warts
Punctate	Central umbilication, or dimpling	Basal cell carcinoma, molluscum
Telangiectasias	Dilated blood vessels within lesion blanch completely; may be markers of systemic disease	Basal cell carcinoma, actinic keratosis

Table 28.1	**Morphologic Criteria of Rashes and Skin Lesions—cont'd**

NATURE OF LESION	DESCRIPTION	EXAMPLES
	PIGMENTATION	
Flesh		Neurofibroma, some nevi
Pink		Eczema, pityriasis rosea
Erythematous		Tinea eruptions, psoriasis
Salmon		Psoriasis
Tan-brown		Most nevi, pityriasis versicolor
Black		Malignant melanoma
Pearly		Basal cell carcinoma
Purple		Purpura, Kaposi sarcoma
Violaceous		Erysipelas
Yellow		Lipoma
White		Lichen planus

Table 28.2	**Descriptive Dermatologic Terms**[a]

LESION		CHARACTERISTICS	EXAMPLES
Annular		Ring shaped	Ringworm
Arcuate		Partial rings	Syphilis
Bizarre		Irregular or geographic pattern not related to any underlying anatomic structure	Factitial dermatitis
Circinate		Circular	
Confluent		Lesions run together	Childhood exanthems
Discoid		Disc-shaped without central clearing	Lupus erythematosus
Discrete eczematoid		Lesions remain separate; Inflammation with tendency to vesiculate and crust	Eczema
Generalized grouped		Widespread; lesions clustered together	Herpes simplex
Iris		Circle within circle; bull's-eye lesion	Erythema multiforme (iris)

Continued

Table 28.2	**Descriptive Dermatologic Terms[a]—cont'd**		
LESION		**CHARACTERISTICS**	**EXAMPLES**
Keratotic		Horny thickening	Psoriasis
Linear		In lines	Poison ivy dermatitis
Multiform papulosquamous reticulated		More than one type of shape or lesion Papules or plaques associated with scaling; lacelike network	Erythema multiforme psoriasis Oral lichen planus
Serpiginous		Snakelike, creeping	Cutaneous larva migrans
Telangiectatic		Relatively permanent dilation of superficial blood vessels	Osler-Weber-Rendu disease
Universal zosteriform[b]		Entire body involved Linear arrangement along nerve distribution	Alopecia universalis; herpes zoster

[a]Examples of different configurations of skin lesions and their descriptions are contained within Table 28.1.
[b]Also known as dermatomal.
From Swartz MH: *Textbook of physical diagnosis: history and examination*, ed. 6, Philadelphia, 2009, Saunders.

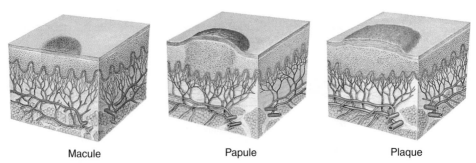

Macule   Papule   Plaque

FIGURE 28.1 Types of skin lesions. (From, Ball JW, Dains JE, Flynn J, et al: *Seidel's guide to physical examination*, ed. 8, St. Louis, 2015, Elsevier.)

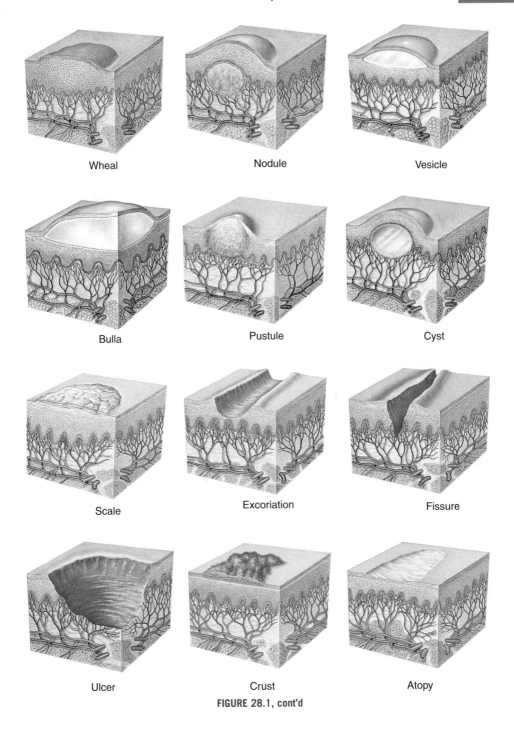

Wheal

Nodule

Vesicle

Bulla

Pustule

Cyst

Scale

Excoriation

Fissure

Ulcer

Crust

Atopy

FIGURE 28.1, cont'd

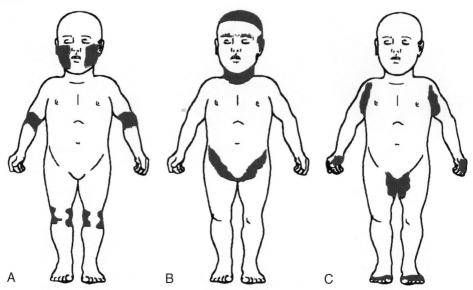

FIGURE 28.2 Typical distribution of papulosquamous eruptions in children. **A,** Atopic dermatitis: usually located on the cheeks, creases of elbows, and knees. **B,** Seborrheic dermatitis: usually located on the scalp, behind the ears, in thigh creases, and in eyebrows. **C,** Scabies: usually located on the axillae, webs of fingers and toes, and intragluteal area. (From Berkowitz C: Pediatrics: *A primary care approach,* ed. 2, Philadelphia, 2000, Saunders.)

- Do you have difficulty swallowing?
- Is the rash tender, and does it involve mucous membranes?

Fever

Fever is common in viral exanthems (rashes), and the accompanying condition is usually not life threatening. However, fever, irritability, hypotension, and a macular or petechial rash may indicate meningococcemia. Treatment needs to be immediate to be lifesaving.

Allergic Reaction

Urticarial allergic reactions may be associated with angioedema (swelling) of the extremities, face, lips, tongue, or airway. Other symptoms include cough, wheezing, shortness of breath, and heart palpitations. The sooner symptoms occur after the exposure to the allergen, the more severe the reaction will be. Treatment needs to be instituted immediately.

Rash with Mucosal Involvement

Toxic epidermal necrolysis (TEN), and Stevens-Johnson syndrome are severe mucocutaneous reactions, most often to medications, characterized by extensive necrosis, and epidermis detachment. These conditions are considered variants of a continuum, based on the percentage of body surface involved. TEN is a more severe condition involving more than 30% of the body surface. Reactions include a tender, morbilliform, erythematous rash accompanied by fever, conjunctivitis, oral ulcers, and diarrhea. Immediate hospitalization is required to treat exfoliation of large areas of skin.

Is the rash acute or chronic (recurrent)?

Key Questions
- How long have you had this rash?
- Have you ever had a rash like this before?

Onset

The diagnosis of skin lesions is initially aided by categorizing the lesion as acute, chronic, or recurrent. Acute eruptions, such as urticaria or various fungal rashes (tinea), are classified as such because they have a tendency to be self-limiting with no recurrence after effective

Box 28.1	**Duration of Rash**

ACUTE	CHRONIC
• Allergic or contact dermatitis	• Acne vulgaris
• *Candida* dermatitis (diaper rash, intertrigo)	• Bullous pemphigus
• Erythema infectiosum (fifth disease)	• Eczema
• Erythema multiforme	• Erythema nodosum
• Fixed drug eruptions	• Kaposi sarcoma
• Folliculitis	• Mycosis fungoides
• Herpes simplex virus	• Polyarteritis nodosa
• Herpes zoster/varicella zoster	• Psoriasis
• Impetigo	• Rosacea
• Infestations (scabies, pediculosis)	• Seborrheic dermatitis
• Insect bites	• Systemic lupus erythematosus
• Kawasaki disease	
• Pityriasis rosea	
• Septicemia (meningococcal)	
• Scarlet fever	
• Tinea (corporis, pedis, versicolor)	
• Urticaria	
• Viral exanthems (measles)	

treatment. Chronic rashes, such as psoriasis or eczema, may persist or be recurrent with exacerbations and remissions. Box 28.1 shows common rashes categorized by duration. Ascertain the duration of the eruption when symptoms are described by the patient; however, the initial occurrence of a chronic rash may be an acute presenting symptom. Conversely, an acute eruption not optimally treated may become a chronic problem.

Where is the rash in its evolution?

Key Questions
• What did this look like initially?
• Has the rash changed? If so, how?
• Has it spread? Where?

Initial Presentation

Most skin lesions evolve over time, although this varies from minutes with urticaria to weeks or even months with psoriasis or cutaneous T-cell lymphoma.

Change in Lesion

Determining whether there has been a change from the initial appearance of a lesion provides diagnostic clues. The eruption of pityriasis rosea classically begins with a "herald patch," a single, scaly, erythematous patch usually on the trunk followed within days by a regional outbreak of numerous smaller erythematous patches, thus providing a key diagnostic clue. The rash may look like that of ringworm, but it appears too quickly to be ringworm. Another example of evolutionary change is the eruption of herpes simplex virus (HSV), which begins with a prodrome of burning, tingling, or itching, followed by the development of small vesicles that later umbilicate, possibly ooze, and eventually crust before healing. A rash may appear in different ways, depending on the point at which evaluation is sought.

Spread

The way in which a rash spreads is helpful in diagnosing the specific rash. There are three general ways in which a rash can spread: centripetal, or moving to the center; centrifugal, or moving away from the center; and caudal, or moving down.

What does the presence of pruritus tell me?

Key Questions
• Does it itch?

Itching

All dermatoses can be classified into three groups: a small group that always itches, those that never itch, and an intermediate group in which itching is variable (Box 28.2). Pruritus is often reported to be worse at night; during the day, pruritus is less troublesome because the patient is distracted by daily routines. At bedtime the slightest sensation of pruritus may become overwhelming because the patient is focusing on trying to sleep. When the patient scratches the area, histamine is released from the inflammatory cells (especially mast cells), and this causes more pruritus, and an itch–scratch cycle is established.

Swimmer's itch, also called cercarial dermatitis, occurs in areas unprotected by a swimsuit. It is an allergic reaction to a microscopic parasite that burrows under the skin. Seabather's itch occurs in areas under the swimsuit. Nocturnal pruritus most typically occurs in scabies infestations. Itching in the absence of a rash may be an important clue to internal disease.

What does associated pain tell me?

Key Questions
• Is it painful or sore?
• Does it burn?

Pain

Pain is a rare symptom with skin rashes. Skin lesions that ulcerate or are associated with swelling can be painful. The classic painful rash is associated with herpes zoster (HZ), including postherpetic neuralgia. Severe psoriasis or eczema with fissures and bleeding may also be described as painful by some patients. Soreness is a more common symptom and is associated with numerous rashes. Tender erythema may be associated with TEN.

Burning

Burning is infrequently reported. It is most notable preceding the rash in herpes virus infections (e.g., HSV or HZ).

What do associated symptoms tell me?

Key Questions
• Do you have a fever? Sore throat? Headache?
• How are you feeling in general?

Fever, Sore Throat, and Headache

Fever is a common presenting complaint in infectious diseases accompanied by rash, such as HZ, erythema infectiosum, scarlet fever, endocarditis, or Kawasaki disease. Malaise, sore throat, nausea, or vomiting can occur with mononucleosis.

General Health

In a patient with a maculopapular eruption, the two most common causes are drug reaction and viral illness. Inquire about viral symptoms, such as fever, malaise, and upper respiratory tract or gastrointestinal symptoms.

Are there possible contacts or sources of contagion?

Key Questions
• Does anyone with whom you live or have close contact have something similar? If so, how long have they had it?
• Have you traveled recently? Where?
• What do you do for a living? What are your hobbies or leisure activities?
• Do you have any pets? Have you been around animals?

Living Situation

Explore the patient's living situation. The geographic details of his or her daily activities

---

Box 28.2	**Itching Comparison**

ALWAYS ITCH	MAY ITCH	NEVER ITCH
• Atopic dermatitis	• Psoriasis	• Warts
• Urticaria	• Impetigo	• Neurofibro- matosis
• Insect bites	• Tinea	• Vitiligo
• Scabies	• Pityriasis rosea	• Nevi
• Pediculosis		
• Lichen planus		
• Chickenpox		

may help provide diagnostic clues, particularly for rashes caused by infectious or infestation mechanisms. Children, in particular, may contract scabies, pediculosis (lice), or impetigo by direct contact in school or daycare.

Travel

A patient may develop a rash weeks or months after travel exposure. Diseases endemic to other parts of the world may have presenting symptoms of rash, including erythema nodosum, which is common in Southeast Asia, or leprosy, which is common in many parts of the world, especially in tropical and subtropical climates. Both eruptions may also occur secondary to tuberculosis. About 40% of erythema nodosum is idiopathic and can be related to inflammatory disease and malignancy. Leishmaniasis is a parasitic infection spread by the bite of phlebotomine sand flies. It is seen in the tropics, subtropics, and southern Europe. Camping trips to wooded areas, especially in the Eastern and upper Midwestern United States, may result in a bite by a deer tick, causing Lyme disease, the leading vector-borne infectious disease. The resultant skin eruption in Lyme disease is known as erythema chronicum migrans, which begins 4 to 20 days after the bite of the tick; only one third of patients remember being bitten. Rocky Mountain spotted fever *(Rickettsia rickettsii)* is transmitted by a tick bite and is common in the south Atlantic region of the United States. Initial symptoms are nonspecific; later symptoms are a petechial rash and fever, usually requiring hospitalization.

Other Exposures

Outdoor occupations or leisure activities may expose individuals to a variety of sources for rashes and lesions, including insect bites as well as allergic or contact dermatitis from poison ivy, excessive sun exposure, and chemical substances. People exposed to animal skins contaminated with *Bacillus anthracis* may develop cutaneous anthrax, which is characterized by lesions that evolve from a papule through a vesicular stage to a depressed eschar. Sun exposure can also worsen chronic eruptions such as rosacea or the malar butterfly rash in systemic lupus erythematosus. Ringworm is common in farmers and ranchers who work with cattle.

Pets

Flea bites produce an urticarial lesion with a central punctum. The reaction is an immunologic one, making it different in each individual. Bites are usually on the legs; infants may have bites on the arms or trunk. New lesions may appear daily, and itching is variable but sometimes intense. Fleas on a cat or dog are usually the culprits. An atypical form of scabies can be transmitted from dogs to humans; the presenting symptom is usually a single lesion in an area under occlusion and it lasts about 1 to 2 weeks.

Is there anything that exacerbates or triggers the reaction?

Key Questions
- Does anything seem to make this worse?
- Do you have any known allergies?

Triggers

Patients often easily identify aggravating factors. Any rash involving vasodilation will become more vivid and likely more pruritic with heat exposure, whether via sunlight, sweating, or a hot shower. Localized eruptions, especially on the hands or forearms, prompt many patients to consider chemicals or other products as causes. People with eczema whose hands are frequently exposed to water are vulnerable to the development of irritant eczema on the exposed skin. Some foods occasionally exacerbate skin lesions. Rosacea is a vasomotor instability disorder characterized by exacerbation with dietary consumption of vasodilators such as coffee, tea, alcohol, or spicy foods. Stress, whether physiological (e.g., menstruation, pregnancy) or psychological, is widely believed to trigger or worsen many chronic rashes, especially eczema, acne, and psoriasis. Stress also may facilitate recurrent eruptions of HSV.

> **EVIDENCE-BASED PRACTICE** *What Is the Evidence About the Prevention and Diagnosis of Melanoma?*

This review summarizes findings from 17 systematic reviews and two guidelines on skin cancer between April 2008 and 2009. Melanoma primary-prevention measures, such as education, are more likely to be successful in younger children than adolescents. The evidence does not currently support population screening for melanoma by whole-body examination. Sunburn later in life increases the risk of melanoma as much as sunburn early in life. Superior diagnostic accuracy of dermoscopy over naked-eye examination for melanoma was mixed.

Reference: Macbeth et al, 2011.

Could this rash be caused by a medication?

Key Questions

- Are you taking any medications (prescription or over-the-counter medications)?
- Do you have any medication allergies?
- Have you had a recent vaccination?

Medication and Medication Allergies

There are four types of dermatologic side effects of drugs: light sensitivity (e.g., photodermatitis), allergic reactions (e.g., urticaria, fixed drug eruptions, morbilliform eruptions), commensal skin eruptions (e.g., pityriasis versicolor in a patient on systemic corticosteroids), and worsening of existing skin eruptions (e.g., tinea eruptions mistakenly treated as eczema with topical corticosteroids). Medications used after the onset of a rash may be irritants or sensitizers and worsen the condition.

Recent Vaccination

Infants and children who have recently had a measles vaccination may display a rash 10 to 14 days after immunization.

Is there a significant dermatologic family history?

Key Questions

- Does anyone in your family have chronic skin problems?

Family History

A family history of dermatologic problems may add insight to the diagnosis. Atopic disease (eczema, asthma, hay fever) tends to cluster in families. Psoriasis, seborrheic dermatitis, and rosacea are also frequently noted to have a familial inheritance pattern. Multiple café-au-lait spots with a positive family history for neurofibromatosis can help identify children with this autosomal dominantly inherited disease.

DIAGNOSTIC REASONING: FOCUSED PHYSICAL EXAMINATION

Look at All the Skin and Mucous Membranes

A "peephole" diagnosis should be avoided; the whole organ should be examined. If the patient is not fully undressed, relevant lesions could be missed. However, it is useful to select one typical well-defined lesion to describe in detail followed by an orderly and sequential system of examination so that no areas of the body are missed. The feet should always be examined in the presence of hand dermatitis so that a hypersensitivity reaction to a tinea infection or a concomitant hand tinea will not be missed. Erythema in dark-skinned people may be difficult to appreciate; it often is seen as postinflammatory hyperpigmentation.

Inspect for Distribution

Determine if the lesion is widespread or localized, unilateral or bilateral, symmetrical or asymmetrical. Symmetrical lesions commonly have internal causes (e.g., eczema, psoriasis); asymmetrical lesions have external causes (e.g., bacterial or fungal infections, allergic contact eczema). Is the lesion predominantly on the flexor (as in atopic dermatitis) or extensor (as in psoriasis) surfaces? A rash on the soles or palms occurs with erythema multiforme, secondary syphilis, and rickettsial infections. Determine if the distribution is confined either to protected areas or to light-exposed areas such as in collagen-vascular diseases, photosensitive reactions to drugs, and airborne contact dermatitis. Is the lesion predominantly centrifugal (affecting the extremities), as seen in erythema multiforme, Rocky Mountain spotted fever, and insect bites, or centripetal (sparing the extremities and concentrated on the trunk)? Intertriginous distribution (neck, axilla, groin) is found in candidiasis, some inflammatory fungal infections, and some forms of psoriasis.

Inspect the Mouth

Drug eruptions from sulfonamides, penicillin, streptomycin, quinine, and atropine often have associated mucosal erosions (enanthems) and crusts. Mucosal involvement is common in hand and foot lesions (e.g., hand, foot and mouth disease), herpes, and syphilis. Oral lesions occur in lichen planus, autoimmune blistering diseases, and malignancies such as squamous cell carcinoma.

Inspect the Hair

In children, a triad of hair loss, scaling, and lymphadenopathy is diagnostic of tinea capitis. A high index of suspicion is warranted in inner-city urban areas, where the condition is common.

Evaluate for hair loss that is diffuse or localized and compare areas such as the temporal and crown region to the occiput. Psoriasis and seborrheic dermatitis may present as scaling and desquamation. A hair pull test will reveal any increased hairs shed with a gentle pull.

Palpate the Skin

Palpate skin lesions to assess for tenderness, texture and consistency, firmness, fluctuance, and depth. Smooth skin has no irregularity. Uneven skin has fine scaling or some warty lesions. Rough skin feels like sandpaper and is characteristic of keratin (horn) or crusts. Assessing the superficial skin for texture is done by palpation with the fingertips. Deeper palpation is done using the thumb and index fingers. Soft skin feels like the lips, normal skin like the cheeks, firm skin like the tip of the nose, and hard skin like the forehead. The depth of the lesion determines if it is on the surface or located within the dermis or subcutaneous tissue. An indurated base is a thickening in the depths of the lesion rather than on the surface.

Palpate the Regional Lymph Glands

Many viral exanthems present with rash and lymphadenopathy. Palpation of the regional lymph glands may be of assistance in the diagnosis if neoplasm is suspected.

Perform an Abdominal Examination

The detection of hepatic or splenic enlargement may assist in the diagnosis of a systemic cause of skin disorders.

LABORATORY AND DIAGNOSTIC STUDIES

Diascopy

Diascopy is used to assess for blanching on pressure and is accomplished by pressing a glass or clear plastic slide on the lesion and observing for color changes. It is used to determine whether a lesion is vascular (inflammatory or congenital), nonvascular (nevus), or hemorrhagic (petechia or purpura). Diascopy is most helpful in evaluating purpuric lesions; blood that is outside vessels (as in petechiae) will not blanch, but blood that is entrapped within dilated vessels (as in telangiectasias) will blanch.

Dermoscopy

Dermoscopy uses a skin surface microscope (dermatoscope) with or without the application of oil on a skin lesion to illuminate and magnify a lesion. This technique allows a more detailed inspection of the surface of pigmented skin lesions to confirm a diagnosis of melanoma and to determine which skin lesions require biopsy or removal. Dermoscopy requires special training and expertise.

Wood's Light

Long-wave ultraviolet (UV) light is used in the diagnosis of lesions caused by fungal infections. Many but not all fungal rashes fluoresce different colors. *Trichophyton* organisms and *Tinea tonsurans,* dermatophytes that are frequently identified in tinea eruptions in the United States, do not fluoresce; *Microsporum* organisms, which can cause tinea eruptions, do fluoresce.

Skin Scraping and Potassium Hydroxide Preparation

Microscopically examine a sample of cells retrieved from a lesion, assessing for the presence of fungal or dermatophytic spores and hyphae. The lesion should be gently scraped using a scalpel (collect cells from an active area such as the border of the lesion); the cells are treated with a drop of 20% potassium hydroxide (KOH) and then warmed or allowed to stand a few minutes to soften the keratin. The addition of 40% dimethyl sulfoxide (DMSO) to the KOH solution accelerates diagnosis. Chlorazol black E stain highlights fungal hyphae as dark, blue-black against a light gray background.

Tzanck Smear

In a Tzanck smear, an indirect test for herpes virus infections (herpes simplex virus, herpes zoster), cells are retrieved by swabbing the base of a lesion (usually a vesicle), smearing it onto a glass slide, and then staining it with Giemsa or Wright solution. Examined microscopically, the presence of multinucleated giant cells confirms the presence of herpes virus but cannot differentiate between herpes simplex virus or varicella-zoster virus infections. Viral culture is diagnostic.

Bacterial or Viral Culture

For a bacterial culture, exudate from a lesion is collected on a sterile swab and cultured for growth. Gram staining may also be done. When a bacterial isolate is known, antibiotic sensitivity testing is performed.

For a viral culture, cells from the base of a lesion (usually a vesicle) are collected on a Dacron swab and cultured for identification of viral infections, particularly HSV or HZ.

Punch Biopsy

In a punch biopsy, a cylindrical-shaped tissue sample is assessed histopathologically for identification. Select a punch size about 3 to 4 mm larger than the lesion or sample an active area if the lesion is large. First the skin is cleansed and local anesthesia is administered. While stretching the skin with the other hand, gently rotate the biopsy instrument while exerting slight downward pressure. When well into the dermis, remove the punch and excise the sample at its base. The defect may be closed using electrocautery, with suture(s), or left open to heal by second intention. Place the fresh specimen on gauze with normal saline for immediate transport to pathology to be processed. If the specimen is being sent for culture or immunofluorescent staining, place in a preservative such as formaldehyde solution.

Excisional Biopsy

In excisional biopsy, a tissue sample is assessed histopathologically for identification. Excise the entire lesion, usually making an elliptical incision around the lesion beyond its margins. Excise the base and close the defect with sutures or cauterize bleeding vessels. Handle the specimen in the same manner used for a punch biopsy.

DIFFERENTIAL DIAGNOSIS

The following conditions represent many of the most common skin eruptions observed in primary care.

Follicular Eruptions

Acne vulgaris

Acne presents as a chronic eruption of the pilosebaceous unit, with noninflammatory lesions (open or closed comedones) or inflammatory lesions (e.g., papules, pustules, cysts), and is most commonly a problem of adolescents. Its distribution follows that of the sebaceous glands: face, neck, chest, back, and upper arms. Neonatal acne first occurs between 2 and 4 weeks of age, lasting until 4 to 6 months of age. Persistence beyond 12 months may indicate endocrine dysfunction. Dark-skinned individuals need aggressive treatment to prevent postinflammatory hyperpigmentation.

Rosacea

Rosacea is a vasomotor instability disorder characterized by sebaceous gland hypertrophy, papules, pustules, persistent erythema, and telangiectasias. It shows a predilection for the face.

Infectious Eruptions

Impetigo

Impetigo presents as a superficial pustular, bullous, or nonbullous eruption followed by crusting (often honey colored). The causative organism is usually staphylococci or streptococci. Contagion occurs via direct inoculation. It is typically a localized eruption that can occur anywhere on the body, with a predilection for the face and trunk.

Folliculitis

Folliculitis is a superficial pustular infection of the hair follicles. Causative organisms are usually staphylococci and occasionally streptococci or gram-negative organisms, including *Pseudomonas, Klebsiella,* and *Proteus* spp. It is typically a localized eruption that can occur anywhere on the body, with a predilection for hairy areas and flexural regions.

Furuncle

A furuncle, often referred to as a boil, is a more extensive infection secondary to folliculitis (see Folliculitis).

Carbuncle

A carbuncle is an abscess of conjoined or adjacent furuncles (see Furuncle).

Macular and Papular Eruptions

Erythema infectiosum (fifth disease)

Fifth disease, also known as slapped cheek disease, is a systemic illness of sudden onset characterized by a coalescing, red, maculopapular eruption on the face. A reticular eruption occurs on the extremities 2 to 3 days later. The causative organism is parvovirus B19. This is a self-limiting condition.

Children with underlying hemolytic anemia may experience an aplastic crisis.

Measles (rubeola)

Measles are caused by a viral exanthem, and the systemic illness that results is characterized by a fine, erythematous, morbilliform eruption on the face that spreads to the trunk over 4 to 7 days, and becomes confluent and reticulate. White patches on red mucosa (Koplik spots) appear on the buccal mucosa. Cough, purulent coryza, photophobia, and fever precede the rash. This is a self-limiting condition and less common with widespread childhood immunization.

Rubella

Rubella results from a viral exanthem similar to measles, starts as fine macules and papules on the face, and progresses caudally within 24 hours. Lymphadenopathy of postauricular nodes is characteristic of this disease.

Pityriasis rosea

The presenting symptom of pityriasis rosea is a rapidly evolving papulosquamous eruption of possible viral etiology. An initial "herald patch" is characteristic followed within days by numerous faintly erythematous patches on the trunk and upper extremities ("T-shirt and shorts" distribution). The lesions follow the lines of cleavage and have a "Christmas tree" pattern on the back. The patches demonstrate fine scaling, and mild to severe pruritus may be present. It is more common in the spring and fall and among adolescents. In African American children, the eruption may consist only of occasional oval lesions along the cleavage lines. The remaining lesions are discrete, scattered follicular or nonfollicular papules over the trunk and proximal extremities. The face may also be involved.

Scarlet fever

Scarlet fever is a systemic illness associated with group A β-hemolytic streptococci (GABHS) (strep throat) and is easily treatable with antibiotics. It is characterized by a macular erythema of the face (flushing), except around the mouth (circumoral pallor), followed by a disseminated fine papular erythema (scarlatiniform), which may then desquamate. The rash is intensified in the flexor folds (Pastia lines). Associated symptoms are sore throat, malaise, fever, circumoral pallor, and a white or strawberry tongue. Scarlet fever is a rarely occurring infectious disease in the United States.

Roseola

Roseola is a viral infection caused by human herpesvirus 6. It is characterized by 2 to 3 days of sustained fever in an irritable infant who otherwise appears well. Mild edema of the eyelids and posterior cervical lymphadenopathy are occasionally seen. After the patient's temperature decreases, a pink, morbilliform, cutaneous eruption appears transiently and fades within 24 hours. This is a self-limiting condition.

Vesicular and Bullous Eruptions

Hand, foot, and mouth disease

Coxsackievirus A16 is the causative organism of this viral exanthem and systemic illness. Painful mouth ulcers followed by painful white vesicles with a surrounding erythema on the fingers, palms, toes, and soles characterize the condition. Patients usually have a low-grade fever, sore throat, and malaise for 1 to 2 days. Some develop submandibular or cervical lymphadenopathy. This is a self-limiting condition.

Insect bites

Mosquito and horsefly bites can cause a common blistering reaction that is surrounded by faint erythema, central pallor if swollen, and usually a visible central punctum. The bites may be arranged in groups if they are multiple. The lesions are pruritic or sore; the condition is self-limiting. The deer tick bite causes a bull's-eye rash at the site of the bite.

Bed bugs

The bed bug, *Cimex lectularius,* is a pest that feeds on blood, causes itchy bites, and generally irritates their human hosts. The Environmental Protection Agency, Centers for Disease Control and Prevention, and United States Department of Agriculture all consider bed bugs a public health pest. However, bed bugs are not known to transmit or spread disease.

Bites on the skin are a poor indicator of a bed bug infestation. Bed bug bites can look like bites from other insects (e.g., mosquitoes, spiders), rashes (e.g., eczema, fungal infections), or even hives. Some people do not react to bed bug bites at all. Bed bug bites can be misidentified, which gives the bed bugs time to spread to other areas of the house.

A more accurate way to identify a possible infestation of bed bugs is to look for physical signs of the pest. For example, noting spots on bedding (about this size: •) that are bed bug excrement is one of the earliest and most accurate methods. The increase in bed bugs in the United States may be caused by more travel, lack of knowledge about preventing infestations, increased resistance of bed bugs to pesticides, and ineffective pest control practices.

Herpes simplex virus

Herpes simplex virus lesions have grouped vesicles that are surrounded by an erythematous base, with discrete, well-demarcated areas that later crust. The condition is associated with soreness or pain and may be preceded by tingling. There is a predilection for lips and genitalia. Recurrences in the same location are common and usually milder.

Herpes zoster (shingles)

Herpes zoster lesions present as clustered vesicles that follow a dermatome. Lesions are surrounded by an erythematous base, with discrete, well-demarcated lesions that later crust. Intense burning and pain often precede the eruption. Herpes zoster along the ophthalmic branch of the trigeminal nerve requires an immediate ophthalmology visit, as this can lead to zoster of the eye and resultant blindness.

Varicella zoster (chickenpox)

Varicella lesions are discrete vesicles with a disseminated distribution; lesions develop in crops or in succession. Vesicles later crust, and occasionally secondary impetigo develops. The illness is associated with malaise and fever. This is a self-limiting condition. Varicella zoster can later be reactivated as shingles in patients over 50 or those who are immunosuppressed. A shingles vaccination is recommended for all adults 60 years and older to reduce the risk of shingles.

Fungal Infections

Candidiasis

Candidiasis is a yeast that produces rashes at a variety of sites; these rashes are called vulvovaginitis, thrush, intertrigo (groin, axilla, gluteal), and diaper dermatitis. The lesion is an erythematous maculopapular eruption that is well demarcated, occasionally with satellite lesions (pinpoint papules) at the periphery with maceration in moist areas. It is associated with mild to intense pruritus; the causative organism usually is *Candida albicans*.

Tinea

Tinea is a fungal eruption that causes rashes at a variety of sites: body (corporis), foot (pedis), beard (barbae), groin (cruris), and scalp (capitis). Lesions have erythematous scaling areas with a discrete border and central clearing that is often associated with pruritus or soreness. The causative organisms are *Trichophyton, Microsporum,* and *Epidermophyton* spp.

Pityriasis (tinea) versicolor

Pityriasis versicolor is a yeast infection characterized by a macular eruption of many colors, hypopigmentation to hyperpigmentation,

and fine scaling. Macules begin insidiously, may take weeks to months to fully develop, and may coalesce. The condition is usually asymptomatic but occasionally pruritic. There is a predilection for a sebaceous gland distribution (neck, trunk). The causative organism is *Pityrosporum orbiculare (Malassezia globosa).* Repigmentation may take years or may never occur. Recurrences are common.

Immunologic and Inflammatory Eruptions

Eczema

Eczema is a chronic relapsing inflammatory condition that can take several forms (atopic, nummular, or dyshidrotic). Erythematous macules, papules, and vesicles that occasionally weep or crust characterize eczema. When severe, eczema may produce fissuring and bleeding. It is associated with mild to intense pruritus. In dark-skinned people, scaling and dryness associated with eczema give an "ashy" appearance to the skin.

Contact or allergic dermatitis

Contact dermatitis is an inflammatory reaction to many substances (e.g., poison ivy, nettles, rubber, nickel). Papulovesicular or bullous eruptions surrounded by erythema, with weeping of exudate (noncontagious), are characteristic of the condition. It may be associated with moderate to intense pruritus.

Psoriasis

Psoriasis is a chronic, relapsing autoimmune disorder characterized by well-demarcated erythematous plaques, patches, and papules, which typically present with silvery scales. There is a predilection for the elbows, knees, hands, nails (pitting), scalp, and gluteal cleft. The condition may be pruritic or sore. The lesions may demonstrate Auspitz sign: pinpoint bleeding when the surface is scraped.

Seborrheic dermatitis

Seborrheic dermatitis is a chronic, relapsing disorder characterized by erythematous scaling patches, which are poorly demarcated and may be pruritic. There is a predilection for the scalp, nasolabial folds, ears, face, central chest, and genitals. The condition is aggravated by cold weather, dry skin, and stress.

Allergic Reactions

Erythema multiforme

Erythema multiforme is an immune complex disorder involving the skin and occasionally the mucous membranes. Iris (target) lesions appear on the extremities and desquamation often follows. Common causes include medications (especially sulfonamides, penicillins, barbiturates, salicylates), histoplasmosis, *Mycoplasma*, HSV, mononucleosis, hepatitis B, and malignancies. Erythema multiforme minor is often self-limited. More severe forms are Stevens-Johnson syndrome, characterized by widespread involvement with vesicobullous lesions and TEN. Both involve the mucous membranes, conjunctiva, and urethra. The more severe forms can involve the lungs, gastrointestinal tract, and kidneys.

Urticaria

Urticaria is characterized by a well-demarcated, usually disseminated eruption that is evanescent over minutes to about 24 hours. The condition usually has an asymmetrical distribution.

Neoplastic Eruptions

Malignant melanoma

Melanoma is an aggressive cancer with a tendency to spread rapidly and metastasize early. Characterized by asymmetry (half of a mole or lesion does not look like the other half), melanoma has an irregular, scalloped, or not clearly defined border with a color that varies or is not uniform (whether the color is tan, brown, black, white, red, or blue). The diameter is usually larger than 6 mm. However, any change in the size of a mole should be viewed with suspicion. The three most significant risk factors for the development of melanoma include a history of melanoma in a first-degree relative, a large number of moles (>50–100), and atypical moles as designated by biopsy. Other factors that increase the risk of melanoma include adulthood, blond or red hair, blue or light-colored eyes, changed or persistently changing mole, white race, fair complexion, freckles, personal history of melanoma, immunosuppression, inability to tan, severe sunburns in childhood, and presence of a congenital mole. In addition, UV light from tanning beds can both cause melanoma and increase the risk of a benign mole progressing to melanoma.

Basal cell carcinoma

Basal cell carcinoma usually appears as a small, fleshy bump or nodule on the head, neck, or hands. Occasionally, these nodules may appear on the trunk of the body, usually as flat growths. These basal cell tumors do not spread quickly. It may take many months or years for one to reach a diameter of 1/2 inch. Untreated, the carcinoma will begin to bleed, crust over, and then repeat the cycle. Although this type of cancer rarely spreads to other parts of the body, it can extend below the skin and cause considerable local damage. The cure rate for basal cell carcinoma (sometimes referred to as nonmelanoma carcinoma) is 95% when properly treated.

Squamous cell carcinoma

Squamous cell carcinoma presents as an indurated papule, plaque, or nodule with a thick scale that is often eroded, crusted, or ulcerated. It can be found on sun-exposed skin surfaces, in areas of radiodermatitis, or on old burn scars. Although slow growing, squamous cell carcinomas arising on the lip, mouth, or ears may be associated with regional lymphadenopathy and metastasis. If promptly and properly treated, it has a cure rate of 95%.

DIFFERENTIAL DIAGNOSIS OF *Common Causes of Rashes and Skin Lesions*

CONDITION	CHARACTERISTICS	DISTRIBUTION OR PROGRESSION	ASSOCIATIONS	DIAGNOSTIC STUDIES
FOLLICULAR ERUPTIONS				
Acne vulgaris	Comedones and/or papules, pustules, cysts	Face, neck, back, chest, upper arms	Onset of puberty, topical steroids, anabolic steroids, systemic corticosteroids, lithium, phenytoin	Usually none
Rosacea	Flushing, persistent redness, sebaceous hyperplasia, erythematous papules, telangiectasias, ocular involvement in up to 40%	Symmetrical, usually face only; may involve eyes	Topical steroids, systemic corticosteroids	Usually none
INFECTIOUS ERUPTIONS				
Impetigo	Vesicular infection; honey-colored crusts and erosions	Face; any area of body with a minor wound, especially excoriated lesions	Scratching as a result of insect bites, atopic dermatitis, scabies	Bacterial culture
Folliculitis	Superficial perifollicular papules and pustules	Any hair-bearing body surface, but especially scalp, beard, legs, axillae	Shaving, hot tubs, contact with mineral oils, occlusive dressings	Bacterial culture
Furuncle	Very tender, deep-seated inflammatory nodule that develops from folliculitis	Same as folliculitis	May have fever	Incision and drainage for bacterial culture
Carbuncle	Multiple coalescing furuncles	Same as furuncle	Same as furuncle	Same as furuncle
MACULAR OR PAPULAR ERUPTIONS				
Erythema infectiosum	Bright-red rash or "slapped cheeks," followed by diffuse maculopapular rash on trunk and extremities, leading to a lacy appearance as exanthem fades	Cheeks, then trunk and extremities	Aplastic anemia in children with underlying hemolytic anemias; fetal hydrops has been reported in pregnant women infected with parvovirus B19	IgM, IgG can be measured

Continued

> **DIFFERENTIAL DIAGNOSIS OF** *Common Causes of Rashes and Skin Lesions—cont'd*

CONDITION	CHARACTERISTICS	DISTRIBUTION OR PROGRESSION	ASSOCIATIONS	DIAGNOSTIC STUDIES
Measles	Patient develops three Cs: cough, coryza, and conjunctivitis; Koplik spots are evident on buccal mucosa; rash begins with spike of convalescent fever; rash is centripetal in distribution, possibly becoming hemorrhagic in severe cases	Rash starts on neck and ears faintly, then covers face, arms, and chest; on second day rash covers lower torso and legs; on third day rash is on feet and face; rash begins to fade on the fourth day	Abdominal pain, otitis media, and bronchopneumonia are commonly associated; severe cases can cause encephalomyelitis	IgM can be measured for measles as well as acute and IgG titers
Rubella	Tender lymphadenopathy of postauricular, posterior occipital nodes; maculopapular and confluent rash that is lacy and not pruritic; rash lasts 3 days	Rash begins on face and spreads to trunk and extremities within first 24 hr	Infection with virus while pregnant results in congenital rubella	Confirmation by acute and convalescent IgG titers, or by direct measurement of rubella IgM antibody
Pityriasis rosea	Multiple oval erythematous lesions with an inner fine circle of scale; ovals line up along skin cleavage lines on trunk, producing a Christmas tree–like pattern	Trunk, proximal extremities, rarely on face; rash is preceded by a "herald patch," appearing from a few days to 3 wk before generalized eruption	More common in spring and fall	If present on palms and/or soles and history warrants, check RPR to rule out secondary syphilis
Scarlet fever	Fine, mildly erythematous papules and sandpaper-like rash found on trunk	Rash begins in axillae, groin, and neck; it avoids face, but there is circumoral pallor	Strawberry tongue; Pastia lines: areas of linear hyperpigmentation in deep creases	Culture for group A streptococci
Roseola	High fever for 3–4 days in infants and young children; as fever returns to normal, a diffuse maculopapular rash erupts	Rash begins on trunk and quickly spreads to arms, face, neck, and legs	Posterior cervical lymphadenopathy	None

▶ **DIFFERENTIAL DIAGNOSIS OF** *Common Causes of Rashes and Skin Lesions—cont'd*

CONDITION	CHARACTERISTICS	DISTRIBUTION OR PROGRESSION	ASSOCIATIONS	DIAGNOSTIC STUDIES
VESICULAR AND BULLOUS ERUPTIONS				
Hand, foot, and mouth disease	Systemic illness caused by coxsackievirus A16; painful white vesicles with surrounding red halo	Painful mouth ulcers followed in 24 hr by painful vesicles on fingers, palms, toes, and soles	Low-grade fever, sore throat, and malaise; cervical and submandibular lymphadenopathy possible	None
Insect bites	Flea, tick bites most common; intensely pruritic eruption, usually in groups of three; bull's-eye rash	Lower legs, but may appear anywhere on body if pets allowed on furniture or beds	Exposure to dogs or cats, or to carpeted areas previously in contact with infected animals; outdoor exposure	Confirmatory biopsy occasionally needed
Bed bugs	Bites may be present, examine bed for small reddish brown spots	General distribution	Travel, sleeping in a different bed	Observe environment for bugs, stains; implement eradication measures
Herpes simplex virus	Primary infection with grouped vesicles on an erythematous base at site of inoculation; regional lymphadenopathy; may be preceded by prodrome of tingling, itching, burning, or tenderness	Can occur anywhere on body, but most common areas are genitals, thighs, mouth, lips, and chin; may be disseminated in patients who are immunocompromised	Other STIs, HIV; triggered by sun, stress, fatigue, fever, trauma	Viral culture Tzanck smear; screen for STIs, HIV if history warrants
Herpes zoster	Unilateral pain, itching, or burning preceded by 3–5 days of eruption of vesicles or bullae; followed by crusting and erosions	Can occur anywhere on body but is unilateral, following a dermatomal pattern; requires prompt referral to ophthalmologist if eye involved (Note: See lesion on tip or side of nose for indication.)	Immunosuppression, older age, local trauma in children	Viral culture, Tzanck smear

Continued

▶ **DIFFERENTIAL DIAGNOSIS OF** *Common Causes of Rashes and Skin Lesions—cont'd*

CONDITION	CHARACTERISTICS	DISTRIBUTION OR PROGRESSION	ASSOCIATIONS	DIAGNOSTIC STUDIES
Varicella zoster	Generalized pruritic vesicular lesions that are in different stages of healing; erythematous vesicles, ruptured vesicles, and crusted vesicles with scabs	Lesions usually begin on trunk and spread to face and proximal extremities	Herpes zoster occurs with reactivation of virus	ELISA titers can confirm acute infection
FUNGAL INFECTIONS				
Candidiasis	Beefy-red, well-demarcated plaques, often with scaling edge and satellite lesions; intertriginous areas may also show erosions and maceration	Diaper area in infants, body folds, mucosal surfaces, nails, and nail folds	Immunocompromised, diabetes, steroid inhalants, pregnancy, oral contraceptives, antibiotics, systemic and topical steroids	KOH, culture
Tinea	Variable, depending on body part affected; hair: scaling, hair loss, pustules; skin: red, scaly patch that may develop central clearing; feet: vesicles or bullae	Skin, hair, feet, nails	Immunocompromised, systemic corticosteroids, farmers and others with animal contact, hot humid weather with tight clothing or occlusive footwear	KOH, culture
Pityriasis (tinea) versicolor	Variably colored white to pink to brown scaling, round or oval macules of varying sizes; often coalescing to form large areas of discoloration	Upper trunk, axillae, neck, upper arms, abdomen, thighs, genitals	Heat, humidity, tropical climates, exercise, systemic corticosteroids, seborrheic dermatitis	KOH shows hyphae and spores in "spaghetti and meatballs" pattern

> DIFFERENTIAL DIAGNOSIS OF *Common Causes of Rashes and Skin Lesions—cont'd*

CONDITION	CHARACTERISTICS	DISTRIBUTION OR PROGRESSION	ASSOCIATIONS	DIAGNOSTIC STUDIES
IMMUNOLOGIC OR INFLAMMATORY ERUPTIONS				
Eczema or atopic dermatitis	Erythema, papules, vesicles, scaling, excoriations, crusts, pruritus always present	Symmetrical; infant: face, flexures; children: flexural creases; adults: may be discrete round patches or be regionalized to specific area	Personal or family history of asthma, seasonal allergies, and eczema; secondary colonization with *Staphylococcus aureus* or HSV	Serum IgE; culture for bacteria or HSV if indicated
Contact or allergic dermatitis	Vesicles and erosions with edema and inflammation, giving way to crusts and lichenification; pruritus	Localized, often asymmetrical; may be generalized with airborne allergens or poison ivy; linear pattern with plant dermatitis	Occupational, recreational pursuits	Patch testing
Psoriasis	Well-demarcated, ham-colored plaques and papules with silvery scale; chronic, recurrent pruritus is common	Favors elbows and knees, scalp; intertriginous areas may involve nails	Streptococcal infection, arthritis, HIV infection, medications, alcohol, family history	ASO titer or strep culture if indicated; HIV if indicated; biopsy
Seborrheic dermatitis	Chronic scaling, flaking, erythematous dermatitis; variable pruritus	Areas where sebaceous glands are most active: face, scalp, eyebrows, eyelashes, body folds, ear folds, presternal area, mid and upper back, genitalia	Atopic history, HIV infection	HIV if indicated
ALLERGIC REACTIONS				
Erythema multiforme	Hypersensitivity reaction seen as annular target or iris lesions	Begins on upper extremities and trunk	Herpesvirus, *Mycoplasma pneumoniae* infections, drugs (especially sulfonamides)	Skin biopsy may assist in diagnosis; chest film for Mycoplasma

Continued

▶ **DIFFERENTIAL DIAGNOSIS OF** *Common Causes of Rashes and Skin Lesions—cont'd*

CONDITION	CHARACTERISTICS	DISTRIBUTION OR PROGRESSION	ASSOCIATIONS	DIAGNOSTIC STUDIES
Urticaria	Transient wheals that may be acute or chronic (lasting >6 wk); individual lesions tend to come and go within hours; pruritic	Localized, regional, or generalized	Angioedema may also be present, may be life threatening; chronic infection, SLE, lymphoma	Biopsy; general medical workup to rule out underlying systemic disease in chronic urticaria
NEOPLASTIC ERUPTIONS				
Malignant melanoma	Asymmetrical border, irregular, has color variation within lesion and is >6 mm	Anywhere on body, including scalp	Usually asymptomatic, unless bleeding, ulceration, discharge present	Skin biopsy, excisional biopsy
Basal cell carcinoma	Papular or nodular lesions, with raised pearly borders, and numerous superficial telangiectases	Sun-damaged areas; also seen in covered areas when there is genetic predisposition to basal cell carcinoma	Usually asymptomatic	Skin biopsy
Squamous cell carcinoma	Indurated papule, plaque, or nodule; may be eroded, crusted, or ulcerated	Sun-damaged areas, areas of radiodermatitis, old burn scars; can occur anywhere on body	Usually asymptomatic; can be associated with HPV, immunosuppression, topical nitrogen mustard, oral PUVA, chronic ulcers, industrial carcinogens, arsenic	Skin biopsy, excisional biopsy

ELISA, enzyme-linked immunosorbent assay; *HIV,* human immunodeficiency virus; *HPV,* human papillomavirus; *HSV,* herpes simplex virus; *IgG,* immunoglobulin G; *IgM,* immunoglobulin M; *KOH,* potassium hydroxide; *PUVA,* psoralen plus ultraviolet A (light therapy); *RPR,* rapid plasma regain; *SLE,* systemic lupus erythematosus; *STI,* sexually transmitted infection.

Rectal Pain, Itching, and Bleeding

Anorectal problems can cause significant discomfort and anxiety. Because patients are often embarrassed by pain or problems in the anorectal area, they may delay seeking care and present with a more advanced disease or condition. Anorectal disorders can range from minor problems to those with significant morbidity. Rectal bleeding can be frightening for patients in every age group.

Rectal concerns include pain, irritation, discomfort, itching, soreness, discharge, and bleeding. Rectal tenesmus is painful sphincter contraction with an urgent desire to evacuate the bowels, or involuntary straining with ineffectual effort to defecate. The causes may be infectious or noninfectious. Rectal pain can be caused by tears, infection, or hemorrhoids. Itching can be caused by inflammation from hemorrhoids, parasites, or hypersensitivity to substances in the environment. Because colorectal cancer is common in adults and may be present with a benign condition, a high index of suspicion for cancer should be maintained when investigating all anorectal symptoms. See the Evidence-Based Practice box for screening recommendations for colorectal cancer.

The anatomy of the anorectal area is important in describing the occurrence of various disorders. The anus is the most distal portion of the gastrointestinal (GI) tract and is approximately 4 cm long. Whereas its distal end is lined by stratified squamous epithelium, the proximal component is lined by simple columnar epithelium. The two components are divided by the dentate line—the line where the distal end of the anal columns and the crypts of Morgagni meet. The dentate line, also known as the anorectal junction and pectinate line, denotes the boundary between the somatic (sensory) and the visceral nerve supply. Proximal to the dentate line, the rectum is supplied by stretch nerve fibers without pain nerve fibers. Below the dentate line, the area is extremely sensitive because it is supplied with pain nerve fibers. The columns of Morgagni are longitudinal columns of mucosa located in the proximal anus. These columns fuse in a ring distally to form the anal papillae at the level of the dentate line. The crypts are the invaginations of the columns of Morgagni. Anywhere from four to eight anal glands drain into the crypts of Morgagni at the level of the dentate line. Most rectal abscesses and fistulas originate in these glands. Figure 29.1 shows the anatomy of the anus and rectum.

DIAGNOSTIC REASONING: FOCUSED HISTORY

Might This Condition Require Immediate Hospitalization or Referral?

Key Questions

- If the patient is bleeding: How much bleeding is there? Are there clots? Are you receiving anticoagulation therapy? Do you have a bleeding disorder?
- Is the patient an infant?
- Do you have HIV/AIDS?
- Are you on chemotherapy?
- Is there purulent discharge?

Bleeding

A patient presenting with significant passage of clots, dark blood, or loose bloody stools needs urgent evaluation to rule out GI bleeding. Melena, blood that is black, tarry, and odorous from partial digestion of the blood, is from the upper GI tract. Melena stool is differentiated from dark stool by a positive guaiac test result. Melena can be seen in children with Meckel diverticulum, a congenital anomaly of the GI tract. When blood is bright red, the source is usually in the more distal GI tract or the rectum. Bleeding from the rectum is a red flag for colorectal cancer but could also represent bleeding hemorrhoids.

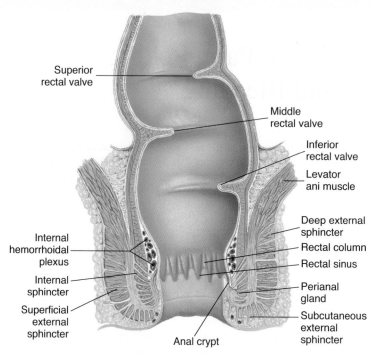

FIGURE 29.1 Anatomy of the anus and rectum. (From Ball JW, Dains JE, Flynn J, et al: *Seidel's guide to physical examination,* ed. 9, St. Louis, 2018, Elsevier.)

Infant

Newborns with melena (black, tarry stool) or hematemesis may have a vitamin K deficiency. Newborns who have not received vitamin K and have a prolonged prothrombin time may have hemorrhagic disease of the newborn. Infants who present with rectal bleeding could have necrotizing enterocolitis (NEC), which is life threatening. All premature infants with lower GI bleeding must be referred and evaluated for NEC. Intussusception, which is also potentially life threatening, is seen in children younger than 1 year old and may cause currant jelly stool (see Chapter 3).

Anticoagulation Therapy or Bleeding Disorder

A patient with a coagulopathy or on anticoagulation therapy with a bleeding internal hemorrhoid may require hospitalization. Bleeding with diverticular disease can be massive and life threatening.

Immunocompromised with an Infection

A perirectal abscess in a person who is immunocompromised may necessitate hospitalization owing to the increased likelihood of the infection spreading systemically.

What do the presenting symptoms tell me?

Key Questions
- If there is bleeding: When does it occur? Describe the color of the blood. Is the blood on the stool, in the toilet, or on the toilet paper? What color is the stool?
- If a child: How old is this patient?
- Do you have pain? When does it occur? Can you describe the pain?
- Specifically, do you have pain on defecation? If a child: Does the child cry on defecation?
- Do you have itching? When does it itch?
- Can you feel a lump?

- Have you had any stains on your underwear? Can you describe the stains (e.g., blood, stool, pus)?
- Do you have diarrhea or constipation?

Bleeding

Anorectal bleeding is usually minor and self-limiting. The bleeding usually comes from internal hemorrhoid veins or from a tear in the anal canal. Excoriations of the perianal skin can also cause bleeding, as can eroded skin overlying a thrombosed external hemorrhoid. Bleeding associated with defecation is characteristic of hemorrhoids. Bleeding from hemorrhoids typically occurs after defecation and is noted on the toilet paper or coating the stool. The blood is bright red and may vary from a few spots on the toilet paper to a thin stream or coating on the stool (hematochezia). Painless hematochezia can also be a presentation of a diverticular bleed. A painful tearing pain with bright red blood during defecation can be indicative of an anal fissure. Spontaneous rectal bleeding can occur with proctitis. Condyloma acuminata may grow to a size sufficient to occlude the rectal opening and will bleed on defecation. Significant pathological conditions such as carcinomas and polyps can bleed intermittently. A loose stool that has bright red blood mixed with mucus may indicate chronic ulcerative colitis.

Some foods such as fruit juices and drinks, food coloring, and beets can make the stool appear reddish. Spinach, blueberries, and grape juice may darken the stool; iron supplementation may also make the stool appear dark. Guaiac testing will differentiate these colorings from blood.

Age of the Child with Bleeding

Newborns

The most common cause of blood in the stool is from swallowing maternal blood during delivery. Neonatal stress can cause gastritis and gastroduodenal ulceration. Another cause of neonatal rectal bleeding is gastroduodenal ulceration from sepsis.

Infants younger than 6 months

Nonspecific colitis or allergic colitis caused by milk allergy can cause blood-streaked stool. Bleeding can also have a bacterial etiology (see Chapter 12). Occasionally, infants who are fed cow's milk protein develop rectal bleeding. After the diet is modified, the isolated bleeding resolves.

Age 6 months to 5 years

Intussusception is seen in children younger than 1 year old and may cause currant jelly stool (see Chapter 3). Meckel diverticulum that ulcerates because of acid secretion onto the gastric mucosa can cause painless, sometimes significant, bleeding resulting in black or maroon stool. Henoch-Schönlein purpura may first manifest as lower GI bleeding (see Chapter 12).

Juvenile colonic polyps are seen in children ages 2 to 5 years. These are benign hamartomatous lesions. Bleeding occurs with defecation because of the sloughing of the polyps.

Anal tears resulting from constipation and stool holding can cause bleeding as well as pain. Blood may be visible on the stool or in the underwear (see Chapter 10).

Age 5 to 18 years

Ulcerative colitis presents in children as acute bloody diarrhea, cramping, and tenesmus. The child may have skin lesions, arthralgia, and growth retardation. Crohn disease may present with bloody diarrhea, abdominal pain, and fever. In mild stages, rectal bleeding may be minor with only small amounts of blood. Blood increases with proximity of the lesion to the anus (see Chapter 12).

Pain

Pain with defecation is characteristic of anal fissures. The pain may be so severe that the patient avoids defecating to avoid the pain. Children will cry with defecation. The pain may last for several hours and then subside until the next bowel movement. Patients with anal fissures complain of cutting or tearing anal pain during defecation and of gnawing, throbbing discomfort after defecation.

Hemorrhoids rarely cause severe pain unless they are ulcerated or thrombosed. Thrombosed

Prolonged Sitting

Occupations that require prolonged periods of sitting predispose people to the development of hemorrhoids, pruritus ani, and pilonidal cysts.

Hygiene

Inadequate hygiene practices are a risk factor for development of pruritus ani and pinworms. Improper cleaning can result in excessive moisture around the canal, which causes breakdown of the epidermal layer of skin. Organisms and parasites can then invade the damaged skin.

Another risk factor in the development of pruritus ani is overzealous cleansing. Pruritus ani can result from excessive use of soaps containing chemical irritants or from excessive rubbing.

Pregnancy and Childbirth

The increased pressure and trauma from pregnancy and childbirth predispose to development of hemorrhoids.

HIV, Chemotherapy, and Diabetes Mellitus

Immunocompromised individuals are at greater risk for proctitis. Herpes simplex infection is common in immunocompromised individuals. Diabetes mellitus places the individual at risk for development of pruritus ani with secondary yeast infections.

History of Colon Polyps

Adenomatous colon polyps in the patient or in first-degree relatives places the patient at higher risk for developing colorectal cancer.

History of Hereditary Colon Cancer Syndrome

Familial adenomatous polyposis or HNPCC in family members places the patient at risk for inheriting the gene mutations that lead to colon cancer. Patients with a mutation for FAP have a 100% chance of developing colorectal cancer in their lifetime. Patients with a mutation for HNPCC have an 80% chance of developing colorectal cancer.

Inflammatory Bowel Disease

Patients with ulcerative colitis or Crohn disease are at higher risk for developing colorectal cancer and proctitis.

Diverticulosis

In diverticulosis, erosion of blood vessels at the site of the diverticulum can cause GI bleeding.

DIAGNOSTIC REASONING: FOCUSED PHYSICAL EXAMINATION

Obtain Vital Signs

Infants who present with rectal bleeding should first be assessed to determine if they are hemodynamically stable. Children have a smaller blood volume, which makes blood loss more significant. Children maintain blood pressure with tachycardia and vasoconstriction, and when this compensation is exhausted, severe shock develops rapidly.

Palpate the Abdomen

Patients with diverticular disease may have abdominal tenderness, typically in the left lower quadrant, which may be accompanied by localized guarding or rebound tenderness. A sausage-shaped mass may be felt in the abdomen of a child with intussusception.

Inspect the Perirectal Area and Anus

Look for scars, warts, petechiae, bruising, fissures, and skin tags. Skin tags and fissures may cause painful defecation, as can skin excoriation, strictures, tears, or hemorrhoids. Midline skin tags immediately anterior to the anus that have been present from birth are seen in some children. Skin tags may also develop when tears or hemorrhoidal bleeding resolves. Hemorrhoids are very uncommon in children, and their presence should heighten suspicion of sexual abuse. Perirectal erythema is common with streptococcal cellulitis, and you may occasionally see vesicles surrounding the anus. Perianal ulceration sometimes can be seen with Crohn disease.

The knee–chest position affords the best visualization in both adults and children. A side-lying position can also be used. Spread the buttocks to reveal the mucocutaneous junction of the anus and carefully inspect the rectum first in the resting position and then as the patient bears down. As the patient bears down, an additional 1 to 2 cm of anorectal tissue is visible.

Look for inflammation, swelling, and erythema that characterize inflammation or infection. These signs may be present with a fissure, fistula, abscess, or proctitis.

Note any lesions or discharge. Condyloma acuminata present as warty growths that are pink or white with a papilliform surface. In the anal region, they tend to grow in radial rows around the anal orifice, forming a confluent mass that can obscure the anal opening. Examination of the entire genital region, including the anal canal, is important because they can extend 1 or 2 cm above the dentate line. Purulent discharge may be present with proctitis or an infected fissure or fistula. An external mass, verrucous growths, polyps, or ulcers may indicate malignancy.

Look carefully around the periphery to see small longitudinal ulcers or tears that characterize anal fissures. Early fissures have the appearance of superficial erosions. More advanced lesions are linear or elliptical breaks in the skin. Long-standing fissures are deep and indurated. Internal fissures are seen when the anal sphincter relaxes as the examining finger is withdrawn. A sentinel tag may be visible.

External hemorrhoids, if present, will be visible as bluish swellings. Internal hemorrhoids may or may not become visible as the patient bears down. A thrombosed hemorrhoid appears as a purple elliptical mass.

Perform a Digital Rectal Examination

A thorough, gentle digital rectal examination (DRE) is essential. Palpate for tenderness. Hemorrhoids are generally not tender unless thrombosed. Pain from an abscess, fissure, or fistula may preclude digital examination.

Palpate for the presence of a mass. Masses from anal or colorectal cancer are usually painless and may be so soft that they are easily missed on palpation.

Feel for foreign bodies, which might be present as the result of insertion of objects. Foreign bodies can also be present as a result of ingestion; for example, children may swallow chicken bones or small objects.

Perform Anoscopy if Indicated

Anoscopy is essential in the evaluation of all patients with rectal pain. It enables a view of the immediate internal anal canal that is not possible on manual DRE. A warmed and lubricated handheld anoscope is eased slowly into the anus while the patient bears down to relax the external sphincter. A light source, preferably a headlamp, is necessary. Anoscopy may not be possible initially in patients with a fissure or abscess because of the pain. However, it should be performed on a follow-up visit to detect inflammatory bowel disorder or rectal cancer.

LABORATORY AND DIAGNOSTIC STUDIES

Fecal Occult Blood Testing

Fecal occult blood testing (FOBT) should be performed on all patients with rectal pain. A positive test result indicates blood in the stool that may be the result of benign conditions such as hemorrhoids or fissures or from ulcerative or malignant lesions. The sensitivity of this test in detecting colorectal cancers and adenomas ranges from 50% to 90%. It is an inexpensive and noninvasive method to screen for bleeding lesions. Serial testing (three samples) can be performed through the use of stool cards at home that are returned by mail for analysis.

Fecal Immunochemical Test

Also called immunochemical FOBT, the fecal immunochemical test (FIT) uses antibodies to human globin to detect a specific portion of a human blood protein. FIT does not react with nonhuman hemoglobin or peroxidase, so food restrictions before the test are not necessary. Immunochemical FOBTs are also more specific for lower GI tract bleeding because they target the globin portion of hemoglobin, which does not survive passage through the upper GI tract. This test is done essentially the same way as conventional FOBT but is more specific and reduces the number of false-positive results. Vitamins and foods do not affect the FIT, and some forms require only one or two stool specimens.

Fecal or Stool DNA

Cells from precancerous polyps and cancerous tumors are shed in the stool and contain recognizable DNA markers. A stool DNA test can identify several of these markers, indicating the presence of precancerous polyps or colon cancer.

Abdominal Radiography

An abdominal flat plate and either upright or cross-table lateral radiography is done to screen for intestinal obstruction or pneumatosis intestinalis (see Chapter 40).

Colonoscopy

Colonoscopy should be performed for unexplained rectal bleeding and when inflammatory bowel disease, polyps, carcinoma, or diverticular disease is suspected. Screening colonoscopy is particularly important for adult patients older than 50 years and for those with a history of FAP, HNPCC, colon polyps, or inflammatory bowel disease.

Computed Tomography

Computed tomography can be useful for evaluating suspected perianal abscesses and inflammation.

Gram Stain Rectal Discharge

Place a smear of rectal discharge on a glass slide for Gram staining. Gram-positive organisms stain purple, and gram-negative organisms stain red. *Neisseria gonorrhoeae*, a common cause of rectal discharge in proctitis, is a gram-negative organism.

Cultures for Infectious Organisms

When discharge or lesions are present, collect a specimen to culture for *Neisseria gonorrhoeae* and herpes simplex virus (HSV). Collect the specimen on a sterile swab and place in the medium provided. Bacterial culture confirms the identity of the causative organism and its sensitivity to antibiotics. A swab specimen of the perianal cellulitis usually yields a heavy growth of group A streptococcus. Viral culture is also used for the diagnosis of HSV. Results may take from 1 to 7 days, with maximum sensitivity achieved at 5 to 7 days. The HSV culture probably will not identify the causative agent if the specimen is taken from a lesion that is 5 or more days old.

Molecular Testing for Infectious Organisms

Molecular testing using a sample of the rectal discharge provides rapid, sensitive, and specific results. Tests include DNA probes, nucleic acid amplification tests, and polymerase chain reaction assays. Tests are available for *Chlamydia trachomatis, N. gonorrhoeae,* herpes virus, and other organisms.

Herpes Virus Antigen Detection Test

This test detects antigens on the surface of cells infected with the herpes virus. Cells from a fresh sore are scraped off and then smeared onto a microscope slide. This test may be done in addition to or in place of a viral culture.

 EVIDENCE-BASED PRACTICE *When Should Screening for Colorectal Cancer Stop?*

The US Preventive Services Task Force (USPSTF) recommends routine screening for colorectal cancer in adults age 50 to 75 years (A recommendation). However, the task force gives a C recommendation for screening adults between 76 and 85 years, taking into account the patient's overall health and prior screening history. The Task Force concludes that the net benefit of screening for colorectal cancer in adults aged 76 to 85 years who have been previously screened is small and that adults who have never been screened are more likely to benefit. The USPSTF does not recommend routine screening for colorectal cancer in adults 86 years and older. In this age group, competing causes of mortality preclude a mortality benefit that would outweigh the harms.

Reference: United States Preventive Services Task Force, 2016.

Testing for Syphilis

Serologic tests are used for screening and diagnosing syphilis and are recommended if other sexually transmitted infections (STIs) are found or suspected. The screening tests are nontreponemal and include Venereal Disease Research Laboratory, rapid plasma reagin, and enzyme immunoassay tests. Diagnostic tests are *Treponema pallidum*-specific and include fluorescent treponemal-antibody absorption test and *T. pallidum* particle agglutination assay. Detection of *T. pallidum* can also be done using DNA testing.

Alum-Precipitated Toxoid Test

The alum-precipitated toxoid (APT) test is performed to identify maternal blood ingestion in newborns. The neonate's gastric contents are mixed with 1% sodium hydroxide. A brown or rusty color indicates that the infant swallowed maternal blood.

Meckel (Technetium-99m) Scan

To confirm Meckel diverticulum, a nuclear substance, technetium-99m pertechnetate, is administered intravenously and the patient is scanned to identify ectopic gastric mucosa on diverticula. This is the hallmark of Meckel diverticulum.

Microscopic Examination of Stool

Stool examination should be considered in patients with symptoms of enterocolitis to rule out infection from common causes. Fecal leukocyte detection is an easy and inexpensive test that is 75% specific for bacterial diarrhea. Leukocytes are found in inflammatory diarrheal disease and are present in bacterial infections that invade the intestinal wall (*Escherichia coli, Shigella* spp., and *Salmonella* spp.). Microscopic white blood cells and red blood cells indicate the presence of Shigella, enterohemorrhagic *E. coli*, enteropathogenic *E. coli, Campylobacter* spp., *Clostridium difficile,* or other inflammatory or invasive diarrhea. Leukocytes are also present in diarrhea from ulcerative colitis and Crohn disease, as well as antibiotic-related diarrhea. They are not seen in viral gastroenteritis, parasitic diarrhea, *Salmonella* carrier states, or enterotoxigenic bacterial diarrheas. Obtain a small fleck of mucus or stool. Do not allow the specimen to dry. Place the specimen on a slide with two drops of Löffler alkaline methylene blue stain and wait 2 minutes before viewing under the microscope.

Stool for Ova and Parasites

Stool examination for ova and parasites should also be considered in patients with symptoms of enterocolitis and in those who have been traveling and have blood in their stool. Fresh stool is required to preserve the trophozoites of some parasites. Use this test in patients with symptoms of diarrhea to rule out infection from *Campylobacter, Shigella, Giardia,* and *Cryptosporidium* spp. and *Entamoeba histolytica.* Usually three serial samples are obtained.

Scotch Tape Test

Use this test when you suspect pinworms, which occur most commonly in children. Instruct the adult to apply clear adhesive cellophane tape to the child's perianal region early in the morning on awakening and bring in the tape. Place it on a glass slide and examine under a microscope for the presence of eggs. Parents may also be able to see the worms in the external anus of the child at night with a flashlight. A female worm is about 10 mm long.

DIFFERENTIAL DIAGNOSIS

Pain

Anal fissure

Anal fissures are longitudinal ulcers that extend from just below the dentate line to the anal verge. They occur most often in the posterior midline. Acute fissures are cracks in the epithelium, but chronic fissures may result in the formation of a skin tag at the outermost edge that is visible on examination. In the chronic stage, fissures can suppurate and extend into the surrounding tissue, causing perirectal abscess.

Patients with anal fissures complain of cutting or tearing anal pain during defecation and of gnawing, throbbing discomfort after

> ## EVIDENCE-BASED PRACTICE *How Effective Is Nonsurgical Therapy for Anal Fissure?*
>
> In this Cochrane review of 75 randomized controlled trials, 17 nonsurgical agents were evaluated for their ability to relax the anal smooth muscle and heal fissures in adults and children. In children with acute and chronic anal fissure, medical therapy with topical nitroglycerin, botulinum toxin injection, or topical calcium channel blockers nifedipine or diltiazem was marginally better than placebo. For chronic fissure in adults, all medical therapies were far less effective than surgery. The authors conclude that a few of the newer agents investigated (clove oil, sildenafil, and a "healer cream") show promise based only on single studies but lack comparison to more established medications.
>
> Reference: Nelson et al, 2012.

defecation. Digital and visual examinations reveal the presence of the fissure. Early fissures have the appearance of superficial erosions. More advanced lesions are linear or elliptical breaks in the skin. Long-standing fissures are deep and indurated. Internal fissures are seen when the anal sphincter relaxes as the examining finger is withdrawn. A sentinel tag may be visible at the anal verge.

Risk factors for the development of fissures include straining at stool, chronic constipation, and anal intercourse. Anal fissures are the most common cause of constipation and bright red rectal bleeding in children up to 2 years old.

Perirectal abscess or fistula

The most common source of infection is the anal glands, located at the base of the anal crypts at the level of the dentate line. Infection may also result from fissures, Crohn disease, trauma, or anal surgery.

Acute infection presents as an abscess, and chronic infection results in a fistula. The patient complains of swelling, throbbing, and continuous progressive pain. On examination, erythema and swelling in the perirectal region of ischiorectal fossa are found. Pain may preclude examination.

Proctalgia fugax

Proctalgia fugax is fleeting pain in the anus. It is sudden and severe, lasting several seconds or minutes and then disappearing completely.

The spasmlike pain often occurs at night. Proctalgia fugax may occur only once a year or may be experienced in waves of three or four times a week. Each episode is transient, but the pain is excruciating and may be accompanied by sweating, pallor, and tachycardia. The patient has an urgency to defecate yet does not pass stool. No specific cause has been found, but proctalgia fugax may be associated with spastic contractions of the rectum or the muscular pelvic floor in irritable bowel syndrome. A few patients report attacks after sexual activity. Other unproven associations are food allergies, especially to artificial sweeteners or caffeine.

Proctitis or proctocolitis

Anorectal infection is common in individuals who engage in anal intercourse, both heterosexuals and homosexuals. Most causes of proctitis are sexually transmitted through the anal sphincter via direct invasion of the infectious agent through the mucous membrane.

Proctitis is characterized by anorectal pain, mucopurulent or bloody discharge, tenesmus, and constipation. Proctitis from an STI may be associated with intense pain. On examination, inflamed mucopurulent mucosa is present. The most common pathogens are *N. gonorrhoeae,* Chlamydia, *T. pallidum,* and herpes virus. Herpes simplex infection can occur above or below the anal sphincter and is common in immunocompromised individuals. Proctitis can also occur in patients with ulcerative colitis and Crohn disease or with patients who have an intact rectum with a colostomy or ileostomy in place. Immuno-compromised patients are at greater risk for proctitis.

Proctocolitis implies involvement beyond the rectum to include the sigmoid colon. The causes may be the same as those of proctitis but are usually caused by *Shigella, Campylobacter,* or *Giardia* spp. Symptoms of proctocolitis may be the same as those of proctitis but may also include diarrhea, fever, and abdominal cramping. On examination, an inflamed mucopurulent rectal mucosa is visible. Gram stain, serology to rule out syphilis, cultures, and molecular testing for infectious organisms assist in diagnosis.

Pilonidal disease

Pilonidal disease refers to an abscess or draining sinus that occurs from subcutaneous infection in the sacrococcygeal area. Hairs that penetrate the subcutaneous tissue instigate a foreign body reaction and initiate formation of a cyst or a sinus. Infection by skin organisms occurs, causing rupture of the sinus into the surrounding adipose tissue. The most common manifestation of pilonidal disease is a painful fluctuant mass in the sacrococcygeal region. Pilonidal disease may present as an abscess, as an acute, recurrent, or chronic pilonidal sinus, or as a perianal pilonidal sinus. Pilonidal disease occurs most often in hirsute young men. Risk factors include a sedentary lifestyle, prolonged sitting, obesity, poor hygiene, and increased sweating.

Perianal streptococcal cellulitis

Separation of the buttocks reveals erythema and, occasionally, vesicles surrounding the anus. The patient usually has a history of group A β-hemolytic streptococcal infection. Pain, erythema, proctitis, and blood-streaked stool are common.

Itching

Pruritus ani

Pruritus ani is a symptom complex consisting of discomfort and itching. It is most often idiopathic. Discomfort is exacerbated by friction or a warm, moist perineal environment. Poor anal hygiene or, conversely, overcleansing is often a contributing factor.

Examination may reveal mild erythema and excoriation of the perirectal skin. In later stages, the skin may be red, raw, and oozing or pale and lichenified with exaggerated skin markings.

Pinworms

Pinworms are nematodes that infect the intestine and cause perianal irritation. The pinworm eggs are ingested and migrate to the duodenum, where they hatch and mature and then travel to the cecum. The adult females emerge at night through the anus, deposit eggs in the perianal region, and die. The eggs stick to the skin and cause perianal pruritus and scratching. The worms may be visible at night, and the ova may be visible under the microscope.

Bleeding

Hemorrhoids

Hemorrhoids are dilated veins located beneath the lining of the anal canal. Internal hemorrhoids are located in the upper anal canal proximal to the dentate line and are covered by rectal mucosa and supported by longitudinal muscle fibers. Internal hemorrhoids are graded by size (Table 29.1). External hemorrhoids are located in the lower anal canal distal to the dentate line and covered by skin, but they lack muscle support.

Bleeding from hemorrhoids is usually painless; the blood is bright red and varies in quantity from a few drops coating the stool to a spattering at the end of defecation. Patients also report a dull aching and itching with prolapse. Itching occurs with chronic prolapse of internal hemorrhoids.

External hemorrhoids can also cause itching but produce pain only when they become thrombosed. With thrombosis, patients report an acute onset of constant burning and throbbing pain and a new rectal lump. A thrombosed external hemorrhoid is an easily visible, purple, elliptical mass that is painful to palpation.

Table 29.1	Classification of Internal Hemorrhoids	
GRADE	DESCRIPTION	SYMPTOMS
1	No prolapse	Minimal bleeding or discomfort
2	Prolapse with straining, reduce spontaneously	Bleeding, aching, pruritus when prolapsed
3	Prolapse with straining, require manual reduction	Bleeding, aching, pruritus when prolapsed
4	Cannot be reduced, or manual reduction ineffective	Bleeding, aching, pruritus when prolapsed

Modified from Metcalf A: Anorectal disorders: Five common causes of pain, itching, and bleeding. *Postgrad Med* 98:81, 1995.

External hemorrhoids are visible on examination as bluish skin-covered lumps at the anal verge. Internal hemorrhoids may become visible when the patient bears down. Risk factors for the development of hemorrhoids include pregnancy, childbirth, straining during defecation, and occupations requiring prolonged sitting.

Diverticular disease

Painless hematochezia is the typical presentation of diverticular bleeding. In most patients with minor bleeding, it is self-limited; however, if the bleeding is massive, it could be life threatening. The bleeding is usually painless except for mild abdominal discomfort and cramping caused by colonic spasm from intraluminal blood. Risk factors for diverticular bleeding include aspirin and nonsteroidal antiinflammatory drug use and a low-fiber diet. Diagnosis is made with colonoscopy.

Condyloma acuminata

Genital warts are a common STI caused by the human papillomavirus. Patients with small lesions usually have few symptoms. When the lesions become large, patients experience bleeding, discharge, itching, and pain. On examination, warts are pink or white with a papilliform surface. They may obscure the anal opening. Examination of the entire genital region, including the anal canal, is important because the warts can extend 1 or 2 cm above the dentate line.

Colorectal cancer

Anal or colorectal cancer can cause many different symptoms or be an incidental finding on rectal examination. Pain is usually absent, and rectal bleeding is inconsistent. The patient may have the sensation of a mass or lump. An external or internal mass may be palpable. Some lesions are so soft that they are missed on palpation. Anal cancer can take several forms, such as ulcers, polyps, and verrucous growths.

Ingestion of Maternal Blood

Newborns may swallow water and maternal blood, and this can appear as upper GI bleeding. To differentiate maternal blood from the newborn's blood, perform an APT test. Fetal blood remains pink, whereas maternal blood turns yellow-brown. Diagnosis is best made with an APT test.

Allergic Colitis

Allergic colitis of infancy is a diagnosis of exclusion. It is seen in infants 3 weeks to 10 months old. The infant presents with loose bowel movements that are streaked with blood and mucus but is otherwise healthy with normal growth. History may show early introduction of milk or a recent episode of gastroenteritis. Laboratory studies are performed to rule out other causes such as diarrheal disease and include stool studies for leukocytes, culture, eosinophils, and complete blood cell count. All milk and soy products are eliminated from the infant's diet. If the mother is breastfeeding, milk and soy products are eliminated from her diet. The infant generally outgrows the problem by the age of 1 year.

Necrotizing enterocolitis

This bowel inflammation may involve only the innermost lining or the entire thickness of the bowel and varying lengths of the bowel. It is seen in premature infants who have fragile and immature colons, but it may also be seen in full-term newborns. The usual presentation may include abdominal distention, lethargy, and bloody stool; however, the signs range from feeding intolerance to sepsis. **This is a life-threatening condition and needs immediate referral.**

Meckel diverticulum

Meckel diverticulum is a congenital abnormality that affects approximately 2% of the population, most of whom are asymptomatic. The diverticulum is thought to be what is left of the fetus's umbilical cord and intestines that were not fully reabsorbed and may contain gastric or pancreatic tissue. Painless rectal bleeding is the usual chief complaint in symptomatic cases in children younger than 2 years.

Intussusception

Intussusception is a telescoping of the intestines. It occurs most commonly in infants between 5 and 9 months of age. The infant experiences severe colicky pain. The child may become pale and limp, and then after the attack, which usually lasts for a few minutes, he or she calms down and appears well. The child may vomit. The stool may contain blood and mucus typically described as currant jelly in appearance. **Emergent intervention is necessary to prevent strangulation of the bowel.**

Juvenile polyps

Benign inflammatory polyps of the colon are found in children between the ages of 2 and 8 years. The patient experiences painless bleeding that occurs during or immediately after defecation. There is no risk of malignancy from these polyps. Colonoscopy is used to diagnose the condition.

> ▶ **DIFFERENTIAL DIAGNOSIS OF** *Common Causes of Rectal Pain, Itching, and Bleeding*

CONDITION	HISTORY	PHYSICAL FINDINGS	DIAGNOSTIC STUDIES
PAIN			
Anal fissure	Cutting or tearing pain during defecation and gnawing, throbbing discomfort afterward	Early fissures appear as superficial erosions; more advanced lesions are linear or elliptical breaks in skin; long-standing fissures are deep and indurated; internal fissures are seen when anal sphincter relaxes as examining finger is withdrawn; sentinel tag may be visible at anal verge	Anoscopy
Perirectal abscess	Swelling, throbbing, continuous progressive pain	Erythema and swelling in perirectal area; pain may preclude examination	Anoscopy, CT scan

Continued

> **DIFFERENTIAL DIAGNOSIS OF** *Common Causes of Rectal Pain, Itching, and Bleeding—cont'd*

CONDITION	HISTORY	PHYSICAL FINDINGS	DIAGNOSTIC STUDIES
Proctalgia fugax	Sudden, severe, transient pain in rectum often occurring at night; may be accompanied by sweating, pallor, tachycardia; may occur once a year or in waves of 3–4 times/wk	Normal rectal examination findings	Diagnosed by clinical history and negative physical examination findings
Proctitis or proctocolitis	Anorectal pain; mucopurulent discharge, tenesmus, constipation with proctitis; also diarrhea, abdominal pain, and fever with proctocolitis; history of anal intercourse, immunocompromised	Purulent discharge, inflamed mucopurulent rectal mucosa	Cultures, DNA testing, Gram stain, syphilis testing; stool examination, stool O&P
Pilonidal disease	Pain in sacrum, superior to rectum; history of sedentary occupation	Erythema, swelling over sacrum, which can be fluctuant	None
Perianal streptococcal cellulitis	History of GABHS, local itching, pain	Erythema, proctitis, blood-streaked stool	Culture of perianal area
Sexual abuse	History of abuse, perianal pain, itching	Large irregular anal fissures, bruising, rectal tone decreased, warts, presence of semen	Syphilis testing; culture (gonorrhea, *Trichomonas vaginalis*, herpes); molecular testing, (herpes, Chlamydia, gonorrhea) HIV testing
ITCHING			
Pruritus ani	Discomfort and itching exacerbated by friction; history of poor anal hygiene or overcleansing	Mild erythema and excoriation over perirectal skin; in later stages red, raw, oozing, pale, lichenified perirectal skin	None
Pinworms	Itching, especially at night	Use flashlight to visualize white-yellow worms 8–13 mm long at night	Scotch tape test positive for eggs

> **DIFFERENTIAL DIAGNOSIS OF** *Common Causes of Rectal Pain, Itching, and Bleeding—cont'd*

CONDITION	HISTORY	PHYSICAL FINDINGS	DIAGNOSTIC STUDIES
BLEEDING			
Hemorrhoids	Bright red rectal bleeding with defecation or blood on stool; burning or itching; straining at stool; prolonged sitting; pregnancy and childbirth	External hemorrhoids: bluish, skin-covered lumps; internal hemorrhoids: may be visible when patient bears down	FOBT or FIT; colonoscopy, fecal or stool DNA to exclude carcinoma
Diverticular disease	Painless hematochezia; may have mild abdominal discomfort and cramping often in LLQ; use of aspirin and NSAIDs and a low-fiber diet	Brisk rectal bleeding; red, or black stool	Colonoscopy
Condyloma acuminata	Few symptoms with small lesions; bleeding, discharge, itching, and pain with large lesions	Pink or white warty lesions with papilliform surface; may extend into anal canal	Syphilis testing to distinguish from condyloma lata caused by syphilis
Cancer of the colon, rectum, anus	Feeling of lump; usually painless; may or may not bleed; may have family or personal history of polyps or colorectal cancer syndromes	Polyp, internal or external mass, ulcers, verrucous growths	Colonoscopy
Ingestion of maternal blood	Newborn	Hematemesis	APT test
Allergic colitis	Infant 0–6 mo, milk formula or breast-feeding mother who has intake of milk	Blood-streaked stool	None
NEC	Preterm newborn, infant	Ileus, abdominal distention, GI bleeding, bilious vomiting	Immediate referral
Meckel diverticulum	Preschool child, painless GI bleeding	Black or maroon stool	Technetium-99m scan and referral
Intussusception	Colicky abdominal pain, vomiting, currant jelly stool	Sausage-shaped mass may be felt in abdomen	Refer
Juvenile polyps	Painless bleeding with stool, ages 2–5 yr	None	Colonoscopy

APT, alum-precipitated toxoid; *CT*, computed tomography; *FIT*, fecal immunochemical test; *FOBT*, fecal occult blood testing; *GABHS*, group A β-hemolytic streptococcal infection; *GI*, gastrointestinal; *LLQ*, left lower quadrant; *NEC*, necrotizing enterocolitis; *NSAID*, nonsteroidal antiinflammatory drug; *O&P*, ova and parasites.

30 Red Eye

The term *red eye* is used to denote a cardinal sign of ocular inflammation. The anatomical location in and around the eye and the
probable cause of the disorder provide an
important framework to use in assessment.
General anatomical locations are the ocular
adnexa (i.e., orbit, conjunctiva, ocular muscles and eyelids), cornea, and anterior and
posterior eye segments (Fig. 30.1).

The eye has two major defense mechanisms. The first is tears, which contain immunoglobulin A and lysozymes; these provide an important washing action. The second
defense mechanism is a conjunctival immune
system of lymphocytes, plasma cells, and
neutrophils. Trauma or inoculation of the eye
with virulent organisms disrupts these normal
defense mechanisms, leading to a red eye.

Although most cases of red eye are caused
by viral or bacterial conjunctivitis, other possibilities include trauma, glaucoma, systemic
disease, and congenital anomalies. Determining the etiology is an important step in assessing the condition.

DIAGNOSTIC REASONING: FOCUSED HISTORY

Is this a chemical emergency?

Key Questions
- Did you get anything in your eye? Did any
  liquids splash in your eye?

Chemical Injury

Chemical burns of the conjunctiva and cornea
represent true ocular emergencies. Alkali
burns usually result in greater damage to the
eye than acid burns because alkali compounds
penetrate ocular tissues more rapidly.

All chemical burns require immediate and
profuse irrigation and immediate referral to

an ophthalmologist. Irrigate the eye with
water or a saline wash for at least 15 minutes
while obtaining a history of the incident and
possible chemical contact.

Could this be caused by an orbital infection?

Key Questions
- Do you notice any swelling or tightness
  around the eye(s) or the eyelid(s)?
- Does it hurt to move your eye?
- Do you have a fever?
- Have you had a recent sinus infection?

Swelling, Redness, and Fever

The orbital septum is a continuation of the
periosteum of the bones of the orbit. It extends to the margins of both the upper and
lower eyelids. Any conditions occurring in
these areas can cause swelling. Secondarily,
the skin of the eyelids is a very thin subcutaneous tissue that is musculofibrous and contains no fat. Thus, the eyelid can allow a
considerable amount of fluid to accumulate in
a short period of time. Swelling and erythema
under and associated with the medial canthus
of the affected eye may indicate dacryocysti-
tis. Swelling of the eyelids may be associated
with inflammation, local infection, or trauma.
Periorbital swelling may indicate cellulitis.
Orbital or periorbital cellulitis can present
with conjunctivitis and signal a medical emergency. They can occur as complications of
sinusitis. Reports of swelling, redness, and
fever should alert you to these conditions.
Both conditions require immediate referral;
orbital cellulitis can be life threatening.

Pain with Attempted Motion of the Eye

Orbital cellulitis causes pain with movement
because of the collection of pus between
the periosteum and the wall of the orbit. The

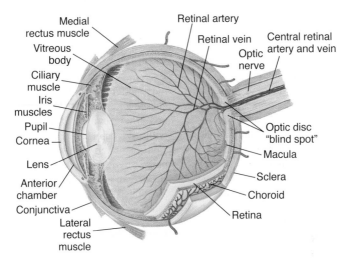

Medial rectus muscle
Vitreous body
Ciliary muscle
Iris muscles
Pupil
Cornea
Lens
Anterior chamber
Conjunctiva
Lateral rectus muscle

Retinal artery
Retinal vein
Central retinal artery and vein
Optic nerve
Optic disc "blind spot"
Macula
Sclera
Choroid
Retina

FIGURE 30.1 Anatomical structures of the human eye. (From Ball JW, Dains JE, Flynn J, et al: *Seidel's guide to physical examination,* ed. 8, St. Louis, 2015, Elsevier.)

inflammation continues to all tissues in the orbit, leading to proptosis and impairment of ocular motility.

Recent Sinus Infection

Sinusitis is a predisposing condition in 86% to 98% of patients with orbital cellulitis. The ethmoid sinuses are most commonly involved, with the maxillary sinus the next most common site of infection.

Can I rule in or rule out trauma?

Key Questions

- How was your eye injured (e.g., foreign body, chemical substance, blow, stab, cut)?

Blunt trauma to the ocular adnexa can cause eyelid swelling or discoloration. Rupture of the globe, fractures of the orbital bones, and internal bleeding may also be possible. Sharp trauma to the area can cause lacerations of the eyelid and underlying lacerations of the globe. Internal bleeding may be subconjunctival (between the conjunctiva and sclera) or intraocular (hyphema). The cornea may have a foreign body or abrasions.

History of forceful trauma causing laceration or perforation of the globe is a surgical emergency and should be referred immediately without manipulation of the eye or eyelid.

Is this an acute or chronic condition?

Key Questions

- How long has the eye been red?
- Did the redness start abruptly, or was it gradual?
- Is this redness different from previous episodes? How often does it recur?

Onset

An abrupt onset of redness typifies trauma, chemical burn, foreign body, ultraviolet exposure, or contact lens problems. Onset over a few hours may indicate infection from adjacent structures (periorbital, orbital, or sinuses). Onset over a few days is characteristic of conjunctivitis. Acute redness can be caused by infection of the conjunctiva or eyelids. Common causative organisms include *Staphylococcus aureus,* *Streptococcus pneumoniae,* group A streptococci, *Haemophilus influenzae,* and *Neisseria gonorrhoeae.*

Recurrence

Recurrent redness is often the result of allergic conjunctivitis from a hypersensitivity reaction to a specific antigen. Iritis from systemic causes can also produce recurrent redness because of collagen destruction.

Key Question

- Does one eye (or do both eyes) bother you?

Whereas unilateral redness is more likely to indicate trauma or infection, bilateral redness is more likely to indicate an allergy or an underlying systemic process. Blepharitis, inflammation of the eyelids, causes itching and crusting of the lash line and is usually bilateral. A hordeolum (stye) produces redness at the base of eyelashes and is usually unilateral. A chalazion is a chronic granulomatous inflammation of the meibomian gland, which is in the middle of the eyelid, often on the conjunctival side, and is usually unilateral. Some conditions can present with either unilateral or bilateral symptoms. Conjunctivitis often starts in one eye and then spreads to the other, sparing the limbal area of the eyes. Subconjunctival hemorrhage is often unilateral but may involve both eyes. Herpetic infection may be unilateral or bilateral.

A unilaterally painful, inflamed eye with photophobia and often a foreign body sensation and without a history of significant trauma may indicate acute glaucoma or keratitis with corneal ulceration.

What does the presence or absence of pain tell me?

Key Questions

- Do you have pain in your eye?
- How severe is the pain?
- Does it feel like there is something in your eye?

Location of Pain

Decide whether the pain is coming from the eye itself or is referred from surrounding structures. A nonverbal child who is light sensitive and in pain may be observed for rubbing the eye, excessive blinking, and irritability. The ophthalmic nerve innervates the eyelid, conjunctiva, cornea, and uveal tract. The retina, vitreous, and optic nerve are less well innervated and seldom a source of pain. Referred pain can originate from contiguous structures or from inflamed structures innervated by the meningeal branches of the ophthalmic nerve.

Severity of Pain

Bacterial conjunctivitis causes minimal pain; most patients report discomfort from the discharge and matting. There may be an itching or burning pain with allergy, moderate pain with iritis, and severe pain with corneal abrasion or ulcer. Constant, boring, throbbing pain, often severe enough to interfere with sleep, can result from ocular inflammation associated with iritis, acute glaucoma, and scleritis.

Foreign Body Sensation

A foreign body in an eye is a likely cause of pain. Viral causes of conjunctivitis produce a gritty sensation in the eye. A scratchy sensation often accompanies conditions that lead to dry eye, such as Sjögren syndrome. Patients who overwear contact lenses frequently report pain in the eye, caused by corneal hypoxia, several hours after removing the contacts.

Key Questions

- Have you noticed any change in or loss of vision?
- Have you had any blurred vision, double vision, halos, or floaters?

Vision Loss

Distinguish vision loss from blurry vision caused by the discharge associated with conjunctivitis. No decrease in vision is seen with bacterial and allergic conjunctivitis, beyond that reasonably related to blurring from the heavy discharge. Vision is mildly decreased in iritis but markedly decreased with acute glaucoma, corneal abrasions, or ulcers. Box 30.1 lists symptom patterns of pain and vision loss (also see Chapter 38).

Sudden diminution in or loss of visual acuity is an ocular emergency and may indicate corneal or uveal tract disorders, retinal tears or detachment, acute glaucoma, or orbital cellulitis.

| Box 30.1 | Symptom Patterns of Pain and Vision Loss | |

Box 30.1 Symptom Patterns of Pain and Vision Loss

RED EYE (NO PAIN OR VISION LOSS)	RED EYE (PAINFUL)	
	VISION IMPAIRED	VISION NORMAL
• Conjunctivitis	• Keratitis	• Glaucoma
• Subconjunctival hemorrhage	• Cluster headache	• Orbital cellulitis
• Episcleritis	• Corneal abrasion	• Scleritis
	• Corneal ulcer	• Corneal abrasion
		• Keratitis
		• Corneal ulcer

Blurring

True blurring is caused by an ocular problem. When the cornea, lens, aqueous humor, or vitreous is hazy, vision blurs and often there is dazzle in bright light. Some patients describe both refractive errors and double vision as blurred vision. Heavy discharge associated with conjunctivitis can also produce perceived blurring of vision.

Double Vision

True double vision becomes single vision when one eye is covered. Sudden onset usually indicates a neurological problem. Chronic diplopia may be caused by muscular problems. Monocular diplopia usually indicates either corneal or lens changes.

Halos

Halos result from prismatic effects. They can be visual signs of corneal edema caused by an abrupt rise in corneal or intraocular pressure (acute glaucoma). Less serious causes are water drops in the cornea or lens (seen in corneal edema or cataract).

Floaters

Floaters or flashing lights occur with vitreoretinal traction. The traction may progress to a retinal tear or detachment. With a tear, patients may report spaghetti-like strands floating in their vision. With a detachment, patients will give a history of blurred or blackened vision over several hours that progresses to complete or partial monocular blindness, often described as a curtain dropping.

What does the presence or characteristic of the discharge tell me?

Key Questions

• Do you have any discharge from your eye?
• Is the discharge from one eye or both eyes?
• What are the color, consistency, and characteristics of this discharge?

Presence and Characteristics of Discharge

A watery, nonpurulent, or mucoid discharge usually indicates allergic conjunctivitis. In allergic conjunctivitis, the discharge is usually bilateral. Discharge that is purulent or mucopurulent may indicate bacterial conjunctivitis and often affects both eyes. Copious purulent discharge may be caused by *N. gonorrhoeae* infection. Viral conjunctivitis discharge is watery and may affect only one eye. Corneal abrasions and ulcers also produce watery or purulent discharge and are usually unilateral.

A neonate who is 24 hours old with mucoid or purulent ocular discharge indicates chemical conjunctivitis from prophylactic instillation of erythromycin ophthalmic ointment and other medications. Severe, bilateral purulent conjunctivitis 3 to 7 days after birth may indicate gonococcal infection of the eye. Discharge 5 to 30 days postpartum may indicate chlamydial conjunctivitis.

What does the presence of photophobia tell me?

Key Questions

• Does light bother you or hurt your eye(s)?

Photophobia usually indicates ocular inflammation or irritation. Intraocular inflammation (iritis or generalized uveitis) causes pain on pupillary changes and thus leads to the avoidance of bright light. This symptom may be mild and often is not reported unless the patient is questioned specifically about this symptom. There is no photophobia with bacterial conjunctivitis. In infants and young children, photophobia signals a serious condition, such as juvenile arthritis, intraocular tumors, congenital glaucoma, keratitis, or trauma.

What other things do I need to consider?

Key Questions
- Do you have excessive tearing?
- Do your eyes itch?
- Does the itching occur at different times of the year?
- Have you had a cough or fever?
- Where have you traveled recently?

Tears

The lacrimal gland, which is situated in the upper lateral orbit, produces tears that are then carried across the eye to the puncta on the nasal side of the upper and lower eyelids. Obstruction of the passage of tears via the nasolacrimal duct to the nose causes regurgitation of fluid down the cheek (tearing). Epiphora (excessive production of tears) is common with viral conjunctivitis, corneal abrasions, infantile glaucoma, and nasal lacrimal duct stenosis.

Itching and Tearing

The hallmark of an allergic conjunctivitis is itching and tearing disproportionate to findings. Vernal conjunctivitis is seasonal, recurrent, and bilateral. Itching is intense in the spring and fall months.

Cough and Fever

Bacterial conjunctivitis is not associated with fever; however otitis-conjunctivitis syndrome begins with a low-grade to moderate fever, mucopurulent rhinorrhea, and cough. Three or four days after the onset of fever, the individual wakes up with the eyelashes crusted together. Ear complaints begin the same day as eye symptoms. Viral conjunctivitis, seen as slight crusting along the eyelid margins, may be seen with upper respiratory tract infections.

Travel

The Centers for Disease Control and Prevention maintains health alerts for various regions of the world at http://cdc.gov. Zika virus has emerged as an infection contracted in warmer climates and may appear as viral conjunctivitis, often accompanied by fever, rash, and arthralgia.

DIAGNOSTIC REASONING: FOCUSED PHYSICAL EXAMINATION

Before conducting specific assessment procedures, perform an overall assessment of the patient to determine if there is visible injury, asymmetry of eyes and eyelids, or other abnormality, such as exophthalmia, to aid in timely assessment and referral.

Test Visual Acuity

In literate, verbal, and English-speaking adults and school-age children adults and children older than 3½ years, use a Snellen or Sloan chart. For young children or adults not able to use the Snellen or Sloan chart, use HOTV characters or LEA symbols. Use a Snellen, Tumbling E, or Lippman chart for children older than 3½ years and adults. In children, the referral standard is 20/40 or worse in both eyes or a two-line difference between eyes. Retesting children before referral is suggested because they may perform better (within normal limits) on the second examination.

For children younger than 3½ years, use an ophthalmoscope. Darken the room. Stay at arm's length from the child and look at the eyes at a distance of 1 m or greater. When the child looks at the light, look at both red reflexes simultaneously and compare them. They should be red and equal in coloration. This indicates that the vision and binocular alignment are good and that no major pathologic condition of the cornea, lens, vitreous, or retina is present. If the reflexes are not equal, refer the child to an ophthalmologist.

Test Visual Fields

Testing of visual fields assesses the function of the peripheral vision and the central retina, optic pathways, and cortex. The visual fields confrontation test provides a gross assessment of peripheral vision. The peripheral field is damaged in glaucoma and by tumors or vascular lesions involving the visual fibers from the chiasm to the occipital cortex.

Assess extraocular movements by testing the six cardinal positions of gaze, assessing the corneal light reflex, and performing the cover-uncover test.

Inspect the Eyelids, Eyelid Margins, Periorbital Tissues, and Orbital Tissues

Note redness or swelling of the eyelids. Look for eyelid lesions. Inspect the eyelid margins. Evert the eyelids and note appearance.

Unilateral inflammation of the eyelids and periorbital tissues without proptosis or limitation of eye movement characterizes periorbital cellulitis. If proptosis or limitation of eye movement is present, orbital cellulitis is a likely cause.

Erythematous swelling without systemic signs may be caused by contact dermatitis. All exposed skin should have the same coloring. A eyelid that is injected, swollen, and irritated may be so because of an underlying disease process in the conjunctiva, cornea, sclera, or intraocular area.

Examine for the presence of focal or diffuse inflammation. Blockage of the glands along the lash line may produce localized or diffuse redness or flaking of the skin as a result of staphylococcal or seborrheic causes.

With viral conjunctivitis, eyelids appear to have follicular changes (small aggregates of lymphocytes) in the palpebral conjunctiva. Eyelids that have large, flattened, cobblestone-like papillary lesions of the palpebral conjunctivae are characteristic of vernal conjunctivitis.

Inflammation of the eyelid margins in all four eyelids with associated loss of eyelashes is common in children; this condition is known as blepharitis. The lash line is waxy, scaling, red, and irritated, and the eyes have slightly swollen eyelid margins.

Eye pain with no external inflammation suggests referred causes, such as sinusitis, carotid artery aneurysm, temporal arteritis, migraine or cluster headache, or trigeminal neuralgia. Optic neuritis can also cause eye pain without inflammation.

Observe for Entropion and Ectropion

The lacrimal puncta are turned backward slightly to catch the pool of tears in the inner canthus and to prevent tears spilling over the cheeks. Anatomical changes of the eyelid margins can develop into entropion, when the eyelid margin turns inward. The eyelashes contact the corneal and conjunctival surfaces, and the patient reports discomfort. Scarring can occur.

Ectropion occurs when the eyelid margin turns outward. A pool of stagnant tears results and does not allow proper mechanical protection of the cornea and conjunctiva. The exposed tarsal conjunctiva is also susceptible to repeated trauma.

Evert the Eyelid

If there is a history of trauma, eversion of the eyelid is necessary to detect a possible foreign body. This is done by first having the patient look down. Hold the upper eyelashes straight forward. Push down on the upper tarsal border with a cotton-tipped applicator. The eyelid everts. Hold the eyelid in this position by moving fingers to the brow. To undo, hold the lashes and pull gently forward while asking the patient to look up.

Inspect the Conjunctiva

Note bilateral or unilateral redness and the location of redness on the conjunctiva. Distinguish between peripheral or circumcorneal injection (ciliary flush). Ciliary flush is the deep conjunctival or episcleral blood vessel injection around the limbus (junction between the cornea and conjunctiva), dilating in response to corneal disease or injury. It is frequently associated with keratopathy, uveitis, and episcleritis or scleritis. Abrasions and ulcers of the cornea cause increased redness of the globe around the corneal limbus, appearing as a reddish ring surrounding the cornea. Note any discharge. Look for visible lesions or foreign bodies on the conjunctiva.

Conjunctival inflammation as a result of infection causes a red eye with peripheral injection that is maximal toward the fornix (the fold between globe and eyelid). Peripheral injection involves the bulbar conjunctiva without edema or exudate, and the cornea is spared.

Look for swelling of the conjunctiva (chemosis). Fluid can accumulate beneath the loosely attached bulbar conjunctiva, causing it to balloon away from the globe. Chemosis occurs most frequently and dramatically with hyperacute bacterial conjunctivitis.

Subconjunctival hemorrhage causes a bright red splash of blood that is visible on the conjunctiva and sclera. Without a history of trauma or bleeding diathesis and no presence of retinal hemorrhage, the cause may be intravascular pressure from coughing, sneezing, or straining.

Systemic autoimmune processes, such as juvenile rheumatoid arthritis, serum sickness, and Stevens-Johnson syndrome, may cause conjunctivitis. Conjunctivitis around the limbus of the eye is seen in juvenile rheumatoid arthritis.

A localized degenerative process of the substantia propria of the conjunctiva, known as pinguecula, may invade the superficial cornea. These are yellow, elevated nodules of fibropathic material that are usually adjacent to the cornea on the nasal side.

Look at the palpebral conjunctiva and the fornices for foreign bodies and pterygia, which are neovascularized structures that can encroach on the cornea and form a pannus, an abnormal layer of fibrous tissue or granulation tissue, which interferes with vision.

Inspect the Sclera

Note the color. The sclera gives the eye its white appearance. Inflammation (scleritis) causes a dusky red color.

Examine the Cornea

Test the corneal light (red) reflex. Note if the cornea is hazy or has opacities. Look for visible foreign bodies.

The normal cornea is transparent, with blood vessels only at the limbus (the junction between cornea and conjunctiva). Illumination of the cornea tangentially may show abnormalities, such as abrasions or foreign bodies. These imperfections of the corneal surface will produce an abnormal light reflex or a break in the image as the light reflects off the cornea. The blood vessels around the limbus dilate in response to corneal disease or injury.

When topical application of fluorescein to the cornea reveals dendrite ulcers, you should suspect herpes simplex virus.

Examine the Iris, Pupil, and Lens

Note pupil size and equality. Note transparency of lens. Test pupillary reaction (direct and consensual). Note any photophobia.

The anterior chamber should contain only clear aqueous humor. Trauma may cause blood to accumulate in the chamber; this is known as a hyphema. The shock wave produced by the sudden compression and decompression of the cornea is transmitted through the eye and may result in a tear in the ciliary body. Disruption of the anterior arterial circle of this structure produces bleeding that accumulates. The hyphema appears as a bright red or dark red fluid level between the cornea and iris or as a diffuse murkiness of the aqueous humor. Pus may also accumulate in this space in association with corneal infection. This is known as hypopyon. All hyphemas are abnormal and must be referred to an ophthalmologist.

The pupil is the central aperture of the iris. It floats in the aqueous humor and divides the anterior segment into anterior and posterior chambers, which communicate throughout the pupillary aperture. It slides freely on the anterior surface of the lens when dilating and contracting. Conditions that affect this anatomy cause pupil abnormalities. Inflammation of the iris (iritis) causes reduction in the reactive capacity of the iris and inequality of pupils. Acute increased intraocular pressure causes the space in the anterior chamber to become very shallow, resulting in a dilated, fixed, oval pupil.

The lens is normally transparent and not visible on inspection; however, any visible clouding of the lens seen through the pupil is indicative of cataract formation.

Perform Ophthalmoscopy

When looking for the red reflex, note any corneal opacity as well as the depth of the opacity. Corneal opacities move in the opposite direction of the ophthalmoscope, lens opacities stay still, and vitreous opacities move in the same direction as the ophthalmoscope. Corneal clouding (edema) is seen with glaucoma.

Look for a large and deepened cup if you suspect glaucoma. Early in the course of the disease, the ophthalmoscopic examination may be normal. Do not use mydriatic agents if you suspect glaucoma.

Test Extraocular Movements

Test eye movement in all six fields of gaze. Note pain or restriction. Inflammation or underlying periostitis and impaired venous drainage as a result of reactive inflammation cause restrictive eye movement and proptosis (exophthalmia). Decreased range of motion can also occur with orbital cellulitis.

Palpate the Eyelid and Lacrimal Puncta

Note if gentle palpation of each lacrimal sac produces any material that regurgitates into the eye. Unilateral swelling over the lacrimal sac on the eyelid margin at the side of the nose because of infection or obstruction of the lacrimal drainage system is common. Infection of the meibomian glands of the eyelids (hordeolum or internal stye) and the glands of Zeis or Moll (hordeolum or external stye) produces pain on palpation. Internal styes are generally large and very tender and may point to the conjunctiva or epidermis portion of the eyelid. External styes are small and superficial and point only to the epidermis side.

Granulomatous inflammation of a meibomian gland nodule that is firm and not tender and has no inflammatory signs is a chalazion.

Examine the Tympanic Membranes

Examination of the tympanic membrane is necessary because of the frequent association with atypical *H. influenzae* acute otitis media (otitis-conjunctivitis syndrome).

Palpate Preauricular Nodes

The preauricular nodes are usually palpable with a viral infection of the eyes. Palpable adenopathy is uncommon in acute bacterial conjunctivitis but may occur in hyperacute infection caused by *N. gonorrhoeae* or *Neisseria meningitidis*.

LABORATORY AND DIAGNOSTIC STUDIES

Fluorescein Staining

This is a test that uses orange dye (fluorescein) and a blue light to detect foreign bodies in the eye. This test can also detect damage to the cornea. Under a blue light, a corneal abrasion and foreign body will stain bright green with fluorescein. Dendrite etchings on the anterior portion of the cornea are seen in herpes infection. Nodules near the limbus with surrounding hyperemia are seen in keratoconjunctivitis. Hypertrophy of the dorsal conjunctiva with elevated grayish areas near the limbus is consistent with vernal conjunctivitis.

Culture

Cultures are not usually required in patients with mild conjunctivitis of suspected viral, bacterial, or allergic origin. However, bacterial cultures should be obtained in patients with severe, chronic, or recurrent conjunctivitis. Moisten a sterile alginate (not cotton) swab with sterile saline and wipe the eyelid margin or conjunctival cul-de-sac. The culture medium is then inoculated directly with the swab tip. Place on solid medium, writing *R* for right eye, *L* for left eye, and *Z* for another culture site. The tip of the applicator may then be broken off and dropped into the tube of liquid culture medium.

Cultures should be taken before instilling topical anesthetics because preservatives will reduce the recovery of some bacteria.

Gram Stain

Obtain a culture of any discharge. Gram-positive cocci in pairs may indicate *Streptococcus pyogenes*. Gram-negative diplococci indicate *N. gonorrhoeae*. Large gram-negative diplobacilli indicate *Moraxella catarrhalis*; *H. influenzae* stains as gram-negative coccobacilli.

Complete Blood Count

A complete blood count with differential can be done to establish the presence of a systemic infection. An increase in white blood cells and bands is seen with systemic infection.

Blood Cultures

Blood cultures are obtained for any suspected orbital cellulitis or when there is reason to suspect a clinically significant bacteremia. *H. influenzae, S. pneumoniae, Staphylococcus aureus, Streptococcus pyogenes*, or anaerobes are possible infecting organisms.

Computed Tomography

A computed tomography scan can determine the presence and extent of an abscess or localize the site of infection in the periorbital region as well as in the sinuses.

Intraocular Pressure

Intraocular pressure can be measured using a variety of tonometry instruments. It can also be used to screen for open-angle glaucoma; however, many patients with open-angle glaucoma do not have increased intraocular pressure. Diagnosis is based on a combination of tests showing characteristic degenerative changes in the optic disc and defects in visual fields (often loss in peripheral vision). Intraocular pressure is measured by a specialist using dilated ophthalmoscopy and a slit lamp to assess intraocular changes.

DIFFERENTIAL DIAGNOSIS

Lacrimal Sac

Dacryocystitis

Infection of the lacrimal sac occurs secondary to obstruction. In infants, it is a complication of congenital dacryostenosis. In adults, duct obstruction results from nasal trauma, deviated septum, hypertrophic rhinitis, and mucosal polyps. The patient experiences pain, swelling, and redness around the lacrimal sac with tearing. Conjunctivitis, blepharitis, and leukocytosis are associated with an acute condition; with a chronic condition, the only symptom may be slight swelling of the sac. Pus may regurgitate through the punctum.

Eyelids

Blepharitis

Blepharitis is the most common inflammation of the eyelids associated with bacterial infection, dry eyes, or a skin condition called acne rosacea. It usually involves the eyelid margins (anterior blepharitis) but can also affect the meibomian glands in the eyelid (posterior blepharitis) and frequently is associated with conjunctivitis. It is bilateral and not painful and has no associated photophobia. The eyelids are inflamed, and scaling of the eyelid margins is seen. Loss of eyelashes occurs late. Visual acuity is unimpaired.

 EVIDENCE-BASED PRACTICE *Is Antibiotic Treatment Needed for Acute Infective Conjunctivitis?*

The purpose of this meta-analysis was to determine the benefit of antibiotic treatment for acute infective conjunctivitis in primary care and which subgroups benefit most. Three eligible trials were identified, and data were available for analysis in 622 patients. Eighty percent of patients who received antibiotics and 74% of control participants were cured at day 7. There was a significant benefit of antibiotics versus control for cure at 7 days in all cases combined. Subgroups that showed a significant benefit from antibiotics were patients with purulent discharge and patients with mild severity of red eye. The type of control used (placebo drops versus nothing) showed a statistically significant interaction ($P = .03$). The authors concluded that acute conjunctivitis seen in primary care is a self-limiting condition, with most patients getting better regardless of antibiotic therapy. Patients with purulent discharge or a mild severity of red eye may obtain a small benefit from antibiotics.

Reference: Jefferis et al, 2011.

Hordeolum

Hordeolum is caused by infection of the glands of Zeis or Moll along the lash line. It develops acutely and manifests as a palpable indurated area along the eyelid margin, with a purulent center and surrounding erythema. It spontaneously drains within 1 to 2 weeks. Patients experience swelling of the eyelid and localized eyelid pain.

Chalazion

A chalazion is a granulomatous reaction in the meibomian gland on the tarsal plate of the eyelid. This is usually a chronic condition. The lesion is usually painless and indurated. When symptoms are present, they include pruritus and redness of the involved eye and eyelid.

Conjunctiva

Bacterial conjunctivitis

S. aureus, S. pneumoniae, group A streptococci, H. influenzae, and N. gonorrhoeae most commonly cause bacterial conjunctivitis. The onset is gradual, begins unilaterally, and often becomes bilateral. The patient usually reports a scratchy sensation instead of pain. There is generally no photophobia. Examination reveals peripheral injection, purulent discharge, and matted eyelids. Visual acuity is not affected, although the presence of discharge may produce "blurring" of vision.

Viral conjunctivitis

Occurring most commonly in young adults, viral conjunctivitis is caused by such viruses as adenovirus, picornavirus, rhinovirus, and herpesvirus. The onset is gradual and unilateral early in the course and then may become bilateral. The patient reports a scratchy, rather than painful, sensation. On examination, peripheral injection with watery discharge is apparent. Visual acuity is intact. The eyelids may have follicular changes (small aggregates of lymphocytes) in the palpebral conjunctiva.

Allergic conjunctivitis

Allergic conjunctivitis is a chronic, seasonal condition caused by a hypersensitivity reaction to a specific allergen. It is bilateral, itchy, and painless. The conjunctival injection is peripheral. There is ropy, mucoid discharge. The palpebral conjunctiva has a cobblestone appearance. Visual acuity is unaffected.

Neisseria gonorrhoeae conjunctivitis

The N. gonorrhoeae organism can produce a bacterial conjunctivitis in newborns. It is bilateral, with very purulent discharge 48 to 72 hours after birth. Although rare in adults, it can occur through direct transmission via finger contact or via contact of the eyes with water in a nonchlorinated swimming pool. The infection has an abrupt onset and is characterized by copious purulent discharge that reaccumulates after being wiped away. In addition to redness and irritation, the patient has marked conjunctival injection, chemosis, eyelid swelling, and tender preauricular adenopathy. The condition warrants immediate ophthalmic referral.

Chemical conjunctivitis

Chemical conjunctivitis occurs with instillation of chemical prophylaxis in the neonate. A bilateral reaction occurs within the first 24 hours.

Subconjunctival hemorrhage

Subconjunctival hemorrhage is usually the result of a small blood vessel rupture in the conjunctival tissue and frequently develops after episodes of coughing or straining. It is painless, although often frightening to the patient. Visual acuity is not impaired.

Anterior Chamber

Hyphema

Hyphema is caused by blood in the anterior chamber of the eye, usually produced by trauma to the eye. The patient has a marked decrease in vision, with red blood cells present diffusely throughout the anterior chamber. A settled layer of blood present inferiorly or a complete filling of the anterior chamber is possible, obscuring the visual examination of the posterior chamber. The pupil is irregular and poorly reactive.

Sclera

Episcleritis

Often a benign inflammatory condition of the covering of the sclera, episcleritis is bilateral, with mild stinging. Peripheral injection is present. There is no discharge, but some lacrimation and photophobia may be present. Visual acuity is unimpaired.

Scleritis

Inflammation of the sclera can result in severe destructive disease. It is usually a unilateral inflammatory condition associated with rheumatoid arthritis, systemic immunologic disease, or other autoimmune disorders. There is pain and ciliary injection. Lacrimation is present and visual acuity is variable.

Cornea

Keratitis

Bacterial, fungal, and viral organisms can cause infection of the cornea, which leads to corneal ulceration and potential destruction of the cornea. Moderate to severe eye pain is present, there is some discharge, and visual acuity is decreased. Pupils are equal and normal, but the cornea appears cloudy. Peripheral injection is present and diffuse. A ciliary flush is also present. All corneal ulcers require immediate ophthalmology referral. A history of contact lens wear increases risk.

Corneal abrasion

Corneal abrasion may be superficial, lying on top of the anterior surface of the cornea, or it may be subtarsal and become implanted on the palpebral conjunctiva, causing the cornea to become irritated when the patient blinks. The patient usually has a history of a foreign body on the anterior surface of the eye. The abrasion causes moderate to severe pain with discharge present. Visual acuity may be normal

or decreased, photophobia is present, and pupil size and reaction are normal. Fluorescein stain is taken into the ulcer and can be seen under a Wood lamp.

Herpetic infection

Caused by the herpes simplex virus, this infection occurs unilaterally or bilaterally. The patient's presenting symptoms are pain, photophobia, and diffuse or ciliary injection. Discharge is variable, and visual acuity is markedly decreased. Dendritic lesions are seen on fluorescein staining.

Herpes zoster can cause inflammation and scarring of the cornea with conjunctivitis and iritis. In some cases the retina and optic nerve are involved. Severe or chronic outbreaks of herpes zoster may cause glaucoma, cataract formation, double vision, and scarring of the cornea. Patients with suspected ocular herpes infection (simplex or zoster) should be referred to an ophthalmologist.

Orbit

Periorbital cellulitis

The patient's presenting symptoms include unilateral eyelid swelling, redness, fever, and hotness. The conjunctiva is clear, the eye moves freely, and vision is not impaired.

Orbital cellulitis

The patient's symptoms include unilateral eyelid swelling, fever, and pain. Examination reveals proptosis, chemosis, and conjunctivitis. There is limitation of eye motion on testing of extraocular movements. The patient appears ill. This is a life-threatening condition and requires immediate intervention.

Uveal Tract

Iritis

Characterized by inflammation of the iris and ciliary body, iritis may be idiopathic and develop in response to coexistent conjunctivitis, keratitis, or eye trauma, or it may occur with chronic inflammatory or infectious processes. Eye pain is moderate and aching, visual acuity is decreased, and photophobia is present. There is minimal eye discharge, the affected pupil is smaller, and the cornea appears normal. There is central redness of the eye, with ciliary flush present.

Glaucoma

The two main types of glaucoma are open-angle glaucoma, which is a chronic condition, and angle-closure glaucoma, which may be a sudden (acute) condition or a chronic disease.

Open-angle glaucoma is the most common type; its frequency increases greatly with age. In acute closed-angle glaucoma, the patient's presenting symptoms include unilateral, deep eye pain and photophobia. There may be a report of halos around visualized objects. There is ciliary injection with tears and decreased visual acuity. The pupil is mid-dilated and has decreased reactivity to light. The cornea is cloudy. There is diffuse redness of the eye with an intraocular pressure of greater than 21 mm Hg. This condition requires emergency referral.

► DIFFERENTIAL DIAGNOSIS OF *Common Causes of Red Eye*

CONDITION	HISTORY	PHYSICAL FINDINGS	DIAGNOSTIC STUDIES
EYELIDS OR LACRIMAL SAC			
Dacryocystitis	Unilateral, acute onset; pain	Swelling and redness around lacrimal sac; tearing; may have pus through punctum	CBC, leukocytosis
Blepharitis	Bilateral, gradual onset; no pain	Lids inflamed; scaling on visual acuity okay; loss of margins, lashes (late)	None
Hordeolum/stye	Unilateral; pain	Swelling of eyelid; indurated lesion with central pus and surrounding erythema	None initially; if repeated, screen for diabetes
Chalazion	Unilateral, chronic; painless	Indurated lesion on tarsal plate of eyelid; may have pruritus and redness of involved eye and eyelid	None
CONJUNCTIVA			
Bacterial conjunctivitis	Gradual onset, unilateral early, bilateral late; scratchy (no pain); photophobia	Peripheral injection; purulent discharge; matted eyelids; visual acuity okay	None initially; if not better with treatment, obtain culture and sensitivities; Gram stain
Viral conjunctivitis	Gradual onset, unilateral early, bilateral late; scratchy (no pain)	Peripheral injection; watery discharge; visual acuity okay; follicular changes (small aggregates of lymphocytes) in palpebral conjunctiva	Same as for bacterial conjunctivitis
Allergic conjunctivitis	Chronic; seasonal; bilateral; itchy (no pain)	Peripheral injection; ropy, mucoid discharge; cobblestone-like mucosa; visual acuity okay	Fluorescein staining; hypertrophy of dorsal conjunctiva with elevated gray areas near limbus with vernal conjunctivitis

Continued

> **DIFFERENTIAL DIAGNOSIS OF** *Common Causes of Red Eye—cont'd*

CONDITION	HISTORY	PHYSICAL FINDINGS	DIAGNOSTIC STUDIES
Neisseria gonorrhoeae conjunctivitis	Bilateral; newborn	Purulent discharge 48–72 hr after birth	Culture on Thayer-Martin plate; Gram stain
Chemical conjunctivitis	Bilateral	Neonate: within first 24 hr	None
Subconjunctival hemorrhage	Unilateral; painless; coughing or straining	Splash of blood in conjunctiva or sclera; visual acuity okay	None
ANTERIOR CHAMBER			
Hyphema	Unilateral; trauma to eye	Red blood cells in anterior chamber; visual acuity decreased; pupil irregular and poorly reactive	Refer to ophthalmologist
SCLERA			
Episcleritis	Bilateral; mild stinging	Peripheral injection; no discharge; visual acuity okay	None
Scleritis	Unilateral; deep, boring pain	Ciliary injection, teary; visual acuity variable; photophobia	Associated with systemic immunologic disease
Keratitis	Unilateral or bilateral; moderate to severe pain; photophobia; contact lens wear	Discharge; ciliary flush; cornea cloudy; visual acuity decreased	Refer to ophthalmologist
Corneal abrasion or foreign body	Unilateral; pain; photophobia	Diffuse injection; tears; visual acuity variable	Fluorescein stain positive
Herpetic keratitis	Unilateral or bilateral; pain; photophobia	Ciliary flush; discharge; visual acuity markedly decreased	Fluorescein stain shows dendritic lesions
ORBIT			
Periorbital cellulitis	Unilateral	Swelling of eyelid; fever, redness; conjunctiva clear; eye moves freely; vision not impaired	CBC, leukocytosis, blood cultures
Orbital cellulitis	Unilateral; pain	Proptosis; eyelid swelling; chemosis; conjunctivitis; limitation of eye motion	CBC, blood cultures; CT scan; life threatening
UVEAL TRACT			
Iritis	Unilateral; moderate aching pain; photophobia	Tearing; affected pupil smaller; cornea normal; ciliary flush	Refer
GLAUCOMA			
Acute closed-angle glaucoma	Unilateral; deep pain; photophobia; halos	Ciliary injection; tears; visual acuity decreased	Tonometry; emergency referral

CBC, complete blood count; *CT,* computed tomography.

31 Sleep Problems

Each year more than 10 million Americans seek medical help for sleep problems. Patients report insufficient or nonrestorative sleep, despite adequate opportunity, that results in some form of daytime impairment. Insomnia is prevalent in 30% to 40% of the adult population, with 10% to 15% reporting that it is chronic, severe, or both. More than 40% of parents report sleep problems in their children, and 20% of these are considered significant. The consequences of chronic sleep problems include difficulty with concentration, fatigue, lack of energy, and irritability. Sleep disturbances in an older adult can result in increased falls and accidents. In children, sleep disturbances can produce learning and behavior problems, alter physical development, and affect family functioning.

Sleep has two separate stages: rapid eye movement (REM) sleep, which is linked to dreaming, and non-REM (NREM) sleep, which is a deeper sleep state. NREM is further divided into four sleep stages. In each stage the sleep is progressively deeper. An individual generally moves through NREM sleep from stage 1 to stage 4. Stages 3 and 4 are the deepest stages. At the end of stage 4, a person goes backward in stages toward the progressively lighter sleep of stage 1. The first REM sleep stage then follows. Movement from stage 1 to the end of REM is termed a sleep cycle. This cycle usually lasts 90 minutes in adults and approximately 50 minutes in infants. In one night, five cycles are usually completed. As an adult goes through the sleep cycles, the REM period increases in length from 10 minutes to occupying most of the 90-minute cycle. Also, the proportion of stage 2 increases, with stages 3 and 4 decreasing in length. The total amount and composition of sleep change throughout life. Sleep quality is often judged by the amount of time spent in stage 4 sleep. People who do not have adequate REM sleep feel they have had too little sleep.

Newborns fall directly into REM sleep. This REM sleep in infancy is thought to provide the brain stimulation necessary for maturation. At age 5, REM sleep in children decreases to that of the adult, which is approximately 20% of total sleep. The REM portion of sleep is constant through all age ranges; however, stages 3 and 4 of NREM sleep begin to decline in adolescents, and older adults, stages 3 and 4 disappear. An older adult may experience more frequent awakenings during the night; some need to compensate for this with rest periods during the day. Some older patients view their pattern of diminished sleep with frustration, but others accept it as an opportunity to have more time for other activities.

Sleep is regulated by two primary processes: the body's circadian rhythm, which causes an increase in sleepiness twice during a 24-hour period (usually between midnight and 7 AM and for a brief period in the midafternoon), and the physiologic need for sleep, which is increased by sleep loss and sleep disruption.

DIAGNOSTIC REASONING: FOCUSED HISTORY

Define the nature of the problem.

Key Questions
- How would you describe your (or the child's) sleep problem?
- Are you having difficulty falling asleep?
- Are you having difficulty staying asleep?
- Are you having difficulty staying awake during the day?
- Have you taken medications for sleep? If so, what are they?
- How long has the problem existed?

Nature of the Problem

Sleep disorders include sleeplessness (insomnia), episodic disturbance of behavior associated with sleep (parasomnias), and excessive sleepiness (hypersomnia). The most common childhood sleep disorders are night awakening, inability to fall asleep, problems going to bed, circadian rhythm problems, and parasomnias. Often it is the caregiver, not the child, who perceives the sleep disturbances to be a problem. The BEARS instrument (Table 31.1) provides a comprehensive screening tool to identify sleep disorders in children.

Table 31.1	**BEARS Sleep Screening**		
	The "BEARS" instrument is divided into five major sleep domains, providing a comprehensive screen for the major sleep disorders affecting children in the 2- to 18-yr-old range. Each sleep domain has a set of age-appropriate "trigger questions" for use in the clinical interview.		
	EXAMPLES OF DEVELOPMENTALLY APPROPRIATE TRIGGER QUESTIONS		
	TODDLER OR PRESCHOOLER (2–5 YR)	**SCHOOL AGE (6–12 YR)**	**ADOLESCENT (13–18 YR)**
1. **B**edtime problems	Does your child have any problems going to bed? Falling asleep?	Does your child have any problems at bedtime? (P) Do you have any problems going to bed? (C)	Do you have any problems falling asleep at bedtime? (C)
2. **E**xcessive daytime sleepiness	Does your child seem overtired or sleepy a lot during the day? Does he or she still take naps?	Does your child have difficulty waking in the morning, seem sleepy during the day, or take naps? (P) Do you feel tired a lot? (C)	Do you feel sleepy a lot during the day? In school? While driving? (C)
3. **A**wakenings during the night	Does your child wake up a lot at night?	Does your child seem to wake up a lot at night? Any sleepwalking or nightmares? (P) Do you wake up a lot at night? Do you have trouble getting back to sleep? (C)	Do you wake up a lot at night? Have trouble getting back to sleep? (C)
4. **R**egularity and duration of sleep	Does your child have a regular bedtime and wake time? What are they?	What time does your child go to bed and get up on school days? Weekends? Do you think he or she is getting enough sleep? (P)	What time do you usually go to bed on school nights? What time do you awake in the morning? Weekends? How much sleep do you usually get? (C)
5. **S**noring	Does your child snore a lot or have difficult breathing at night?	Does your child have loud or nightly snoring or any breathing difficulties at night? (P)	Does your teenager snore loudly or nightly? (P)

From Mindell JA, Owens JA: *A clinical guide to pediatric sleep: diagnosis and management of sleep problems*, Philadelphia, 2003, Lippincott Williams & Wilkins.
C, Child-directed question; *P*, parent-directed question.

Difficulty Falling Asleep

Difficulty in falling asleep is often related to poor sleep hygiene practices, use of medications or stimulants, or disruption in circadian rhythms. Difficulty falling asleep also can occur as a result of pain, nocturia, or as a symptom of anxiety.

Difficulty Staying Asleep

Difficulty staying asleep occurs when the sleep cycle is disrupted; this may be related to physiological factors, illness, depression, pain, or use of medications or alcohol.

Daytime Sleepiness

Nighttime insomnia and daytime sleepiness are not isolated symptoms. Daytime sleepiness may be related to an increased need for sleep because of nighttime sleep loss, or it may represent narcolepsy. Daytime sleepiness could also be medication induced or due to psychological causes.

Medications

Over-the-counter (OTC) and prescription medications used to promote sleep can have side effects, such as daytime sleepiness and headaches. Long-term use of sleep medications often produces tolerance and a need for an increased dosage. Some agents, particularly the benzodiazepines, are habituating with long-term use; stopping them may cause withdrawal symptoms.

Duration of the Problem

Sleep disorders can be transient (lasting a few days), short term (lasting weeks), or chronic (lasting months to years). An acute problem, lasting a few days to a few weeks, can be caused by stress, acute illness, environmental disturbance, or jet lag. A chronic problem may be due to a specific sleep disorder, a mood disorder, or the use of medications or stimulants. Primary insomnia is diagnosed when no underlying cause can be identified.

Is this a specific sleep disorder?

Key Questions
- Do you have a creeping, crawling, or uncomfortable feeling in the legs that is relieved by moving your legs?
- Does your bed partner report that your arms or legs jerk during sleep?
- Do you (or the child) snore loudly, gasp, choke, or stop breathing during sleep?
- Do you (or the child) have difficulty staying awake during the day or do you fall asleep during routine tasks (for adults, especially driving)?
- Do you have episodes of muscle weakness?

Limb Sensation

Restless legs syndrome includes the sensation of crawling, pulling, and tingling with an irresistible urge to move the legs. Symptoms increase in the evening, especially when the person is lying down and remaining still. Patients often have coexisting periodic limb movements in sleep.

Limb Jerking

Periodic leg movements during sleep are common in people older than 65 years. Bilateral, repeated, rhythmic jerking or twitching movements, primarily in the legs, characterize periodic limb movement disorder. Less frequently, movement occurs in the arms. Full-body movements are an early sign of Lewy body dementia.

Snoring

Obstructive sleep apnea (OSA) is characterized by loud snoring, mouth breathing, and restless sleep patterns. The patient may report insomnia but more commonly notes excessive daytime sleepiness.

Parental smoking can be a risk factor for snoring in children. Passive smoke inhalation can provoke mucosal edema and inflammation, resulting in a narrowing of the pharynx and causing snoring. In addition, allergic respiratory diseases may cause snoring.

Daytime Dozing, Excessive Daytime Sleepiness, and Muscle Weakness

Excessive daytime sleepiness may be caused by narcolepsy. Adults with narcolepsy report falling asleep while driving or performing routine tasks. Initially, children with narcolepsy have great difficulty getting up in the mornings. When awakened, the child may appear to be confused or may be aggressive or verbally abusive. The child may fall asleep at school, in the vehicle on the way home from school, or while watching television. Cataplexy is common in adults with narcolepsy. This disorder is identified as episodes of sudden muscular weakness and atonia generally instigated by an emotional trigger. The patient will have to lean against a wall for support because his or her legs feel rubbery.

The degree of daytime sleepiness can be quantified using the Epworth Sleepiness Scale (Box 31.1).

Could the sleep problem be secondary to a health condition?

Key Questions

- Have you been ill recently?
- Do you have a chronic health condition?
- What medications (prescription and OTC) do you take?
- Do you have depression or anxiety?

Illness: Acute or Chronic

Acute illness can be a cause of sleep disturbance. Nocturnal pruritus, associated with chronic eczema, may also cause awakening.

In children, otitis media and chronic serous otitis, even without acute infection, can disturb sleep. Some believe that middle ear pressure rises when the child is supine at night and report sleep improvement with treatment of otitis. In children, enlarged adenoids and upper airway obstruction may cause awakening. Children with asthma have a greater incidence of night awakening.

Gastroesophageal reflux disease (GERD) may cause night awakening but produces few symptoms during the day. GERD, chronic obstructive pulmonary disease, peptic ulcer disease, and congestive heart failure are associated with paroxysmal nocturnal dyspnea,

---

Box 31.1   The Epworth Sleepiness Scale

The Epworth Sleepiness Scale may be used to evaluate daytime sleepiness. The scale is a simple questionnaire that measures the general level of daytime sleepiness by gauging the probability of falling asleep in a variety of situations. On a scale of 0 to 3, the patient rates the likelihood that he or she would doze in each of eight different situations as part of his or her "usual way of life in recent times."

The patient's responses are added together, and the total score can range from 0 to 24. The normal range is from 2 to 10, with a modal score of 6. Scores increase linearly in patients with obstructive sleep apnea syndrome according to the severity of the apnea. Any score higher than 10 is considered significant.

The Epworth Sleepiness Scale has high test-retest reliability in normal subjects ($r = 0.82$, $p < .001$). It is a unitary scale with high internal consistency (Cronbach coefficient alpha = 0.88). It is simple, easy to understand, and a very inexpensive measurement of daytime sleepiness.

On a scale of 0 to 3, indicate the likelihood that you would fall asleep in the following situations, taking into account your usual way of life in recent times. Using the scale below, choose the most appropriate number for each situation:

0 = Would never doze
1 = Slight likelihood of dozing
2 = Moderate likelihood of dozing
3 = High likelihood of dozing

SITUATION: LIKELIHOOD OF DOZING

Reading while seated	_____
Watching TV	_____
Sitting, inactive, in a public place such as a theater or meeting	_____
As a passenger in a car for an hour without a break	_____
Lying down to rest in the afternoon when circumstances permit	_____
Sitting and talking to someone	_____
Sitting quietly after a lunch during which you did not drink alcohol	_____
In a car, while stopped for a few minutes in traffic	_____
Total:	_____

Modified from Johns MW: Daytime sleepiness, snoring and obstructive sleep apnea. The Epworth Sleepiness Scale, *Chest* 103:30, 1993. Permission conveyed through Copyright Clearance Center, Inc.

which frequently disturbs sleep and is often interpreted by the patient as insomnia. Prostatic hypertrophy may cause nocturia and thus disturb sleep.

Medications

Many medications can have stimulating effects and cause sleep disruption. Common offenders include antidepressants, decongestants, bronchodilators, β-blockers, thyroid preparations, phenytoin, methyldopa, and corticosteroids. The potential sedating effects of medications should also be considered in patients who report excessive daytime sleepiness. Medications such as antihistamines often cause sleep disturbances. In older adults, paradoxical reactions to antihistamines are common and may contribute to sleep disruption.

Pain

Pain may interfere with sleep onset or contribute to early awakenings. Patients with chronic pain may have mood and cognitive disturbances that contribute to insomnia and early morning awakening.

Psychological Causes

Psychological conditions causing insomnia include depression, anxiety disorder, panic disorder, mania, and acute psychosis. People with depression tend to have early morning awakening, whereas those with anxiety disorder have trouble falling asleep (see Chapter 4).

Could this be related to sleep hygiene?

Key Questions
- What is your bedtime routine?
- What else do you do in your bedroom?
- Do you consume alcohol, nicotine, or caffeine before bedtime?
- Do you exercise before bedtime?
- How do you put your child to sleep?
- Where does your child sleep?

Bedtime Routine

Sleep hygiene is related to health practices and environmental influences on sleep. It is important to consistently go to bed at the same time and wake up at the same time.

Environment

Using the bedroom for other activities, such as work or watching television, can produce an environment that disrupts sleep. Lights and a television produce awakening cues. Routinely using the bedroom for other activities may also condition the patient to an arousal state while in the bedroom. Noise may affect sleep by leading to increasing amounts of wakefulness, increase in light sleep, and decrease in REM sleep, causing daytime sleepiness. Room temperatures above or below normal may disrupt the ability to stay asleep.

Consumption of Stimulants

Caffeine, diet pills (with ephedrine), and nicotine are stimulants that can cause sleep disruption. Although the consumption of alcohol before bedtime promotes sleep onset, alcohol tends to shorten total sleep time and exacerbate other conditions, such as GERD and sleep apnea. Alcohol withdrawal in a heavy drinker may be associated with restlessness and sleep disturbance that can continue for a prolonged period after alcohol cessation.

Exercise

Vigorous exercise is a stimulant; it should be avoided for 1 to 2 hours before bedtime.

Child's Routine

A child who is put to bed while still awake and learns to fall asleep using self-comforting measures is often able return to sleep when he or she rouses in the middle of the night, as do most children and adults. Toddlers are fearful of separation, and routines need to be established before bedtime. A routine gives the toddler a sense of predictability and security; having a nightly routine is helpful.

Infant Sleeping Environment

The sleep environment should be quiet and dark, and the room temperature should be comfortable. Infants in waterbeds, on very soft bedding, on couches with pillows, or in any situation in which their heads may slip between the mattress and a wall or bedpost are at risk of suffocation. In many cultures, infants sleep with their parents; however, some infants who sleep with parents have sleep problems. As parents arise or move from the bed, the infant awakens because of the lighter sleep state.

Key Questions
• Are you a shift worker?
• Do you sleep in the same bed each night?
• Do you travel frequently?
• Are you a caregiver?

Shift Work

Shift work, particularly periodic shift work, can cause sleep disruption. It may interrupt the usual circadian rhythm or alter usual sleeping patterns and habits.

Sleep Environment

Sleeping in unfamiliar surroundings affects the quality of sleep and increases sleep latency. It is associated with more wakefulness, an increased amount of light sleep, and a shorter REM sleep stage.

Travel

Jet lag is a common cause of sleep disruption. It may interrupt the usual circadian rhythm or alter usual sleeping patterns and habits. Even 1 to 2 hours of time zone change can disrupt the usual sleep–wake pattern.

Caregiver

Sleep wake patterns can be disturbed if the caregiver needs to get up during the night to attend to the child or adult being cared for.

Could this be related to age?

Key Questions
• How old is the patient (e.g., child, adolescent, older adult)?
• At what age did the problem begin?
• Does the child have problems going to bed?
• Does the child refuse to go to sleep?
• Does the child wake up screaming at night?

Age: Child

Newborns wake every 20 minutes to 4 hours during a 24-hour period, reflecting their sleep–wake cycle. This cycle changes between 3 and 6 months with the establishment of a diurnal sleep–wake rhythm. During this time, an initial "settling" period that typically takes 10 to 20 minutes begins to occur. Daytime sleep decreases over the next 3 years and consolidates at night. At age 4 years, most children no longer nap. School-age children sleep approximately 8 hours a night.

Problems going to sleep and sleep refusal

Toddlers have a strong attachment to their caregiver, and separation from this person at bedtime causes distress and sleep problems. Older toddlers who are in the preoperational stage are developing a sense of autonomy and use going to bed as an issue of control or a general pattern of oppositional behavior. Examination of the child's naptime is important. In school-age children and adolescents, problems going to sleep may be caused by anxiety,

---

▌EVIDENCE-BASED PRACTICE *Is Bed Sharing with Infants Safe?*

Eleven case-control studies were included in this meta-analysis. Data from a total of 2464 cases and 6495 control participants were included, with bed sharing in 710 cases (28.8%) and 863 control participants (13.3%). All studies found an increased risk for sudden infant death syndrome (SIDS) with bed sharing. The summary odds ratio (OR) for bed sharing was 2.89. Four studies reported the risk of SIDS and bed sharing with smoking mothers. In this subgroup analysis, the risk of SIDS with maternal smoking and bed sharing was almost six times that of the risk with nonsmoking mothers. In addition, in three studies reporting the infant's age, the risk was 10 times higher in infants younger than 12 weeks old; the risk for infants older than 12 weeks old was not elevated. The authors concluded that bed sharing strongly increases the risk of SIDS. This risk is greatest when parents smoke and when infants are younger than 12 weeks of age.

Reference: Vennemann et al, 2012.

negative conditioning, delayed sleep phase (often caused by caffeine), or a bedtime that is too early. Vigorous activity before bedtime may delay sleep onset.

Waking up screaming at night

Night terrors are nocturnal episodes in which the child sits straight up in bed, screams, and is inconsolable. Most episodes last 1-2 minutes but it can take up to 30 minutes to settle a child back to sleep. This occurs within the first few hours of sleep. The child is not readily awakened, although he or she may seem to be awake, and has no recollection of the event the next day.

Nightmares are bad dreams that awaken the dreamer. They occur later at night than night terrors. Unlike night terrors, the dream is remembered and the child is awake and may be consoled by the caregiver.

Age: Adolescent

The diurnal circadian rhythm of infancy and childhood changes during adolescence, causing a change toward later sleep and wake times. Adolescents therefore require an increased amount of sleep; about 9.5 hours per night. Many adolescents do not get this amount, leaving them with a concomitant sleep debt. To recover from the debt, the adolescent usually sleeps later on weekends. In a policy statement, the American Academy of Pediatrics (AAP) recommends that middle and high schoolers start school no earlier than 8:30 AM.

Age: Menopause

Menopause-related changes may contribute to or cause sleep disturbance. Hot flashes promote arousal from sleep. Menopause is associated with reduced total sleep time, prolonged time to initiate sleep, and reduced REM sleep.

Age: Older Adult

Total sleep time generally remains the same or is slightly decreased (6.5–7 hours/night). However, older adults may take longer to initiate sleep, spend more time in the lighter stages of sleep, and experience increased fragmentation of the entire sleep cycle. Older adults have more nighttime arousals and

awakenings and may feel sleep deprived even if the total sleep time remains the same.

If the onset of sleep is not correspondingly earlier, excessive daytime sleepiness may result. Daytime napping may compound the problem by reducing the drive for sleep at the usual bedtime hour.

Could this be conditioned insomnia?

Key Questions

- Are you able to fall asleep easily in places other than the bedroom?
- If a child: What does the child do when he or she awakens at night?
- If a child: What actions do you take to get the child back to sleep?

Sleep Location

Most cases of insomnia develop initially in response to a psychosocial stressor. As sleeplessness persists, the patient begins to associate the bed with wakefulness and heightened arousal rather than sleep. The patient may fall asleep easily outside the bedroom (e.g., while watching television or reading in another room) but feels wide awake in bed.

Child's Need for Comfort or Food

Infants who are soothed and cuddled and placed in bed when they are asleep do not learn how to settle themselves; when these infants are aroused at night, they require the same routine to fall back asleep. Children who do not have self-comforting behaviors will be unable to fall asleep on their own. They awaken, cry, and want to be held or rocked before they can go back to sleep. An infant older than 6 months who continues to wake during the night is considered a trained night crier.

Children who need to be fed after they are awakened at night are trained night feeders. The child does not need the additional nutrition but becomes conditioned to a feeding to go back to sleep. Caregivers often bottle feed or breastfeed the child until the child falls back to sleep. The intake of nighttime feeding after 7 or 8 months of age may prevent the development of a more mature circadian rhythm. This rhythm is a digestive-endocrine-sleep–wake cycle that adjusts to a day–night cycle, resulting in a consolidation of sleep.

Could this be somnambulism?

Key Questions
- Do you (or does the child) sleepwalk?

Sleepwalking usually occurs only once a night and lasts about 15 minutes. The person gets out of bed and moves about slowly and in an automatic manner with a blank facial expression. The person may mumble. After a great deal of effort, the person can be awakened and will have little or no memory of the episode.

DIAGNOSTIC REASONING: FOCUSED PHYSICAL EXAMINATION

Obtain Growth Parameters and Body Mass Index

Children with OSA may present with failure to thrive. In adults, obese middle-age men are most often affected by sleep apnea.

Inspect the Ears

Otitis media and serous otitis may cause wakefulness in infants and children, especially when they are in the supine position, because of the pressure of fluid accumulation in the middle ear.

Inspect the Nose

Obstruction of the nose by secretions may cause sleep apnea in infants younger than 6 weeks. In children older than 6 weeks or in adults, nasal obstruction may cause OSA.

Inspect the Mouth, Throat, and Nose

Look for a narrow pharyngeal space, a long or edematous uvula, and enlarged tonsils and adenoids. Enlarged tonsils may cause obstruction while the person is sleeping. In adults, increased neck circumference (>17 inches in men, >16 inches in women), lateral peritonsillar narrowing, macroglossia, tonsillar hypertrophy, elongated or enlarged uvula, high arched or narrow hard palate, or nasal abnormalities (polyps, deviation, turbinate hypertrophy) may be found with OSA.

Auscultate the Lungs and Heart

Nighttime wheezing in patients with asthma often causes sleep disturbances. Congestive heart failure is a risk factor for sleep apnea.

Palpate the Abdomen

Gastroesophageal reflux disease may elicit upper abdominal pain on palpation.

LABORATORY AND DIAGNOSTIC STUDIES

Sleep Diary

A sleep diary should be kept for 1 to 2 weeks. Have the patient record bedtime, total sleep time, time until sleep onset, number of awakenings, use of sleep medications, time out of bed in the morning, rating of quality of sleep, daytime symptoms, daytime naps, number and time of alcoholic drinks, and life stresses.

Sleep Studies

Objective assessment of sleep uses polysomnography (PSG) to assess sleep apnea, specific sleep stage abnormalities, nocturnal myoclonus, and unusual nocturnal behaviors. It is not recommended for routine evaluation of chronic insomnia. PSG includes an electroencephalogram (EEG), electrooculogram, electromyelogram, electrocardiogram (ECG), measures of oxygen saturation, carbon dioxide values, nasal and oral airflow, thoracic and abdominal respiratory movements, and leg muscle activity. The PSG is taken during sleep, usually for the entire night. A multiple sleep latency test is a series of four or five nap opportunities, each separated by a 2-hour interval. The 15- to 20-minute naps are used to assess sleep disorders such as OSA and narcolepsy.

Home Sleep Studies

Home medical devices to assess for OSA are available. A home testing device should be validated against an in-laboratory PSG to ensure that it functions at an adequate level.

Actigraphy

Actigraphy is a technique to record activity during waking and sleeping without application of any electrodes. An actigraph is worn on the wrist and is about the size of a watch.

It records movement and nonmovement data plotted against time for 1 or 2 weeks. The patient wears the device continuously during sleep and daily routine activities. Actigraphy is suitable for extended examination of the sleep–wake cycle.

Ferritin Level

Serum iron stores (measured by serum ferritin) have been shown to correlate inversely with restless legs syndrome. Iron is a cofactor in tyrosine hydroxylase, the rate-limiting enzymatic step in the conversion of tyrosine to dopamine.

DIFFERENTIAL DIAGNOSIS

Restless Legs Syndrome

Restless legs syndrome includes the sensation of crawling, pulling, and tingling with an irresistible urge to move the legs. Symptoms increase in the evening, especially when the person is lying down and remaining still. The symptoms occur before sleep, causing a delay in sleep onset. Patients often have coexisting periodic limb movements in sleep. Restless legs syndrome may also be associated with iron deficiency, Parkinson disease, kidney failure, diabetes, peripheral neuropathy, and pregnancy.

Periodic Leg Movement

Periodic leg movements during sleep are common in adults older than 65 years. Bilateral repeated, rhythmic jerking or twitching movements, primarily in the legs, characterize periodic limb movement disorder. Less frequent movement can occur in the arms. The movements occur every 20 to 90 seconds and can cause brief arousal that disrupts sleep and decreases the amount of time in the deep stages of sleep. The patient may not report waking up but reports that sleep was not refreshing. The condition commonly coexists with restless legs syndrome.

Obstructive Sleep Apnea

Clinically, OSA is defined by the occurrence of daytime sleepiness, loud snoring, witnessed breathing interruptions, or awakenings caused by gasping or choking, in the presence of at least five obstructive respiratory events (apneas, hypopneas, or respiratory effort-related arousals) per hour of sleep. OSA hypopnea syndrome is characterized by daytime somnolence, snoring, difficult-to-control hypertension, refractory arrhythmias, angina, and heart failure.

During sleep, the normal tone of the airway muscles is relaxation, especially during REM sleep cycles. However, the diaphragm during this time is active. The activity of the diaphragm unchecked by the airway muscles leads to collapse of the upper airway. Associated with this is any anatomic barrier, such as enlarged adenoids, with resulting obstruction. The signs, symptoms, and consequences of OSA occur as a result of repetitive collapse of the upper airway, sleep fragmentation, hypoxemia, hypercapnia, marked swings in intrathoracic pressure, and increased sympathetic activity.

Risk factors for sleep apnea include obesity, congestive heart failure, atrial fibrillation, treatment of refractory hypertension, type 2 diabetes, stroke, nocturnal dysrhythmias, and pulmonary hypertension. Physical findings that may suggest the presence of OSA include increased neck circumference (>17 inches in men, >16 inches in women), body mass index greater than 30 kg/m^2, lateral peritonsillar narrowing, macroglossia, tonsillar hypertrophy, elongated/enlarged uvula, high arched or narrow hard palate, and nasal abnormalities (polyps, deviation, turbinate hypertrophy).

In children, OSA is generally the result of enlarged tonsils and adenoids after age 6 weeks. Children ages 4 to 6 years are most prone to this condition. Most children presenting with OSA have failure to thrive and may also exhibit nocturnal enuresis, hyperactivity, learning problems, and morning headaches.

The patient may report insomnia but more commonly notes excessive daytime sleepiness. Hundreds of apneic episodes occur during the night. The frequent interruptions coupled with repeated drops in blood oxygen saturation may cause a marked decline in daytime alertness and performance. The patient should be evaluated in a sleep laboratory (see the Evidence-Based Practice box).

Narcolepsy

Narcolepsy is a disorder of excessive daytime sleepiness. It is characterized by sudden, irresistible attacks of daytime sleepiness that last 10 to 30 minutes. Most adults with narcolepsy also experience cataplexy, a sudden loss of muscle tone in response to sudden emotional stimuli. Although the episodes are typically brief, the person is at risk for falls or other accidents because he or she cannot move or speak. Cataplexy is not commonly seen in children. People with narcolepsy usually experience sleep paralysis once or twice a week at the time of sleep onset. There is a period of mental alertness, but the person is paralyzed except for respiratory and eye musculature. Hypnagogic (brief, vivid, dreamlike) hallucinations typically occur at sleep onset. Involuntary daytime sleep attacks may begin in adolescence or young adulthood, and people may have symptoms for years before the disorder is diagnosed. Not all people with narcolepsy experience all symptoms. Narcolepsy is uncommon in children.

Delayed Sleep Phase Syndrome

This is an extreme shift in sleep–wake schedule seen in adolescents. The adolescent goes to bed but does not fall asleep for many hours and is then awakened for school, having had only a few hours of sleep. On the weekend, the adolescent, when allowed to sleep, will sleep at least 8 hours.

Secondary to a Health Condition or Medications (Comorbid Insomnia)

Gastroesophageal reflux disease, chronic obstructive pulmonary disease, peptic ulcer disease, and congestive heart failure are associated with paroxysmal nocturnal dyspnea. Sleep disturbance is often interpreted by the patient as insomnia. Prostatic hypertrophy may cause nocturia and thus disturb sleep.

Many medications can have stimulating effects and cause sleep disruption. Common offenders include antidepressants (activating selective serotonin reuptake inhibitors), decongestants, bronchodilators, β-blockers, thyroid preparations, phenytoin, methyldopa, and corticosteroids.

Pain may interfere with sleep onset or contribute to early awakenings. Patients with chronic pain may have mood and cognitive disturbances that contribute to insomnia and early morning awakening.

Psychological conditions that cause insomnia include depression, anxiety disorder, panic disorder, mania, and acute psychosis.

Poor Sleep Hygiene

Sleep hygiene is related to health practices and environmental influences on sleep. Bedtime routines, environmental distractors, and stimulants affect the ability to fall asleep. Lights and televisions produce awakening cues. Routinely using the bedroom for other activities may also condition the patient to an arousal state while in the bedroom. Noise may reduce the amount of REM sleep and lead to daytime sleepiness.

Caffeine, diet pills, and nicotine are stimulants that can cause sleep disruption. Alcohol consumed before bedtime tends to shorten total sleep time and exacerbate other conditions, such as GERD and sleep apnea.

A child who is put to bed still awake and learns to fall asleep using self-comforting measures is often able to return to sleep when he or she rouses in the middle of the night, as do most children and adults. Toddlers are fearful of separation, and bedtime routines need to be established.

> ## EVIDENCE-BASED PRACTICE *Diagnosing Obstructive Sleep Apnea*
>
> In this review of the evidence the authors concluded that questionnaires, physical examination, and clinical prediction rules estimate the pretest probability of obstructive sleep apnea (OSA) hypopnea syndrome, but they are not specific enough to make the diagnosis. The Epworth Sleepiness Scale is a reliable measure of daytime sleepiness. Physical examination offers clues: decreased visibility of the posterior pharynx when the patient opens the mouth and sticks out the tongue, truncal obesity, and a waist-to-hip ratio greater than 1 in men and greater than 0.85 in women make the occurrence of OSA more likely, but they are not sufficient to make a diagnosis. The bottom line is that in patients with suspected OSA, additional evaluation is required for diagnosis.
>
> Reference: Jacobs and Coffey, 2009.

Infants who sleep with their parents may have sleep problems. As parents arise or move from the bed, the infant awakens because of the lighter sleep state.

The AAP recommends that all infants sleep on their backs for the first 6 months of life to decrease the risk of sudden infant death syndrome. The sleep environment should be quiet and dark and the room temperature should be comfortable.

Lifestyle

Shift work, particularly periodic shift work, has been reported to cause sleep disruption. It may interrupt the usual circadian rhythm or alter usual sleeping patterns and habits.

Sleeping in unfamiliar surroundings affects the quality of sleep and increases sleep latency. It is associated with more wakefulness, an increased amount of light sleep, and a shorter REM sleep stage.

Jet lag is a common cause of sleep disruption. It may interrupt the usual circadian rhythm or alter usual sleeping patterns and habits. Even 1 to 2 hours of time zone change can disrupt the usual sleep–wake pattern.

Age-Related Sleep Disorders

Night awakening

Newborns wake every 20 minutes to 4 hours during a 24-hour period, reflecting their sleep–wake cycle. This cycle changes between 3 and 6 months of age when a diurnal sleep–wake rhythm is established. During this time, an initial "settling" period, which typically takes 10 to 20 minutes, begins to occur. The infant drifts from stage 1 NREM sleep to stage 3 or 4. The infant may return to stage 1 and cycle again. After one or two cycles of NREM sleep, the infant enters REM sleep at about 60 to 90 minutes. The initial one third of the night is mostly deep sleep (NREM stages 3 and 4). The last half of the night is predominantly stage 2 NREM and REM. Daytime sleep decreases over the next 3 years and consolidates at night. At age 4, most children no longer nap. School-age children sleep approximately 8 hours a night. Stage 4 sleep decreases to 75 to 80 minutes. This decline is associated with an increase in stage 2 sleep. The onset of REM sleep decreases

from about 140 minutes in the 6- to 7-year-old to 124 minutes in the 10- to 11-year-old child.

Sleep refusal

Toddlers are emerging from a sensory-motor period to a preoperational period. They have a strong attachment to their caregiver, and separation from this person at bedtime causes distress and sleep problems. Furthermore, older toddlers who are in the preoperational stage are developing a sense of autonomy and use going to bed as an issue of control or a general pattern of oppositional behavior. Examination of the child's naptime is important. In school-age children and adolescents, anxiety, negative conditioning, delayed sleep phase (often caused by caffeine), or a bedtime that is too early may be the cause. Also, vigorous activity before bedtime may delay sleep onset.

Night terrors

Night terrors are nocturnal episodes in which the child sits straight up in bed, screams, and is inconsolable for up to 30 minutes before relaxing and falling back to sleep. It occurs within the first few hours of sleep. Children at around the age of 3 years have NREM occurring more in the first part of the night; this may account for the night terror. The child is not readily awakened, although he or she seems to be awake and has no recollection of the event the next day. Night terrors occur between the ages of 3 and 10 years.

Nightmares

Nightmares are bad dreams that awaken the dreamer. They occur later at night than night terrors and occur during REM sleep, which in children is near the end of the sleep cycle. Unlike night terrors, the dream is remembered and the child is awake and may be consoled by the caregiver. Nightmares occur at any age.

Adolescent patterns

Adolescents have an increase in slow-wave sleep with an increase in the amount of sleep required. However, most adolescents are in a sleep debt because they tend to leave less time for sleep. Repeated changes in the sleep cycle (short sleep periods followed by occasional long sleep periods) may disrupt the circadian rhythm, causing a delayed sleep phase syndrome.

Menopausal patients

Menopause-related changes may contribute to or cause sleep disturbance. Evidence that sleep difficulties are related to the hormonal changes of menopause is mixed. Hot flashes and night sweats promote arousal from sleep.

Older adult patterns

Sleep in older adults is characterized by more nighttime awakenings and reduced or nonexistent deep states of NREM sleep. However, REM sleep tends to be preserved. That older adults sleep less than younger adults may reflect their ability to sleep, not their need to sleep. Although a mild deterioration in sleep quality may be normal in the aging process, significantly disrupted nighttime sleep or excessive daytime sleepiness is not considered part of normal aging. Older adults have a circadian rhythm disruption and tend to awaken earlier in the morning. If the onset of sleep is not correspondingly earlier, excessive daytime sleepiness may result. Daytime napping may reduce the drive for sleep at the usual bedtime hour. In the night owl pattern, bedtime is delayed until the early morning hours, and the condition may progress to day–night reversal, in which sleep does not begin until dawn and continues until midday.

Conditioned Insomnia

Trained night crier

Children who do not have self-comforting behaviors will be unable to fall asleep on their own. They awaken, cry, and want to be held or rocked before they can go back to sleep. An infant older than 6 months who continues to wake during the night is considered a trained night crier.

Trained night feeder

A child who needs to be fed when awakened at night is considered a trained night feeder. The child does not need the additional nutrition but becomes conditioned to requiring a feeding to go to sleep. Caregivers often bottle feed or breastfeed the child until the child falls back to sleep. Nighttime feeding in an infant older than 7 or 8 months may prevent development of a more mature circadian rhythm. This rhythm is a digestive-endocrine sleep–wake cycle that adjusts to a day–night cycle, resulting in consolidation of sleep. Continued nocturnal feeding keeps the infant in a recurrent interruption pattern of frequent night awakening and prevents consolidation of sleep.

Somnambulism

Sleepwalking occurs during NREM stages 3 and 4, which occur in the initial third of the night. Sleepwalking usually occurs only once a night and lasts about 15 minutes. The person gets out of bed and moves about slowly and in an automatic manner with a blank look on the face. Sometimes the person is mumbling; after a great deal of effort, he or she can be awakened but will have little to no memory of the episode. Providing a safe environment is important because there is a genuine risk of injury during the sleepwalking episode. Sleepwalking in an older adult may be a sign of dementia.

▶ **DIFFERENTIAL DIAGNOSIS OF** *Common Causes of Sleep Disorders*

CONDITION	HISTORY	PHYSICAL FINDINGS	DIAGNOSTIC STUDIES
SPECIFIC DISORDERS			
Restless legs syndrome	Irresistible urge to move legs while in bed	Normal	Sleep studies; serum ferritin
Periodic limb movement	Older than 65 yr; reports of rhythmic jerking of legs or arms while asleep	Normal	Sleep studies

DIFFERENTIAL DIAGNOSIS OF *Common Causes of Sleep Disorders—cont'd*

CONDITION	HISTORY	PHYSICAL FINDINGS	DIAGNOSTIC STUDIES
Obstructive sleep apnea	Apneic episodes, loud snoring, restless sleep patterns	Decreased oxygen; enlarged adenoids, tonsils	Sleep studies: polysomnography, home testing
Narcolepsy	Excessive sleepiness, cataplexy	Normal	Referral to sleep specialist
Delayed sleep phase syndrome	Adolescent with extreme shift in sleep–wake cycle; unable to fall asleep for many hours	Normal	Referral to sleep specialist
Secondary to medical condition or medications	GERD, COPD, PND, CHF, enlarged prostate or nocturia, depression, or anxiety Medications: antidepressants, decongestants, bronchodilators, β-blockers, thyroid preparations, phenytoin, methyldopa, corticosteroids	Consistent with medical condition	Consistent with underlying medical condition; trial off or change of medication(s)
Poor sleep hygiene	Routine, habits, environment not conducive to sleep; use of alcohol, caffeine, diet pills, nicotine	Normal	Sleep diary
Lifestyle	Shift work, travel, jet lag	Normal	Sleep diary
AGE-RELATED SLEEP DISORDERS			
Night awakening	Single to repeated awakenings at night	Initial physical examination to eliminate associated medical illness	As directed by examination
Sleep refusal	Refusal of child to go to sleep	Normal	None
Night terrors	Inconsolable awakening occurring early in sleep, lasting 15 min, no memory of event	Normal	None
Nightmares	Occur later in sleep cycle; dream is remembered	Normal	None
Adolescent patterns	Decrease in amount of sleep obtained	Normal	Sleep diary
Menopause	Hot flashes	Consistent with menopause	Sleep diary
Older adult patterns	Nighttime arousals and awakenings; night owl pattern; early wakening; daytime napping	Physical examination to rule out underlying medical condition	Sleep diary
Conditioned insomnia	Identify initial trigger with persistent problem	Physical examination to rule out underlying medical condition	Sleep diary
Trained night crier	Child unable to soothe self	Normal	None
Trained night feeder	History of frequent feedings on awakening at night	Normal	None
Somnambulism	Sleepwalking in early sleep cycle	Normal	None

CHF, congestive heart failure; *COPD,* chronic obstructive pulmonary disease; *GERD,* gastroesophageal reflux disease; *PND,* paroxysmal nocturnal dyspnea.

32 Sore Throat

Sore throat, or pharyngitis, is one of the most common concerns of patients in primary care. It is most often a transient condition of viral origin (adenoviruses, coxsackie A viruses, influenza, or parainfluenza virus). Throat pain is the result of an inflammation of the mucosa of the oropharynx, secondary to an infectious cause (e.g., viral, bacterial, fungal, or spirochetal). Less commonly, sore throat may be a symptom of systemic illness, such as mononucleosis. The posterior pharynx is also vulnerable to environmental irritants and drainage from the nose and sinuses. Thus pharyngitis begins as an inflammation of the mucous membranes with secondary involvement of the lymph node drainage system, rarely progressing to deep neck and mediastinal involvement. Throat pain can also be referred from other structures, most commonly the ears and thyroid gland.

Sore throats can be classified according to whether or not pharyngeal ulcers are present. This will sort out those relatively few sore throats caused by specific viral or fungal infections that produce pharyngeal ulcers and those caused by agents and processes characterized by an absence of pharyngeal ulcers.

The goals of assessment and diagnosis are to identify those patients with group A β-hemolytic streptococcus (GAS) infection and those with epiglottitis. Patients with GAS infection are at risk for rheumatic fever and glomerulonephritis, and timely treatment can reduce the possibility of sequelae of peritonsillar and retropharyngeal abscess. GAS is the most common bacterial cause of acute pharyngitis, responsible for 10% of sore throat visits in adults and 30% in children, especially during winter months.

DIAGNOSTIC REASONING: FOCUSED HISTORY

Is this an emergency?

Key Questions
- Have you been drooling?
- Have you been unable to swallow?
- Have you been unable to lie down?
- Have you been restless, unable to stay still?
- Have you been unable to talk?

History

The previous symptoms signal acute epiglottitis. The history is usually elicited from another individual because the patient is either a child or too ill to talk. Acute epiglottitis is rare: its incidence is 10 in 100,000 in children younger than 15 years and 1 to 8 in 100,000 in adults. The morbidity and mortality that result from airway obstruction, however, are significant.

Associated Symptoms

Symptoms and signs of epiglottitis are sore throat, difficulty swallowing, dyspnea, drooling, and inspiratory stridor. *Haemophilus influenzae* type b (Hib) is the most common pathogen, although it is decreasing in vaccinated children. The incidence of *H. influenzae* type B (Hib) epiglottitis is highest in children ages 2 to 5 years. Epiglottitis is a rapidly progressive illness with a potentially fatal outcome and must be recognized and referred immediately.

Severe throat pain with trismus and refusal to speak indicates severe peritonsillitis, which may lead to peritonsillar abscess formation (quinsy). Peritonsillar abscess is also an acute infection that needs to be identified immediately for referral and treatment. The symptoms of peritonsillar abscess and cellulitis include a severe sore throat, odynophagia, trismus (spasm of the masticatory muscles and difficulty opening the mouth), and medial deviation of the soft palate and peritonsillar fold. These symptoms are caused by infection penetrating the tonsillar capsule and surrounding tissues. About 30% of patients with peritonsillar abscess require an emergency tonsillectomy.

What does the presence of fever tell me?

Key Questions
- Have you had a fever?
- When did it start?
- How high has it been?

Patterns of Fever

Fever is almost always present with GAS and is the most commonly occurring symptom in children. The fever is of sudden onset and the temperature rises above 38.5°C (101.5°F) with malaise, headache, and painful swallowing. Fever is also present in children and adults with epiglottitis. Influenza is characterized by the abrupt onset of fever, with temperatures typically ranging from 37.8° to 40°C (100° to 104°F). Children with adenoviral infection can be afebrile or have a fever greater than 40°C (104°F). Patients with Epstein-Barr virus (EBV) have a low-grade fever.

Fever, followed by an interval of several days without fever and then recurrent fever, or a continuing fever for several days may indicate peritonsillar abscess.

The absence of fever may also suggest a noninfectious cause, such as candidiasis and aphthous stomatitis.

Is the sore throat related to an infectious cause?

Key Questions
- Is anyone else at home sick?
- Are any of your friends or coworkers sick?
- When did the pain start?
- How severe is the pain?

Exposure

Exposure to other ill individuals increases the likelihood of viral or bacterial infection. Respiratory illness caused by GAS is spread within families, with approximately 20% of family members becoming infected. EBV is not highly contagious and requires intimate contact between susceptible individuals and symptomatic shedders of the virus. Transmission is primarily through saliva.

Onset

The sudden onset of sore throat is often caused by GAS. The organisms invade the pharyngeal epithelium, where they multiply and cause an intense immune response. Gradual onset is more common in infectious mononucleosis. The EBV infects B lymphocytes of the pharynx with resultant dissemination throughout the lymphoreticular system (also referred to as the reticuloendothelial system or the mononuclear phagocytic system), causing an immune response that is more gradual in onset.

In viral pharyngitis, a sore throat begins a day or two after the onset of other illness symptoms, reaching its peak by the second or third day.

Noninfectious causes of sore throat typically have an insidious onset. The patient often is not able to pinpoint when the sore throat started but notes that it has been persistent.

Severity

Throat pain associated with streptococcal infection is usually intense. Throat pain associated with influenza and adenovirus is severe, with prominent edema of the throat. The throat pain produced by noninfectious causes tends to be less severe and may be described as "scratchy" or "annoying."

Young children may not be able to express the sensation of a sore throat or the severity of it. Instead, they may refuse to eat or drink.

What does the presence of upper respiratory tract symptoms tell me?

Key Questions
- Do you have a cough?
- Have you had a runny nose? If so, what color is the drainage?
- Do you have postnasal drip?

- Do you have eye redness or discomfort?
- Have your eyes been itchy or watery?
- Have you been hoarse?
- Have you been sneezing?
- Have you been wheezing?

Cough and Rhinorrhea

Cough, rhinitis, conjunctivitis, and hoarseness rarely occur with streptococcal pharyngitis, and the presence of two or more of these signs or symptoms most often suggests a viral infection.

Influenza is often associated with several days of fever, cough, and rhinorrhea. Viral pharyngitis is characterized by a sore, scratchy throat, nasal congestion, rhinorrhea, and cough. Clear nasal discharge is common in allergic pharyngitis and may produce postnasal drip that causes a sore throat.

Conjunctivitis

Conjunctivitis rarely occurs with streptococcal pharyngitis. Mild conjunctivitis is common with viral infection. Watery or itchy eyes are also associated with exposure to allergens.

Hoarseness

Hoarseness is not uncommon in allergy-associated sore throat and may be present with viral infection as well. Inflammation produces laryngeal edema that results in hoarseness. Hoarseness is not typically associated with GAS infection.

Sneezing

Sneezing is common with both viral infection and allergen exposure. The sneezing associated with allergic pharyngitis is more persistent and is often seasonal.

Wheezing

Wheezing can occur with exposure to allergens. When the body detects an allergen, it views it as a foreign body and tries to reject it by producing antibodies and histamine. Histamine causes a person's airways to become inflamed and produce mucus. As a result, the airways become narrower. Air forced through a smaller space causes a whistling or wheezing sound.

What do the associated symptoms tell me?

Key Questions
- Do you have muscle aches?
- Have you had nausea, vomiting, or diarrhea?

Systemic Symptoms

Systemic symptoms, such as myalgia, are common in influenza and GAS infection. Streptococcal pharyngitis or influenza in children older than 2 years is associated with headache, abdominal pain, and vomiting. Fatigue, especially if prolonged, may indicate mononucleosis.

Influenza is often associated with several days of fever and systemic symptoms, such as myalgias, cough, and rhinorrhea. Common cold viruses associated with pharyngitis can also produce systemic symptoms such as myalgia.

Does the presence of risk factors help me narrow the cause?

Key Questions
- How old are you?
- What is your smoking history?
- What kind of work do you do?
- Do you engage in oral sex?
- Are you taking medications?
- Do you have any chronic health problems?
- Are your immunizations up to date?

Age

Group A streptococcal infection is primarily a disease in children 5 to 15 years of age. Influenza affects all ages; whereas parainfluenza and respiratory syncytial viruses (RSV) primarily affect children. Almost all children younger than 2 years of age will have RSV, and 25% to 40% will develop bronchiolitis or pneumonia.

Adenoviruses, the major viral agents isolated in exudative pharyngitis in younger children, are endemic. In military populations, adenovirus type 4 and, to a lesser extent, types 3, 7, and 21 are the most common causes of pharyngitis.

Adolescents and young adults are more likely than children and older adults to have a sore throat associated with mononucleosis caused by EBV. In older adults, mononucleosis often occurs without pharyngitis, adenopathy, or splenomegaly.

Irritant Exposures

Agents such as tobacco smoke, smog, dust, and allergens can irritate the throat. These agents cause mucosal irritation and set up the inflammatory process. People who work outdoors may have greater exposure to environmental allergens. Housekeepers have an increased risk of exposure to dust mites and chemical irritants.

Sexual Behavior

Pharyngitis from *Chlamydia trachomatis* or *Neisseria gonorrhoeae* is more prevalent in people with a history of orogenital sexual activity. Gonococcal pharyngitis is present in about 10% of patients with anogenital gonorrhea.

Medications and Chronic Health Problems

Immunosuppression increases susceptibility to viral agents that produce pharyngeal ulcers (e.g., herpangina, herpes simplex). People with diabetes and those taking broad-spectrum antibiotics are more susceptible to candidiasis. People with a history of gastroesophageal reflux disease may have a sore throat secondary to reflux of gastric contents.

Immunizations

Infants receive the DTaP (diphtheria, tetanus, pertussis) and Hib vaccines as part of routine immunization. DTaP prevents diphtheria, tetanus, and pertussis. Hib prevents Hib responsible for epiglottitis in children. Adults should get a booster dose of Td every 10 years. Unimmunized children and adults are at higher risk for infection.

DIAGNOSTIC REASONING: FOCUSED PHYSICAL EXAMINATION

Assess Severity of Illness

Assessment of the patient begins with general observation about the severity of illness. Severe illness with signs of upper airway obstruction such as restlessness, stridor, difficulty breathing, drooling, inability to swallow, and high fever signals epiglottitis and requires immediate referral. Further physical examination with a tongue blade could trigger laryngospasms and lead to airway obstruction.

Inspect the Mouth

Examine the buccal mucosa, tongue, and sublingual area for the presence of ulcers. Note the location, number, size, and appearance of any lesions.

The lesions produced by the group A coxsackievirus (herpangina) first appear as small, grayish, papulovesicular lesions on the soft palate and pharynx. They progress to shallow ulcers, usually less than 5 mm in diameter.

Vincent angina (necrotizing ulcerative gingivostomatitis) is a fusospirochetal infection of the gingiva. The gingiva appears inflamed and ulcerated, often covered with a gray slough. As the infection spreads, ulcers may appear on the oral mucosa and posterior pharynx.

Aphthous stomatitis, or canker sores, are lesions that affect about 20% of the general population and are associated with immunological mechanisms. They occur most often on the buccal mucosa, tongue, and soft palate. The lesions first appear as indurated papules and then progress to shallow ulcers. The ulcers have a yellow membrane and red halo.

Herpes simplex lesions involve the anterior oral mucosa and the gums. Herpetic pharyngitis is manifested by vesicles, ulcers, or exudate of the oral and pharyngeal mucosa. Specifically, the lesions involve the tonsils, pharynx, uvula, and edges of the soft palate. Vesicular lesions may or may not be intact.

Streptococcal infection in children may cause enlarged papillae on the tongue, which gives the tongue a strawberry appearance.

Inspect the Posterior Pharynx and Observe Swallowing

Examine for edema, color, and exudate of the posterior pharynx, and determine the presence, size (Table 32.1), and condition of the palatine tonsils. Good visualization is critical for accurate diagnosis. Use a good light source and ask the patient to open wide and say "ah" but not to protrude the tongue. If you cannot

Table 32.1	**Grading Tonsillar Size**
GRADE	**TONSIL LOCATION**
1	Behind pillars
2	Between pillars and uvula
3	Touching uvula
4	Extending beyond midline of oropharynx

view the pharynx, depress the tongue firmly with a tongue blade, far enough back to have a good view but not enough to cause the patient to gag. Use two tongue depressors to retract tissues medially and laterally when examining such areas as the retromolar region, the floor of the mouth, and the orifices of Wharton and Stensen ducts (Fig. 32.1). The best visualization is achieved with a headlight.

Drooling may indicate peritonsillar abscess or epiglottitis partially occluding the pharynx and esophagus. Only occasionally can the red, swollen epiglottis be visualized above the base of the tongue. If you suspect epiglottitis, do not examine the pharynx because manipulation may precipitate laryngospasms and airway obstruction. Refer the patient immediately for specialist evaluation

and further tests, which may include soft tissue radiography of the head and neck and laryngoscopy.

Edema of the affected tonsil, with movement of the tonsil toward midline, indicates peritonsillar abscess. Diphtheria may appear as a thick, gray tonsillar exudate or pseudomembrane, spreading to the tonsillar pillars, uvula, soft palate, posterior pharyngeal wall, and larynx. The exudate is not easily removable and bleeds easily.

Pharyngeal or tonsillar exudate can be present with either a bacterial or a viral infection. A yellowish exudate of GAS pharyngitis is often present. Generally, the exudate of viral agents tends to be whiter than that from GAS.

A bright red uvula and the presence of petechiae on the posterior pharynx and palate indicate group A streptococcal pharyngitis. "Doughnut lesions," or red, raised hemorrhagic lesions with a yellow center, are diagnostic of streptococcal pharyngitis.

Postnasal drainage can irritate the posterior pharynx and should be observed for color. Purulent drainage that is yellow or greenish is associated with infectious sinusitis. White curdlike patches that bleed on scraping are characteristic of oral candidiasis.

When examination reveals normal findings, suspect a systemic referred cause for the

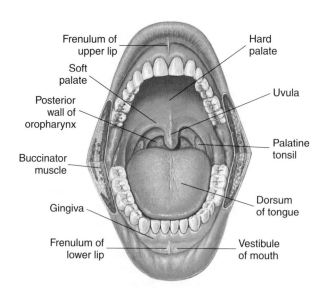

Frenulum of upper lip · Soft palate · Posterior wall of oropharynx · Buccinator muscle · Gingiva · Frenulum of lower lip · Hard palate · Uvula · Palatine tonsil · Dorsum of tongue · Vestibule of mouth

FIGURE 32.1 Anatomical structures of the mouth. (From Ball JW, Dains JE, Flynn J, et al: *Seidel's guide to physical examination*, ed. 8, St. Louis, 2015, Elsevier.)

sore throat, particularly acute otitis media, sinusitis, or thyroiditis.

Palpate the Cervicofacial Lymph Nodes

In streptococcal pharyngitis, the anterior cervical lymph nodes are often enlarged and tender. In viral infections, the posterior cervical nodes are more often enlarged. Lymphadenopathy is a cardinal sign of infectious mononucleosis, with more than 90% of patients having enlarged posterior cervical nodes.

Inspect the Nasal Mucosa

Red, swollen turbinates indicate an infectious process; in contrast, pale, boggy turbinates indicate an allergic process. Mucoid discharge occurs in allergic rhinitis. Purulent discharge suggests infectious sinusitis.

Inspect the Conjunctivae

Injected conjunctivae associated with a sore throat may indicate pharyngoconjunctival fever. It is caused by an adenovirus and is often associated with nonpurulent discharge, fever, and pharyngitis. It frequently occurs in epidemics. Mild conjunctivitis in the presence of itching eyes and clear watery discharge is associated with an allergic process.

Inspect the Tympanic Membrane

Evidence of otitis media with effusion may indicate atypical *H. influenzae* acute otitis media (conjunctivitis-otitis syndrome). Earache can be caused by referred pain, especially from the tonsils.

Palpate the Thyroid

Acute thyroiditis is associated with a sore throat, painful swallowing, and an enlarged or tender thyroid gland on palpation.

Inspect the Skin

Evidence of a fine maculopapular erythema that has a generalized distribution with accentuation in the skinfolds, circumoral pallor, and sparing of the palms and soles indicates scarlet fever. The rash characteristically is followed by a fine desquamation, starting at the hands.

Auscultate the Lungs

Mycoplasma pneumoniae is frequently associated with sore throat in adolescents and young adults. If pneumonia is present, palpation, percussion, and auscultation of the lungs reveal an area of consolidation and adventitious breath sounds (see Chapter 14 for further discussion of the lung examination).

 EVIDENCE-BASED PRACTICE *What Is the Current Evidence on Management of Peritonsillar Abscess?*

This literature review was limited to articles published from 1991 to 2011 and examined areas of controversy about peritonsillar abscess. Findings showed that (1) intraoral ultrasound has a sensitivity and specificity of between 89% and 95% and 79% and 100%, respectively, for correctly diagnosing peritonsillar abscess and is currently underused; (2) steroids can effectively aid recovery, reducing hospitalization time and improving symptom relief; however, further study is needed, especially related to the risk-to-benefit ratio (penicillin and metronidazole are an effective combination in at least 98% of cases of peritonsillar abscess); (3) there is no convincing evidence in favor of either aspiration or incision and drainage; tonsillectomy with an abscess present is safe and reduces overall recovery time when compared with tonsillectomy when symptoms are not present; (4) peritonsillar abscess can be effectively managed on an outpatient basis in many cases; and (5) the recurrence rate of peritonsillar abscess is poorly defined but estimated as 9% to 22%. Interval tonsillectomy may be indicated in patients at high risk of recurrence. The authors concluded that peritonsillar abscess is a common condition with increasing incidence. However, lack of consensus suggests that better evidence is needed for peritonsillar abscess management, especially for recurrence rates and different management strategies.

Reference: Powell and Wilson, 2012.

Palpate the Abdomen

Splenomegaly is found in about half the cases of mononucleosis, although hepatomegaly is rare. Gastroesophageal reflux disease may be associated with palpable upper epigastric tenderness.

LABORATORY AND DIAGNOSTIC STUDIES

The laboratory evaluation of sore throat is generally limited to the identification of GAS. Other infectious causes, such as gonorrhea or diphtheria, are rare, and testing is conducted only if the history indicates exposure. It is important to diagnose streptococcal pharyngitis so it can be treated promptly with antibiotics, avoiding serious sequelae, such as peritonsillar abscesses, rheumatic fever, or glomerulonephritis.

Rapid Screening Tests

A throat swab is a rapid screen for streptococcal antigens and should be done if GAS is suspected. If it is positive, the patient is treated without follow-up cultures. If the swab result is negative, a throat culture is obtained. The test has a sensitivity of 75% to 85% and a specificity of 95% to 98%.

The Monospot is a rapid slide test that detects heterophil antibody agglutination; it is not specific for EBV. It is most sensitive 1 to 2 weeks after symptoms appear and remains positive for up to 1 year. If chronic fatigue syndrome is being considered as a differential diagnosis, specific EBV antibody tests should be considered.

Culture

A throat culture to detect GAS is the gold standard of diagnosis, with a 10% or lower false-negative rate. When obtaining a culture, first remove crusts from lesions, taking care to touch only the throat or tonsils with the sterile swab. Avoid touching the tongue. Roll the throat swab over one tonsil, proceed across the posterior pharynx, and then swab the other tonsil. A culture can confirm a diagnosis of gonococcal pharyngitis.

Antistreptolysin O Titer

Group A β-hemolytic streptococcus produces enzymes that include streptolysin. An antistreptolysin O (ASO) titer is a serology test that detects the presence of a previous streptococcal infection. This titer does not increase until 1 to 6 months postinfection, so it is of no diagnostic value. It is used to aid in the diagnosis of streptococci-associated infections, such as rheumatic fever, glomerulonephritis, and pericarditis. A caution, however, is that in as many as 50% of positive streptococcal cultures, an elevated ASO titer will not be found postinfection.

Potassium Hydroxide Smear for Wet Mount

Obtain a sample of pharyngeal discharge using a cotton-tipped applicator. Using a microscope, examine the potassium hydroxide slide for branching and budding hyphae that are characteristic of yeast infection (see Chapter 37).

Complete Blood Count with Differential

Test results of 50% lymphocytes and at least 10% atypical lymphocytes support a diagnosis of mononucleosis; a positive monospot test result is diagnostic.

Computed Tomography Scan

Suspicion of an obstruction or swelling of the throat should be referred for further evaluation with computed tomography.

Nasal Smear

Nasal cytology can be performed on secretions obtained by having the patient blow his or her nose into a paper or by using a cotton-tipped swab to obtain secretions from the nose. The presence of eosinophils on a nasal smear stained with Wright stain viewed under a high-power microscope suggests an allergic, inflammatory process.

DIFFERENTIAL DIAGNOSIS

Pharyngitis without Ulcers

Epiglottitis

Epiglottitis is caused by infection with Hib that produces inflammation and edema of the epiglottis and the surrounding areas, obstructing the flow of air. The edematous epiglottis may be pulled into the larynx during inspiration and can completely occlude the airway. Symptoms are respiratory distress, sore throat, difficulty with secretions, drooling, pain on swallowing, and a toxic appearance. The infection occurs in both children and adults.

Peritonsillar or retropharyngeal abscess

A peritonsillar abscess, also called quinsy, is a collection of pus between the tonsil and the capsule of the tonsillar pillar. This condition occurs in children but is more common in adults, especially in people with a history of recurrent tonsillitis. The patient's presenting concerns usually include a history of respiratory symptoms, difficulty swallowing, otalgia, malaise, fever, and cervical lymphadenopathy. On examination, there may be trismus; asymmetrical swelling of the uvula, tonsils, or posterior pharynx; or a visible abscess. Children's presenting symptoms typically include fever, toxic appearance, refusal to swallow, drooling, and stridor. Children with retropharyngeal abscess are usually under the age of 4 and need immediate referral.

Viral pharyngitis

Most sore throats are caused by viral infections. Patients usually have symptoms of malaise, fever, headache, cough, and fatigue. The pharynx is usually erythematous, or it may be pale, boggy, and swollen. There usually is no tonsillar enlargement or pharyngeal exudate, although infection with an adenovirus may produce exudate. The presence of concomitant upper respiratory tract symptoms such as cough and congestion makes the diagnosis of viral pharyngitis more likely than that of streptococcal pharyngitis. Common cold viruses cause sore throats most frequently during the colder months of the year.

Streptococcal pharyngitis

The major differential diagnoses for sore throat will be viral or bacterial infection. About 10% of adults and 30% of children who seek care for sore throat symptoms, especially during winter

months, have streptococcal tonsillopharyngitis. However, reliance on clinical impression to arrive at a specific diagnosis is problematic. The symptoms most likely to occur with streptococcal pharyngitis include a fever with a temperature of 38.5°C (101.5°F) or higher, tonsillar exudate, anterior cervical adenopathy, and a history of recent exposure. The incidence of streptococcal pharyngitis increases from 10% in the summer and fall to 40% during the winter and early spring. GAS cannot be reliably diagnosed on the basis of signs and symptoms, and even when cultures are obtained, a causative agent may not be identified in 50% of patients. Table 32.2 shows the groups at risk for GAS.

Mononucleosis

Mononucleosis causes about 5% of sore throats. It occurs most often in young adults, and the causative agent is EBV in more than 90% of cases. History typically reveals a gradual onset, low-grade fever, mild sore throat, posterior cervical lymphadenopathy, weight loss, and pronounced malaise and fatigue. Diagnosis can be confirmed with a positive Monospot test and a complete blood count that shows greater than 50% lymphocytosis. Splenomegaly occurs in about 50% of cases, and palatine petechiae are a less common symptom. GAS occurs concomitantly in 10% to 20% of cases.

Gonococcal pharyngitis

This form of pharyngitis can occur in patients with a history of orogenital sexual activity. The patient may have no symptoms. Examination shows an exudative pharyngitis with bilateral cervical lymphadenopathy. Gram staining or culture will confirm the diagnosis.

Inflammation

Inflammatory sore throat occurs in the presence of sinusitis or exposure to local irritants. The patient often reports postnasal drip and allergic symptoms (itchy, watery eyes, runny nose) that may follow seasonal patterns. On examination, the patient may have sinus

Table 32.2	Groups at Risk for Group A β-Hemolytic Streptococcus (GAS) Pharyngitis	

RISK FACTORS	DIAGNOSTIC TESTS
HIGH RISK	
Tonsillar exudate	None; treat on basis of risk factors
Temperature >38.5°C (101.5°F)	
Cervical lymphadenopathy	
Absence of cough	
Existing valvular rheumatic heart disease	
PRESUMED STREP	
Scarlet fever	None; treat
Strep epidemic	
Antibiotics already started	
MEDIUM RISK	
Exudate, nodes, or fever present	Rapid strep screen; if positive, treat; if negative,
Prior rheumatic fever	culture; treat if culture positive; do not treat
"Low risk" by PE but younger than 25 yr old and no URI	if culture negative
Person with diabetes	
Recent "strep" exposure	
LOW RISK	
No exudate, nodes, or fever	Rapid strep screen; if positive, treat; if negative, do not culture; do not treat if culture negative

PE, physical examination; URI, upper respiratory tract infection.

tenderness. The pharynx may be swollen or pale with posterior drainage present. The patient does not have fever or lymphadenopathy.

Pharyngitis with Ulcers

Herpangina

Herpangina is an infection caused by the coxsackievirus. The patient reports a painful sore throat, fever, and malaise. Headache, anorexia, and neck, abdomen, and extremity pain may occur. Within 2 days of onset, small, grayish, papulovesicular lesions appear on the soft palate and pharynx. These progress to shallow ulcers, usually less than 5 mm in diameter. Outbreaks occur during the summer months. Coxsackie virus peaks in August, September, and October, although some cases occur during the winter months. It is more common in children and in immunosuppressed patients. Diagnosis is based on symptoms and characteristic oral lesions. An antibody titer can confirm diagnosis.

Vincent angina

Vincent angina is caused by a fusospirochetal infection that results in necrotizing ulcerative gingivostomatitis. The patient's symptoms include painful ulcers, foul breath, and bleeding gums. Without secondary infection, there usually is no fever. On examination, gray, necrotic ulcers without vesicles are apparent on the gingivae and interdental papillae. Gram staining shows spirochetes and confirms the diagnosis.

Aphthous stomatitis

Aphthous stomatitis, or "canker sores," appears as discrete ulcers without preceding vesicles. The ulcers are located on the inner lip, tongue, and buccal mucosa. Lesions last about 1 to 2 weeks.

The cause of the lesions is unknown, but immunologic mechanisms play a major role.

Herpes simplex virus type 1

An infection from herpes simplex virus type 1 (HSV-1) is associated with fever, headache, sore throat, and lymphadenitis. Characteristic clusters of yellow vesicles appear on the palate, pharynx, and gingiva. Lesions last 2 to 3 weeks. Recurrent lesions are characterized by prodromal symptoms of burning, tingling, or itching. Active lesions are usually painful.

Recent studies indicate that HSV-1 infections afflict about 30% to 90% of the US population.

Candidiasis

Candidiasis is a yeast infection that produces white plaques over the tongue and oral mucosa with erythema; the plaques bleed when scraped. *Candida* infection occurs commonly in otherwise normal infants in the first weeks of life; in immunocompromised people, including those with diabetes; and in people taking antibiotics or using inhaled steroids.

▶ DIFFERENTIAL DIAGNOSIS OF *Common Causes of Sore Throat*

CONDITION	HISTORY	PHYSICAL FINDINGS	DIAGNOSTIC STUDIES
PHARYNGITIS WITHOUT ULCERS			
Epiglottitis	Sore throat, difficulty with secretions, odynophagia (seen in pediatric patients younger than 2 yr), unable to lie flat, unable to talk	Respiratory distress, drooling, toxic appearance; do not examine the pharynx	Refer immediately
Peritonsillar or retropharyngeal abscess	History of recurrent tonsillitis; sore throat, difficulty swallowing, respiratory tract symptoms, fever, malaise	Orthopnea, dyspnea, symmetrical swelling, abscess, trismus	Refer immediately: CT scan; head and neck radiographs; laryngoscopy
Viral pharyngitis	Scratchy, sore throat, malaise, myalgias, headache, chills, cough, rhinitis	Erythema, edema of throat, tender posterior cervical nodes	None
Group A β-hemolytic streptococcal pharyngitis	Most common in people 5–15 yr old; known exposure; fall and winter season; sudden onset of fever, severe sore throat, and malaise; absence of cough and upper respiratory tract symptoms	Temperature >38.5°C (101.5°F); exudate; anterior cervical lymphadenopathy	Positive rapid strep antibody screen; strep culture
Mononucleosis (Epstein-Barr virus)	Young adults; slow onset of malaise, low-grade fever, mild sore throat	Presence or absence of pharyngeal exudate, posterior cervical lymphadenopathy, splenomegaly	Positive Monospot; CBC with differential; >50% leukocytes
Gonococcal pharyngitis	History of orogenital sexual activity; may be asymptomatic	Pharyngeal exudate; bilateral cervical lymphadenopathy	Gram stain; gonorrhea culture

Continued

▶ DIFFERENTIAL DIAGNOSIS OF *Common Causes of Sore Throat—cont'd*

CONDITION	HISTORY	PHYSICAL FINDINGS	DIAGNOSTIC STUDIES
Inflammation	Exposure to irritants; postnasal drip; allergic symptoms	Sinus tenderness, pale or swollen pharynx, postnasal drainage visible, no fever or lymphadenopathy	Eosinophils in nasal secretions with allergies
PHARYNGITIS WITH ULCERS			
Herpangina (coxsackievirus)	More common in children; immunosuppressed; painful throat; fever, malaise	Lymphadenopathy; small grayish papulovesicular lesions on soft palate and pharynx, progressing to shallow ulcers, usually <5 mm in diameter	Serology
Fusospirochetal infection (Vincent angina)	Poor oral hygiene; painful ulcers, foul breath, bleeding gums	Gray necrotic ulcers without vesicles on gingival margins and interdental papillae	Gram stain reveals spirochetes
Aphthous stomatitis	Oral trauma, ill-fitting dentures; painful ulcers varying in size; absence of other symptoms	Shallow ulcers, no vesicles; indurated papules that progress to 1-cm ulcers; ulcer has yellow membrane and red halo; no fever or nodes	None
Herpes simplex infection	History of trauma to mucosa; pain, fever, headache	Perioral lesions; lymphadenitis; vesicles on palate, pharynx, gingiva	Viral culture
Candidiasis	Immunosuppressed; people taking antibiotics or with diabetes; sore mouth or throat	Curdlike white plaques that bleed when scraped off	Potassium hydroxide smear shows hyphae; culture

CBC, complete blood count; *CT*, computed tomography; *STI*, sexually transmitted disease.

CHAPTER
33   Syncope

Syncope is the transient loss of consciousness and postural tone that results from a sudden decrease in cerebral perfusion. It is distinct from coma, seizures, shock, vertigo, and other states of altered consciousness. It is a symptom that about 10% of adults of any age will experience at least some time during their lives, and the incidence increases exponentially in people older than 70 years old. It is less common in children except when there is a seizure disorder, primary cardiac arrhythmia, or a breath-holding incident.

The causes of syncope can be difficult to determine because patients generally are seen after the event has occurred. Syncope can be quite benign, such as a vasovagal response, or it can indicate serious disease. However, even benign syncope can place the patient at risk for falls or injury. Cardiogenic syncope has high associated morbidity and mortality, and the emphasis in diagnosis is to rule out the most serious causes through a careful history and physical examination, with a few laboratory and diagnostic tests to establish a possible diagnosis.

DIAGNOSTIC REASONING: FOCUSED HISTORY

Is this really syncope?

Key Questions
- Did you lose consciousness?
- If you lost consciousness, how long did it last?
- Did you have any warning symptoms?
- What were you doing when the event occurred?
- Did your limbs jerk during the event?
- Did anyone see you faint?

Loss of Consciousness

Distinguish syncope from other symptoms. Dizziness, vertigo, and presyncope do not cause loss of consciousness or postural tone. Episodes of syncope lasting longer than 10 minutes are rarely physiologic.

Prodromal Symptoms

Sweating, vertigo, nausea, and yawning are prodromal symptoms that are associated with syncope; seizures may be associated with an aura or tongue biting. Aura also suggests migraine etiology.

Pre-event Characteristics

Characterize what precipitated the episodes. Loss of consciousness precipitated by pain, exercise, urination, defecation, or stressful events is probably not a seizure. Breath-holding spells commonly cause syncope in children and are usually precipitated by pain, anger, a sudden startle, or frustration. Obtain information about when the patient last ate or drank, as dehydration or fasting may cause reflex syncope. Syncope occurs with rest or when supine during a seizure or arrhythmia. Syncope that occurs without warning symptoms is highly suspect to have a cardiovascular origin.

Event and Postevent Characteristics

Rhythmic movements of extremities during the event usually indicate a seizure, although they can occur with syncope. Disorientation after the event, slowness in returning to consciousness, and unconsciousness lasting longer than 5 minutes indicate seizure. Often children with breath-holding spells have associated cyanosis, clonic jerks, opisthotonos, and bradycardia.

EVIDENCE-BASED PRACTICE *Diagnosing Syncope*

MORE OFTEN ASSOCIATED WITH CARDIAC CAUSES OF SYNCOPE	MORE OFTEN ASSOCIATED WITH NONCARDIAC CAUSES OF SYNCOPE
• Older age (older than 60 yr of age) • Male sex • Presence of known ischemic heart disease, structural heart disease, previous arrhythmias, or reduced ventricular function • Brief prodrome, such as palpitations, or sudden loss of consciousness without prodrome • Syncope during exertion • Syncope in the supine position • Low number of syncope episodes (one or two) • Abnormal cardiac examination • Family history of inheritable conditions or premature sudden cardiac death (younger than 50 yr of age) • Presence of known congenital heart disease	• Younger age • No known cardiac disease • Syncope only in the standing position • Positional change from supine or sitting to standing • Presence of prodrome: nausea, vomiting, feeling warmth • Presence of specific triggers: dehydration, pain, distressful stimulus, medical environment • Situational triggers: cough, laugh, micturition, defecation, deglutition • Frequent recurrence and prolonged history of syncope with similar characteristics

Reference: ACC et al, 2017.

Witness

The patient is unconscious when the syncopal event takes place and therefore is a poor historian. A careful history is needed from both the patient and a witness to help in the diagnosis. Adolescents who have psychogenic syncope episodes generally have an audience when the event occurs and are able to describe details of the event that would not be known to an unconscious patient.

Does this require immediate referral?

Key Questions

• Do you have a history of heart disease? What is it?
• Do you have a congenital heart problem?
• Are you having chest pain or shortness of breath?
• Do you have palpitations?
• Did this occur during or after exercise?

History of Heart Disease or Congenital Heart Problem

The presence of structural heart disease increases the risk of sudden death. Patients with a history of coronary artery disease, congestive heart failure, or ventricular arrhythmia should be hospitalized. Cardiac syncope may

be either arrhythmic or mechanical in origin. Cardiac outflow obstruction from aortic or mitral stenosis or a prosthetic valve may cause syncope. Complete heart block, the result of interruption of atrioventricular conduction, is a leading cause of syncope. Children who have had cardiac surgery to correct severe congenital heart disease are at risk for arrhythmias.

Palpitations

Supraventricular or ventricular tachycardia are associated with syncope and sudden death. Ventricular tachycardia with a heart rate of 200 beats per minute may be asymptomatic or cause syncope. Chaotic ventricular activity of ventricular fibrillation is always fatal unless it is reversed with electrical defibrillation (see Chapter 26 for Palpitations).

Chest Pain or Shortness of Breath

Obstructive mechanical blockage may be caused by pulmonary embolism, cardiac ischemia, or myocardial infarction with pump failure.

After Exercise

Syncope that accompanies exercise should be considered of cardiac origin unless it is proven

EVIDENCE-BASED PRACTICE *Is the Valsalva Maneuver Effective for Stopping an Abnormal Heart Rhythm?*

Supraventricular tachycardia (SVT) is a common heart rhythm disturbance that can occur in healthy individuals and includes symptoms of chest pain, palpitations, dyspnea, sweating, feeling faint, and loss of consciousness. Treatment is usually a combination of Valsalva maneuver, medications, and electro reversion. The Valsalva maneuver stimulates the vagus nerve (cranial nerve X), which in turn leads to slowing of the heart rate. This maneuver is performed by having a patient blow into a syringe while lying prone for 15 seconds to generate increased pressure within the chest cavity and a slowing of heart rate that may stop the abnormal rhythm.

Three studies involving a total of 316 participants were included in a systematic this review. Results showed that reversion is between 19.4% and 54.3%. Potential side effects reported include hypotension and syncope. No side effects were reported in the three studies reviewed, and within the three studies, reversion was achieved on completion of each Valsalva maneuver. The authors concluded that the Valsalva maneuver is a simple, noninvasive method of stopping an abnormal heart rhythm, but its safety and overall effectiveness are difficult to quantify. Further research is required to improve the evidence surrounding this practice.

Reference: Smith et al, 2015.

otherwise. Syncope after exertion in a well-trained athlete who has no heart disease is likely vasovagal in origin.

What do associated symptoms tell me?

Key Questions

- Do you have headaches?
- Have you experienced vertigo, dizziness, or visual changes?

Headaches

The pain of migraine headaches and the effect of the migraine on the brainstem can cause syncope. Generally, the patient has associated symptoms, such as vomiting, photophobia, severe headache (often unilateral), and a strong family history of migraines. The headache continues after consciousness is regained. Consider the possibility that the headache may indicate a head injury secondary to the syncopal episode.

Vertigo, Dizziness, and Visual Symptoms

The presence of vertigo, dizziness, diplopia, or other visual changes may accompany migraine headache. Interruption in cerebral perfusion, such as with a transient ischemic attack (TIA), also must be considered.

Is this neurocardiogenic in origin?

Key Questions

- Did this occur in response to a specific situation (e.g., stressful event, urination, defecation)?
- Do you have a history a slow heart rate?

Situational Fainting

Vasovagal syncope is the most common type seen in adults and healthy children. Syncope can occur in response to urination, defecation, cough, swallowing, or emotional stress. It is neurocardiogenic and tends to occur in families. It is often precipitated by emotional stress, fear, extreme fatigue, or injury. It can occur without any obvious antecedent cause. Warm temperature, anxiety, blood drawing, and crowded rooms may cause peripheral vasodilation. Lack of large muscle activity prevents the venous return that is needed for cardiac filling with consequent bradycardia and fainting. When supine, venous return to the heart occurs, awakening the patient. Rapid standing will cause recurrence of the episode. Mental alertness is present.

Posttussive syncope follows paroxysmal coughing caused by increased intrathoracic pressure, which is then transmitted to the intracranial circulation, increasing intracranial pressure and decreasing cerebral blood flow.

Bradycardia

Postmicturition syncope, occurring during or after urination, is caused by the release of intravascular pressure on urination, which triggers vasodilation and vagally mediated bradycardia.

Key Questions

- Did you experience symptoms with rapid standing, sitting, or lying down?
- What medications are you taking?
- Have you recently started blood pressure medicine or has the dose changed?
- What other health problems or conditions do you have?

Rapid Standing

Syncope upon rapid standing is a vasovagal response caused by a drop in blood pressure, however it can also occur while sitting. It often is triggered by a stressful event, prior illness, or dehydration.

Medications

About 10% of syncopal episodes are caused by prescribed medications. Medications include antidepressants, antiarrhythmics, β-blockers, diuretics, anticholinesterase inhibitors, over-the-counter medications, and recreational drugs (e.g., alcohol, cocaine) that produce orthostasis, bradycardia, or prolonged QT interval. Adolescents may use drugs such as amyl nitrite and butyl nitrite as aphrodisiacs and euphoriants. These drugs lead to vasodilation, and syncope may occur.

Children may ingest medications that belong to family members, and a history of such activity must be investigated as a cause of the syncope.

Key Questions

- Do you have any chronic health conditions?
- Are you pregnant?

Other Health Problems or Conditions

Diabetes may induce hypoglycemia, causing a gradual syncope. Anemias and chronic gastrointestinal bleeding from an ulcer or another source may cause syncope.

Patients who are pregnant or dehydrated or who have been on prolonged bed rest are at risk for orthostatic hypotension and syncope.

Key Questions

- Have you had this before? How often?
- Did it occur with sudden head turning?
- If a child: Has the child had Kawasaki disease?
- Do you have Lyme disease?

Frequent Syncope with No Heart Disease

Psychogenic syncope is often associated with repeated episodes in which unpredictable motor reflexes appear with a lack of pathological reflexes. Blood pressure and pulse rate measurements show normal readings, and skin and mucous membranes do not change color. Panic attacks or hyperventilation are often interpreted as feeling faint, but the patient does not usually appear pale, nor are the symptoms relieved when recumbent.

After Sudden Head Rotation

Carotid sinus hypersensitivity produces a cardioinhibitory response that results in a profound drop in heart rate or may induce an abrupt vasopressor response with a drop in blood pressure.

History of Kawasaki Disease

Syncope can occur in children who have had Kawasaki disease. These children are at risk for coronary heart disease, which may present as chest pain associated with exercise.

Lyme Disease

Lyme disease can cause arrhythmia in the form of heart block, which may result in syncope.

Key Questions

- Do you have a family history of sudden death?
- Do you have a family history of fainting?

- If a child: Did the mother have systemic lupus erythematosus while pregnant?

Family History of Sudden Death

A family history of idiopathic hypertrophic subaortic stenosis is a risk factor for sudden death, and referral is necessary to rule out this condition. A history of a family member who had a myocardial infarction before age 30 years is a significant risk factor for sudden death.

Family History of Fainting

Neurocardiogenic syncope is common in families.

Prenatal Systemic Lupus Erythematosus

Systemic lupus erythematosus in a pregnant patient may cause autoimmune injury, resulting in congenital complete atrioventricular block.

DIAGNOSTIC REASONING: FOCUSED PHYSICAL EXAMINATION

Measure Blood Pressure and Pulse Rate

Obtain blood pressure readings in supine, sitting, and standing positions. Orthostatic hypotension occurs as a result of a decrease in systolic blood pressure of at least 20 mm Hg or symptoms such as fainting, weakness, or lightheadedness, which prevent continued standing.

Compare blood pressure readings in the two arms. Unequal measurements may indicate a cardiac cause of the syncope.

Bradycardia of 35 to 40 beats/min usually does not compromise cerebral blood flow. Rates below this, however, will impair cerebral circulation and function. Tachycardia up to 180 beats per minute does not usually compromise cerebral circulation.

Observe Hydration Status

Poor hydration status secondary to diuretic use, poor nutrition, or loss of fluids from vomiting and diarrhea may be associated with syncope.

Perform Heart and Lung Examination

Observe for jugular venous distention. Palpate the precordium to assess the point of maximal impulse to estimate the size of the left ventricle. Feel for lifts. Listen to the heart as the patient moves from a squat to a standing position. This maneuver may reveal a systolic ejection murmur related to dynamic left ventricular outflow obstruction. Listen for heart rate and murmurs and for radiation of murmurs. Listen for an abnormally loud second heart sound (S_2) or the presence of a third heart sound (S_3). Auscultate for carotid bruits and pericardial rub. Listen to the lungs to assess for rales associated with congestive heart failure.

Perform a Neurologic Examination

Begin with a brief mental status examination. Assess cranial nerves, deep tendon reflexes, and motor function. Perform a Romberg test as well as gait and proprioception evaluation. Assess pupillary asymmetry and look for nystagmus (see Chapter 13).

Perform an Abdominal Examination

Auscultate and observe for signs of aortic aneurysm.

Examine the Extremities

Observe lower extremities for signs of thrombophlebitis, a source of pulmonary embolism.

LABORATORY AND DIAGNOSTIC STUDIES

Suspected or Known Cardiac Cause

Electrocardiogram

The usefulness of the electrocardiogram (ECG) usually lies in identifying abnormalities that provide clues to underlying cardiac causes of syncope. These findings include evidence of conduction disorder or signs of coronary artery disease or left ventricular hypertrophy. A 12-lead ECG is used for the basic evaluation. This should be evaluated for rhythm and rate first. Hand-measured interval measurement should be made. A Q wave found in the anterolateral lead may indicate abnormal placement of the left coronary artery. A patient with a prolonged QT interval or the presence of Q waves must be referred.

Complete heart block requires immediate referral for pacemaker insertion evaluation.

Event monitoring or continuous-loop monitoring

These measures are used in patients with suspected cardiac arrhythmias as the cause of the syncope. Holter (24 hours) or long-term (weeks, months) event monitoring is used to document electrocardiographic recordings. Holter monitoring is a continuous, 24-hour ECG recording to evaluate the type and amount of irregular heartbeats during regular activities, exercise, and sleep. The patient keeps a 24-hour diary to record daily activities and any symptoms experienced.

Cardiac event monitoring is a continuous-loop, digital memory recorder worn for extended periods of time (up to 30 days or longer) that saves and records transient events felt by the patient. These monitors are patient activated, as symptoms occur or may be triggered automatically by a predefined high or low heart rate. Loop monitors save information for a predetermined period before the patient trigger and therefore can help identify the initiation sequence for arrhythmias. These stored events can be transmitted through a telephone for review.

Doppler studies

Transcranial Doppler and carotid ultrasonography are used to detect hemodynamically significant stenosis in the major intracranial or extracranial arteries.

Exercise stress test

Cardiac stress testing is performed to evaluate exercise-associated arrhythmias and syncope. It can confirm the presence of coronary artery disease.

Echocardiography

Echocardiography is used if underlying structural cardiac disease is suspected. This may include valvular disease, hypertrophic cardiomyopathy, tumor or thrombus, or left ventricular failure.

Electrophysiological studies

Electrophysiological studies are invasive tests that use electrical stimulation and monitoring to diagnose conduction disorders or the propensity for the development of tachyarrhythmia. Electrodes are threaded through arm or leg veins and placed at strategic positions in the ventricles, atria, or both. The electrodes record electrical signals and allow mapping of electrical impulses. The electrodes also can electrically stimulate the heart at programmed rates to trigger latent ventricular tachycardia.

Suspected Neurologic Cause

Baseline blood testing

Routine blood tests (electrolyte levels, renal function, blood glucose level, complete blood count) rarely yield useful diagnostic information. Most patients with abnormalities in these areas have seizures rather than syncope.

Electroencephalography

Electroencephalography may be useful in patients whose history suggests seizure.

Computed tomography scanning

Computed tomography may be useful if the patient has focal neurological findings.

Unexplained Syncope

Toxicology screen

Toxicology screening may be indicated on the basis of the history.

Tilt-table testing

Tilt-table testing is used to provoke vasovagal syncope in susceptible patients. Provocative agents such as isoproterenol or nitroglycerin may be used. Using the table, the patient is tilted upright while continuous minute-to-minute blood pressure, heart rate, and oxygen saturation measurements are recorded. Patient symptoms are recorded in each position.

Patients with neurocardiogenic syncope develop a sudden drop in heart rate or blood pressure after their body has been tilted up for several minutes. If symptoms of lightheadedness or fainting occur during this test, the test result is considered positive for neurocardiogenic syncope.

DIFFERENTIAL DIAGNOSIS

Cardiac Causes

Cardiac causes have a higher rate of mortality than do other causes of syncope. Cardiac causes include coronary artery disease, congenital and valvular disease, cardiomyopathy, arrhythmias, and conduction system disorders. Coronary artery disease, congestive heart failure, and ventricular hypertrophy can result in arrhythmias and syncope. Patients with organic heart disease may have chest pain, dyspnea, and syncope with exertion. Patients with arrhythmias may have palpitations or sudden syncope without other physical symptoms. On physical examination, murmurs or carotid bruits may be present. Other findings might include a loud S_2, precordial lift, S_3 pericardial rub, or unequal blood pressure measurements in the arms. ECG testing is indicated; other cardiac testing may be helpful.

Neurocardiogenic Causes

Vasovagal syncope is the most common type in young people, but it can occur at any age. It usually occurs in a standing position and is precipitated by fear, emotional stress, or pain. Autonomic symptoms such as nausea, sweating, blurred or fading vision, epigastric discomfort, lightheadedness, and a feeling of warmth may precede syncope by a few minutes. The syncope occurs secondary to efferent vasopressor reflexes resulting in decreased peripheral vascular resistance. Physical examination usually has normal findings. Tilt-table testing may be useful in establishing a diagnosis.

Situational syncope is vasovagal syncope with a known precipitant. It is commonly related to conditions that produce a Valsalva maneuver. Micturition, defecation, and cough are types of situational syncope. These stimuli result in autonomic reflexes with a vasopressor response, ultimately leading to transient cerebral hypotension. The physical examination has normal findings.

Carotid sinus hypersensitivity produces a cardioinhibitory response or vasopressor response that produces syncope with head turning.

Orthostasis

Orthostatic (postural) syncope indicates variable or unstable vasomotor reflexes. A drop in blood pressure when one assumes an upright position is caused by loss of vasoconstriction reflexes in the lower extremities. Sudden standing or rapid movement after assuming a standing position can trigger syncope; the prevalence of this type of syncope increases with age. The syncope is caused by hypotension that occurs as a blunted baroreceptor response and inability of the cardiovascular system to respond to hypotensive stresses. It may also occur from age-related physiological changes, volume depletion, medication, and autonomic insufficiency. Orthostatic hypotension is produced with testing.

Medication-Related Causes

Use of prescribed medications or recreational drugs can produce syncope. Medications that can cause syncope include antidepressants, antidysrhythmic medications, β-blockers, and diuretics. Recreational drugs (e.g., alcohol, cocaine) can produce orthostasis, bradycardia, or prolonged QT interval. Amyl nitrite and butyl nitrite cause vasodilation and syncope. Physical findings depend on the underlying physical condition of the patient. Syncope is a contraindication for a patient taking anticholinesterase inhibitors.

Neurologic Causes

Neurologic causes include TIAs, migraines, and seizures. Prodromal symptoms may include vertigo, diplopia, and loss of balance. Syncope results from vertebrobasilar insufficiency. In an acute syncopal attack, circulation is briefly obstructed to the reticular activating system in the brainstem, resulting in loss of consciousness. Neurological findings, such as diplopia, pupillary asymmetry, nystagmus, ataxia, and gait instability, may be present.

Psychiatric Causes

Syncope of unexplained origin may be psychogenic. Panic and anxiety disorders, somatization, major depression, and substance abuse are the main psychiatric problems associated with syncope. Physical examination usually has normal findings. Psychiatric evaluation may reveal the underlying disorder.

Unknown Causes

Syncope from unknown causes accounts for about one-third of all episodes of syncope. The workup has normal results.

▶ DIFFERENTIAL DIAGNOSIS OF *Common Causes of Syncope*

DISORDER	HISTORY	PHYSICAL FINDINGS	DIAGNOSTIC STUDIES
CARDIAC CAUSES			
Organic heart disease	Shortness of breath, chest pain, palpitations, exercise-associated syncope	May have bradycardia or tachycardia, cyanosis	Refer
Arrhythmias	Palpitations; absence of other symptoms	Loud S_2, S_3; murmur, lift	Electrocardiogram, Holter monitor, echocardiogram Doppler studies, cardiac stress testing
NEUROCARDIOGENIC CAUSES			
Vasovagal	Emotional event, standing for long periods, crowded room, warm environment	None	Tilt-table testing, CSM
Situational	Occurs with cough, micturition, defecation, swallowing	None	None
Breath holding	Children 6 mo–5 yr; associated with anger, pain, brief cry; breath-holding LOC; may have twitching	Cyanosis or pallor	None
Hyperventilation	Anxiety- or fear-induced event, shortness of breath	None	None
Cough syncope	History of asthma; coughing paroxysm awakens child from sleep, becomes flaccid with clonic muscle spasm, LOC	Wheezes	None
ORTHOSTASIS			
Orthostatic hypotension	Position change from lying or sitting to standing, pregnancy, prolonged bed rest	Hypotension on testing orthostatic blood pressure	20–mm Hg drop in systolic pressure on standing

DIFFERENTIAL DIAGNOSIS OF *Common Causes of Syncope—cont'd*

DISORDER	HISTORY	PHYSICAL FINDINGS	DIAGNOSTIC STUDIES
MEDICATION-RELATED CAUSES			
Prescribed medications	History of antidepressants, antiarrhythmic agents, β-blockers, or diuretics	Depends on underlying condition	None
Drug-induced causes	History of use of illicit drugs	Arrhythmia may be present	Toxicology screen
NEUROLOGIC CAUSES			
Migraine	Headache, vomiting, photophobia, positive family history	Usually none; nystagmus, photophobia	None
Seizures	Convulsions, incontinence, postictal phase	Usually none; nystagmus	Electroencephalogram
PSYCHIATRIC CAUSES			
Mental disorder	Symptoms consistent with depression, anxiety, panic	None	Psychiatric evaluation
Hysterical reaction	Adolescent, event occurs with audience present; gentle fall, memory of incident exact	None	None
Unknown Causes	No diagnostic characteristics	None	Workup normal results

CSM, cardiac sinus massage; *LOC,* loss of consciousness.

CHAPTER

34 Urinary Incontinence

Urinary incontinence is any involuntary loss of urine. It occurs as a result of pathological, anatomical, psychological, or physiological factors that produce obstruction, bladder irritability, or interference with neurologic functioning. Environmental factors such as decreased mobility or inaccessibility of toilet facilities may also produce periodic incontinence.

Urinary incontinence is a common problem, particularly in older adults. It is so common in older women that some think of it as normal. The prevalence in the United States is 30% to 40% in postmenopausal years. In noninstitutionalized older adults, the prevalence is 8% to 30%. In older adults in nursing homes, the rate rises to almost 50%.

Urinary incontinence in adults is categorized according to the underlying anatomical or physiological impairment. There are five main categories of urinary incontinence: stress incontinence, urge incontinence (overactive bladder), overflow incontinence, mixed incontinence, and incontinence from reversible causes.

Stress incontinence is leakage of urine during activities that increase intraabdominal pressure, such as coughing, sneezing, laughing, or other physical activities. It is caused by hypermotility at the base of the bladder and urethra associated with pelvic floor relaxation or intrinsic urethral weakness.

Urge incontinence is an abrupt and strong desire to void with the inability to delay urination and is caused by detrusor muscle hyperactivity or hypersensitive bladders, which are both caused by neurologic impairment. Detrusor muscle overactivity occurs when pathological brain disorders interfere with central inhibitory centers and fail to prevent detrusor muscle contractions.

Patients with features of both stress and urge incontinence are considered to have mixed incontinence. This occurs when incontinence is produced as the result of several anatomical or physiological factors.

Overflow incontinence occurs with overdistention of the bladder caused by an underactive or acontractile detrusor muscle; by sphincter-detrusor dyssynergia, which is loss of the synergistic urinary sphincter relaxation that normally occurs with bladder detrusor muscle contraction; or from bladder outlet or urethral obstruction. Sphincter weakness can occur from damage to the urethra or its innervation or from pelvic floor muscle relaxation.

Incontinence from reversible factors originates outside of the lower urinary tract and is caused by mental status impairment, immobility, or medication. This is also called functional or transient incontinence.

In children, involuntary discharge of urine is abnormal beyond the age of 4 years for daytime wetting and beyond the age of 6 years for nighttime wetting. Daytime wetting is diurnal enuresis while nighttime wetting is known as nocturnal or sleep enuresis. In children, enuresis may be nonorganic or organic. Nonorganic enuresis can be primary or secondary. Primary nonorganic enuresis occurs in 75% to 90% of children with enuresis. This enuresis is defined as wetting that has continued since infancy without an established pattern of dryness. Secondary nonorganic enuresis occurs in 10% to 25% of children with enuresis and is defined as recurrence of wetting after continence has been established for at least 6 months. The possibility of abnormal urinary anatomy is high in young children who present with urinary tract symptoms.

Reversible Factors That Can Cause Urinary Incontinence in Adults

D	Delirium, dementia, depression
I	Infection
A	Atrophic vaginitis/urethritis
P	Pharmaceuticals
E	Endocrine/excess urine production
R	Restricted mobility, retention
S	Stool impaction

Modified from Resnick NM: Initial evaluation of the incontinent patient, *J Am Geriatr Soc* 38:311, 1990.

DIAGNOSTIC REASONING: FOCUSED HISTORY

Adults

Could this be the result of reversible factors? (Box 34.1)

Key Questions
- What medications are you taking?
- Do you have any of the following urinary symptoms: urgency, frequency, burning, pain, blood, or flank pain?
- Do you have vaginal dryness or itching?
- Do you have pain or discomfort with sexual activity?
- Have you had changes in bowel function?
- When was your last bowel movement?

- Are you feeling depressed or "blue"?
- Are you aware of any urinary incontinence?
- How active are you?
- Are you able to get to the toilet easily?
- Do you have any chronic health problems?

Medications

Hypnotic–sedatives, diuretics, anticholinergic agents, adrenergic agents, and calcium channel blockers can cause incontinence. α-Adrenergic agonists and β-adrenergic agonists increase sphincter tone and may cause retention. Anticholinergics, prostaglandin inhibitors, calcium channel blockers, and narcotic analgesics decrease detrusor tone. Diuretics can cause incontinence because of increased production of urine. Central nervous system (CNS) depressants, such as hypnotic-sedatives, can interfere with functional ability.

Table 34.1 lists categories of medications and their mechanism of action in urinary incontinence.

Urinary Tract Infection, Vaginal Dryness, and Dyspareunia

Urinary tract infection (UTI) and atrophic vaginitis can cause incontinence through local irritation and loss of muscle tone. Pain with sexual intercourse and vaginal dryness can be a sign of atrophic vaginitis.

Table 34.1   Medications That Can Cause or Contribute to Urinary Incontinence

TYPE OF INCONTINENCE	MECHANISM OF ACTION	MEDICATION CATEGORY
Overflow	Decreased detrusor muscle tone	Anticholinergics, antidepressants, antipsychotics, sedative–hypnotics, antihistamines, narcotics, alcohol, calcium channel blockers, β-adrenergic agonists
Overflow	Sphincter contraction with outflow obstruction	α-Adrenergic agonists
Stress	Lax sphincter	α-Adrenergic antagonists
Urge	Detrusor muscle irritability from high urine volume	Diuretics
Urge	Diuretic effect	Caffeine
Urge	Functional effect of CNS depressant	Sedative–hypnotics
Urge	Diuretic effect and functional effect of CNS depressant	Alcohol

CNS, central nervous system.

Bowel Function

Fecal impaction can cause incontinence through mechanical obstruction of the urethra. Chronic constipation reduces bladder capacity.

Mental Status, Mobility, and Chronic Health Problems

Excessive urine production may be a problem if mobility is restricted, health is poor, or orientation is variable. Chronic health problems, psychological factors, and restricted mobility can result in incontinence because of loss of functional ability or mentation.

What do the presenting symptoms tell me?

Key Questions
• What is symptom most concerns you (e.g., urgency; dribbling; lack of sensation; nocturia; abdominal discomfort; burning; leakage with laughing, coughing, or sneezing)?
• How often do you urinate?
• How much urine is voided each time?
• Do you have difficulty starting to urinate?
• Does your urine stream start and stop while you are urinating?
• Do you urinate involuntarily when you cough, sneeze, or exercise?

Primary Symptom

Urgency incontinence is the primary symptom of detrusor overactivity. Symptoms of urgency incontinence are involuntary leakage with the sense of urgency to urinate.

The symptoms of stress incontinence are leakage of urine associated with increased intraabdominal pressure commonly caused by sneezing, laughing, coughing, or working out. Stress incontinence is caused by sphincter dysfunction. The severity of provoked symptoms varies based on the level of sphincter dysfunction.

Overflow incontinence is often described by urinary dribbling, urinary leakage, and the feeling of incomplete bladder emptying. Overflow incontinence is caused by dysfunctional detrusor contractility or bladder outlet obstruction. Men often report nocturia and dribbling with overflow incontinence. Abdominal discomfort often occurs with overflow incontinence because of bladder distention. A decrease in urine frequency can

be caused by overflow incontinence. This can lead to a buildup of urine in the bladder that may result in a secondary stress incontinence.

Frequency of Voiding

Increase in frequency of voiding occurs with detrusor instability or hyperactivity and may occur with some transient causes such as use of diuretics or large-volume fluid intake. Decreased frequency is common in overflow incontinence.

Amount of Urine Lost with Each Episode

Involuntary loss of small amounts of urine occurs with stress incontinence and overflow incontinence.

Character of Stream

Voiding a small-caliber or intermittent stream or difficulty in starting the stream indicates obstructive uropathy. This may be secondary to an enlarged prostate or other obstruction such as a bladder tumor or kidney stone.

Are there any other symptoms that will point me in the right direction?

Key Questions
• How much fluid do you drink in a day?
• How much caffeine and alcohol do you drink in a day?
• What time of day do you drink fluids?
• How thirsty are you?
• Have you lost or gained weight recently?
• In older adults, is the incontinence associated with gait disturbance and dementia?

Fluid Intake

A significant increase in the amount of fluid intake or an unusually large volume may indicate diabetes. Caffeine and alcohol can act as diuretics and may be a cause of reversible incontinence. Artificial sweeteners and caffeine can also be bladder irritants and either produce or exacerbate urge incontinence. A large volume of fluid intake may produce enuresis secondary to a large urine volume, particularly if fluids are consumed in the evening before bedtime.

Thirst

Unusual thirst accompanied by a large intake of fluid may indicate diabetes.

Weight Loss or Gain

Weight loss may indicate a chronic health problem, tumor, or dementia. Weight gain may indicate congestive heart failure or loss of mobility.

Dementia and Gait Disturbance

In order adult the triad of incontinence, dementia, and an abnormal gait could represent normal pressure hydrocephalus (NPH).

Children

Is this primary or secondary enuresis?

Key Questions

- Has the child ever had consistent dryness for at least 6 months?

Primary enuresis occurs when a child has never achieved consistent dryness. Secondary enuresis is involuntary voiding of urine in a child who has had a period of dryness of more than 6 months. Secondary enuresis is often indicative of some other form of voiding dysfunction or significant underlying pathology. In children, daytime urinary incontinence beyond the age of 4 years may indicate congenital abnormalities in the urinary tract or nervous system.

Is this organic enuresis?

Key Questions

- Does the child have pain on urination?
- Does the child have intermittent daytime wetness?
- Does the child seem thirsty and urinate a lot?
- Has the child had nervous system trauma?
- Does the child have constipation or encopresis?
- Does the child have constant wetness or dribbling throughout the day?
- Does the child have an abnormal stream such as dribbling or hesitancy?
- Has the child had a change in gait?
- Has the child had a recent lumbar puncture?
- Does the child snore or have apnea at night?
- Does the child report rectal itching at night?

Organic explanations of enuresis focus primarily on the genitourinary and nervous systems.

Genitourinary System

Fifteen percent of children with a UTI present with enuresis. It is unclear whether UTI causes the enuresis or vice versa. A wet perineum predisposes to ascending infection, and prompt treatment of the infection cures the enuresis in about one-third of cases. Asymptomatic bacteremia in school children is associated with enuresis.

Fecal retention that is chronic or intermittent is responsible for the production of functional bladder neck obstruction. Displacement of the bladder and posterior urethra by the full rectum in the fixed and limited space of the bony pelvis causes detrusor perineal dyssynergia, which is thought to be the mechanism responsible for urinary stasis and interference with micturition produced by constipation.

Abnormal daytime voiding suggests urologic abnormality. Dribbling suggests the presence of an ectopic ureter, labial fusion, a deeply positioned meatus, or a hymen covering the meatus. Chronic leakage of urine may indicate an ectopic ureter that terminates in the vagina. Partial distal urethral obstruction can cause straining to urinate. Polyuria from glucose-induced osmotic diuresis can be seen in patients with diabetes. Renal tubules lose their ability to concentrate urine, resulting in the production of large volumes of very dilute urine.

Nervous System

Lumbosacral disorders affect bladder innervation and may cause enuresis. Head injury or brain tumor can cause polyuria and polydipsia. If the kidneys are unable to concentrate urine because of deficiency in the hypothalamic production of antidiuretic hormone (ADH), central diabetes insipidus (DI) develops; renal unresponsiveness to ADH causes nephrogenic DI.

Interference with the nerve supply to the bladder causes a neurogenic bladder and obstruction. This can be functional, resulting from an imbalance between detrusor muscle contraction and urethral sphincter relaxation. It can also be congenital or acquired such as with meningomyelocele or spinal cord injury. Gait disturbance may suggest lower spinal cord dysfunction.

Children who snore demonstrate a decreased arousability that may contribute to the increased frequency of nocturnal enuresis. Often the snoring is a result of Obstructive Sleep Disorder. Sleep apnea interferes with the child's ability to wake appropriately in response to stimuli to void.

Other

Pinworms *(Enterobius vermicularis)* primarily inhabit the cecum and lower bowel and are the most common cause of rectal itching in children. Pinworms have been implicated in incontinence in children, although the reason is not clear.

> *What risk factors does this child have for nonorganic enuresis?*

Key Questions
- Is the child a boy or a girl?
- Is there a history of bedwetting in the family?
- Is the child a twin?
- What is the child's birth order?
- Has the child been institutionalized?
- Does the child have sickle cell disease?
- What is the child's daily fluid intake?

Gender

Boys are more likely to have nocturnal enuresis. Girls are more likely to have diurnal enuresis related to UTI.

Family History

Children with nonorganic enuresis often have a very strong family history of fathers who had nocturnal enuresis as a child.

Twin or Birth Order

Nocturnal enuresis is most common in the firstborn and in twins.

Institutionalization

Institutionalized children have a greater tendency for enuresis because of developmental delay.

Sickle Cell Disease

Children with sickle cell anemia may have a concentrating defect and excrete low-specific-gravity urine in large volumes, which may make the child wet the bed.

Fluid Intake

A large volume of fluid intake may produce enuresis secondary to a large urine volume, particularly if the fluids are consumed in the evening before bedtime.

DIAGNOSTIC REASONING: FOCUSED PHYSICAL EXAMINATION

Perform Mental Status Examination

Assess orientation and cognitive function. In adults, incontinence can occur as the result of disorientation, delirium, or dementia.

In children, secondary enuresis can be caused by the presence of stress factors during the developmental period from 2 to 4 years of age. Separation from family, death of a parent, birth of a sibling, a move, marital conflict, and other stress-related causes may produce transient and intermittent enuresis.

Observe Gait

The urinary bladder receives extensive autonomic as well as somatic innervation. Gait abnormalities can be a marker for lesions along the neuraxis from the cortex to peripheral nerves that produce abnormalities of micturition. Gait disturbance is the most prominent clinical feature of NPH. The gait disturbance features a broad-based, small-step, magnetic gait with the feet turning outwards.

Take Vital Signs

Blood pressure readings in children are important to rule out nephrotic causes of enuresis. When chronic renal failure is the result of an inadequate amount of normally functioning renal tissue, the clinical presentation may be enuresis. Fever in infants without any other signs is likely caused by UTI.

Examine the Abdomen

Palpate for masses, suprapubic tenderness, or fullness. Palpate the bladder. Abdominal distention or palpable bladder is suggestive of urinary retention and overflow incontinence.

Examine Male Genitalia

Look for abnormalities of the foreskin, glans, meatus, penis, and perineal skin that might contribute to or produce incontinence.

Perform Pelvic Examination

Note signs of pelvic prolapse (cystocele, rectocele). Palpate for a pelvic mass and perivaginal muscle tone. Note the condition of the vaginal mucosa and look for atrophic vaginitis, which will produce incontinence in adults.

Examine the Vaginal Area in Girls

Place the child on the caretaker's lap in a frog leg position. Examine the labia and vagina. Reddened labia and vagina may signal vaginitis, which can cause urinary incontinence in children.

Observe for evidence of sexual abuse such as abrasions, tears, or bruising. Urethral irritation, especially if discharge is present, may indicate sexual abuse in children.

Perform Provocative Stress Testing

During the pelvic examination, ask the patient to relax and then cough vigorously (or perform a Valsalva maneuver). Watch for urine loss from the urethra, which indicates stress incontinence.

Perform Digital Rectal Examination

Assess for perineal sensation, resting and active sphincter tone, rectal mass, fecal impaction, and fissures. A lax sphincter suggests spinal cord involvement. Use the fifth digit for rectal examination in children, feeling for stool in the rectal vault.

In men, assess the consistency and contour of the prostate. Prostate enlargement or masses suggest the possibility of overflow incontinence from obstruction.

Conduct a Neurologic Examination

Assess the intactness of the neurologic system. Note focal deficits, test deep tendon reflexes, and test for sensation in the perineal and perirectal areas. Assess spinal nerve roots S2 to S4 by testing anal reflex and sphincter tone. To test the anal reflex, lightly stroke the circumanal skin and watch for contraction of the external anal sphincter (anal wink). Test for muscle tone and strength. Deficits may point to a neurologic cause of the incontinence.

Examine and Palpate the Spine in Children

Look for an undetected birth defect that may be causing a neurologic disturbance. A spinal dimple or hair tuft may alert you to a potential problem.

Perform Musculoskeletal Examination

Assess mobility, strength, and functional ability. In many older adults, the inability to get to a toilet causes incontinence.

An easy assessment of mobility is the timed get-up-and-go test. Time the patient getting up from a chair, walking 10 feet, and sitting back down. Although the time required to perform this test will vary, an older adult who is mobile and independent can perform this activity in about 10 seconds.

Additional Procedures

Postvoid residual

Have the patient void without straining and then catheterize or perform bedside ultrasound. A residual volume greater than 100 mL suggests either bladder weakness (stress incontinence) or outlet obstruction (overflow incontinence).

Observe voiding

Note hesitancy, dribbling, interrupted stream, and decreased force or caliber of stream. These symptoms suggest outlet obstruction and overflow incontinence.

LABORATORY AND DIAGNOSTIC STUDIES

Urinalysis

Dipstick urinalysis (U/A) can rule out or point to infection or systemic disease as a cause of the incontinence. Note hematuria, pyuria, bacteriuria, or the presence of leukocyte esterase or nitrites as indicators of UTI. Glycosuria or proteinuria may indicate diabetes or renal disease.

Specific Gravity

A specific gravity greater than 1.015 rules out diabetes insipidus as the cause of incontinence.

Urine Culture

A culture can be used to determine the organism(s) producing a UTI and can confirm the diagnosis.

Urine Cytology

Urine for cytology is indicated if microscopic or gross painless hematuria is present in the absence of infection.

Bladder Diary

A 24-hour bladder diary (3-day voiding diary for children) can provide an accurate record of urine output, average voided volume, frequency of voiding, frequency and nature of incontinent episodes, as well as the type and volume of fluid intake. Patients or parents can use a measuring cup to catch and measure urine output.

Blood Urea Nitrogen and Creatinine

Use these indicators of renal function if you suspect obstruction or urinary retention.

Vaginal Specimen Microscopy, Molecular Testing, or Culture

These tests can confirm vaginal infection. See Chapter 37 for the procedures for these tests.

Office Cystometrography

Have the patient void and empty the bladder. Have men lie supine and place women in the dorsal lithotomy position. Insert a sterile 12 to 14 French (nonballooned) catheter and empty the bladder. (Measure the postvoid residual and collect urine for U/A at that time.) Insert a 50-mL syringe with the plunger removed into the end of the catheter and position it about 15 cm above the urethra. Fill the syringe by pouring sterile water into it in 25- to 50-mL increments. Record cumulative total fluid instillation in the bladder and note the volume at which the patient first reports the urge to void. Continue adding fluid slowly until the fluid level in the syringe rises, indicating an increase in intrabladder pressure and contraction of the detrusor muscle. The rise may be gradual or sudden. Detrusor contraction at less than 300 to 350 mL of bladder volume indicates detrusor instability (urge incontinence). Have the patient void at the end of the procedure. The amount instilled minus the amount voided will also provide a measure of postvoid residual.

Urodynamic Testing

Complete urodynamic testing includes uroflowmetry, cystometrography, perineal electromyelography, and voiding cystourethrography. It is indicated when patient symptoms do not correlate with objective physical findings, when results may change management, after treatment failure, or if more

information is needed to plan further therapy (see the Evidence-Based Practice box, Urodynamic Testing).

Cystoscopy and Contrast Radiography

These procedures are indicated for detection of neoplasms or stones.

Ultrasound

Ultrasonography may be useful in determining the presence of an obstruction.

Magnetic Resonance Imaging

Although not diagnostic, magnetic resonance imaging (MRI) can be useful in evaluating patients with possible NPH to determine ventricular and sulcal size.

DIFFERENTIAL DIAGNOSIS

Incontinence from Anatomical Causes

Stress incontinence

Stress incontinence is associated with activities that increase intraabdominal pressure, such as coughing, sneezing, running, or laughing. The underlying abnormality is typically urethral hypermotility as a result of inadequate pelvic support of the bladder neck (urethrovesical junction). Normally, increased intraabdominal pressure is transmitted evenly across the bladder neck and body. When adequate support is lacking, an increase in intraabdominal pressure displaces the bladder neck outside the abdominal cavity. The subsequent disproportionate increase in bladder pressure as compared to urethral pressure results in urine loss. Poor urethral sphincter function also contributes to stress incontinence. The amount of urine lost with each episode is small. The patient usually has a history of childbirth. On examination, pelvic floor relaxation may be evident with the presence of a cystocele or rectocele. The urethral sphincter may appear lax, and there is loss of urine with provocative testing. Atrophic vaginitis is a common finding in postmenopausal women. U/A and culture may be performed to rule out infections or urinary tract problems. Postvoid residual is normal.

> ## EVIDENCE-BASED PRACTICE *Urodynamic Testing*
>
> A Cochrane systematic review compared outcomes in women with urinary incontinence based on urodynamic testing. The authors concluded that women assessed using urodynamic testing in addition to clinical methods were more likely to receive medication or surgical treatment. However, there was insufficient evidence to show whether they were less likely to be incontinent after treatment than women who did not have urodynamic tests. The authors concluded that larger definitive trials are needed to determine if performance of urodynamics results in higher continence rates after treatment. No data were available to evaluate the use of urodynamics in other patient groups.

Reference: Clement et al, 2013.

Urge incontinence

Urge incontinence is characterized by an uncontrolled urge to void, secondary to detrusor muscle irritability or hyperactivity or to a hypersensitive bladder. Most cases result from an idiopathic inability to suppress detrusor contraction. The urine volume lost is large. Physical examination results are usually normal. Postvoid residual is normal. Diagnostic testing includes U/A and culture to rule out infection and determination of blood urea nitrogen and creatinine levels to rule out nephropathy. On office cystometrography, the urine volume is less than 300 to 350 mL before the urge to void occurs. Complete urodynamic testing can confirm the diagnosis.

For more information, see the Evidence-Based Practice box: Determining the Type of Urinary Incontinence.

Mixed incontinence

Patients who experience symptoms of both stress and urge incontinence are considered to have mixed incontinence. It is important to determine which symptom is predominant and most bothersome to the patient and treat it first.

Overflow incontinence

Overflow incontinence occurs in the presence of obstruction or interruption in the nervous system. It is a result of overdistention of the bladder from an underactive or acontractile detrusor muscle, from sphincter-detrusor dyssynergia (loss of the synergistic urinary sphincter relaxation that normally occurs with bladder detrusor muscle contraction), or from bladder outlet or urethral obstruction. Sphincter weakness can occur from damage to the urethra, errors in its innervation, or from pelvic floor muscle relaxation. Interference with the nerve supply to the bladder can result in neurogenic bladder obstruction, and consequent overflow incontinence caused by an imbalance between detrusor muscle contraction and urethral sphincter relaxation. Overflow incontinence can also be congenital or acquired, such as with meningomyelocele or spinal cord injury, or can be a surgical complication from radical prostatectomy. On examination, the anal sphincter may be lax. Neurologic testing may reveal deficits.

Overflow incontinence is small-volume incontinence, with symptoms of dribbling and hesitancy. In men, symptoms of an enlarged prostate may be present (i.e., nocturia, dribbling, hesitancy, and decreased force and caliber of stream). On examination, look for a distended bladder, prostate hypertrophy, evidence of spinal cord disease, or neuropathy. Postvoid residual is more than 100 mL. Diagnostic testing includes U/A, urine culture, and determination of blood urea nitrogen and creatinine levels.

Incontinence from Reversible Factors (Functional Incontinence)

Medications

Sedatives, hypnotics, diuretics, anticholinergic agents, α-adrenergic agents, and calcium channel blockers can cause incontinence.

α-Adrenergic agonists and β-adrenergic agonists increase sphincter tone and may cause retention; they can also cause urge incontinence. Anticholinergics, prostaglandin inhibitors, calcium channel blockers, and narcotic analgesics decrease detrusor tone and can produce incontinence. Diuretics can cause incontinence because of increased production of urine, and CNS depressants such as hypnotic-sedatives can interfere with functional ability.

Urinary tract infection

The patient with a UTI has symptoms of lower or upper tract infection such as burning, dysuria, frequency, urgency, flank pain, and fever. The urine may have a foul odor. The patient may exhibit suprapubic or costovertebral angle (CVA) tenderness. In infants, a fever with no localizing signs frequently indicates UTI. U/A and culture can confirm the diagnosis of a lower UTI (see Chapter 35). Older adults are prone to recurrent UTI and may present atypically (no fever or dysuria).

Vaginitis

Vaginitis produces incontinence as a result of local irritation. Atrophic vaginitis indicates a loss of estrogen and a concomitant loss of the vesicourethral angle, which predisposes women to stress incontinence. Provocative stress testing can demonstrate stress incontinence. Microscopy, DNA testing, or culture can confirm vaginal infection (see Chapter 37).

Constipation and fecal impaction

Constipation or fecal impaction can produce obstructive overflow incontinence by mechanical pressure on the urethra. The patient may experience abdominal pain and fecal soiling. On examination, stool may be felt in the colon or ampulla.

Change in mental or functional status

Depression, dementia (late middle to late stage) and delirium can all produce incontinence (see Chapter 9). Restricted mobility can result in incontinence because of loss of functional ability.

Diabetes insipidus

In DI, the kidneys are unable to concentrate urine because of a deficiency in the hypothalamic production of ADH (central DI) or a renal unresponsiveness to ADH (nephrogenic DI). The result is polyuria, which may cause incontinence. The patient also exhibits polydipsia. Urine specific gravity will be less than 1.015.

Diabetes mellitus

Diabetes often presents with excessive fluid intake and urination. The excess fluid volume may result in incontinence, particularly in older adults with chronic health problems, restricted mobility, or compromise in mental or functional health. U/A can screen for glycosuria. Follow-up testing should include fasting blood glucose level and hemoglobin A_{1C} measurement.

Hyperthyroidism

Patients with hyperthyroidism may report urgency, urge incontinence, nocturia, and enuresis.

Incontinence from Organic Causes

Genitourinary causes

Genitourinary disorders that can produce enuresis include UTI, ectopic ureter, iatrogenic damage to the external sphincter, and urethral obstruction. Physical examination findings are usually normal. Fever and abdominal tenderness may be present with a UTI. Anatomical genitourinary abnormalities may signal an ectopic ureter. Diagnostic testing includes urinalysis, urine culture, and specific gravity to rule out infection and diabetes. Referral for further evaluation may be necessary.

Neurologic causes

Nervous system involvement can also produce enuresis. Lumbosacral disorders affect bladder innervation and may cause enuresis. Head injury or brain tumor can cause polyuria and polydipsia. Interference with the nerve supply to the bladder causes neurogenic bladder and obstruction, which can result in enuresis. Interference in innervation can occur from congenital or acquired causes. Diagnostic testing includes urinalysis, urine culture, and specific gravity to rule out infection and diabetes. Referral for further evaluation may be necessary. Some children with sleep apnea have been found to have an increased atrial natriuretic factor, inhibiting the renin–angiotensin–aldosterone pathway, causing enuresis.

In older adults NPH may result in the classic triad of urinary incontinence, dementia and gait disturbance. Urinary urgency rather than incontinence may be present at early stages. Detrusor muscle instability is compounded by the gait disorder which may interfere with the patient's ability to reach the bathroom in time. In later stages urinary incontinence is accompanied by indifference, reflecting its probable origin in frontal lobe impairment.

Enuresis from Nonorganic Causes in Children

Primary enuresis

Primary enuresis occurs when a child has never achieved consistent dryness. The normal developmental patterns of micturition follow a characteristic pattern in children, but at an individual rate. The usual progression depends on the maturation of the CNS. Generally, the following stages are seen:

Birth to 6 months: Bladder emptying is an uninhibited reflex action.

6 to 12 months: Bladder emptying is less frequent because of CNS inhibition of reflex action.

1 to 2 years: Child consciously perceives bladder fullness; CNS inhibition increases.

3 to 5 years: At age 5 years, most children are aware of bladder fullness; they develop the ability to inhibit the need to void, both voluntarily and unconsciously.

Primary enuresis may represent a developmental delay or maturational lag. Often there is a family history of enuresis. The enuresis usually is only nocturnal. The incidence is higher in boys than in girls and usually resolves as the child matures. Physical examination findings are normal. Diagnostic testing includes urinalysis, urine culture, and specific gravity to rule out other causes.

Developmental (secondary) enuresis

Developmental enuresis that is secondary may be related to changes or stresses in a child's life. It can also occur as the result of genital trauma, infection, distended colon, or fecal impaction. The enuresis occurs in a child who has had a period of dryness of more than 6 months. Diagnostic testing includes urinalysis, urine culture, and specific gravity to rule out other causes.

Small bladder

An anatomically small bladder can also produce enuresis. The child voids frequently but not an excessive volume. Physical examination findings are normal. Diagnostic testing includes urinalysis, urine culture, and specific gravity to rule out other causes.

Sickle cell anemia

Children with sickle cell anemia have a concentrating defect and may experience enuresis because of volume excess. Physical examination findings are consistent with the sickle cell disorder. Diagnostic testing includes urinalysis, urine culture, and specific gravity.

▶ DIFFERENTIAL DIAGNOSIS OF *Common Causes of Urinary Incontinence*

CONDITION	HISTORY	PHYSICAL FINDINGS	DIAGNOSTIC STUDIES
INCONTINENCE FROM ANATOMICAL CAUSES			
Stress incontinence	Small-volume incontinence with coughing, sneezing, laughing, running; history of prior pelvic surgery	Pelvic floor relaxation; cystocele, rectocele; lax urethral sphincter; loss of urine with provocative testing; atrophic vaginitis	U/A and culture; PVR normal
Urge incontinence	Uncontrolled urge to void; large-volume incontinence; history of CNS disorders, such as stroke, multiple sclerosis, parkinsonism	Normal examination; may have neurologic deficits	U/A and culture; PVR normal; office cystometrography: <300- to 350-mL volume; BUN, creatinine, urodynamic testing
Mixed incontinence	Symptoms of both stress and urge incontinence	Finding related to stress and urge incontinence	U/A and culture; PVR; office cystometrography
Overflow incontinence	Small-volume incontinence, dribbling, hesitancy; in men symptoms of enlarged prostate: nocturia, dribbling, hesitancy, decreased force and caliber of stream; in neurogenic bladder: history of bowel problems, spinal cord injury, or multiple sclerosis	Distended bladder; prostate hypertrophy, stool in rectum; fecal impaction; in neurogenic bladder: evidence of spinal cord disease or diabetic neuropathy; lax sphincter; gait disturbance	U/A and culture; PVR >100 mL; BUN, creatinine; in neurogenic bladder, refer for testing
INCONTINENCE FROM REVERSIBLE FACTORS (FUNCTIONAL)			
Medications	Hypnotics, diuretics, anticholinergic agents, α-adrenergic agents, calcium channel blockers	Normal except for findings related to other physical conditions	U/A to rule out urinary tract problems; blood chemistry to rule out systemic problem
Urinary tract infection (UTI)	Dysuria, urgency, daytime accidents	Frequency, odor, fever	U/A and culture
Vaginitis	Itching, odor	Discharge, atrophic vaginitis, evidence of sexual abuse	Gram stain, KOH, culture, molecular testing
Constipation/fecal impaction	Abdominal pain	Soiling; stool felt in colon or ampulla	None
Change in mental or functional status	Change in mental status; impaired mobility; new environment	Impaired mental status; impaired mobility	U/A and culture; blood chemistry

▶ DIFFERENTIAL DIAGNOSIS OF *Common Causes of Urinary Incontinence—cont'd*

CONDITION	HISTORY	PHYSICAL FINDINGS	DIAGNOSTIC STUDIES
Diabetes insipidus (DI)	History of trauma to head; thirst, frequency	Weight loss	U/A specific gravity >1.015
Diabetes	Thirsty, increased frequency	Weight loss	U/A; serum glucose
INCONTINENCE FROM ORGANIC CAUSES			
Genitourinary causes	UTI history; dribbling; urine leakage	Fever, abdominal tenderness; anatomical abnormalities (ectopic ureter); examination may be normal	U/A and culture; specific gravity; referral for testing
Neurologic causes	Head injury; spinal cord injury; polydipsia, polyuria; sleep apnea; NPH	Lax sphincter, spinal tuft, neurologic deficits; altered gait; examination may be normal	U/A and culture; specific gravity; referral for evaluation
ENURESIS FROM NONORGANIC CAUSES IN CHILDREN			
Primary enuresis	Child has never been dry; may have family history	Normal examination; developmental delay	U/A and culture; specific gravity to rule out other causes
Developmental (secondary) enuresis	Child has been dry for 6 mo in a row; changes or stresses in child's life	Examine for genital trauma or abuse, infection, distended colon, fecal impaction	U/A and culture; specific gravity to rule out other causes; screen for glycosuria
Small bladder	Void frequently, not in excessive volume	None	Bladder capacity = child's age + 2 yr, for children < 11 yr
Sickle cell anemia	Family history	Findings related to sickle cell disease	U/A and culture; specific gravity

BUN, blood urea nitrogen; *CNS,* central nervous system; *KOH,* potassium hydroxide; *NPH,* normal pressure hydrocephalus; *PVR,* postvoid residual; *U/A,* urinalysis.

Urinary Problems in Patients with Female Genitalia

Common adult urinary concerns include changes in usual urination patterns (frequency, urgency, nocturia, incontinence), changes in urine appearance (color, cloudiness), and pain (dysuria, flank pain, or suprapubic pain).

Urinary problems in adults can be caused by infection, inflammation, calculi (stones), congenital malformation, or trauma. The majority of urinary tract infections (UTIs) are caused by gram-negative bacteria, predominantly *Escherichia coli*. The sexually transmitted pathogens *Chlamydia trachomatis, Neisseria gonorrhoeae,* and herpes simplex are common causes of urethritis. Vaginitis can also cause urinary symptoms. Urinary stones can occur anywhere in the urinary tract and are common causes of pain, bleeding, obstruction, and secondary infection.

In children, UTI is the second most common clinical disorder after respiratory tract disorders. The symptoms of urinary tract disorder may be vague or absent, making the diagnosis easily overlooked. Infection may be present without symptoms, with symptoms that are obviously related to the urinary system, or with symptoms that may divert attention to another organ system problem. Abdominal masses in newborns are most frequently caused by renal enlargement, specifically dysplastic kidney, or congenital hydronephrosis. Vesicoureteral reflux (VUR) is the major structural abnormality associated with UTI and renal damage.

DIAGNOSTIC REASONING: FOCUSED HISTORY

Are there systemic or upper urinary tract symptoms present?

Key Questions
- Have you had a fever, body aches, or chills?
- Have you had nausea or vomiting?

- Have you had acute pain in the abdomen or back?
- Are you positive for HIV infection? Are you receiving chemotherapy? or immunosuppressant therapy?
- In an infant: Has the infant been irritable or had anorexia or lethargy?

Fever, Body Aches, and Chills

The presence of fever and chills suggests a systemic inflammatory response and indicates an acute condition that should be treated aggressively. Suspect pyelonephritis or lithiasis of the upper urinary system. UTI is the most common bacterial infection in febrile infants and children who have no obvious source of infection.

Nausea and Vomiting

Nausea and vomiting often accompany upper UTI, pyelonephritis, or lithiasis. Like fever and chills, these symptoms suggest a systemic inflammatory response and indicate that the patient may be acutely ill. In newborns and infants, nonspecific symptoms such as vomiting, diarrhea, and feeding difficulties may indicate UTI.

Acute Pain

Acute pain in the back or abdomen suggests upper UTI and pyelonephritis. Flank pain occurs with stretching of the renal capsule associated with parenchymal swelling and may indicate infection, obstruction, or primary renal disease.

Urinary tract stones may produce localized back pain or excruciating pain that often radiates to the thigh.

Immunocompromised Patients

Immunocompromised patients are susceptible to overwhelming infections by both common and atypical organisms, and aggressive investigation is warranted.

Irritable Infant

Urinary tract infection in neonates and infants is manifested in subtle ways such as irritability, anorexia, and weight loss. Some infants with UTI present with bacteremia.

Is there hematuria?

Key Questions

- Have you had blood in your urine? When in the stream does it occur?
- Do you have pain with urination?
- Do you have bleeding without urination?
- Have you done any strenuous exercise recently?

Hematuria

Red to brown discoloration is commonly caused by infection, trauma, or urinary tract stones. It may also be caused by parenchymal renal disease, systemic disease, medications, coagulopathies, or bladder cancer.

Pyelonephritis or urinary tract stones are common causes of gross (macroscopic) hematuria. Neoplasm, trauma, and some medications can also produce gross hematuria. Gross hematuria occurs in 60% to 90% of bladder tumors. Hematuria can be produced by local irritation in cystitis. Platelet disorders and hemophilia can cause both gross and microscopic bleeding. Urinary frequency or urgency, dysuria, or suprapubic pain suggests that the origin of hematuria is confined to the lower urinary tract.

Whereas initial hematuria (at the beginning of urination) suggests the urethra is the source, terminal hematuria (at the end of urination) suggests posterior urethra or bladder base involvement. Total hematuria means red blood cells are dispersed throughout the urinary stream, characterizing origination in the kidney, ureter, or bladder.

Pain

Hematuria without pain is usually caused by renal disease or cancer of the bladder or kidney. Other causes of painless hematuria include stones, polycystic kidney disease, renal cysts, sickle cell disease, and hydronephrosis. When discomfort such as renal colic accompanies hematuria, suspect a ureteral stone.

Hematuria with dysuria suggests bladder infection or lithiasis.

Bleeding Without Urination

Bladder lesions may produce bleeding independent of micturition.

Strenuous Exercise

Transient hematuria occasionally occurs after strenuous exercise. The amount of bleeding is proportional to the amount of exercise and the trauma sustained by the urinary tract. Exercise-related hematuria is caused by direct trauma to the kidneys and bladder as well as by ischemic injury. It is caused by the shifting of blood flow from the renal circulation to the heart, lungs, and skeletal muscles during periods of high oxygen demand.

Can the symptoms be localized to the lower urinary tract?

Key Questions

- What are your primary symptoms (e.g., pain, frequency, urgency, small amounts of urine, nausea, nocturia, itching)?
- Have you had any suprapubic pain?
- Do you have involuntary urination?

Primary Symptoms

Dysuria suggests inflammation of the bladder neck or urethra, which is usually caused by bacterial infection or irritation that injures the bladder mucosa and leads to inflammatory changes, infiltration, and edema. These changes, from mild stretching of the bladder to a loss of bladder elasticity, can result in urgency and frequency.

Dysuria is the cardinal symptom of uncomplicated lower UTI (acute bacterial cystitis). In children, it may also be the first indication of an anatomical lesion such as obstruction of the urinary tract or vesicoureteral reflux (VUR). Other common symptoms include frequency, mild nausea, nocturia, urgency, and voiding small amounts. Fever is notably absent. Infants may have strong-smelling urine and continuously damp diapers.

Dysuria also suggests urethritis, especially if accompanied by vaginal discharge. External dysuria, a burning sensation as the urine passes the inflamed labia, suggests vulvo-vaginitis. Patients with vulvovaginitis may also report discharge, odor, or itching. Patients with active herpes lesions may also experience external dysuria. Young children with pinworms *(Enterobius vermicularis)* may have dysuria and vaginitis because of the abrasions that result from periurethral and perivaginal itching and scratching.

Interstitial cystitis produces diminished bladder capacity along with symptoms of frequent painful urination. Hematuria may be present. Increased frequency can also occur as a result of stones or a tumor.

Suprapubic Discomfort and Urinary Incontinence

Discomfort in the suprapubic area is indicative of bladder involvement and urinary incontinence and is characteristic of bladder neck irritability caused by inflammation. Local causes of incontinence can also include pelvic relaxation and impaired bladder muscle activity. Preschool-age children with UTIs frequently have enuresis (see Chapter 34).

Could this be the result of trauma?

Key Questions
- Have you had any recent injury?
- Have you been hit recently?
- If a child: Have you noticed the child putting foreign objects in his or her genitourinary tract?

Recent Injury

An injury or a blow to the flank area can produce hematuria originating from the kidney. Straddle injury may result in abrasions and local inflammation, causing pain on urination. About 5% of childhood trauma involves the kidney, making it a relatively uncommon event. About 10% of the injured kidneys have underlying abnormalities, such as hydronephrosis or a horseshoe shape, making them more vulnerable to injury.

Trauma

Physical injury to the trunk, including trauma from domestic violence, may cause blood in the urine. Trauma may or may not be associated with pain. Active children may not remember trauma to the area.

Foreign Objects

Children have a propensity to put foreign objects in any orifice. Placing foreign objects in the vagina can cause dysuria and pyuria.

Could this be genitourinary in origin?

Key Questions
- Are you sexually active? How frequently do you engage in sexual activity?
- Have you had a new sexual partner recently?
- How many sexual partners do you have?
- Does your sexual partner have any symptoms?
- Do you use spermicidal gel?
- Do you use a diaphragm?
- Do you have vaginal discharge?
- If a child: Have parents noticed masturbation?
- Are you taking hormones?

Sexual Activity

Factors that contribute to the development of acute bacterial cystitis include frequent sexual intercourse, use of a diaphragm, and use of spermicidal gel for contraception. Urethritis is associated with a history of a new sexual partner, a partner with urethritis, and multiple sexual partners. Masturbation may also cause dysuria as a result of either local irritation or the introduction of organisms that produce a lower UTI.

Organisms from sexually transmitted infections (STI) can cause urethritis when they are present in large numbers in the urethra, which may result in a local inflammatory response. The most common pathogen of urethritis is *C. trachomatis,* but *N. gonorrhoeae, Trichomonas vaginalis,* and herpes simplex are also seen with urethritis. Active herpes lesions may also produce dysuria as the urine passes across the inflamed external mucosa.

Diaphragm Use

Some patients who use a diaphragm experience mechanical compression of the urethra, with subsequent urine retention that predisposes them to the development of cystitis.

Vaginal Discharge and Hormone Therapy

Vaginal infections are a common cause of dysuria. Atrophic vaginitis can also cause dysuria. Postmenopausal patients who are not on hormone therapy are more likely to have atrophic vaginitis. Transgender men on testosterone therapy are likely to have atrophic vaginitis.

Are there any specific risk factors to point me in the right direction?

Key Questions
- Have you had this or similar problems before? If yes, when and how many times?
- Have you had recent catheterization or urinary tract procedures performed?
- Is there a family history of kidney or urinary problems?
- Do you have diabetes?
- How much spicy food, caffeinated beverages/food, carbonated beverages, or alcohol do you consume?
- How much water do you drink?
- Do you suppress the urge to urinate (postpone urination)?
- Do you use bubble baths, shampoos, feminine hygiene products, powders, and soaps?
- Do you have constipation?
- If a child, is there a history of breathing disorder with sleep?

History of Similar Problems

Patients with previous urinary problems are at risk for chronic relapsing conditions such as unresolved infections, resistant strains of organisms, or reinfection.

Recent Instrumentation

Recent instrumentation in the urinary tract places the patient at risk for infections.

Family History of Urinary Problems

A family history of renal or urinary tract problems places the patient at increased risk for urinary tract disorders. A family history of deafness or renal insufficiency suggests hereditary nephritis or Alport syndrome.

History of Diabetes Mellitus

Diabetes mellitus or a history of impaired glucose tolerance is associated with recurrent bacterial cystitis.

Types of Food Consumed

Dysuria without pyuria can be caused by chemical irritants such as spicy foods, caffeine, carbonated beverages, and alcohol.

Decreased or Increased Fluid Intake

Decreased fluid intake and concentrated urine produce an irritant effect on bladder mucosa and may cause dysuria without pyuria. It can also predispose to the development of bacterial cystitis.

Excessive nocturnal fluid intake may cause nocturnal enuresis.

Urge to Urinate

Patients who ignore the urge to urinate or who postpone urination are predisposed to the development of bacterial cystitis. Urine in the bladder for a prolonged period promotes bacterial growth.

Children who have a history of squatting or leg crossing to stop urination may have a UTI. Uncontrolled bladder contractions against a closed bladder sphincter cause the behavior. These children may develop VUR and infection.

Bubble Bath and Hygiene Products

Common chemical irritants can cause dysuria without infection. The most common irritant, particularly for children, is found in bubble baths.

Constipation

Mechanical factors related to compression of the bladder and bladder neck by a hard mass of stool from constipation may cause UTI. There is also a relationship between constipation and dysfunctional voiding accompanied by incomplete bladder emptying.

Breathing Disorder

Sleep disordered breathing such as sleep apnea is a common cause of nocturnal enuresis.

Key Questions
- Have you had recent treatment for an STI?
- Have you been diagnosed with, but not treated for, an STI?
- Have you had excessive urination?
- Have you had a sore throat or been treated for strep throat recently?

Sexually Transmitted Infections

Because vaginitis can cause urinary tract symptoms, a sexually transmitted vaginitis may be producing symptoms. The need for recent treatment of an STI may indicate treatment failure, a coinfection that was not covered by the prescribed drug, or a reinfection (see Chapter 37).

Excessive Urination

The presence of polyuria suggests diabetes mellitus or diabetes insipidus. Patients with diabetes mellitus are also prone to development of UTIs. Polyuria is defined as a volume greater than 3 L of urine/day and depends on fluid intake and the patient's state of hydration. Polyuria may be an early indication of renal disease progression because of the kidneys' inability to concentrate urine. Taking a history of fluid intake is important to identify possible causes of polyuria. Pseudo polyuria results from increased fluid ingestion and may present with certain personality disorders or as a result of excessive water intake as part of a health regimen.

Recent Streptococcal Infection

Poststreptococcal glomerulonephritis may develop after a 1- to 3-week latency period after pharyngeal or skin infections with certain strains of group A β-hemolytic streptococci. The peak incidence is at age 7 years.

DIAGNOSTIC REASONING: FOCUSED PHYSICAL EXAMINATION

Note General Appearance

A patient who appears ill or who is pacing in pain is likely to have an upper urinary tract problem such as pyelonephritis or urolithiasis. Patients with lower urinary tract problems usually do not present with signs of systemic involvement, are not febrile, and generally appear well. Neonates present with malaise, irritability, and difficulty feeding. Toddlers and preschoolers appear ill with nausea, vomiting, and diarrhea.

Obtain Vital Signs, Height, and Weight

Failure to thrive is a common presenting sign of urinary tract disease in neonates and young children. Hypertension is seen in patients with nephritis.

Examine the Skin

Neonates with UTIs may present with jaundice.

Palpate and Percuss for Flank Pain and at the Costovertebral Angle Bilaterally

Pain that is reproducible is indicative of renal capsule distention and characterizes acute pyelonephritis or acute ureteral obstruction.

Palpate and Percuss the Abdomen

Polycystic kidneys may produce abdominal distention. A flank mass may indicate a hydronephrotic kidney. Pain in the lower quadrant indicates lower ureter involvement. Suprapubic tenderness is characteristic of lower UTI. Perform deep palpation to identify kidney or other abdominal masses. Normal kidneys are usually not easily palpated. A distended bladder rises above the symphysis pubis and is characteristic of residual urine resulting from incomplete bladder emptying. Palpation of an enlarged bladder may cause pain. In hypertensive patients, auscultate at the subcostal anterior abdomen for bruits that could indicate a renovascular cause of hypertension.

Inspect the Perirectal Area

Inspect the skin and hair for inflammation, lesions, parasites, and dermatitis. Note inflammation, presence of lesions, or vaginal discharge. Observe for the presence of labial adhesions that might predispose the child to perineal bacterial colonization. Note personal hygiene. External excoriation could be the cause of burning or pain on urination.

Note if there are any abrasions, tears, or bruising present which might indicate trauma or sexual abuse.

Perform a Pelvic Examination if Indicated

A pelvic examination is essential if you suspect vaginitis or vulvovaginitis as a cause of the urinary tract symptom(s). On external examination, observe for bladder or uterine prolapse. On internal examination, note vaginal color, moistness, rugae of vagina, and characteristics of discharge. Pale, dry mucosa with lack of rugae characterizes atrophic vaginitis. Vaginal discharge not characteristic of physiological discharge suggests a vaginal infection. (For a discussion of vulvovaginitis, see Chapter 37.) Determine rectal tone. An atonic anal sphincter suggests a neurogenic bladder. Rectal examination for fecal impaction is indicated if the history suggests significant constipation or encopresis.

Laboratory and Diagnostic Studies

The extent of diagnostic investigation is determined by the history and the findings of the examination. The symptoms reported by the patient are taken into account when ordering diagnostic tests to corroborate or verify the diagnosis. General screening tests can be used to provide additional data for patients with urinary tract problems.

Urine should be freshly voided and preferably taken midstream. If not examined immediately, the specimen should be refrigerated because cells begin to disintegrate after 1 to 2 hours.

Urine Dipstick

Reagent strips can be used to screen urine in the clinical setting. A positive Leukocyte esterase test result is indicative of urethritis (75%–90% sensitivity, 95% specificity). Urine that tests positive for leukocyte esterase may require culture for bacteria. Vaginal infection with *Trichomonas* spp. can produce false-positive results; diets high in vitamin C can produce false-negative results.

Urine that tests positive for nitrites may require culture for bacteria. However, note that some organisms that cause UTIs do not convert nitrates to nitrites (e.g., staphylococci and streptococci).

Proteinuria may indicate kidney involvement. Suspect proximal renal tubular damage if urine glucose is elevated while serum glucose levels are normal.

Hematuria can be caused by urethritis, hemorrhagic cystitis, renal stones, or tumors of the kidney, renal pelvis, ureter, bladder, and urethra.

Urinalysis with Microscopic Examination

Color

The urine should be clear to yellow, depending on the concentration. The precipitation of calcium phosphate or urates can turn the urine milky, especially when stored in the refrigerator. Warming the urine to body temperature causes these precipitated salts to return to solution, removing the milky appearance. Methylene blue and indigo blue can make the urine blue. Vegetable dyes and paint from toys ingested by young children can turn their urine various colors. Brown urine is often observed in glomerulonephritis. Turbidity with a foul odor indicates infection. Color changes of the urine may result from various sources: hemoglobin from systemic red blood cell lysis; myoglobin from damaged muscle cells or rhabdomyolysis; vegetable pigments from food such as red beets; pigments from drugs such as rifampin and phenazopyridine; or porphyrins from porphyria.

Discoloration of the urine should be investigated with microscopic examination to determine if red blood cells (RBCs) or any foreign substances are present. Pyuria results from white blood cell (WBC) debris and leukocytes in the urine, but cloudy urine can also result from other causes.

Sediment

Sediment from casts, blood cells, and bacteria can be detected by microscopic examination. Casts indicate hemorrhage or various conditions of the nephron. RBCs indicate acute inflammatory or vascular disorders of the glomerulus. More than 1 or 2 RBCs per high-power field (HPF) is abnormal and may indicate renal or systemic disease or trauma to the kidney. Sediment is labeled as active when an abnormal number of cells, tubular casts, crystals, or infectious organisms are found.

A healthy person's urinalysis usually contains no cells, although an occasional cell per HPF is seen. More than 1 tubular epithelial and transitional epithelial cell per HPF is suggestive of damage to the tubules or bladder wall. More than 1 RBC or WBC per HPF is considered abnormal. The more cells per HPF, the more active may be the renal disease.

Microscopic examination of the urine resulting in 20 or more organisms per HPF indicates UTI. Fewer than 20 organisms per HPF merits further study such as culture and sensitivity (C&S).

Red blood cells

Hematuria is the presence of more than 3 RBCs/HPF. Distorted, irregularly shaped cells indicate a glomerular problem. The major causes of hematuria include urethritis, hemorrhagic cystitis, renal stones, or tumors of the kidney, renal pelvis, ureter, bladder, and urethra. Hematuria with proteinuria usually suggests a renal origin. Isolated hematuria is usually produced by sites outside the kidneys.

White blood cells

Pyuria (>5 WBCs/HPF) is highly sensitive for the presence of a UTI. However, it may occur with dehydration, renal stones, appendicitis, or other extrinsic ureteral irritation in the absence of demonstrable microbial infection.

Casts

Tubular casts are formed in the distal portion of the nephron. A hyaline cast is a wispy, translucent, cylindrical replica of the tubular lumen. RBC casts are characteristic of glomerular origin. The presence of abnormal cells, protein, hemoglobin, myoglobin, or other debris with a cast helps identify the type of renal disease.

Urine Culture and Sensitivity

A C&S test is indicated in children if you are uncertain of a diagnosis of uncomplicated lower tract UTI based on clinical findings and urinalysis or if the patient has signs and symptoms of an upper UTI or complicated UTI. C&S is typically not indicated in adults suspected of having an uncomplicated lower UTI. Urine cultures are recommended for those with suspected acute pyelonephritis, for symptoms that do not resolve or that recur within 2 to 4 weeks after the completion of treatment, and in those with atypical symptoms.

Potassium Hydroxide and Wet Mount or Preparation

Perform these procedures if you suspect vulvovaginitis as a cause of the urinary tract symptoms (see Chapter 37).

Vaginal Culture or Molecular Testing for Infectious Organisms

Use these testing procedures to diagnose or confirm vaginal infection (see Chapter 37).

Ultrasonography

Ultrasonography is a noninvasive technique that can provide information about the kidneys, ureters, bladder, and vascular structures. Renal ultrasound is a good first test to determine kidney size and contour and the presence of calculi. Urinary bladder sonogram is used to identify tumors of the bladder, thickening of the bladder wall, posterior masses behind the bladder, or obstruction of the lower urinary tract showing residual urine. Renal and bladder ultrasound is indicated in any infant or young child with a second UTI.

Radiography

A flat plate of the abdomen can be used to identify structures of the kidney, ureters, and bladder. Urinary calculi are usually visible on radiographs.

Computed Tomography

Noncontrast helical (spiral) computed tomography (CT) is the gold standard for evaluating kidney stones. It has 95% sensitivity and 98% specificity.

DIFFERENTIAL DIAGNOSIS

Uncomplicated Urinary Tract Infection

Uncomplicated lower UTIs (or bacterial cystitis) are common in women. Uncomplicated UTIs occur in individuals with normal urinary tract anatomy and function. Patients present with symptoms of dysuria, urinary frequency, hematuria, back pain, mild nausea, nocturia, urgency, and voiding of small amounts. Fever is notably absent in adults but may be present in pediatric patients. Symptoms in neonates may include prolonged jaundice and failure to thrive.

The adult patient appears well on physical examination and may or may not have costovertebral angle (CVA) tenderness. Clinical diagnosis is supported by urine dipstick findings, which may include the presence of blood, leukocyte esterase, and nitrites. However, a negative dipstick result does not rule out UTI. Microscopic analysis may show the presence of RBCs and WBCs. No casts will be present. Urine C&S will confirm the diagnosis. See the Evidence-Based Practice boxes for evidence supporting the diagnosis of UTI in adults or children.

Urinary tract infections in older adults are sometimes mistaken as the early stages of dementia or Alzheimer disease because the symptoms may be confusion, delirium, agitation, hallucinations, behavioral changes, poor motor skills or dizziness, and falling.

Urethritis

Dysuria suggests urethritis, especially if accompanied by vaginal discharge. The history often includes a new sex partner, frequent sexual activity, a partner with urethritis, or multiple sex partners. As with uncomplicated UTI, the patient appears well and on physical examination has no CVA tenderness or fever. On urinalysis using a dipstick, findings may include the presence of blood, leukocyte esterase, and nitrites, although the patient may have urethritis in the absence of these findings. Urine culture or DNA testing confirms the presence of the offending pathogens, usually Chlamydia, *N. gonorrhoeae, Trichomonas* spp., and herpes.

Vulvovaginitis

Vulvovaginitis is a common cause of dysuria. The patient often describes the dysuria as "external"—a burning sensation as the urine passes inflamed labia. The patient usually has a history of vaginal discharge, odor, or itching. On physical examination, discharge is usually present in the vagina or from the cervix. Wet mount, KOH, and vaginal culture or DNA testing for infectious organisms can confirm the diagnosis (see Chapter 37).

Atrophic Vaginitis

Atrophic vaginitis may produce urinary tract symptoms. These patients may be perimenopausal or postmenopausal. Patients with atrophic vaginitis may report vaginal dryness or discomfort during sexual intercourse. On physical examination, the vaginal mucosa is thin, pale, and dry with fewer rugae. Diagnosis is made on the basis of clinical findings.

Interstitial Cystitis

Interstitial cystitis produces diminished bladder capacity along with symptoms of frequent, painful urination. Hematuria may be present. The cause is unknown but may be related to collagen disease, an autoimmune disorder, or an allergic manifestation, or it may occur secondary to an unidentified infectious agent. The bladder wall becomes inflamed, with mucosal ulceration and scarring that produce contraction of the smooth muscle and cause the symptoms. Middle-aged women are most often affected. Typically, the patient appears well and has no physical findings. Symptoms include bladder discomfort and suprapubic or pelvic tenderness. Urinalysis findings are usually negative. This is a diagnosis of exclusion, and the patient is often frustrated because no cause will have been found for the long-standing and persistent symptoms. The patient has no evidence of urological disease on radiographic and cystometric studies. Cystoscopic evidence of interstitial disease includes focal ulceration, edema, and perivascular infiltrates.

EVIDENCE-BASED PRACTICE *Diagnosing Uncomplicated Urinary Tract Infections in Adults*

In this systematic review the authors report that the symptoms of dysuria, frequency, hematuria, and back pain along with costovertebral angle tenderness significantly increase the probability of uncomplicated urinary tract infection (UTI). Women with one or more of the symptoms have about a 50% probability of having a UTI. The probability increases to more than 90% in women with specific combinations of symptoms, such as dysuria and frequency without vaginal discharge and irritation. A urine dipstick that has positive results for both nitrites and leukocyte esterase has a sensitivity of 75% and a specificity of 82% in determining UTI. However, a urine dipstick with negative results does not rule out UTI. The absence of dysuria and back pain with the presence of vaginal discharge and irritation significantly decrease the probability of UTI.

Their conclusion: History alone may effectively rule in the diagnosis of uncomplicated UTI, and the likelihood of a correct diagnosis is improved when the urine dipstick has positive results. However, the history, physical examination, and a dipstick urinalysis with negative results cannot reliably rule out UTI.

Reference: Bent S et al, 2002.

 EVIDENCE-BASED PRACTICE *Diagnosing Urinary Tract Infections in Infants and Children*

This meta-analysis offers insight into the diagnosis of urinary tract infection (UTI) in infants and children based on clinical examination and urine dipstick. Although certain signs and symptoms (high fever, fever for 24 hours, history of a previous UTI, abdominal pain, nonblack race, lack of circumcision, back pain, dysuria, frequency, new-onset urinary incontinence, suprapubic tenderness, and absence of another source of fever on examination) increase the probability of UTI, no single sign or symptom has a sufficiently high likelihood ratio to defini-tively diagnose UTI or a sufficiently small likelihood ratio to rule out UTI. A urine dip that is positive for both nitrites and leukocyte esterase substantially increases the likelihood of a UTI. A positive dipstick test should always be followed up with a confirmatory urine culture.

The bottom line: Although no sign or symptom is diagnostic of UTI in children by itself, the absence of several key signs and symptoms in combination can be used to identify infants at low risk for UTI.

Reference: Shaikh et al, 2007.

Pyelonephritis

The patient presents with fever and chills, appears toxic, and reports back pain. Nausea and vomiting may be present. Some patients also report lower urinary tract symptoms, including frequency and dysuria. The patient feels and looks ill. On physical examination, CVA tenderness is usually present. The abdomen may also be tender. On microscopic examination, WBCs are usually present. WBC casts suggest pyelonephritis. Bacterial casts, although rare, are pathognomonic of pyelonephritis. Urine C&S or DNA testing confirms the diagnosis and identifies the pathogen—usually *E. coli,* *Klebsiella* spp., *Proteus mirabilis,* or *Enterobacter* spp.

Urolithiasis

Urinary stones can occur anywhere in the urinary tract and may produce symptoms of acute pain, hematuria, and secondary infection. Many calculi are "silent" and may cause only hematuria, either microscopic or gross. Renal calculi may occur when a stone obstructs the urinary tract. Typical symptoms of renal colic include severe flank pain that radiates along the pathway of the ureter to the inner thigh. Chills, fever, and urinary frequency are common. The patient may have nausea, vomiting, and abdominal distention.

The clinical diagnosis is supported by urinalysis and imaging findings. The urine may be normal; however, gross or microscopic hematuria is common. Pyuria (WBCs) with or without bacteria may be present. Crystalline structures may be present. Noncontrast helical (spiral) CT is the gold standard for evaluating kidney stones.

Poststreptococcal Glomerulonephritis

This condition is an immune-mediated nephritis that occurs after a streptococcal skin or pharyngeal infection in the previous 1 to 3 weeks. It occurs most commonly in elementary school children. The patient reports anorexia, vomiting, fever, abdominal pain, headache, and lethargy. On physical examination, periorbital edema is usually present, as is hypertension. Other presenting symptoms are orthopnea, dyspnea, cough, rales, hematuria, and proteinuria. A positive serum antistreptolysin O titer confirms recent infection. Low serum complement levels are indicative of an antigen-antibody interaction. A depressed serum concentration of complement component 3 (C3) is found in the first few days of the disease.

Chemical Irritation

Bubble baths, body lotions, soaps and sprays can act as local chemical irritants. The patient experiences frequency, burning, and urgency with small volumes of voided urine. Children will frequently suppress voiding because of pain. Physical examination may reveal erythema of the labia and urethral outlet. Laboratory examination may reveal pyuria and bacteriuria as a result of local infection and denudation.

> ▶ **DIFFERENTIAL DIAGNOSIS OF** *Common Causes of Urinary Problems in Children and Patients with Female Genitalia*

CONDITION	HISTORY	PHYSICAL FINDINGS	DIAGNOSTIC STUDIES
Uncomplicated UTI	Dysuria, frequency, mild nausea, nocturia, urgency, voiding small amounts; neonates and young infants present with anorexia and irritability	No fever in adults; appears well; no CVA tenderness; may have suprapubic tenderness; neonates and young infants may present with failure to thrive, bacteremia, and fever	Urine dipstick: may be positive for blood, leukocyte esterase, nitrites; microscopic analysis: RBCs, WBCs, no casts; urine C&S; renal and bladder ultrasound in any infant, young child with a second UTI
Urethritis	Dysuria; vaginal discharge; history of new sex partner, frequent sex, partner with urethritis, multiple sex partners	Appears well; has no CVA tenderness or fever	Urine dipstick: may be positive for blood, leukocyte esterase, nitrites; urine culture; molecular testing
Vulvovaginitis	History of vaginal itching, discharge, burning	Inflamed or atrophic labia; vaginal or cervical discharge	Microscopic examination, vaginal cultures, molecular testing
Atrophic vaginitis	Vaginal dryness; dyspareunia; postmenopausal	Thin, pale, dry vaginal mucosa with loss of rugae	None

Continued

> **DIFFERENTIAL DIAGNOSIS OF** *Common Causes of Urinary Problems in Children and Patients with Female Genitalia—cont'd*

CONDITION	HISTORY	PHYSICAL FINDINGS	DIAGNOSTIC STUDIES
Interstitial cystitis	Frequent painful urination; hematuria; most often middle-aged women; often frustrated because no cause has been previously found for long-standing and persistent symptoms	Appears well and has no physical findings; suprapubic tenderness may be present	Urinalysis usually negative; radiography and cystometric studies to rule out other urologic disease; cystoscopy to diagnose
Pyelonephritis	Fever, chills, back pain, nausea and vomiting, toxic appearance; some patients also have frequency and dysuria	Feels and looks ill; fever; CVA tenderness; abdomen may be tender	Urine dipstick: may be positive for blood, leukocyte esterase, nitrites; microscopic examination: WBCs may have white cell casts or bacterial casts; urine C&S: *Escherichia coli, Klebsiella* spp., *Proteus mirabilis, Enterobacter* spp.; blood cultures
Urolithiasis	Pain, hematuria; may have symptoms of secondary infection; renal colic: pain that radiates to inner thigh; nausea, vomiting	May have CVA tenderness; looks ill during periods of acute pain; may have abdominal distention	Urinalysis: gross or microscopic hematuria; WBCs with or without bacteria; crystalline structures may be present; noncontrast helical CT
Poststreptococcal glomerulonephritis	History of skin or throat infection 1–3 wk earlier; lethargy, anorexia, vomiting, abdominal pain	Hypertension, periorbital edema, CVA tenderness; may have dyspnea, cough, pallor	U/A: proteinuria, hematuria; ASO titer; serum C3 is low, early in disease
Chemical irritation	History of bubble baths, soaps, lotions, sprays; urgency, dysuria	No fever; erythematous labia, urethral opening	Hematuria common, gross hematuria unusual and casts never seen

C&S, culture and sensitivity; *CT,* computed tomography; *CVA,* costovertebral angle; *RBC,* red blood cell; *U/A,* urinalysis; *UTI,* urinary tract infection; *WBC,* white blood cell.

Vaginal Bleeding

The average menstrual cycle is 28 days. It is considered abnormal if the cycle occurs more often than every 21 days (polymenorrhea) or less often than every 35 days (oligomenorrhea). Bleeding at irregular intervals is known as metrorrhagia. Intermenstrual bleeding is bleeding between cycles. The average duration of menses is 4 days; a duration longer than 7 days or blood loss heavier than 80 mL is considered excessive and classified as menorrhagia. Hypomenorrhea occurs when the frequency of periods remains normal but the menstrual flow decreases in amount. Systemic disorders that cause an imbalance in the hypothalamic–pituitary–ovarian (HPO) axis may lead to menses that are too heavy (menorrhagia/hypermenorrhea), too often (polymenorrhea), or too heavy and irregular (menometrorrhagia).

Other systemic reasons for vaginal bleeding include blood dyscrasias, liver and kidney diseases, and medications (e.g., hormones, anticoagulants, nonsteroidal antiinflammatory drugs). Organic causes for aberrant menstrual cycles are multiple and include vaginitis, ectopic pregnancy, fibroids, and polyps. Vaginal bleeding in perimenopausal and postmenopausal patients may indicate cancer.

DIAGNOSTIC REASONING: FOCUSED HISTORY

Is this an acute condition that requires immediate intervention?

Key Questions
- How heavy is the bleeding?
- Do you have a bleeding disorder?
- Are you taking anticoagulants?

Patients who have profuse bleeding, have had substantial blood loss, or are hemodynamically unstable require immediate intervention.

Amount of Bleeding

Saturating one or more sanitary pads or tampons hourly for several consecutive hours likely equates to greater than 80 mL of blood loss. A history of flooding, clots, or leaking, especially overnight, may be associated with a clotting disorder.

Bleeding Disorder or Anticoagulants

Severe acute uterine bleeding in a nonpregnant patient usually occurs as the result of a coagulopathy or from taking anticoagulants. Patients with submucous fibroids can also present with profuse bleeding.

Could this be related to pregnancy?

Key Questions
- Do you have any symptoms of pregnancy (e.g., missed period, breast tenderness, nausea, vomiting)?
- When was your last menstrual period?
- What are you using for birth control?
- Have you recently had a baby?

Pregnancy

A small amount of bleeding can occur at implantation. The blastocyst burrows into the endometrium and invades the maternal blood supply; the formation and implantation of the placenta follow. If bleeding occurs from implantation, it happens about 1 week before the expected menstrual cycle. Regard patients of childbearing age with a uterus as pregnant until pregnancy is ruled out. It is estimated that up to 50% of all fertilized eggs die and are aborted spontaneously, usually before the pregnancy is detected. About 20% of pregnant patients have some vaginal bleeding during the first trimester.

Recent Childbirth

If the patient has recently delivered a baby, the abnormal vaginal bleeding is likely from retained placenta, infection of the uterus (endometritis), or laceration.

If the patient is pregnant, is this a complication?

Key Questions

- How old are you?
- How many weeks pregnant are you?
- Do you have any chronic health problems?
- Are you experiencing pain or cramping?
- Have you passed any tissue?
- Are you having other symptoms?
- Have you ever had a sexually transmitted infection (STI)?
- Have you ever had an infection of your tubes (pelvic inflammatory disease [PID])?
- Have you ever been pregnant before? What were the number of times and outcomes of your pregnancies?

Age

The risk for spontaneous abortion is higher after age 35 years. Most ectopic pregnancies occur in ages 25 to 34 years. However, patients older than age 35 years have a higher mortality rate from ectopic pregnancy.

Weeks of Gestation

Among known pregnancies, the rate of spontaneous abortion is approximately 10% and usually occurs between the 7th and 12th weeks of pregnancy. An estimated 10% to 15% of clinically recognized pregnancies result in first trimester loss. The patient experiencing an ectopic pregnancy typically presents at about 6 to 8 weeks of gestation.

Chronic Health Conditions

The risk for spontaneous abortion is higher in patients with systemic conditions, such as diabetes mellitus, polycystic ovarian syndrome (PCOS), obesity, systemic lupus erythematosus, hypertension, antiphospholipid antibodies, thyroid disease, chronic liver disease, and renal diseases.

Pain

Low back pain or abdominal pain that is dull, sharp, or cramping may indicate spontaneous abortion or ectopic pregnancy. If there is pain associated with ectopic pregnancy, it will usually be described as "crampy," pelvic pressure, or "soreness" in the lower abdomen. In ectopic pregnancy, the pain may lateralize to one side. Severe, sharp, and sudden pain in the lower abdominal area may indicate rupture of the ectopic pregnancy. Ruptured ectopic pregnancy is a surgical emergency.

Passing Tissue

The passage of tissue from the vagina suggests spontaneous abortion. Ectopic pregnancies can be accompanied by sloughing material.

Other Symptoms

Pain referred to the shoulder is suggestive of ectopic pregnancy rupture with peritoneal free fluid and significant hemorrhage. Other symptoms of rupture include feeling dizzy or faint or actually fainting.

Sexually Transmitted Infection

Sexually transmitted infections that have been unnoticed, untreated, or inadequately treated can cause scarring of the fallopian tubes, which is associated with greater risk for ectopic pregnancy. Ectopic pregnancy occurs in about 1 of every 200 pregnancies (Box 36.1). However, if the patient has had PID, the rate is as high as 1 of every 40 pregnancies.

Previous Pregnancies

The risk for spontaneous abortion is higher after age 35 years and in patients with a history of three or more prior spontaneous abortions.

Box 36.1	**Risk Factors for Ectopic Pregnancy**

- History of pelvic inflammatory disease
- Previous ectopic pregnancy
- History of tubal surgery
- Infertility
- In utero diethylstilbestrol exposure
- Present use of intrauterine device
- Smoking

Is this related to age? Where is the patient in the reproductive life cycle?

Key Questions

- How old are you?
- Are you postmenopausal?

Age

Knowing the age can help focus the differential diagnosis. The majority of adolescents with abnormal bleeding experience anovulatory cycles caused when estrogen stimulates the uterine lining with no opposing progesterone. This condition leads to a thicker, more vascular, and less stable endometrium, predisposing the adolescent to dyssynchronous bleeding. A young patient's bleeding is most frequently caused by pregnancy, contraceptive methods, or infection. Patients over age 40 years are more likely to have problems related to polyps, fibroids, or ovarian dysfunction.

Postmenopause

After menopause, the origin of bleeding irregularities is often hormone therapy, endometrial hyperplasia, or endometrial cancer (see section on postmenopausal bleeding).

What does the character of the bleeding tell me?

Key Questions

- When did the bleeding begin?
- How long have you been bleeding?
- What is the flow like?
- How many pads do you use?
- Are there any accompanying problems?

Symptom Analysis

Determine the amount of flow and its duration to establish if there is menorrhagia, metrorrhagia, or menometrorrhagia. Menorrhagia is considered to be 80 mL of menses over the course of the cycle, which is estimated as saturating one or more sanitary pads or tampons hourly for several consecutive hours. Metrorrhagia is defined as bleeding at irregular intervals or intermenstrual bleeding. When the menstruation has an unpredictable schedule and lasts for a prolonged time, it is termed menometrorrhagia.

Associated Symptoms

Patients may experience postcoital bleeding with cervical infections, cervical polyps, or cervical cancer. Accompanying dyspareunia may indicate endometriosis. Dysmenorrhea can be caused by an intrauterine device (IUD) or adenomyosis (presence of endometrial tissue in the myometrium). Pelvic pressure or pain is suspicious for persistent corpus luteum cyst. Uterine prolapse causes pelvic pressure, which is subjectively described as "something falling out of the vagina." Fever is associated with a pelvic infection. Menorrhagia, accompanied by fatigue, weight gain, hair loss, cold intolerance, decreased libido, and constipation, is a symptom of hypothyroidism. Bleeding disorders may become apparent for the first time in a teenager, with severe menorrhagia accompanied by bruising, petechiae, and gingival bleeding.

Is this problem acute or chronic? How does it compare with usual menses?

Key Questions

- Has this kind of vaginal bleeding occurred before?
- Were your periods regular before this episode?
- How long did they last?
- What was the amount and pattern of bleeding?

Irregular Menses

In anovulatory cycles, the endometrium proliferates under the influence of high estrogen levels until it can no longer be supported; then bleeding occurs. This results in a menstrual pattern that is longer than 28 days with a very heavy flow that lasts 7 to 14 days. With fluctuating estrogen levels, the patient may have two periods a month. Both of these patterns are consistent with dysfunctional uterine bleeding. However, organic problems with any component of the reproductive tract must be ruled out.

Acute Bleeding

One episode of acute bleeding in a patient with normally regular menstrual cycles suggests uterine fibroids or a complication of pregnancy, such as threatened abortion. In a postmenopausal patient with an intact uterus, an episode of vaginal bleeding is indicative of endometrial hyperplasia and is suspicious for endometrial cancer.

Chronic Bleeding

Chronic, irregular menstrual cycles coupled with obesity are likely to be caused by PCOS, also known as Stein-Leventhal syndrome. Chronic midcycle spotting can occur secondary to the normal midcycle drop in estrogen levels and usually is not bothersome to the patient because the amount of vaginal bleeding is very scant and the duration is short.

Could this be caused by the patient's birth control method?

Key Questions
- Do you use birth control?
- Which kind(s) of birth control do you use?
- How long have you been using it?

Birth Control

Menorrhagia from IUD contraception is accompanied by increased cramping and pain. If spotting or cramping is not of a usual pattern, ectopic pregnancy or infection must be considered. Displacement or perforation of the uterus by the IUD can be verified by pelvic ultrasound. Patients who have recently discontinued the use of oral contraceptive (OC) pills after several years may experience heavier menstrual bleeding than when they were taking OC pills. Breakthrough bleeding caused by OC pills may occur in the first 2 weeks of the cycle because of low estrogen level or in the last 2 weeks because of low progesterone level. Long-acting progestin contraceptives (Norplant) may cause irregular heavy menses because there is a lack of estrogen to stabilize the endometrium. Changes in bleeding patterns for progestin users necessitate ruling out pregnancy.

Is this prepubertal bleeding?

Key Questions
- How old is the child?
- Is there a family history of early sexual development?

- Is there a family history of bleeding problems or blood dyscrasias?
- Did the child ingest any birth control pills or estrogens?
- Are there any accompanying symptoms?

Pediatric Vaginal Bleeding

In the United States, the average age of menarche is 12 years old. Age of menarche may vary by race and BMI. Vaginal bleeding before age 8 years is abnormal and may indicate a foreign body, injury, or sexual abuse. Secondary sexual characteristics indicate sexual precocity. Newborn girls may experience breast bud enlargement, galactorrhea, and a small amount of vaginal bleeding from maternal exogenous hormones. These symptoms resolve without intervention within a few weeks.

Although uncommon, malignant genital tract tumors can cause vaginal bleeding. Vaginal adenosis and adenocarcinoma are the most common tumor types.

Bleeding Problems

A family history of bleeding problems or a positive review of systems and physical examination indicating the presence of petechiae or bruises suggests a bleeding tendency. Platelet counts or clotting studies are indicated.

Accompanying Symptoms

Vulvovaginitis is the most common pediatric gynecologic problem. Vaginal discharge, vaginal itching, vulvar erythema, and lesions often accompany vulvovaginal bleeding. A foul-smelling discharge is noted with bacterial vaginosis, trichomoniasis, and a foreign body. All vaginal discharges in a child should be tested, including testing for gonorrhea and chlamydia. If an STI or sexual abuse is suspected, syphilis and human immunodeficiency virus testing should be done. Throat and rectal specimens for gonorrhea and chlamydia should also be obtained.

Trauma to the perineum is more common in children because the vulva has less subcutaneous fat. Large lacerations and hematomas warrant referral for examination and repair under anesthesia.

Prolapse of the urethra may cause bleeding. It is accompanied by pain at the meatus and pain with urination.

Is the patient experiencing anovulatory cycles?

Key Questions

- Have you had irregular menstrual cycles?
- Are you having symptoms of menopause (e.g., vaginal dryness, hot flashes, night sweats)?
- At what age did your mother or grandmother go through menopause?

Irregular Menstrual Cycles

Anovulatory cycles are the most common cause of irregular bleeding patterns among females beginning (adolescent) or ending (perimenopausal) their menstrual cycles. It is estimated that 80% of young adolescents will be anovulatory during the first year of menstruation. Regular ovulatory cycles are usually established by the second year of menses but may take up to 5 years. Irregular cycles are common during the perimenopause. During this phase menstrual patterns often change and the patient may experience irregular bleeding or spotting or skipped periods. Periods may be heavier and longer some months and shorter and lighter other months. The interval between periods may increase or decrease.

Menopausal Syndrome

The frequency of monthly ovulation becomes irregular at about 40 years of age, which leads to intermittent symptoms of menopause. The time frame from onset of symptoms to complete cessation of menstruation is termed the perimenopause or climacteric phase. The perimenopause phase can last up to 10 years. The age of menopause is genetically determined and will be similar to those of the patient's mother and grandmother. Menopause is unrelated to age of menarche, pregnancies, or contraceptive methods used.

Is the patient experiencing postmenopausal bleeding?

Key Questions

- How old were you when you stopped menstruating?
- Do you have a uterus?
- Did you have a hysterectomy? Why did you have it? Were your ovaries removed?
- Are you taking hormones (prescription or homeopathic)?

Age at Menopause

The average age for menopause in the United States is 51 years. Menopause is defined as 1 year without menstrual cycles. However, a diagnosis can be made earlier by measuring the rising follicle-stimulating hormone (FSH) and the falling estradiol levels. Postmenopausal bleeding is any bleeding that occurs after the establishment of menopause. Vaginal bleeding after menopause warrants investigation to rule out endometrial cancer. Box 36.2 lists risk factors for endometrial cancer.

Intact Uterus

In postmenopausal patients with an intact uterus, unexplained vaginal bleeding suggests endometrial hyperplasia with a suspicion for endometrial cancer.

Hysterectomy

Any vaginal bleeding after a hysterectomy justifies suspicion of cancer, but the bleeding will most likely be a symptom of atrophic vaginitis. If the ovaries were left in place at

---

Box 36.2 **Risk Factors for Endometrial Cancer**

- Endometrial hyperplasia
- Family history of endometrial cancer
- Hypertension, diabetes mellitus, liver disease
- Obesity
- Chronic anovulatory cycles
- Unopposed estrogen therapy with an intact uterus
- Polycystic ovarian syndrome
- Tamoxifen therapy

the time of the hysterectomy, the patients may not experience menopause until about 8 to 10 years after the surgery. The ovaries become atrophic and nonfunctional over time, probably secondary to altered blood flow resulting from the surgery. Atrophic vaginitis bleeding occurs from the slightest trauma; even wiping the perineum with tissue after urination can cause spotting.

Hormone Therapy

Hormone therapy for menopausal symptoms may cause vaginal bleeding in patients with an intact uterus. Regimens for those with an intact uterus include the cycling of estrogen and progestin and continuous daily doses of both hormones. The cycled hormones produce regular scheduled bleeding. However, the continuous daily combination therapy will often cause amenorrhea after 3 to 6 months of use. After a pattern of amenorrhea has been established, new bleeding should be investigated.

Unopposed estrogen therapy in a patient with an intact uterus predisposes to endometrial cancer from a thick, built-up endometrium. Endometrial hyperplasia accounts for about 20% of postmenopausal patients who report abnormal vaginal bleeding. Endometrial hyperplasia can be diagnosed with endometrial biopsy, ultrasonography, or dilation and curettage (D&C).

Vaginal bleeding can also be caused by a cancerous cervical lesion (diagnosed with colposcopy and biopsy), cervical polyps, or endometrial polyps. Ovarian tumors can excrete estrogens and progestins, causing vaginal bleeding. Fallopian tube cancer more commonly presents with scant vaginal bleeding or watery vaginal discharge and a pelvic mass.

> ### Could this be from infection or inflammation?
>
> **Key Questions**
> - Have you noticed any sores, rashes, or lumps in the vaginal area?
> - Do you have vaginal discharge or vulvar itching or burning?
> - What was the result of your last Pap test?

Lesions and Lumps

Genital warts (condylomata acuminata) can cause bleeding secondary to trauma to the warts. Typically, genital warts are located inferiorly from the fossa navicularis to the fourchette and perineal area and internally on the walls of the vagina and cervix. A painless ulcer that bleeds easily suggests syphilis and classically appears as a solitary lesion; however, there can be more than one chancre, especially if the patient is immunocompromised. Squamous cell carcinoma can also present as a painless ulcer that bleeds. Lesions secondarily infected by bacteria may bleed. Inguinal lymphadenopathy can signal an STI of the genitourinary tract.

 EVIDENCE-BASED PRACTICE *Hormone Therapy and Endometrial Hyperplasia*

One aim of this review of 46 randomized clinical trials of oral hormone therapy was to assess which of the regimens—unopposed estrogen or estrogen plus progesterone administered either continuously or sequentially—provides the best protection against the development of endometrial hyperplasia or carcinoma. After 1 year of treatment, low-dose unopposed estrogen was associated with a marginally nonsignificant increase in endometrial hyperplasia versus placebo. At 2 and 3 years of treatment, unopposed estrogen therapy was associated with a significantly increased risk of endometrial hyperplasia at all doses, and there was evidence of a dose-response and a duration-of-treatment response between unopposed estrogen and risk of hyperplasia. The addition of progesterone to unopposed estrogen therapy in women with intact uteri significantly reduced the risk of endometrial hyperplasia, with either sequential or continuous combined regimens, compared with the unopposed estrogen group.

The authors concluded that unopposed estrogen is associated with increased risk of endometrial hyperplasia at all doses and with durations of therapy between 1 and 3 years. Hormone therapy for postmenopausal women with an intact uterus should comprise both estrogen and progesterone to reduce the risk of endometrial hyperplasia.

Reference: Furness et al, 2012.

Vaginal Discharge

Acute or chronic endometritis and PID may cause heavy menstrual bleeding. An endometrial infection disturbs the clotting properties, resulting in painful, heavy bleeding. Chlamydia and gonorrhea are the most frequent causes of PID.

Last Pap Test

The last Pap test result may provide clues to a chronic vaginal infection showing a predominance of coccobacilli or atrophy with inflammation; a progressive, low-grade, squamous, intraepithelial lesion; or a cancerous condition. However, the accuracy of a Pap test is unreliable if a cervical lesion or abnormal cervical vascular pattern is noted on physical examination.

What other causes of bleeding should I consider?

Key Questions

- Could this bleeding be from the urethra or rectum?
- Are you taking tamoxifen?
- What (other) medications are you taking?
- Do you have a history of anemia, or do you bleed easily with dental work?
- Did your mother take diethylstilbestrol (DES) when she was pregnant with you?

Urinary or Rectal Bleeding

Bleeding from the urethra or rectum can be misinterpreted as vaginal bleeding. A prolapsed cystocele or rectocele might be subject to drying, abrasion, and bleeding. These causes can be documented through physical examination, urinalysis, fecal testing for occult blood, and colonoscopy.

Tamoxifen

Tamoxifen, used for primary or secondary prevention of breast cancer, can cause endometrial hyperplasia and produce vaginal bleeding. Endometrial biopsy is required.

Other Medications

Antibiotics, phenobarbital, rifampin, phenytoin, carbamazepine, and other drugs that induce hepatic microsomal enzymes may produce lower estrogen levels and cause bleeding irregularities. Aspirin can increase menstrual flow.

Blood Dyscrasias

Some women with a coagulation defect have excessive menstrual bleeding as the first symptom of a blood disorder; in addition, most platelet abnormalities will cause vaginal bleeding. If the patient has severe anemia (hemoglobin <10 g/dL) resulting from the vaginal bleeding, it is highly probable that a coagulopathy is present. If this occurs in the perimenarchal or second or third decade of life, suspect von Willebrand disease, which is a congenital bleeding disorder caused by deficiency in factor VIII.

Diethylstilbestrol Exposure in Utero

In utero exposure to diethylstilbestrol (DES) has been associated with adenocarcinoma of the vagina.

DIAGNOSTIC REASONING: FOCUSED PHYSICAL EXAMINATION

Perform a General Assessment

Determine whether the patient's general state of health includes problems of nutrition (e.g., obesity or muscle wasting), hirsutism, or skin or hair changes, which may indicate an imbalance in the HPO axis.

Assess Vital Signs

Determine whether a patient with profuse bleeding is hemodynamically stable. Look for orthostatic changes in blood pressure. In patients who are tachycardic and tachypneic, suspect a ruptured ectopic pregnancy. The patient will show signs of hemorrhage and shock.

Determine Patient Weight and Calculate Body Mass Index

A body mass index greater than 25 corresponds to being overweight, and an index greater than 30 signals obesity. Excess weight and obesity can cause anovulatory cycles as the adipose cell stroma converts androstenedione to estrogen (estrone) as the body fat increases. Obesity also increases sex hormone–binding globulin, thereby increasing free steroid levels. Both processes can cause an imbalance in the HPO axis and increase the probability of an anovulatory cycle and heavy vaginal bleeding. Amenorrhea in anorexia nervosa may precede weight loss by many months.

Perform a Lymph Node Examination

Examine the lymph nodes to assess for leukemia or metastatic gynecologic cancer. Inguinal lymph nodes can be enlarged from an STI or a vulvar infection (e.g., bartholinitis).

Perform a Thyroid Examination

Observe and palpate the thyroid gland. Enlargement may be found in hypofunctioning glands. Hypothyroidism is known to be present in 22% of patients with severe menorrhagia.

Perform a Breast Examination

The finding of spontaneous, bilateral, clear, or nonbloody nipple discharge on breast examination could indicate hyperprolactinemia, which can cause amenorrhea or irregular vaginal bleeding, either from either a pituitary microadenoma or from medications (antipsychotics, tricyclic antidepressants, monoamine oxidase inhibitors, and some antihypertensive agents).

Perform a Pelvic Examination

An external and internal pelvic examination can verify bleeding suspected to be uterine in origin. Examine the external genitalia, noting whether the bleeding is coming from external hemorrhoids or a painless labial lesion, such as a squamous cell cancer or condylomata acuminata. Note bruising, lacerations on the vaginal walls, or other signs of sexual abuse. Observe the introitus for signs of a prolapsed uterus or cystocele or rectocele that might be subject to drying, abrasion, or bleeding. These signs are usually accompanied by pelvic pressure or urinary or bowel symptoms.

Observe the external genitalia for signs of estrogen deficiency: sparse hair distribution; graying or white hair color; clitoral atrophy; and a thin, small labia minora. These signs strongly suggest atrophic vaginitis as the cause of bleeding.

Next, perform a vaginal examination. Note the color and condition of the vaginal walls.

Pale, nonrugated vaginal walls are a sign of an atrophic vagina that is easily abraded to cause bleeding. Pale vaginal mucosa with splotchy red patches is also a sign of vaginal atrophy. Bleeding from atrophic vaginitis most commonly follows intercourse or douching. It often is a whitish-brown discharge with no particular foul odor. The patient may also have pruritus and a burning sensation of the vagina, labia, and urinary tract because of a lack of estrogen.

Note the amount, color, consistency, and odor of the vaginal discharge. Take samples for wet mount examination from the pooled discharge in the lateral fornices. Note cervical friability and discharge from the cervical os. Take samples of the discharge and assess as noted in Chapter 37. Cervical polyps are red, glossy, nontender masses protruding from the cervical os. They are usually benign and can be removed by twisting them off with ring forceps. The specimen should be sent for pathological evaluation.

If a threatened or spontaneous abortion is suspected, check the internal cervical os to determine if it is closed or open.

Ectopic pregnancy will cause adnexal or cervical motion tenderness. However, uterine enlargement is not often appreciated. Uterine size and contour can be grossly assessed via bimanual examination. On pelvic examination, the uterus is enlarged but smaller than anticipated from dates provided. The cervix is tender to motion, and a tender adnexal mass may be palpable. Diagnosis is confirmed by positive human chorionic gonadotropin (hCG) test results and ultrasound. Serial quantitative serum hCG levels may be useful. A ruptured ectopic pregnancy is a surgical emergency.

Uterine leiomyomas (myomas, fibroids) typically feel firm and may make the uterus asymmetrical. These tumors can progress to a size that mimics an advanced pregnant uterus. The uterine size is measured in weeks, just as the uterus is measured in pregnancy. When the uterus reaches a 12- to 14-week size, referral to a gynecologist for surgery (myomectomy or hysterectomy) is appropriate. The patient may experience urinary or bowel problems (e.g., urinary frequency and constipation) because the fibroid is distorting or obstructing those systems. Carcinogenic tumors of the uterus are classically firm, hard, and rapidly growing, becoming fixed masses. Ultrasound is a valuable tool in documenting the size and growth patterns of tumors.

The average-size adult uterus measures 8 cm long, 5 cm wide, and 2.5 cm deep for a nulliparous woman. Add 1 cm to each dimension for the average size of a multiparous uterus ($9 \times 6 \times 3.5$ cm). The uterus with adenomyosis is increased in size to two to three times that of normal, may be globular, and has a uniform consistency. Adenomyosis is accompanied by worsening menorrhagia and dysmenorrhea.

The rectovaginal examination can detect lesions or nodularity of the cul-de-sac, which is present with endometriosis or a primary rectal tumor.

Pediatric Examination: Perform a Breast and Genital Examination

Assess for signs of sexual precocity by determining the presence and stage of secondary sexual characteristics of the breasts and pubic hair. Assess development using Tanner staging (see Chapter 5, Figs. 5.2 and 5.3). Inspect the vulva, noting the hygiene status; presence of smegma in the labial folds, urine, fecal material, or erythema and lesions. Examine the urinary meatus. A prolapsed urinary meatus is noted by the presence of dark red tissue surrounding the urinary opening. This tissue is usually tender. Use an appropriate pediatric-size speculum, long otoscope, or nasal speculum. It may be necessary to refer the patient for a vaginoscopy or cystoscopy under anesthesia for a complete assessment of the vagina and uterus.

Consider the possibility of infection or sexual abuse. See Chapter 37 for assessment of vaginal discharges.

LABORATORY AND DIAGNOSTIC STUDIES

Qualitative Urine and Serum Human Chorionic Gonadotropin Tests

Qualitative urine and serum hCG tests are monoclonal antibody tests using radioimmunoassay to determine or exclude pregnancy. The serum hCG test is more sensitive than the urine hCG test. The serum test can be performed in about 2 hours, and hCG can be detected as early as 6 days after conception. The result is reported as either negative or positive. Because the β-subunits are measured, it is highly specific and does not crossreact with luteinizing hormone (LH).

Depending on the specific test used, urine testing can detect pregnancy from before to several days after a missed period. The results are obtained in minutes. A positive test result (usually a color change) indicates pregnancy.

Quantitative Serum Human Chorionic Gonadotropin Test

A quantitative hCG (β-hCG) test is the first step in determining a complication of pregnancy. The test is a fluorometric enzyme immunoassay that is highly specific for the β-receptors of hCG, with almost no crossreactivity with other hormones. Results are provided as values. The reference ranges for determining an abnormal pregnancy are as follows:

- Not significant: 0 to 5.0 mIU/mL
- Borderline significance: 5.0 to 25 mIU/mL
- Evaluate with serial determinations: >25 mIU/mL

A rapid β-hCG test (with a sensitivity of ≥5 mIU/mL) result of less than 5 mIU/mL is highly predictive in excluding ectopic pregnancy. The β-hCG levels have a doubling time of 58 hours with pregnancy. Ectopic pregnancy causes an increase in hCG levels at the same rate as a normal pregnancy but only up to a certain point. In ectopic pregnancy, that point is usually less than 4 to 6 weeks, at which time the hCG levels plateau or begin to fall. Therefore, serial determinations are more useful than a single determination.

Hematocrit and Hemoglobin Levels

Hematocrit and hemoglobin levels are used to determine anemia caused by blood loss from long-standing menorrhagia. Hematocrit and hemoglobin levels are not useful in evaluating acute blood loss from a single episode of heavy bleeding caused by a spontaneous abortion or ectopic pregnancy.

Complete Blood Count with Indices and Differential

Complete blood count (CBC) with indices will provide information about the degree and cause of anemia. Typically, the hematocrit and hemoglobin levels reflect the degree of anemia, with erythrocyte indices suggesting the cause. Whereas microcytic hypochromic anemia is reflective of chronic blood loss, normocytic normochromic anemia suggests acute hemorrhage. Microcytic hypochromic anemia is indicated by a mean corpuscular volume of less than 80 fL and a mean corpuscular hemoglobin level of less than 27 pg. These values are within reference ranges in normocytic normochromic anemia.

An infectious cause of vaginal bleeding will be reflected by an increased white blood cell (WBC) count with a shift to the left (an increase in the number of bands that are immature neutrophils). Additionally, the CBC can provide evidence for leukemia and thrombocytopenia, both of which can produce abnormal vaginal bleeding.

Prothrombin Time, Partial Thromboplastin Time, and Bleeding Time

If the history, physical examination, or both suggest a bleeding problem, prothrombin time, partial thromboplastin time, and bleeding time can differentiate among blood dyscrasias, hepatic or renal diseases, and iatrogenic causes (e.g., anticoagulants, nonsteroidal antiinflammatory drugs).

Serum Progesterone Levels

A serum progesterone level greater than 25 ng/mL is predictive of an intrauterine pregnancy; a level less than 15 ng/mL suggests an ectopic pregnancy.

Serum Follicle-Stimulating Hormone Levels

Ovarian failure, which causes a reduced secretion of estradiol, will raise the FSH level to greater than 40 mIU/mL. If both the FSH and LH levels are greater than 50 mIU/mL, primary ovarian failure is established. If the patient is older than 30 years, menopause is diagnosed; if younger than 30 years, a chromosomal karyotype should be obtained. An FSH measurement less than 40 mIU/mL denotes a hypothalamic–pituitary dysfunction and secondary ovarian failure.

Serum Luteinizing Hormone Levels

A serum LH level of greater than 35 mIU/mL is frequently seen in patients with PCOS. An LH/FSH ratio higher than 2:1 is suggestive of PCOS, and a ratio greater than 3:1 is diagnostic of PCOS.

Dehydroepiandrosterone-Sulfate Serum Test

Most women with PCOS have elevated dehydroepiandrosterone sulfate (DHEA-S) levels greater than 200 µg/dL.

Serum Estradiol Levels

Serum estradiol levels are less than 15 pg/mL with menopause.

Serum Prolactin Level

About one-third of women with no obvious cause of amenorrhea will have an elevated prolactin level. Prolactin levels are normal in PCOS.

Molecular Testing for Infectious Organisms

Molecular testing using a sample taken from the vagina provides rapid, sensitive, and specific results. A number of products are available. Molecular tests include DNA probes, nucleic acid amplification tests (NAATs), and polymerase chain reaction assays. Tests are available for *Chlamydia trachomatis, Neisseria gonorrhoeae, Trichomonas vaginalis, Gardnerella vaginalis, Candida* spp., and herpes simplex virus. Samples for chlamydia and gonorrhea testing can be obtained by the clinician or by the patient. Urine NAATs can be used to screen for possible STIs in both adults and children. A positive test result must be followed up with a culture for definitive diagnosis.

Fecal Occult Blood Test or Fecal Immunochemical Test

A negative fecal occult blood test or fecal immunochemical test result rules out the colon or rectum as the site of bleeding (see Chapter 29).

Transvaginal and Lower Abdominal Ultrasound

Ultrasonography is used to determine endometrial thickness. Endometrial thickness varies depending on the phase of the menstrual cycle and ranges from 1 to 16 mm. In postmenopausal patients, 5 mm is the cutoff for a normal stripe. Ultrasound is also helpful in identifying cystic enlargement of the uterus, the presence of leiomyomas, and the presence or absence of the products of conception. Ultrasonography is used to determine complications of pregnancy such as ectopic pregnancy, placenta previa, or threatened abortion. When the intrauterine sac is identified within the uterus by ultrasound, an ectopic pregnancy is rarely the diagnosis, even though it is possible to have simultaneous intrauterine and ectopic pregnancies.

Endometrial Biopsy

Endometrial biopsy is used to detect cancer in any perimenopausal or postmenopausal patient who is experiencing abnormal vaginal bleeding. It is used to exclude endometrial cancer in patients taking tamoxifen who experience vaginal bleeding. Endometrial biopsy can be performed on patients in their 30s who are at increased risk for endometrial cancer (see Box 36.2). Endometrial biopsy has a sensitivity of 95% to 97% for endometrial carcinoma. If the test result is abnormal or inadequate in terms of amount of tissue, the next diagnostic test would be D&C. If that test is normal and abnormal bleeding continues, further workup is indicated to exclude neoplasia.

Dilation and Curettage

Dilation and curettage is useful in determining the cause of abnormal uterine bleeding and for the removal of retained products of conception. The curetting of the entire uterus provides specimens to send to pathology to rule out carcinogenic causes for uterine bleeding.

Hysteroscopy

Hysteroscopy allows for visualization of the uterine cavity. Endometrial biopsies, endometrial polyps, and submucosal leiomyomas can be obtained or removed by hysteroscopy.

DIFFERENTIAL DIAGNOSIS

Organic Causes of Vaginal Bleeding

Pregnancy

A small amount of bleeding can occur at implantation. The blastocyst burrows into the endometrium and invades the maternal blood supply; the formation and implantation of the placenta follow. If bleeding occurs from implantation, it happens about 1 week before the expected menstrual cycle. Regard patients of childbearing age with a uterus as pregnant until pregnancy is ruled out.

Spontaneous abortion

A spontaneous abortion (miscarriage) is the natural termination of a pregnancy before fetal viability (before 20 weeks). Approximately 15% of diagnosed pregnancies abort spontaneously. It is a complete spontaneous abortion if the fetus and the placenta are completely expelled and incomplete if partial tissue remains within the uterus. Most often the presenting symptoms are persistent uterine cramping and bleeding that is increasing in severity and amount. There may have been passage of tissue. The typical patient experiencing a spontaneous abortion presents to the clinic at about 10 to 12 weeks of gestation. The pregnancy test may remain positive for weeks after fetal death. A drop in serial hCG levels and an ultrasound that does not identify an intrauterine gestational sac support the diagnosis of spontaneous abortion.

Threatened abortion

Threatened abortion produces menstruation-like cramping and bleeding but the cervical os remains closed. The pain is often midline or suprapubic. Perform a sterile speculum examination to inspect the external cervical os. Only if the facility is prepared to deal with the possibility of surgical intervention should a cotton-tipped applicator or ring forceps be passed through the os to verify its closed status. In addition to bleeding and cramping, if the cervical os is open or if tissue is in the cervical canal, the patient is diagnosed with an inevitable abortion.

Placenta previa

Placenta previa occurs in the third trimester of pregnancy and presents with bright red painless bleeding. The placenta is implanted in the lower segment of the uterus. When the cervix begins to dilate, the placenta is pulled away from the endometrial wall, and bleeding can occur. Any significant bleeding that leads to hemorrhage can endanger the mother and may interfere with uteroplacental sufficiency. Fetal activity is present. The uterus is nontender with a normal resting tone. Diagnosis is made by sonogram. Pelvic examination should not be performed to avoid dislodging any clot that may have formed at the cervix.

Placenta abruptio

Placenta abruptio can occur any time after 20 weeks of gestation. As the placenta detaches from the uterine wall, the patient experiences dark red, painful bleeding. The amount of bleeding varies from scant to profuse. On physical examination, vaginal bleeding is apparent, and the uterus may be tender and demonstrate increased tone. Signs of fetal distress may be apparent. Vaginal examination is not performed until placenta previa is ruled out with ultrasound.

Ectopic pregnancy

Ectopic pregnancy occurs in about 1 of 200 pregnancies. Ectopic pregnancy is a leading cause of maternal death in the United States. Maintain high suspicion for this life-threatening condition. A ruptured ectopic pregnancy is a surgical emergency (see Chapter 3). Ectopic pregnancy symptoms can be the same as normal pregnancy symptoms; therefore, any pregnancy accompanied by bleeding or pain must be considered high risk for ectopic pregnancy and must be evaluated to rule out the condition. Persistent one-sided pain or pain that radiates toward the midline of the abdomen is indicative of ectopic pregnancy. The patient experiencing an ectopic pregnancy

typically presents at about 6 to 8 weeks of gestation. The menstrual pattern for these patients begins with a time of amenorrhea followed by abnormal bleeding. They may have some symptoms of pregnancy (e.g., breast tenderness, nausea, and vomiting), have passed some tissue (decidual cast), or have experienced fainting or dizziness. Ninety percent of ectopic pregnancies are implanted in the fallopian tube. About half of these patients will have an adnexal mass. Diagnosis is made through serial quantitative hCG testing and transvaginal ultrasound.

Leiomyomas (myomas or fibroids)

Fibroids are found in about 25% of patients with a uterus after age 35 years. They are more frequently found in African Americans than in whites, and they usually decrease in size after menopause. Depending on location, they are associated with infertility in 2% to 10% of patients. These benign tumors are estrogen dependent and may grow during hormone therapy. The most frequent symptom of leiomyomas is bleeding, which ranges from slightly heavier menstrual flow to continuous bleeding. Fibroids may occur as single or multiple tumors within the uterine layers or they can be pedunculated. Pain is not a common complaint with fibroids unless there has been strangulation of a pedunculated fibroid, degeneration of a large fibroid, or compression of other organ systems.

Adenomyosis

Adenomyosis is a condition in which there are endometrial glands and stroma within the myometrium of the uterus. It is more common in multiparous patients and occurs in the later reproductive years. The uterus is two to three times its normal size, and there is often dysmenorrhea and infertility. Adenomyosis often coexists with uterine fibroids. Ultrasound may not identify this diffuse intramural lesion. Adenomyosis is found in 20% of hysterectomy specimens.

Uterine or Endometrial Cancer

Endometrial cancer is now the most common female genital cancer in the United States.

The average age at diagnosis is 61 years, but it can occur at any time during the reproductive and postmenopausal years. Uterine cancer risk factors are anovulatory states (e.g., obesity), endometrial hyperplasia (e.g., unopposed estrogen), and family history (see Box 36.2). Classic symptoms include painless vaginal bleeding and a rapidly enlarging uterus. Late symptoms, such as weight loss and weakness, are those of systemic disease.

Systemic Causes of Vaginal Bleeding

Anovulatory cycles

Perimenopause

The perimenopausal years occur from ages 40 to 50 years and last about 7 to 10 years. The perimenopausal patient experiences irregularities in her menstrual flow. Often there is spotting, followed by 1 or 2 days of heavy bleeding or a regular menstrual flow and a few days of spotting at the end of the cycle. These types of irregular patterns are characteristic of a degenerating corpus luteum function. A patient with 1 year of irregular periods and who has missed the past three cycles can be clinically diagnosed as being in perimenopause (a synonymous term is *climacteric*).

The perimenopause progresses to menopause when the FSH level is greater than 40 mIU/mL or there are no periods for 1 full year. An FSH level of 30 mIU/mL is typical of perimenopause.

Perimenarche

With perimenarche, the patient has a history of beginning menstrual cycles and then experiencing months of amenorrhea followed by resumption of regular cycles caused by an immature HPO axis. The menstrual flow may be heavier, more frequent, or longer than normal. The young adolescent has appropriate secondary sexual characteristics and sexual maturity ratings. These symptoms are characteristic of anovulatory cycles.

Newborn

A bloody vaginal discharge may occur normally in female newborns because of maternal estrogen hormone withdrawal during the first few weeks of life.

Endocrinopathies

Polycystic Ovary Syndrome

In PCOS, the patient typically is obese, hirsute, and has oligomenorrhea and large cystic

---

EVIDENCE-BASED PRACTICE *Does This Patient Have an Ectopic Pregnancy?*

This systematic review and meta-analysis evaluated prospective studies of pregnant women with abdominal pain or vaginal bleeding. Patient history, physical examination, laboratory values, and sonography were compared with a reference standard of either direct surgical confirmation of ectopic pregnancy or clinical follow-up. Fourteen studies with 12,101 patients were included. The patient history and symptoms were not helpful in diagnosing ectopic pregnancy. Cervical motion tenderness, adnexal mass on bimanual examination, abdominal pain with cough, or tenderness during light palpation suggested ectopic pregnancy. The absence of cervical motion tenderness, peritoneal findings, adnexal mass, or adnexal tenderness did not decrease the likelihood of an ectopic pregnancy.

No single quantitative serum human chorionic gonadotropin (hCG) value determined ectopic pregnancy. Transvaginal sonography was most useful in diagnosing ectopic pregnancy. The presence of an adnexal mass along with the absence of an intrauterine pregnancy indicated a high likelihood of an ectopic pregnancy. The sensitivity of transvaginal sonography to detect ectopic pregnancy was 88% with specificity at 99%.

The authors concluded that patient history and clinical examination alone are insufficient to determine the presence of an ectopic pregnancy. When the patient is hemodynamically stable, the appropriate evaluation includes transvaginal sonography and serial quantitative serum hCG testing.

Reference: Crochet et al, 2013.

ovaries. However, patients with chronic anovulatory cycles and hyperandrogenemia meet the criteria for PCOS even if slim and without hirsutism. The LH-to-FSH ratio is greater than 3 to 1. DHEA-S levels are elevated.

Thyroid Dysfunction

Both hypothyroidism and hyperthyroidism are associated with abnormal menstrual bleeding. Whereas menorrhagia can occur with hypothyroidism, oligomenorrhea or scant menses may occur with hyperthyroidism.

With hypothyroidism, the patient may also experience delayed growth, weight gain, fatigue, constipation, and cold intolerance. On physical examination, dry skin, coarse hair, and galactorrhea may be noted. The TSH level will be high.

With hyperthyroidism, the patient may experience weight loss, nervousness, heat intolerance, and palpitations. On physical examination, the skin may be moist and sweaty, the hair thin, and the pulse rate may be rapid. The thyroid gland may be enlarged or nodular. The TSH level will be low, with high triiodothyronine (T_3) and thyroxine (T_4) levels.

Hyperprolactinemia

Prolactin inhibits gonadotropin release and causes anovulatory cycles that may be associated with irregular and sometimes heavy bleeding or with amenorrhea (see Chapter 5). Galactorrhea often accompanies hyperprolactinemia. Nipple discharge will be negative for red blood cells. Prolactin levels will be elevated. Thyroid function tests can rule out hypothyroidism. Magnetic resonance imaging of the hypothalamic/pituitary area assists in the diagnosis of pituitary tumor.

Vaginal infection

Atrophic Vaginitis

In atrophic vaginitis, there is a dry (shiny), pale, thin vaginal wall caused by an insufficient amount of endogenous estrogen. During menopause, the vaginal mucosa and vulva, which lack glycogen, become fragile and are susceptible to injury and infection. The patient may experience burning, dryness, irritation,

dyspareunia, or atrophic vaginitis. This also occurs in postpartum women, women who are breastfeeding, and prepubertal girls. The pH is alkaline and ranges from 6.5 to 7.0. Wet mount reveals a few WBCs and is negative for pathogens.

Endometritis

Endometritis is an infection of the endometrium, in which Chlamydia is the cause about 25% of the time. Group A or B streptococci produces puerperal sepsis and may lead to peritonitis, abscess, thrombophlebitis, disseminated intravascular coagulation, septic shock, and infertility. The woman has a slight vaginal discharge (lochia) that is bloody or purulent. The bleeding is accompanied by fever (temperature 39°–39.8°C [102°–103°F]) and uterine tenderness often within the first 24 hours after delivery. Endometritis should be suspected in a woman with these symptoms, especially if she has undergone an emergency cesarean section or an intrauterine manipulative procedure. Other contributing factors for endometritis are premature rupture of membranes and prolonged labor.

Pelvic Inflammatory Disease

Pelvic inflammatory disease is most commonly caused by *C. trachomatis* or *N. gonorrhoeae* (see Chapter 3) and can produce bleeding, abdominal pain, fever, and vaginal discharge. Patients with PID have an increasing amount of vaginal discharge and bleeding after intercourse. Infection begins intravaginally in most cases and then spreads upward, causing salpingitis. In the early stages, patients may be asymptomatic. Patients may have a purulent discharge that originates from the endocervical columnar and transitional cells. With gonorrhea, patients often experience inflammation of Skene glands, Bartholin glands, or the urethra, which causes pain and dysuria. On examination, there is abdominal, cervical motion, and adnexal tenderness. As with peritonitis, patients may also have guarding and rebound tenderness. WBC counts and erythrocyte sedimentation rate are usually elevated. Cultures, molecular testing, and Gram staining can assist with the diagnosis (see Chapter 37).

Genital Warts

Genital warts (condylomata acuminata) are caused by the human papillomavirus and may be precursors to genital cancer. The warts may involve the vagina, cervix, perineum, or perianal areas. Condylomata can be flat or raised verrucous lesions. The patient usually notices a bump on the genital region accompanied by itching and leukorrhea. A wet mount should be performed to rule out any coexisting vaginal infections. An acetic acid test is helpful in identifying flat warts. Refer to a dermatologist or gynecologist for treatment of warts of the urethra or anus.

Foreign Body

In foreign body retention, the presenting symptom is a very malodorous, whitish discharge. In children, the foreign body is as variable as those objects found in the ears and nose. Children younger than 12 months do not have the coordination to insert anything into their vaginas; suspect child abuse in those cases and inspect for bruising or excoriations. Wet mount reveals many WBCs.

Vulvovaginitis

In children with vulvovaginitis, vulvovaginal bleeding may accompany vaginal discharge, vaginal itching, vulvar erythema, and lesions. See Chapter 37 for a more detailed discussion. Vaginal discharge should be tested for gonorrhea and Chlamydia. If an STI or sexual abuse is suspected, syphilis and human immunodeficiency virus testing should be done. Throat and rectal specimens cultures for gonorrhea and chlamydia should also be obtained.

Blood dyscrasias

Von Willebrand Disease

Von Willebrand disease is a congenital autosomal dominant bleeding disorder characterized by altered factor VIII activity and deficient platelet function. The patient has a prolonged bleeding time. Hypermenorrhea may occur at menarche or may begin in women 20 to 30 years of age.

Leukemia

Hypermenorrhea may be one of the chief concerns of the woman presenting with leukemia. Other symptoms may include fatigue, bruising, and lymph node enlargement. The CBC and bleeding times will direct the workup for this diagnosis.

Other

Medications

Drugs such as rifampin, phenytoin, carbamazepine, and phenobarbital reduce the efficacy of oral OCs. If the woman is on a low-estrogen-dose OC, this is likely to be the cause of irregular vaginal bleeding. Changing the OC to a higher estrogenic potency will alleviate the bleeding. Tamoxifen, which acts as an antiestrogen on breast tissue, has estrogenic effects on the endometrium and can cause endometrial hyperplasia or endometrial cancer. The symptom is vaginal bleeding.

▶ DIFFERENTIAL DIAGNOSIS OF *Common Causes of Vaginal Bleeding*

CONDITION	HISTORY	PHYSICAL FINDINGS	DIAGNOSTIC STUDIES
ORGANIC CAUSES OF VAGINAL BLEEDING			
Pregnancy	Implantation bleeding; breast tenderness, nausea and vomiting	Internal cervical os closed; minimal spotting; globular, enlarged uterus; soft, bluish color cervix	Pregnancy test; β-hCG positive
Spontaneous abortion	Vaginal bleeding following time of amenorrhea; cramping, passage of tissue; history of miscarriages	Internal cervical os open; blood from cervical os	Serial declining β-hCG levels; ultrasound negative

Continued

► DIFFERENTIAL DIAGNOSIS OF *Common Causes of Vaginal Bleeding—cont'd*

CONDITION	HISTORY	PHYSICAL FINDINGS	DIAGNOSTIC STUDIES
Threatened abortion	Vaginal bleeding following time of amenorrhea; mild cramping	Fetal activity present; internal cervical os may be open	β-hCG positive; ultrasound positive
Placenta previa	Late pregnancy: bright red, painless bleeding	Fetal activity present; uterus is nontender, normal resting tone	Ultrasound
Placenta abruptio	Dark red, painful bleeding; any time after 20 wk of gestation	Vaginal bleeding; uterus tender with tone; signs of fetal distress	Rule out placenta previa with ultrasound
Ectopic pregnancy	Painless vaginal bleeding; multiparity, older gravida, multiple gestation; history of PID, infertility, STIs	Internal cervical os closed; bloody discharge present	β-hCG positive; ultrasound; laparoscopy
Leiomyomas	Heavier menstrual bleeding; menorrhagia	Enlarged uterine size; firm, spherical masses; nontender	Pelvic examination; ultrasound
Adenomyosis	Worsening menorrhagia; dysmenorrhea	Pelvic enlargement (two to three times normal size)	Pelvic examination; ultrasound not always helpful
Uterine or endometrial cancer	Rapidly enlarging uterus; painless menorrhagia; pelvic pressure; weight loss, weakness	Enlargement of uterus, often symmetrical; fixed with advanced disease	Endometrial biopsy; D&C; ultrasound; CT or MRI

SYSTEMIC CAUSES OF VAGINAL BLEEDING

Anovulatory Cycles

Perimeno- pause	Irregular menses, amenorrhea coupled with heavier and longer menstrual cycles; hot flashes, night sweats, insomnia, mood changes	Pale, dry vaginal mucosa, few rugae	FSH and LH high; estradiol low
Perimenarche	History of beginning menses within past 1–2 yr; amenorrhea followed by irregular menstrual cycles that are heavy, frequent, or of long duration	Physical examination findings normal; secondary sexual characteristics present	History and examination
Newborn	Younger than 2 mo old	Small amount of vaginal spotting	History and examination

▶ **DIFFERENTIAL DIAGNOSIS OF** *Common Causes of Vaginal Bleeding—cont'd*

CONDITION	HISTORY	PHYSICAL FINDINGS	DIAGNOSTIC STUDIES
Endocrinopathies			
Polycystic ovary syndrome	Infertility; irregular menstrual cycles	Hirsute; obese; enlarged ovaries	Pelvic examination; ultrasound; enlarged ovaries with multiple fluid-filled cysts
Thyroid dysfunction	Hypothyroid: menorrhagia, delayed growth, weight gain, fatigue, constipation, cold intolerance	Hypothyroid: dry skin, fine hair, galactorrhea	TSH high
Hyperprolactinemia	Menometrorrhagia, oligomenorrhea	Bilateral, multiduct, clear to white nipple discharge	Serum prolactin level; MRI if indicated
Vaginal Infection			
Atrophic vaginitis	Dyspareunia; vaginal dryness	Pale, thin vaginal mucosa; brown or bloody discharge; pH >4.5	Folded, clumped epithelial cells
Endometritis	History of emergency cesarean section, PROM, prolonged labor, intrauterine manipulative procedures	Tenderness of uterus on bimanual examination; temperature 102°–103°F; discharge or lochia may be purulent	WBC count >10,000/mm^3
Pelvic inflammatory disease	History of PID; chronic vaginitis; STIs	Bilateral abdominal pain following menses; pelvic mass; cervical motion tenderness; vaginal discharge; temperature >100.4°F	WBC, ESR; Gram staining, cultures, molecular testing
Genital warts	Mild to moderate itching; foul vaginal discharge; child: history of sexual abuse; adult: new or multiple partners; history of warts	Moist, pale pink, verrucous projections on base; located on vulva, vagina, cervix, or perianal area; bleeding with trauma	Acetic acid test: white
Foreign body	Red and swollen vulva; vaginal discharge; history of use of tampon, condom, or diaphragm	Foreign body present (tampon, condom); bloody, foul-smelling discharge	Wet mount: many WBCs, no pathogens; history and examination
Vulvovaginitis	Vulvovaginal bleeding with vaginal discharge, and itching. Common in children	Vulvar erythema, possible lesions; discharge	Molecular testing of discharge for gonorrhea and chlamydia; if an STI or sexual abuse is suspected, syphilis and human immunodeficiency virus testing

Continued

> **DIFFERENTIAL DIAGNOSIS OF** *Common Causes of Vaginal Bleeding—cont'd*

CONDITION	HISTORY	PHYSICAL FINDINGS	DIAGNOSTIC STUDIES
Blood Dyscrasias			
von Willebrand disease	Menorrhagia, adolescent	Bruising; petechiae; gingival bleeding	Bleeding time, factor VIII deficiency, decreased platelets
Leukemia	Menorrhagia; fatigue usually <3 mo duration	Fever, bruising, pallor; lymph node enlargement; hepatic or splenic enlargement	WBC count: 1000–400,000/mm^3, leukocytosis with immature blasts or cells; anemia, thrombocytopenia, decreased factor V or VIII
Other			
Medications	Taking rifampin, phenytoin, carbamazepine, or phenobarbital while on low-estrogen-dose OC; tamoxifen	Normal gynecological examination	Bleeding stops with higher estrogen dose OC; endometrial biopsy

CT, computed tomography; *D&C*, dilation and curettage; *ESR*, erythrocyte sedimentation rate; *FSH*, follicle-stimulating hormone; *hCG*, human chorionic gonadotropin; *LH*, luteinizing hormone; *MRI*, magnetic resonance imaging; *OC*, oral contraceptive; *PID*, pelvic inflammatory disease; *PROM*, premature rupture of membranes; *STI*, sexually transmitted infection; *TSH*, thyroid-stimulating hormone; *WBC*, white blood cell.

Vaginal Discharge and Itching

Infectious causes of vaginal discharge or itching include *Trichomonas vaginalis, Candida* spp., and bacterial vaginosis (BV), which account for the majority of all vaginal infections in the United States. Sexually transmitted causes of lower genital tract infections include *Chlamydia trachomatis, Neisseria gonorrhoeae,* and *Trichomonas vaginalis.*

Postmenopausal patients often have discharge, itching and irritation related to atrophic vaginitis, caused by the deficiency of estrogen in the vaginal tissues. Chemical vaginitis in adolescents and adults occurs because of the use of scented douches, lubricants, or hygiene sprays

Vulvar itching, burning, and a foul odor often accompany vaginal discharge. Pubic lice, scabies, pinworms, and genital warts (condylomata acuminata) can all cause itching. Common foreign bodies found in the vagina of adult patients are lost or forgotten tampons, which can produce a foul-smelling discharge.

In childhood and adolescence, vulvar itching soreness, and vaginal discharge are common. The lack of estrogen stimulation, neutral pH of the vaginal secretions, lack of protective thick labia and pubic hair, and daily living habits (e.g., wiping, clothing, play activities, environment, and baths) lead to this condition. Additionally, the vaginal mucosa is thin and less resistant to infectious organisms. Chemical vaginitis in a child is usually caused by sensitivity to bubble bath.

DIAGNOSTIC REASONING: FOCUSED HISTORY

What kind of vaginitis might this be?

Key Questions
- What is the amount, color, and consistency of your discharge?
- Do you have itching, swelling, or redness?
- Is there an odor?

Characteristics of Discharge

Copious amounts of greenish, offensive-smelling discharge are most consistent with *T. vaginalis.* Mucopurulent or purulent discharges are associated with gonorrhea and chlamydia. A moderate amount of white, curd-like discharge is consistent with candida vulvovaginitis. BV typically produces a discharge that is thin and white, green, gray, or brownish. Although characteristic symptoms associated with each type of vaginal discharge can be helpful in arriving at a diagnosis, they are not diagnostic in and of themselves. Microscopic examination of the vaginal discharge is more sensitive than the clinical picture in confirming the diagnosis (Fig. 37.1).

Itching, Swelling, and Redness

Vaginitis causes inflammation of the tissues, resulting in erythema and edema. Because of the inflammatory process, the amount of discharge will produce a concomitant amount of swelling and redness of the vulva and vagina. Itching is consistently present with candidiasis. Scratching can lead to excoriations and satellite lesions. BV does not involve an inflammatory process and results in discharge with little vulvovaginal erythema and edema.

Odor

A fishy odor caused by the release of amines from organic acids is prominent with BV. It is accentuated by the addition of potassium hydroxide (KOH) to the wet mount slide and is considered a positive "whiff" test. Odor commonly accompanies trichomonal infections. Retained tampons or other foreign bodies can also cause a foul odor.

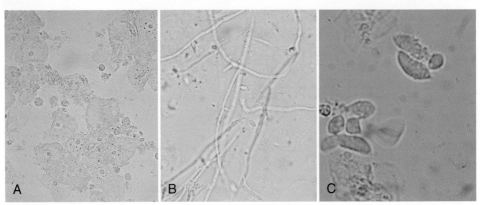

FIGURE 37.1 Microscopic differential diagnosis of vaginal infections. **A,** Clue cells (epithelial cells with clumps of bacteria) are evident in bacterial vaginosis. **B,** Budding, branching hyphae characterize candidiasis. **C,** Motile trichomonads are seen with trichomoniasis. (From Zitelli BJ, Davis HW: *Atlas of pediatric physical diagnosis,* ed. 3, St Louis, 1997, Mosby-Wolfe.)

Is this likely a sexually transmitted infection?

Key Questions

- Are you sexually active? Do you have multiple partners? Do you have a new partner?
- Have you had sex against your will? If a child, you might ask, "Has anyone touched your private parts?"
- What form of protection do you use? How often do you use protection?
- Have you or your partner(s) ever been tested or treated for a sexually transmitted infection (STI)?
- Do you have any rashes, blisters, sores, lumps, or bumps in the genital area?

Sexual History

Early-age onset of sexual activity, multiple partners, and nonuse of barrier contraceptives, particularly condoms, increase the risk of vaginal infection. STIs are common in patients of childbearing age (12–50 years) who have acquired a new partner, but the highest prevalence is in sexually active young adults younger than age 24 years. The patient who frequently changes sexual partners or participates in risky sexual practices (e.g., anal intercourse without a condom) is at high risk for STIs.

Do not ignore the possibility of an STI in older adults or children. About half of all children with an STI have been found to be sexually abused. *T. vaginalis* is rare in children but can be transmitted to a neonate from an infected mother.

Recent Treatment for a Sexually Transmitted Infection

Recent treatment for an STI may indicate treatment failure, a coinfection that was not covered by the prescribed drug, or recent exposure.

Lesions

Vesicles usually indicate herpes infection. Patients typically notice them on the external labia and report that they itch or burn. Condylomata lata, condylomata acuminata, and molluscum contagiosum are all papular lesions found on the labia, perineum, and anal regions. Molluscum contagiosum, when occurring in the genital area, may extend to the inner thighs. Typically, condylomata acuminata (genital warts) are rough, verrucous lesions that are usually located inferiorly from the fossa navicularis to the fourchette and perineal area. A painless ulcer suggests syphilis and classically appears as a solitary lesion. However, there can be more than one chancre, especially if the patient is immunocompromised.

Key Questions

- Have you ever been told that you have diabetes, Cushing syndrome, or human immunodeficiency virus (HIV) infection?
- Have you been ill recently?
- Are you taking antibiotics, hormones, or oral contraceptive pills?
- Have you received chemotherapy?
- Does the itching seem to be worse at night?
- Can you describe some of your recent activities?
- If an adolescent: Have you had a menstrual period?

Immunocompromised States

Refractory fungal vulvovaginitis may indicate undiagnosed diabetes or an immunocompromised state.

Recent Illness

Chickenpox, scarlet fever, and measles can cause vaginitis.

Medications or Chemotherapy

Birth control pills, corticosteroids, antibiotics, and chemotherapy are associated with candidal vulvovaginitis. Oral contraceptives can alter the vaginal pH, and antibiotics can alter the normal vaginal flora; both predispose to fungal infection. Corticosteroids and chemotherapy can produce an immunocompromised state and provide the opportunity for fungal infection.

Night Itching

Pinworms are intestinal parasites that inhabit the rectum or colon and emerge to lay eggs in the skinfolds of the anus. Perianal pruritus, especially at night, along with pain or itching of genitals is common (Fig. 37.2).

Activities

Riding a bicycle, using pools or hot tubs, or wearing tight-fitting pants or pantyhose can lead to heat and moisture in the genital area, causing mechanical irritation and such infections as candidiasis or BV.

Premenarche

Children who have not yet reached menarche are prone to vulvovaginal infections because of a nonestrogenized vagina and the lack of labial development and hair growth.

Key Questions

- How long have you had these symptoms?
- Are they getting better or worse?
- Have you ever had these symptoms before?

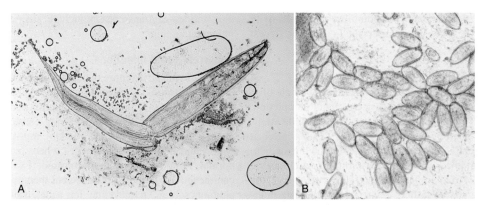

FIGURE 37.2 Pinworms *(Enterobius vermicularis)*. **A,** On this wet mount, a mature worm is shown surrounded by eggs. **B,** Eggs are shown more clearly at higher power. (From Zitelli BJ, Davis HW: *Atlas of pediatric physical diagnosis*, ed. 3, St Louis, 1997, Mosby-Wolfe.)

- How many episodes have you had in the past year?
- Are the episodes related to any particular activity or time?

Chronology of Symptoms

The occurrence of vaginal discharge after having a new sex partner suggests an acute condition, such as an STI. Symptoms associated with use of condoms or spermicidal jelly suggest sensitivity to the product. If the discharge occurs monthly with worsening after menses, suspect a chronic condition, such as vulvovaginitis candidiasis. Recurrent episodes related to bathing activities point to chemical irritation.

If this is acute, could it be related to a previous infection?

Key Questions

- Have you been tested and treated for this condition? What medication was prescribed?
- Did you take all of the medication?
- What other prescriptions were you taking at that time?
- What over-the-counter medications have you taken?

Adequate Diagnosis

Diagnoses made clinically on the basis of the color or appearance of discharge may be incorrect, or a concomitant vaginal infection may have been missed. However, self-diagnosis and treatment are common, especially with the over-the-counter medicines for "yeast infection."

Adequate Treatment

Medication regimens that are not single dose present a challenge to treatment completion. Patients may stop using vaginal medications when menses begins and resume after it ends. They may also discontinue the medication early, as soon as symptom relief occurs, or if they have a drug side effect (e.g., the metallic taste of metronidazole). Drug interactions may account for inadequate therapy, or the intake of certain foods or substances, such as alcoholic beverages, may need to be restricted.

If this is chronic, what should I suspect?

Key Questions

- Have any family members or sexual partners reported itching, rashes, sores, lumps, or bumps with any vaginal or urinary tract infections?
- Do you have a new or untreated partner?
- What are your sexual practices (e.g., vaginal, oral, anal sex)?
- Have you had recurrent yeast infections in the past year?

Transmission

Caregivers, parents, and siblings can spread infections, such as candidiasis, molluscum contagiosum, herpes, lice, and pinworms, to children through poor hygiene practices. Autoinoculation is also possible, especially for herpes, genital warts, and molluscum contagiosum.

New or Untreated Partner

The most common cause of reinfection is intercourse with a new or untreated partner.

Sexual Practices

Possible infection reservoirs are oral and anal cavities, which may need to be cultured for herpes or gonorrhea. Additionally, materials used during intercourse may need to be disinfected (e.g., diaphragm, sex toys). Less common modes of transmission include shared intimate clothing.

Recurrent yeast Infections

If the patient has had more than three separate episodes of candidal vulvovaginitis in 1 year, consider diabetes or the immunocompromised state of HIV/AIDS as the underlying cause. Yeast grows best in areas that are dark, moist, warm, and high in glucose, areas where the normal flora has been compromised. Oral contraceptives, hormone replacement therapy, antibiotics (e.g., tetracycline for acne), steroids, diets high in carbohydrates or artificial sweeteners, and clothing that holds moisture against the vulva (e.g., pantyhose, tight jeans) are risk factors associated with vulvovaginitis.

What are other possible causes for this vaginitis?

- What are your personal hygiene practices?
- Do you douche?
- Have you changed brands of contraceptive products?
- Could you have forgotten to remove your diaphragm or tampon?

Hygiene Practices

Feminine hygiene practices can contribute to vaginitis by causing a local allergic reaction, altered vaginal flora, or contamination of the vagina from the rectum. Perfumes in douches, sprays, lubricants, and bubble baths are frequent offenders in allergic vaginitis.

When a child is out of diapers, toileting is less closely assisted, and wiping techniques may be poor, leading to contamination of the vagina with bowel flora.

Douching

Frequent douching can change the balance of normal vaginal flora by altering the pH and is not recommended. This allows recolonization of the vagina with enteric bacteria, leading to pruritus and discharge. Douching can cause an allergic reaction. Colored or perfumed toilet paper can irritate the perineum, causing redness and itching. Wiping with tissue after urination or defecation in the direction from the anus toward the vagina can inoculate the vagina with rectal microbes.

Contraceptive Products

Contraceptive products (e.g., spermicidal jellies, suppositories, foam, and latex condoms) can cause an allergic inflammation of the sensitive mucosa and produce itching, erythema, tenderness, and an increase in usual vaginal secretions.

Foreign Body

Foul-smelling vaginal discharge can be caused by a lost tampon or condom or a forgotten diaphragm. A child who puts a foreign object into the vagina may have pruritus, burning, or foul, purulent vaginal discharge. Foreign bodies in the vagina are associated with vaginal bleeding or spotting. If the object is left for some time, it can imbed and perforate the vaginal wall.

Are there any associated symptoms that point to a cause?

- Do you have burning or pain with urination? Do you have urinary frequency or hesitation or nighttime urination?
- Is intercourse painful?
- Do you have abdominal or pelvic pain?
- If an infant: Does the infant have an eye infection?
- If an infant: Does the infant have a cough?

Urinary Tract Symptoms

Atrophic vaginitis is often accompanied by dysuria, dyspareunia, and vaginal dryness. Estrogen deficiency affects the patient's entire lower genital tract and may produce symptoms that can be confused with a urinary tract infection. Low estrogen levels may exacerbate stress and urge incontinence. Trichomonas and chlamydia may produce a coexisting urethritis that causes frequency and dysuria.

Dyspareunia and Pain

Vaginal atrophy, genital warts, or vaginal infections can cause dyspareunia. A more likely reason for deep vaginal dyspareunia is endometriosis, pelvic inflammatory disease (PID), or fibroids. STIs such as gonorrhea and chlamydia can cause cervicitis, which, if left untreated, can progress to PID and produce abdominal or pelvic pain (see Chapter 3).

Eye Infection

Eye infections in a newborn may be associated with gonorrhea and chlamydia (see Chapter 30).

Cough

Pneumonia in the newborn may be an indication of chlamydia (see Chapter 11).

DIAGNOSTIC REASONING: FOCUSED PHYSICAL EXAMINATION

Note Vital Signs

The presence of a fever may alert you to a serious infection, such as PID. Fever is uncommon with vaginitis.

Perform an Oral Examination

Oral thrush may accompany vulvar candidiasis, particularly in children. Look for white patches that bleed when you try to scrape them off.

Perform an External Genitalia Examination

Palpate for inguinal lymphadenopathy and tenderness, which can be present with vaginal infections. Inspect the vulva and labia, looking for erythema, excoriations, and induration. The skin is often bright red and swollen with small fissures or excoriations from candidiasis. Also, thick white curds of discharge are often noted in the labial folds. BV often produces a profuse, thin, whitish discharge that will leak out of the vagina onto the perineum. Palpate Bartholin and Skene glands and milk the urethra for discharge. Palpable Bartholin glands often coexist with STIs. If purulent discharge is seen, consider the diagnoses of gonorrhea or chlamydia and obtain specimens for diagnostic tests.

Condylomata lata, condylomata acuminata, and molluscum contagiosum are all papular lesions found on the labia, perineum, and anal regions. Molluscum contagiosum, when occurring in the genital area, may extend to the inner thighs. Herpes lesions are usually ulcerative in nature when seen clinically and need to be differentiated from other similar lesions (e.g., syphilitic chancre can be more than one lesion and tender if secondarily infected). Herpetic lesions—painful vesicles on an erythematous base—are found in clusters and can extend from the labia into the vagina. Typically, condylomata acuminata (genital warts) are rough, verrucous lesions that are located inferiorly from the fossa navicularis to the fourchette and perineal area.

In an overweight patient, vulvovaginitis candidiasis is frequently accompanied by intertriginous candidiasis (e.g., under the breasts and the abdominal apron).

In a young child, it is important to tell her in simple terms what you are about to do. A common position for examination is the frog leg position. Have the parent sit on a chair and then have the patient sit on her parent's lap for the examination. The most common problem (vulvovaginitis) of the younger child requires only the lower third of the vagina to be visualized. A more detailed visual examination requires labial separation and labial traction.

Perform an Internal Vaginal Examination

Note the condition of the vaginal walls. A plastic speculum makes vaginal wall inspection easy and helps in the identification of a foreign body for removal. In children, the knee–chest position is useful for inspecting the vagina. If a foreign body is suspected in children, removal is done using sedation. Pale or mottled red splotches of the vaginal mucosa with a sticky, yellow-brown discharge are associated with atrophic vaginitis. In severe cases of atrophic vaginitis, the pale, thin mucosa may have adhered to the opposing vaginal wall, and the speculum examination often causes an oozing bloody discharge.

The appearance of the cervix should be noted. A friable or "strawberry" appearance of cervical petechiae with a frothy, foul-smelling discharge is descriptive of a trichomonas infection. A mucopurulent discharge from the cervical os requires an endocervical sample for gonorrhea and chlamydia testing. This discharge is yellowish-green when collected on an endocervical swab. The character of the discharge does not consistently identify common infectious causes of vaginitis. Treat vaginal infections before the Papanicolaou test is obtained because BV and trichomoniasis may cause inflammatory atypia results.

Obtain a sample for testing. The wet mount is a valuable diagnostic tool, and a sample of vaginal discharge is best obtained from the lateral vaginal fornices. Three positive characteristics for any one etiology can correctly identify the causative agent (e.g., increased pH; the presence of "clue cells," which are epithelial cells full of bacteria that obscure the cell border; and a thin gray discharge seen in

BV) (see Differential Diagnosis). Molecular testing or culture may also be indicated (see Laboratory and Diagnostic Studies). Cultures for BV, fungal infections, and *T. vaginalis* are not routinely recommended and are usually reserved for determining resistant organisms.

Perform a Bimanual Examination

Assess the condition of the uterus, fallopian tubes, and ovaries by checking for uterine and cervical motion tenderness (CMT), ovarian size, and presence of masses. CMT or pain on palpation of the uterus and adnexa confirms the spread of vaginitis or cervicitis to the upper genital tract and results in PID. This warrants immediate evaluation and treatment or referral to prevent tubal scarring, ectopic pregnancy, and infertility.

Perform a Vaginal-Rectal Examination

Vaginal-rectal examination is a technique in assessing the posterior uterus and condition of the cul-de-sac as well as the rectum. The internal examination glove must be changed before rectal insertion to prevent contamination of the rectum with vaginal discharge organisms. A rectal examination, using the fifth digit, is used to palpate a foreign body and to check pelvic anatomy in the child.

LABORATORY AND DIAGNOSTIC STUDIES

Potassium Hydroxide and Wet Mount or Preparation

Obtain a discharge sample from the lateral fornices of the vagina using a cotton-tipped applicator. There are several acceptable techniques for preparing a diagnoses and wet mount. One is to prepare two slides with a smear of vaginal discharge. To one slide, add 1 drop of 10% KOH and put a coverslip in place. To the other slide, add 1 drop of normal saline and put a coverslip in place. The result of the whiff test is positive when the addition of the 10% KOH produces a fishy odor, which is caused by the release of amines. The whiff test has a positive predictive value of 76% for BV. Look under the microscope at the KOH slide for the presence of branching and budding hyphae that are characteristic of yeast

infection. Examine the saline wet mount microscopically for motile trichomonads that signal the presence of trichomonas. Clue cells are characteristic of BV (see Fig. 37.1).

Test for pH

Most litmus paper reads the pH range from 3.0 to 9.0. This is a simple inexpensive test to aid in determining the cause of the vaginal discharge. Normal vaginal secretions have a pH less than 4.5. A pH greater than 4.5 is consistent with BV, trichomoniasis, or atrophic vaginitis.

Fungal Culture or Sabouraud Agar Culture

Fungal culture may be needed in the diagnosis of non–*Candida albicans* (e.g., *C. glabrata*, *C. tropicalis*, *C. krusei*) that are refractory to medication regimens.

Herpes Viral Culture

Viral culture is the most specific method of diagnosing herpes. Results may take from 1 to 7 days, with maximum sensitivity achieved at 5 to 7 days. The herpes culture will probably not be able to identify the causative agent if the specimen is taken from a lesion that is 5 or more days old. It is important to document positive genital herpes infections in the pregnant patient and in skin lesions of the newborn. Collect cells or fluid from a fresh sore with a cotton swab and place them in the culture container. You may need to unroof a vesicle to obtain a specimen.

Herpes Virus Antigen Detection Test

This test detects antigens on the surface of cells infected with the herpes virus. Cells from a fresh sore are scraped off and then smeared onto a microscope slide. This test may be done in addition to or in place of a viral culture.

Tzanck Smear

Characteristic findings of a Tzanck smear are multinucleated giant cells that are likely to be found if the specimen is from an intact herpes lesion. Prepare the Tzanck smear by removing the roof of the vesicle and scraping the skin with a scalpel blade. Make sure that the base and the margins of the vesicle are scraped. Do not use the vesicular fluid for this specimen. The cellular material is spread onto a glass slide, fixed with absolute alcohol for 1 minute, and then stained with Wright stain. Alternative staining methods are available, and guidelines can be obtained from local laboratories.

Modified Diamond Culture

Diamond culture can be used to identify *Trichomonas* spp., but it is seldom needed to make the diagnosis.

Thayer-Martin Culture

Thayer-Martin medium is a bacterial culture that identifies gonococcal infections. A culture is taken from the endocervical canal of the uterine cervix. First remove excess mucus from a portion of the cervix using a cotton ball held in ring forceps or a large cotton-tipped procto-swab. Insert a sterile cotton-tipped applicator (Q-Tip) into the endocervical canal and allow it to absorb the mucus for 10 to 30 seconds before inoculating the medium. Inoculate the medium bottle or plate in a zigzag manner while simultaneously rolling the small cotton-tipped applicator. When opening the Thayer-Martin culture bottle, avoid holding the bottle totally upright, which will allow for the loss of the carbon dioxide from the specimen collection bottle.

Molecular Testing for Infectious Organisms

Molecular testing using a sample taken from the vagina provides rapid, sensitive, and specific results. Molecular testing has largely replaced the need for culture methods. A number of products are available. Tests include DNA probes, nucleic acid amplification tests (NAATs), and polymerase chain reaction (PCR) assays. Tests are available for *C. trachomatis, N. gonorrhoeae, T. vaginalis, Gardnerella vaginalis, Candida* spp., and herpes simplex virus. Samples for chlamydia and gonorrhea testing can be obtained by the clinician or by the patient. Urine NAATs can be used to screen for possible STIs in both adults and children.

Syphilis Testing

Serology tests are used for screening and diagnosing syphilis and are recommended if other STIs are found or suspected. The screening tests are nontreponemal and include Venereal Disease Research Laboratory, rapid plasma reagin, and enzyme immunoassay tests. Diagnostic tests are *T. pallidum*-specific and include FTA-ABS (fluorescent treponemal antibody absorption test) and *T. pallidum* particle agglutination assay. Detection of *T. pallidum* can also be done using PCR molecular testing.

 EVIDENCE-BASED PRACTICE *Self-collected Vaginal Swabs Compared with Clinician-Collected Swabs*

A meta-analysis of 21 studies and more than 6100 paired samples estimated the accuracy of self-collected samples compared with clinician-collected samples for diagnosing chlamydia and gonorrhea. Six studies compared self-collected vaginal samples with clinician-collected cervical samples. When the studies were pooled, sensitivity was 0.92 (95% confidence interval [CI], 0.87–0.95), and specificity was 0.98 (95% CI, 0.97–0.99). Taking into account that urine samples may be less sensitive than cervical samples, eight chlamydia studies that compared urine self-collected versus clinician-collected cervical samples had a sensitivity of 87% (95% CI, 81–91) and high specificity of 99% (95% CI, 0.98–1.00).

For gonorrhea in women, three studies compared self-collected urine samples with clinician-collected cervical swabs. The pooled sensitivity was 0.79 (95% CI, 0.70–0.88), and specificity was 0.99 (95% CI, 0.99–1.00). One cross-sectional study (*n* = 309) compared self-collected vaginal samples with clinician-collected cervical samples. The reported sensitivity was 0.98 (95% CI, 0.88–1.00), and the specificity was 0.97 (95% CI, 0.94–0.99).

The authors concluded that the high sensitivity and specificity of vaginal self-collected swabs compared with swabs collected by clinicians supports the use of vaginal swab self-collection for chlamydia and gonorrhea testing in women.

Reference: Lunny et al, 2015.

Urinalysis

Urinalysis should be obtained if the patient has dysuria. However, external pain on urination may originate from urine on inflamed vulvar tissue, eliminating the need for urinalysis.

Microscopy and Skin Scraping

Viewing a skin scraping under the microscope is used to assist with the differential diagnosis of scabies and pubic lice (see Chapter 28).

Scotch Tape Test

Use this test when you suspect pinworms *(Enterobius vermicularis),* which occur most commonly in children. Instruct the adult to apply clear adhesive cellophane tape to the child's perianal region early in the morning when the child awakens. The tape is then removed, placed in a plastic bag, and brought into the clinic. Place it on a glass slide and examine it under a microscope for the presence of eggs. Parents may also be able to see the worms by shining a flashlight on the external anus of the child at night. A female worm is about 10 mm long (see Fig. 37.2).

Acetic Acid Test (Acetowhite)

The acetic acid test is best used to detect subclinical lesions caused by human papillomavirus (HPV) when a genital wart has been identified, when there has been sexual contact, or when the Pap test indicates dysplasia. The application of 5% acetic acid (vinegar) to the cervix, labia, or perianal area causes the lesion to turn white (acetowhite). Saturate a gauze pad with vinegar and place it on the lesion for 5 to 10 minutes. After this soaking, the white wart will have a sharp circumscribed macular or papular border. The surface will appear verrucous. False-positive results can occur with candidiasis, psoriasis, lichen planus, and sebaceous glands.

Follicle-Stimulating Hormone

Follicle-stimulating hormone levels that are greater than 30 mU/mL are diagnostic of perimenopause, and levels of 40 mU/mL or higher represent menopause. This test is particularly helpful in establishing the hypoestrogenic status of a young patient

who is experiencing premature menopause and atrophic vaginitis (see Evidence-Based Practice box).

DIFFERENTIAL DIAGNOSIS

Discharges

Physiological discharge

Normal vaginal discharge, produced by the cervical and vulvar glands, is mucoid, clear or white in color, and has no foul odor. Throughout the menstrual cycle it varies in consistency and amount from scant to profuse, depending on the amount of estrogen stimulation to the tissues. On occasion, physiological discharge can lead to slight vulvar irritation and mild itching secondary to wetness. The vaginal pH is less than 4.5. Wet mount reveals up to 3 to 5 white blood cells (WBCs)/high-power field (HPF) and the presence of epithelial cells and lactobacilli.

Bacterial vaginosis

Bacterial vaginosis is the most common cause of vaginal discharge and is considered a disturbance in normal vaginal flora. Many patients are asymptomatic. BV is often found after intercourse with a new partner or in conjunction with other STIs. Infection is associated with increased preterm labor in patients who are pregnant. The diagnosis of BV in premenopausal women is usually based on the presence of at least three Amsel criteria: characteristic homogeneous, thin, grayish-white vaginal discharge, and a vaginal pH greater than 4.5; fishy odor (whiff test) when a drop of 10 % KOH is added to a sample of vaginal discharge; and the presence of clue cells on saline wet mount (see Fig. 37.1).

Candida vulvovaginitis

Ninety percent of patients with candida vulvovaginitis present with vulvar pruritus. In children, it may be accompanied by oral thrush. The discharge is often thick, white, and "curdy"; the labia are erythematous and edematous. Vaginal pH is 4.0 to 4.7. A KOH wet mount shows pseudohyphae and spores (see Fig. 37.1).

> **EVIDENCE-BASED PRACTICE** *Clinical Diagnosis of Vaginitis*
>
> According to this systematic review, approximately 33% of patients with vaginal discharge will have bacterial vaginosis (BV), 25% will have candidiasis, and 10% will have trichomoniasis. The lack of a perceived odor makes candidiasis more likely (likelihood ratio, 2.2), but the absence of the symptom is not conclusive. No symptoms reliably identify trichomoniasis. A thick or "curdy" discharge is compatible with yeast but does not rule out additional infection. Microscopic evaluation is required to identify clue cells (BV), yeast forms (vaginal candidiasis), or trichomonads (vaginal trichomoniasis). The authors concluded that diagnosis is best established by measuring the pH of the discharge, performing the whiff test, and using microscopic examination.
>
> Reference: Piscitelli and Simel, 2009.

Trichomoniasis

Trichomoniasis is often asymptomatic. It is usually transmitted via sexual contact but can also be spread by fomites. Patients with chronic infections will have copious amounts of discharge and little or no inflammation of the vaginal tissues. When there is an acute infection, they will report vulvar itching, swelling, and redness. The pH is greater than 5; the discharge is white, grayish-green, or yellow and sometimes frothy; infrequently, there will be a "strawberry cervix" (cervical petechiae). If the patient has douched within the past 24 hours, the sensitivity of tests will be greatly decreased. Wet mount shows "gyrating" motile protozoa and often greater than 10 WBCs/HPF (see Fig. 37.1).

Atrophic vaginitis

In atrophic vaginitis, there is a dry (shiny), pale, thin vaginal wall caused by an insufficient amount of endogenous estrogen. During menopause, the vaginal mucosa and vulva, which lack glycogen, become fragile and are susceptible to injury and infection. Patients may experience burning, dryness, irritation, or dyspareunia. This also occurs in postpartum patients, those who are breastfeeding, and prepubertal adolescents. The pH is alkaline and ranges from 6.5 to 7.0. Wet mount shows a few WBCs and is negative for pathogens.

Allergic vaginitis

The causes of allergic vaginitis are different in children and adults. In children, the most common offending agents are bubble baths and perfumed soaps. Vulvovaginitis in adults involves any harsh or caustic substance that has direct contact with the area. Often a new brand of vaginal lubricant, douche, spermicide, or condom will cause the inflammation and edema. Vinegar douches stronger than 1 to 2 tablespoons per quart of water may also irritate tissues. The wet mount is positive for WBCs and negative for pseudohyphae.

Foreign body

The presenting symptom in foreign body retention is a very malodorous, whitish discharge. In children, the foreign body is as variable as objects found in the ears and nose. However, children younger than 12 months do not have the coordination to insert anything into their vaginas, so suspect child abuse in such cases and inspect for bruising or excoriations. Wet mount reveals many WBCs.

Chlamydia

Chlamydia is the most prevalent STI in the United States. About 30% of infected patients are asymptomatic. Gonorrhea and chlamydia coexist in up to 60% of patients. Women with chlamydia have an increasing amount of vaginal discharge and bleeding after intercourse. Those at greatest risk for infection are younger than 25 years, sexually active with three or more partners, and not using barrier methods of contraception. Wet mount shows greater than 10 WBCs/HPF and few microscopic bacteria. molecular testing confirms the diagnosis. Except for perinatal syndromes, nonsexual transmission has not been reported;

therefore, suspect child abuse in children with chlamydia infection.

Gonorrhea

Gonorrhea is one of the most common reportable diseases. Patients are asymptomatic 50% to 80% of the time. However, the patient may have purulent discharge that originates from the endocervical columnar and transitional cells. Patients often experience inflammation of Skene glands, Bartholin glands, or the urethra, which causes pain and dysuria. Molecular testing or culture confirms the diagnosis. A finding of gonorrhea in children is considered specific evidence of sexual abuse.

Pelvic inflammatory disease

Pelvic inflammatory disease is most commonly caused by *C. trachomatis* and *N. gonorrhoeae* (see Chapter 3) and can produce bleeding, abdominal pain, fever, and vaginal discharge. Patients with PID have an increasing amount of vaginal discharge and bleeding after intercourse. Infection begins intravaginally in most cases and then spreads upward, causing salpingitis. In the early stages, patients may be asymptomatic. Patients may have a purulent discharge that originates from the endocervical columnar and transitional cells. With gonorrhea, patients often experience inflammation of Skene glands, Bartholin glands, or the urethra, which causes pain and dysuria. On examination, abdominal tenderness, CMT, and adnexal tenderness are present. As with peritonitis, patients may also have guarding and rebound tenderness. WBCs and erythrocyte sedimentation rate are usually elevated. Cultures, Gram staining, and molecular testing can assist with diagnosis. Patients with suspected PID should have a pregnancy test to rule out ectopic pregnancy and complications of an intrauterine pregnancy. All patients diagnosed with acute PID should also be tested for HIV infection.

Itching and Lesions

Syphilis

The chancre of primary syphilis is an ulcerative lesion that most often develops at the site of initial inoculation. The syphilitic chancre begins as a papule and progresses to a painless, tender, hard, indurated ulcer. The infection causes inguinal lymphadenopathy. Even without treatment, the lesion will heal in 3 to 6 weeks. Many chancres go unnoticed until the appearance of condylomata lata, the warty papule of secondary syphilis, or a maculopapular rash on the palms of the hands and soles of the feet. The diagnosis is confirmed with serological or molecular testing for syphilis.

Genital warts

Genital warts (condylomata acuminata) are caused by the HPV and may be precursors to genital cancers. The warts may involve the vagina, cervix, perineum, or perianal areas. Condylomata can be flat or raised verrucous lesions (Fig. 37.3). The patient usually notices a bump in the genital region accompanied by itching and leukorrhea. A wet mount should be performed to rule out any coexisting vaginal infections. An acetic acid test is helpful in identifying flat warts. Referral to a dermatologist or gynecologist is indicated for treatment of warts of the urethra or anus. High-risk HPV testing of genital warts is not recommended.

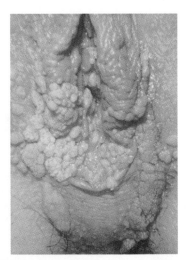

FIGURE 37.3 Condylomata acuminata. (From Morse SA, Holmes KK, Ballard R: *Atlas of sexually transmitted diseases and AIDS,* ed. 3, St Louis, 2003, Mosby.)

Herpes

Herpetic lesions can be difficult to distinguish from ulcerative lesions. The most typical presentation is that of grouped vesicles on an erythematous base that rupture and erode (Fig. 37.4). A prodrome of tingling or itching occurs before the outbreak of the vesicles. On the vulva, the erosions are covered with a whitish, exudative layer. Herpetic outbreaks can involve the cervix, vagina, vulva, anus, or extragenital organs, such as the pharynx. Molecular testing, culture, antigen test, or Tzanck smear confirms the diagnosis.

If the mother has an active primary herpes simplex virus infection at the time of birth, the infant has a 50% risk of becoming infected. Recurrent maternal infections impart a less than 5% risk of transmission. Clinical signs of the infant's infection become apparent in the first week of life and pose the possibility of death.

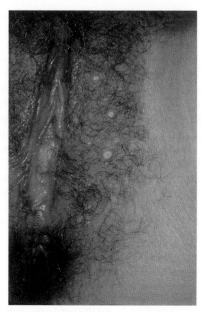

FIGURE 37.5 Molluscum contagiosum. (From Black M, Ambros-Rudolph C, Edwards L, et al: *Obstetric and gynecologic dermatology,* London, 2008, Mosby.)

Molluscum contagiosum

Molluscum are small (2–5 mm in diameter), umbilicated, flesh-tone papules (Fig. 37.5). These characteristic lesions are the hallmark of the diagnosis. Scratching can spread them. Molluscum is an STI of adults and a likely finding in HIV-infected patients. When children are found to have genital molluscum, suspect child abuse.

Vulvar intraepithelial neoplasia

A premalignant condition of the vulvar skin, is a condition associated with a high risk of recurrence and the potential to progress to vulvar cancer. The condition is complicated by its multicentric and multifocal nature. The incidence appears to be rising, particularly in the younger age group.

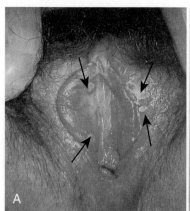
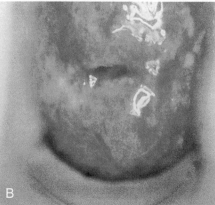

FIGURE 37.4 Herpes. (*Left* from Habif. TP: *Clinical dermatology,* ed 4, St. Louis, 2004, Mosby. *Right* from Morse SA, Holmes KK, Ballard R: *Atlas of sexually transmitted diseases and AIDS,* ed. 3, St Louis, 2003, Mosby.)

> ## DIFFERENTIAL DIAGNOSIS OF *Common Causes of Vaginal Discharge and Itching*

CONDITION	HISTORY	PHYSICAL FINDINGS	DIAGNOSTIC STUDIES
DISCHARGES			
Physiological discharge	Increase in discharge; no foul odor, itching, or edema	Clear or mucoid; pH <4.5	Up to 3–5 WBCs/ HPF; epithelial cells, lactobacilli
Bacterial vaginosis	Foul-smelling discharge	Homogeneous thin white or gray discharge; pH >4.5	Presence of KOH "whiff" test; presence of clue cells; few lactobacilli (see Fig. 37.1)
Candida vulvovaginitis	Pruritic discharge	White, curdy discharge; pH 4.0–5.0	KOH prep: mycelia, budding, branching yeast, pseudohyphae (see Fig. 37.1)
Trichomoniasis	Watery discharge; foul odor	Profuse, frothy, greenish discharge; red friable cervix; pH 5.0–6.0	Round or pear-shaped protozoa; motile "gyrating" flagella (see Fig. 37.1)
Atrophic vaginitis	Dyspareunia; vaginal dryness	Pale, thin vaginal mucosa; yellow-brown discharge pH >4.5	Folded, clumped epithelial cells
Allergic vaginitis	Examples: new bubble bath, soap, douche	Foul smell, erythema, "lost tampon," pH <4.5	WBCs
Foreign body	Red and swollen vulva; vaginal discharge; history of tampon, condom, or diaphragm use	Bloody, foul-smelling discharge	WBCs
Chlamydia	Partner with nongonococcal urethritis; asymptomatic; discharge or bleeding after intercourse	May or may not have purulent discharge	Molecular testing; >10 WBCs/HPF
Gonorrhea	Partner with STI; often asymptomatic	Purulent discharge; inflammation of Skene or Bartholin gland	Molecular testing, Gram stain; culture
Pelvic inflammatory disease	Bleeding, abdominal pain, fever, and vaginal discharge; increasing amount of vaginal discharge and bleeding after intercourse	CMT and adnexal tenderness; may also have guarding and rebound tenderness	WBC; Gram stain; DNA testing (chlamydia and gonococcus), culture; syphilis testing; ESR,CRP; pregnancy, HIV

Continued

> DIFFERENTIAL DIAGNOSIS OF *Common Causes of Vaginal Discharge and Itching—cont'd*

CONDITION	HISTORY	PHYSICAL FINDINGS	DIAGNOSTIC STUDIES
ITCHING AND LESIONS			
Syphilis	History of painless ulcerative lesion; rash on palms and soles of feet; warty growth on vagina or anus	Chancre: usually one but can be more, painless ulceration; condylomata lata: flat, whitish papule or plaque; maculopapular rash: palm, soles, body	Syphilis and molecular testing
Genital warts	Mild to moderate itching, foul vaginal discharge; child: history of sexual abuse; adult: new or multiple partners; history of warts	Moist, pale-pink, verrucous projections on base; located on vulva, vagina, cervix, or perianal area	Acetic acid test: white
Herpes	History of prodromal syndrome, paresthesias, burning, itching; may have mucoid vaginal discharge	Grouped vesicles on red base, erode to an ulcer; if on mucous membrane, exudates form; if on skin, crusts form; redness, edema, tender inguinal lymph nodes	Molecular testing; viral culture; Tzanck smear
Molluscum contagiosum	History of contact with infected person; if inflamed: itching	Flesh-colored, dome-shaped papules, some with umbilication; usually 2–5 mm in diameter	None
Vulvar Intraepithelial Neoplasia	Vulvar itching	Usually elevated lesion found on vulva	Refer for biopsy

CMT, cervical motion tenderness; *CRP*, C-reactive protein; *ESR*, erythrocyte sedimentation rate; *HIV*, human immunodeficiency virus; *HPF*, high-power field; *KOH*, potassium hydroxide; *STI*, sexually transmitted infection; *WBC*, white blood cell.

38   Vision Loss

Vision loss is a condition that ranges from vision impairment to total blindness. Most severe vision loss is associated with age, in persons 50 years and older. The most common cause of vision loss in children is refractive error. For vision to occur, light is transmitted through the eye to photoreceptors in the retina that collect light and send neural impulses to the brain. These impulses are then processed to give information on what is being seen. Vision loss occurs with any interruption in this visual pathway, such as opacification of the cornea, lens, or vitreous body (see Chapter 30, Fig. 30.1, for the anatomical structures of the eye). Vision loss also occurs when light energy cannot be converted into neural impulses, such as in glaucoma, retinal detachment, ischemic optic nerve atrophy, and pituitary or occipital tumors. Because vision loss is a self-reported condition, functional causes, formerly called malingering or hysteria, can be considered.

The most common causes of vision loss in adults are refractive errors, cataracts, glaucoma, age-related macular degeneration (AMD), and diabetic retinopathy. Infectious causes of vision loss (i.e., trachoma and onchocerciasis) have dropped dramatically globally. In all cases, impaired vision requires evaluation by an ophthalmologist. However, knowledge of the causes of vision loss can provide important clues to the diagnosis of these conditions.

DIAGNOSTIC REASONING: FOCUSED HISTORY

What is the extent of vision loss?

Key Questions
- What can you see? Can you detect light?
- Is your vision blurred?

- To self: Does the patient look at me?
- If a child: Does the child's eye wander?

Total Absence of Vision

Disease that affects the optic nerve or retina, such as retinal detachment, leads to total loss of vision. Blindness is a complete lack of form and visual light perception.

Blurring of Vision

Distinguish between loss of vision and loss of visual acuity. Vision loss is the absence of vision, completely or partially, in one or both eyes. Blurriness refers to a change in the acuity of vision. The most common cause of visual acuity change is refractive error.

Ability to Focus

Patients who are without sight have no ocular alignment and commonly manifest a gross searching and wandering nystagmus. Nystagmus in the first year of life suggests bilateral vision loss until proved otherwise. In infancy, vision loss is a common cause of nystagmus.

Visual Fixation

Even though the visual system is incompletely developed at birth, most infants can see and demonstrate visual interest when stimulated by a human face. At birth, infants have visual fixation present, and by 2 months of age, fixation is well developed. Any parental concern about a child's visual functioning is an important history finding.

Is this an emergency that requires immediate intervention?

Key Questions
- Was the loss of vision sudden?
- Is the loss in one or both eyes?

- Is the loss complete or partial?
- Is there any pain with the loss of vision?
- Are there other symptoms associated with the loss, such as a flash of light?
- Was the loss momentary or persistent?

Onset and Laterality

Sudden loss of vision suggests a vascular etiology, specifically occlusion of the central retinal artery until proven otherwise. In occlusion of the central retinal artery, the patient notes that vision is lost suddenly, and light cannot be distinguished from dark. Occlusion of the central retinal artery is an emergency and requires immediate treatment. Loss of vision in one eye indicates that the problem is anterior to the chiasm; hemianopic field defects in both eyes suggest a postchiasmal lesion (Fig. 38.1).

Pain

Sudden loss of vision with eye pain and photophobia indicates pathology of the cornea, iris, and ciliary body. Sudden loss of vision with a red painful eye may indicate acute-angle glaucoma (see Chapter 30). Inflammation, demyelinization, or degeneration of the optic nerve causes pain on movement of the eye and is thought to be the result of general inflammation of the posterior portion of the orbit or inflammation of the optic nerve (cranial nerve II). Retrobulbar neuritis is the most common disease in this category.

A common cause of sudden loss of vision without pain is vitreous hemorrhage. The patient describes floaters that begin to drift in front of the eye followed by a red glow. The vision gradually fades until only light and dark are distinguished. Painless

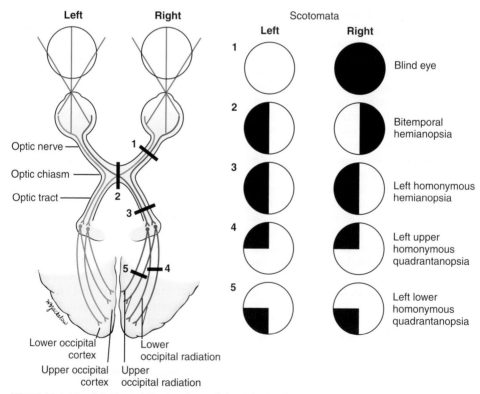

FIGURE 38.1 Visual fields and five locations of visual field defects and associated visual field changes. Examples of visual field defects along the optic nerve, optic chiasm, optic tracts, and optic radiations in the cortex. (From Ferri FF: *Ferri's color atlas and text of clinical medicine,* Philadelphia, 2008, Saunders.)

vision loss is also associated with macular degeneration, retinal detachment, diabetic retinopathy, and anterior ischemic optic neuropathy.

Children

In children, acute optic neuritis rarely occurs as an isolated condition and is usually a manifestation of a neurologic or systemic disease such as meningitis, viral infection, or demyelinating diseases. It may also be associated with lead poisoning and long-term use of certain drugs, most notably chloramphenicol or vincristine.

Flash of Light with Loss of Vision

Patients who have retinal detachment describe a flash of light shortly before loss of vision. Some patients describe a veil over the eye either just before or immediately after the flash. The reason for the flashes is that detachment of the retina causes mechanical stimulation of the rods and cones as it tears away from the pigment epithelium and floats free.

Patients whose retinae pull away or tear but do not detach experience the same flash of light as those with retinal detachment. They may also experience momentary total or partial loss of vision in the affected eye.

Transient Loss of Vision

Some patients with migraine headaches experience a scotoma, or an area of impaired vision within the visual field, before the onset of the headache. The scotoma may be either positive (the patient sees a light spot or scintillating flashes [scintillating scotoma]) or negative (the patient experiences a blind spot). Scotoma may be prodromal to a migraine headache. Profound anxiety can produce a transient loss of vision or a perceived loss of vision.

Can I rule out trauma?

Key Questions
- Is there a history of head trauma?
- Is there a history of eye trauma?
- Has there been a chemical or thermal injury?

Head Trauma

Loss of vision is most likely to occur after trauma to the occiput. The vision loss is sudden and complete, but vision usually returns in a matter of hours. Severe head trauma with skull fracture but without direct damage to the eyeball can result in loss of vision that occurs immediately or shortly thereafter. Occasionally, a patient can have good vision in the affected eye after the accident and subsequently lose vision as a result of severe retrobulbar hemorrhage. In children, trauma is the most common cause of retinal detachment. Abusive head trauma, called shaken baby syndrome, may result in retinal and vitreous hemorrhage.

Eye Trauma

Blunt trauma occurs when an object impacts the bony orbit of the eye. High-velocity injuries to the eye are not always immediately obvious. Small perforations or penetrations of the cornea may appear similar to corneal abrasions. Sharp trauma includes impact from a sharp object that may perforate the cornea, leaking fluid from the eye.

Cataract formation is a result of major trauma to the eye in children. Opacification of the lens can result from a blunt or penetrating injury.

Chemical or Thermal Trauma

Alkaline burns from household cleaners and lawn and garden products can cause irreversible vision loss. Exposure to extreme heat or flames can damage the cornea and eyelids.

Minutes make a difference with chemical trauma to the eye; treat first and examine later. Wash the eye with copious amounts of water or normal saline solution immediately for an alkaline burn.

Is the vision loss because of a chronic problem?

Key Questions
- How long has vision loss been present?
- Has vision decreased over time?

Progression of Vision Loss

Slowly progressive degenerative disease of any part of the eye can cause progressive vision loss. Progressive loss of visual acuity and color vision can be seen with optic gliomas, the most frequently occurring tumor of the optic nerve in childhood. A history of neurofibromatosis can be found in 25% of patients. Children who have surgery for cataracts are especially at risk for glaucoma. Glaucoma may cause chronic loss of vision. AMD is associated with decreased reading vision (see Chapter 30).

Is this related to a genetic, familial, or intrauterine risk?

Key Questions

- Is there a family history of vision or eye problems?
- Is there a history of maternal, intrapartum, or neonatal conditions?

Family History

A family history of retinoblastoma, congenital cataracts, or metabolic or genetic disease is a risk factor for visual and ocular abnormalities. Retinoblastoma occurs in 12% of children with a family history. Hereditary congenital cataracts occur in 10% to 25% of children with a family history. Autosomal dominant inheritance is the most common cause.

Maternal, Intrapartum, and Neonatal Risks

Infants at risk for vision problems are those who are premature, have been on oxygen therapy, have low birth weight, or have mothers who have had infections related to human immunodeficiency virus/acquired immune deficiency syndrome or to toxoplasmosis, rubella, cytomegalovirus, or herpes simplex—known as the TORCH complex of infections. These conditions during pregnancy may produce blindness at birth or vision loss later in life. Down syndrome is associated with cataracts. Children with galactosemia develop cataracts in infancy. Children with galactokinase deficiency develop cataracts in the first decade of life.

Is the loss because of a systemic disease?

Key Questions

- Do you have diabetes or other chronic disease?

Chronic Disease

Diabetic retinopathy is a leading cause of vision loss. It is a progressive condition resulting from incompetent arterioles or microinfarctions and allowing hard exudates to leak into the retina. The risk of retinopathy increases with the duration of uncontrolled diabetes. Neurodegenerative disease and juvenile idiopathic arthritis can cause vision changes. Prolonged treatment with systemic steroids almost invariably results in the formation of posterior subcapsular cataracts. Marfan syndrome may cause dislocated lens.

Could this be an anatomical problem?

Key Questions (to self)

- Do the eyes cross?
- Do the eyes appear symmetrical?
- Are the eyes bulging or sunken?

Key Questions (to the patient or caregiver)

- If a child: Do you notice the child squinting in bright lights?
- Do you notice that an eyelid droops?

Eye Alignment

Amblyopia is impaired vision in an eye that appears to be structurally normal. It is defined in one of the following three ways:

1. **Strabismic amblyopia** occurs when one eye is out of alignment and the fovea of that eye receives an image that is different from that received in the opposite eye. The brain suppresses the image in the deviating eye to avoid diplopia and visual confusion.
2. **Refractive amblyopia** occurs when the refraction of each eye is so different that the child uses the eye that focuses the best, resulting in poor development of the other eye.
3. **Deprivation amblyopia** is anything that prevents an image from being received clearly by the retina. Conditions such as severe ptosis, congenital cataracts, or vitreous opacity may cause this.

Exophthalmos

Bilateral exophthalmos is protrusion of the eyeballs that occurs with hyperthyroidism. Eyelid lag is observed on downward gaze as a lag in the falling of the eyelid with the globe as it moves downward. Unilateral exophthalmos may indicate a tumor located behind the eye.

Enophthalmos

Enophthalmos is the backward displacement of the eyeball in the eye socket, leading to a sunken appearance. It is caused by starvation, dehydration, or trauma.

Squinting

Squinting blocks out the outer rays from the object, resulting in a smaller amount of distortion, and increases the chance of being able to perceive the image on the retina more clearly. This often occurs with strabismus. Excessive squinting in bright light may indicate glaucoma.

Ptosis

With ptosis, the eyelid margin is at or below the pupil. The eyelid appears to be drooping and interferes with vision. Ptosis may indicate a lesion of the oculomotor nerve (cranial nerve III), a neuromuscular weakness, or a congenital condition.

Is there a pattern to the vision loss?

Key Questions
• When does the vision loss occur?

Pattern of Vision Loss

Retinitis pigmentosa is characterized by progressive disorganization of the pigment of the retina, usually accompanied by a decrease in the number of retinal vessels and some degree of optic atrophy. Night blindness is often the first symptom of vision loss. Vitamin A deficiency or the result of retinotoxic drugs, such as quinine, can cause night blindness.

A progressive loss of vision may occur over decades. Dimming of vision upon standing can occur in someone with low blood pressure or impending shock.

Can I associate the vision loss with the age of the patient?

Key Questions
• What is your age?
• If a child: Is there a history of developmental delay?
• If a child: Is there a change in school performance?

Vision Loss with Aging

Age-related macular degeneration is the leading cause of permanent blindness in older adults. The prevalence increases with each decade after 50 years to almost 35% by the age of 75 years. The majority of adults older than 50 years have some degree of visual impairment. The incidence of cataracts increases with age. By age 80 years, more than half of all Americans either have a cataract or have had cataract surgery.

Developmental Delay

Decreased vision can result in developmental delays. Motor development requires good visual cues and depth perception. Poor school performance may be the first indication of vision loss related to refractory errors and progressive myopia in some children. Craniopharyngiomas can compress the optic nerve system, causing a decrease in visual acuity and a decrease in school performance (Box 38.1).

Box 38.1 Development of Vision and Eye Movements

AGE	NORMAL VISION AND EYE MOVEMENTS
Birth (term)	Fixation Poor following Intermittent strabismus frequently present Visual acuity, 20/400–20/600
1 mo	Horizontal following to midline Normal alignment Visual acuity, 20/300
2 mo	Vertical following begins Normal alignment Visual acuity, 20/200
3 mo	Good horizontal and vertical following Normal alignment Visual acuity, 20/100 Accommodation begins Binocularity detectable
6 mo	Visual acuity, 20/20–20/30 Binocularity well developed
8–10 yr	End of sensitive period for amblyopia

From Del Monte M: The eye in childhood, *Am Fam Physician* 60:907, 1999.

DIAGNOSTIC REASONING: FOCUSED PHYSICAL EXAMINATION

Children become increasingly threatened the closer the examiner comes to the face. The least threatening assessment should be done first.

Assess for Visual Acuity

Visual acuity for distance vision in adults and children older than 4 years is tested using the Snellen or Sloan chart. For young children or adults not able to use the Snellen or Sloan chart, HOTV characters or LEA symbols are used. Each eye is tested separately, with and without corrective lenses. Normal visual acuity tested using a Snellen or Sloan chart is 20/20 in the best eye without correction. A Snellen or Sloan of 20/70 indicates visual impairment, and vision that cannot be corrected to better than 20/200 is legal blindness. A Rosenbaum pocket card held 15 inches from the eyes is used to test near or reading vision.

To test for central vision in infants, observe the infant's eyes as they follow large objects, such as the face or hand of the examiner, in various gazes. In children ages 1 to 3 years, use the cover/uncover test and observe the corneal light reflex.

Any child who has a difference of one line between the two eyes must be referred. Vision of 20/50 for 5-year-old children and 20/40 for children 6 years and older requires referral. Retest using the Snellen or Sloan chart before referring because children tend to do better on a second examination (Table 38.1).

Assess Eyelids, Pupils, and Orbits

Note the position of the eyelids. Eyelids that droop (ptosis) may cause vision loss. Assess for the symmetry of each eye and observe for a transparent cornea.

The appearance of a white pupil (leukokoria) may indicate a cataract, retinoblastoma, persistent hyperplastic primary vitreous retinal detachment, vitreous hemorrhage, or intraocular infection, such as by *Toxocara canis,* which is a roundworm that is contracted from dogs and invades the liver, abdomen, and eyes.

Pupil size is smaller in infants and older adults. Five percent of people will have noticeable differences in pupil size (physiological anisocoria). However, many types of central nervous system (CNS) diseases also cause differences in pupil size.

Enlargement of the pupil may be caused by ocular injury, acute glaucoma, systemic parasympatholytic drugs, and dilating drops. Constriction of the pupil is seen in iris inflammation and patients with glaucoma who are treated with pilocarpine. Irregularity of the pupil contour is invariably abnormal, occurring in iritis, syphilis of the CNS, trauma, and congenital defects.

Inspect for Nystagmus

On far lateral gaze, some eyes will develop a rhythmic twitching motion (nystagmus) in the direction of gaze followed by a drift back. This is a normal finding. However, nystagmus is a neurologic sign that may indicate disease or structural changes in the vestibular–cerebellar–oculomotor system (see Chapter 13). Pathological nystagmus is seen when the movement is in the same direction, regardless of the direction of gaze. Nystagmus in the first year of life suggests bilateral vision loss.

Assess Visual Fields

Testing of the visual fields assesses the function of the peripheral vision and central retina, the optic pathways, and the cortex. The peripheral field is damaged in glaucoma and by tumors or vascular lesions involving the visual fibers from the chiasm to the occipital cortex. A central vision loss is decreased visual function surrounded by normal function. Hemianopsia is a visual defect in the right and left halves of the visual field caused by a lesion involving the chiasm. In homonymous hemianopsia, the same half of the visual field of each eye is affected by a lesion posterior to the chiasm (see Fig. 38.1).

Test Corneal Light Reflex

The corneal light reflex test is used to detect strabismus. Alignment of the eyes is most easily demonstrated by observing the reflection of a light on the cornea. The light should fall

| Table 38.1 | Pediatric Eye Evaluation Screening Recommendations for Primary Care Providers, Nurses, Physician Assistants, and Trained Lay Personnel[a] | |

RECOMMENDED AGE FOR SCREENING	SCREENING METHOD	CRITERIA FOR REFERRAL TO AN OPHTHALMOLOGIST
Newborn to 3 mo	Red reflex[b] Inspection	Abnormal or asymmetrical Structural abnormality
6 mo to 1 yr	Fix and follow with each eye Alternate occlusion Corneal light reflex Red reflex[b] Inspection	Failure to fix and follow in cooperative infant Failure to object equally to covering each eye Asymmetrical Abnormal or asymmetrical Structural abnormality
3 yr (approximately)	Visual acuity[c] Corneal light reflex and cover/uncover Red reflex[b] Inspection	20/50 or worse or two lines of difference between eyes Asymmetrical ocular refixation movements Abnormal or asymmetrical Structural abnormality
5 yr (approximately)	Visual acuity[c] Corneal light reflex and cover/uncover Stereoacuity Red reflex[b] Inspection	20/40 or worse or two lines of difference between eyes Asymmetrical/ocular refixation movements Failure to appreciate stereopsis Abnormal or asymmetrical Structural abnormality
Older than 5 yr	Visual acuity[c] Corneal light reflex and cover/uncover Stereoacuity[d] Red reflex[b] Inspection	20/30 or worse or two lines of difference between eyes Asymmetrical/ocular refixation movements Failure to appreciate stereopsis Abnormal or asymmetrical Structural abnormality

[a]Note: These recommendations are based on expert opinion.
[b]Physician or nurse responsibility.
[c]Figures, letters, E, or optotypes.
[d]Optional: Random Dot E Game (RDE), Titmus Stereograms (Titmus Optical, Inc., Petersburg, VA), Randot Stereograms (Stereo Optical Company, Inc., Chicago).
Modified from the American Academy of Ophthalmology Pediatric Ophthalmology/Strabismus Panel. Preferred Practice Pattern® Guidelines. Pediatric Eye Evaluations. San Francisco, CA: American Academy of Ophthalmology; 2007.

 EVIDENCE-BASED PRACTICE *Should Adults Have Routine Screening for Glaucoma?*

The purpose of this systematic review was to measure the diagnostic accuracy of examination findings and risk factors in identifying individuals with primary open-angle glaucoma (POAG) because early identification may prevent associated vision loss. The prevalence of glaucoma in the studies was 2.6% (95% confidence interval, 2.1%–3.1%). Myopia of 6 diopters or greater and family history of glaucoma were risk factors that had the strongest association with glaucoma. Demographic factors associated with an increased risk were Black race and increased age (especially age older than 80 years). Other risk factors included an increased cup-to-disc ratio (CDR), CDR asymmetry, disc hemorrhage, and increased intraocular pressure. The authors found no studies of screening examinations performed by generalist physicians in a routine setting and conclude that the evidence supports examination by an ophthalmologist or optometrist as the most accurate way to detect glaucoma.

Reference: Hollands H, Johnson D, Hollands S, et al: Do findings on routine examination identify patients at risk for primary open-angle glaucoma? The rational clinical examination systematic review. *JAMA* 309:2035, 2013.

in each eye at the same point. An asymmetrical light reflex will be present in a deviating eye or in an eye with an asymmetrical contour.

Perform a Cover/Uncover Test

Have the patient look with both eyes at a specific point. With one eye covered, watch the uncovered eye. If this eye moves to fix on the point, it was not aligned before the other eye was covered, and a heteropsia, or deviation of an eye, is present. If the uncovered eye does not move, alignment is present, and this is referred to as orthophoria. Repeat the test for the other eye.

Perform an Alternating Cover/Uncover Test

Alternate the cover rapidly on each eye and note any movement of the eyes. Perform this test to discover a latent tendency for misalignment of the two eyes, a condition referred to as heterophoria.

Use the Amsler Grid

An Amsler grid is used to test for distortion of central vision. The patient is asked to wear reading glasses, and the chart is held 15 inches from the eyes. Ask the patient to stare at the dot and tell you if the lines around the dot are curved or bent. Distortion, called metamorphopsia, is found in AMD or central vision loss (Fig. 38.2).

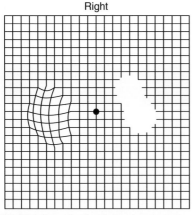

Right

FIGURE 38.2 Example of metamorphopsia and a scotoma projected on an Amsler grid. (From Hampton GR, Nelson PT: *Age-related macular degeneration principles and practice,* New York, 1992, Raven Press.)

Test for Extraocular Movements

Extraocular movements test six pairs of ocular muscles and three cranial nerves (III, IV, and VI). Strabismus is any condition in which the normal binocular alignment of the eyes to a single point in any and all fields of gaze is disturbed; there is an imbalance in neuromuscular sensory and motor control of the extraocular muscles. Half of patients with strabismus also have amblyopia.

Paralytic strabismus is a deviation in the direction opposite the muscle involved. Double vision is usually a symptom but may not be present if the condition occurred at an early age, and the child suppressed the vision in one eye or developed a compensatory head malposition.

Nonparalytic strabismus is present when the angle of deviation is the same in all cardinal fields of gaze.

Obtain a Direct and Consensual Pupillary Response

In monocular blindness, the affected eye will have no direct pupil response but will react consensually to stimulation of the opposite eye. Stimulation of the blind eye, however, will not cause consensual reaction of the opposite normal eye.

Perform an Ophthalmoscopic Examination

Examination of the optic disc can rule out optic atrophy, papilledema, and glaucoma. Death of the optic nerve fibers results in disappearance of the vessels of the disc, leading to pallor or whiteness of the disc.

Observe for a red light reflex, especially in the early days and months of life. If the red reflexes are not equal, refer to an ophthalmologist. To obtain a red reflex in a newborn or young infant, swaddle and then hold the child. Position the ophthalmoscope diopter at 0, direct it to the eye, and gently swing or slightly parachute the infant. The vestibular system usually triggers the infant's eyes to open because of the maneuver.

In older children and adults, darken the room and instruct the patient to stare at an object or a glow sticker in the distance. When the patient looks at the ophthalmoscope light, look at both red reflexes simultaneously and compare them. A uniform red glow equal in color is normal. Absence of a red reflex indicates that some abnormality is blocking the transmission of light through the eye.

The earliest sign of papilledema is a hyperemic disc caused by increased venous pressure. The dilated vessels leak their contents. The fluid leak causes elevation of the disc, which may spread beyond the disc margins, making the edges of the disc appear swollen or indistinct. In glaucoma, one sees a glaucomatous cup. The disc edge appears to be displaced slightly backward, causing a cup shape.

Hemorrhages scattered in the vitreous cavity tend to disperse and absorb light. A red reflex is not seen; only darkness will be seen. This is a common finding in advanced diabetic retinopathy.

LABORATORY AND DIAGNOSTIC STUDIES

Ophthalmoscopy with Pupillary Dilation

Direct ophthalmoscopy allows a view into the retina and optic nerve. More of the peripheral posterior segment is seen when the eye is dilated with a mydriatic drug.

If the iris seems abnormally close to the cornea, dilation is contraindicated because of the risk of inducing acute angle-closure glaucoma.

Tonometry

A tonometer is a device that measures intraocular pressure. Intraocular pressure greater than 21 mm Hg is considered a high-risk factor for glaucoma.

Fluorescein Dye

Fluorescein dye is used to detect the presence of abrasions or a foreign body on the corneal surface. If the corneal epithelium has been disturbed, fluorescein will pool within these areas and stain the hydrophilic stoma. A stain showing a dendritic pattern indicates herpes infection.

DIFFERENTIAL DIAGNOSIS

Early detection and treatment of vision and eye diseases yield immense benefits.

Strabismus and Amblyopia

The most common causes of vision loss in children are amblyopia and strabismus. Amblyopia, or lazy eye, is reduced visual acuity in one eye that is not correctable with lenses. It is caused by incomplete visual system development when a refractive error is not corrected in childhood. Strabismus is a condition in which the two eyes do not point in the same direction when the patient is looking at a distant object. These conditions cause vision loss in 2 of every 100 children. The risk of the development of amblyopia is greatest during the first 2 to 3 years of life, but the potential for recurrence exists until visual development is complete at 9 years of age.

Refractive Errors

Refractive errors are a common visual disorder of childhood, occurring in 20% of children by 16 years of age. Permanent visual impairment may result if optical correction is not provided at an appropriate age.

Myopia (nearsightedness) is when the cornea and lens of the eye focus the image in front of the retina. Hyperopia (farsightedness) is a refractive error in which the focus of an image is behind the retina. Hyperopia can be corrected to some degree by adjustment of the natural lens (accommodation) normally done for near-focusing. The use of accommodation can cause visual fatigue, discomfort, and headache.

Astigmatism

Astigmatism is an irregularity in the refractive system of the eye that prevents light from being focused onto the retina. It can be secondary to the shape of the cornea or lens and is usually correctable with lenses.

Cataracts

A cataract is any opacity of the crystalline lens of the eye. There are many causes of cataracts, and they can be defined by onset, cause, or anatomy.

Congenital cataracts are inherited in an autosomal dominant form and are associated with intrauterine infections by the TORCH complex of organisms. Cataracts of infancy and childhood occur in 1 per 1000 live births, and congenital glaucoma occurs in 1 per 10,000 live births.

Adult cataracts are a major cause of visual impairment in older adults because with time, the human lens begins to develop opacities. Cataracts can be caused by galactosemia, metabolic disorders (e.g., diabetic cataracts), and trauma (e.g., from heat or blunt trauma); steroid-induced cataract formation is also possible. The first signs of opacity are the inability to focus on near objects (presbyopia) and altered color vision.

Optic Neuritis

Optic neuritis occurs more often in younger adults, 20 to 50 years old, and in women; it is typically monocular. It is often idiopathic and may be associated with multiple sclerosis, after viral infection, and with granulomatous inflammatory conditions. Vision loss occurs over a few hours to days and is extremely variable. Visual field loss includes central scotoma in 90% of patients. In the majority of patients, pain precedes the vision loss and is worse with eye movement.

Optic Nerve Hypoplasia

This visual disorder affects the optic nerve, the bundle of fibers that transmits signals from the retina to the brain. It is a nonprogressive disorder in which the optic nerve is 25% smaller than the normal size. Some children have a loss of peripheral vision, and others lose central vision.

Injury

More than 100,000 eye injuries occur annually in the general population of the United States, of which 90% are preventable with the use of protective eyewear. Exposure to long periods of high heat or blunt trauma to the eye globe can result in cataracts.

Retinoblastoma

This is the most common intraocular tumor of childhood; it occurs bilaterally in 30% of cases. A common symptom is strabismus. Retinoblastoma is inherited in an autosomal dominant manner. Early lesions are flat, transparent, or white masses in the retina. The tumor can spread to the brain through the optic nerve or into the bone marrow.

Retinopathy of Prematurity

This condition is seen in premature infants and refers to the changes of ischemia, blood vessel growth, and fibrosis that occur because of inadequate oxygen delivery to the peripheral retina. The vessels of the retina normally complete vascularization by 40 weeks of gestation. Infants who are born before this time may have incomplete vascularization with subsequent poor vessel development and visual impairments. Infants who weigh less than 1500 g are at greatest risk.

Central Retinal Artery Occlusion

Patients with this condition have a sudden onset of severe vision loss in one eye. There is no associated pain. The loss is caused by plaque lodging at the level of the lamina cribrosa. On physical examination a few hours after occlusion, the retina becomes edematous and white or opaque. There is a reddish-orange reflex from the intact choroidal vascular and foveola that creates a "cherry red spot" that contrasts with the surrounding white retina. With time, the retinal artery opens and the retinal edema clears.

Glaucoma

Glaucoma is loss of vision caused by increased pressure in the eye. It is characterized by defects in the visual field and optic nerve damage. Glaucoma is a leading cause of blindness in the United States. Glaucoma can be classified as primary or secondary and as open or closed angle. Secondary glaucoma is associated with another ocular or nonocular event, but primary glaucoma is not. Closed-angle glaucoma is caused when the anterior chamber angle is narrowed, reducing the outflow and removal of aqueous humor. Open-angle glaucoma, the most common type, occurs with a normal anterior chamber angle. The condition is painless, and symptoms appear in late stages of the disease. Ophthalmic examination reveals pathological cupping of the optic disc that may be asymmetrical. Patients with intraocular pressures above 21 mm Hg should be referred to an ophthalmologist (Box 38.2).

Retinal Detachment

This condition occurs when the neurosensory retina is separated from the retinal pigment epithelium. About half of patients will have brief flashes of light (photopsia) or floaters (entopsia). It is caused by a collection of fluid beneath the neurosensory retina, traction from fibrovascular elements associated with diabetic retinopathy, or trauma. Nearly 95% of detachments are treatable.

Macular Degeneration

Age-related macular degeneration may be asymptomatic or associated with gradual loss of central vision. Risk factors include advanced age, family history, cigarette smoking, hyperopia, and hypertension. There are two forms of pathological macular degeneration, wet and dry. The wet (exudative) form results in rapid vision loss caused by the development of abnormal blood vessels that grow from the choroid into the macular portion of the retina. These new blood vessels, called choroidal neovascularization, are very fragile and often leak blood and fluid. Blurred vision is a common early symptom, but vision loss may be rapid and severe. The dry (nonexudative) form is associated with breakdown of the light-sensitive macular cells and gradual loss of central vision. Distortion upon testing with the Amsler grid is found with dry AMD. Both types can occur in the same eye.

Diabetic Retinopathy

Diabetic retinopathy is a retinovascular disease that occurs in two forms. Nonproliferative retinopathy is characterized by microaneurysms, macular edema, lipid exudates, and intraretinal hemorrhages. In proliferative retinopathy, blood vessels regenerate on the retina. The patient may be asymptomatic or have decreased vision or floaters. Diabetic retinopathy progresses with the duration of diabetes.

Uveitis

Uveitis is a general term used to describe inflammatory activity of the iris, ciliary body, and choroid. Symptoms vary according to cause and severity, but most patients experience some decrease in vision, light sensitivity, and tearing. Pain may be variable. Acute uveitis lasts less than 3 months but may have a chronic recurrent pattern.

Keratitis

Keratitis is an inflammation of the cornea that creates pain, redness, and blurred vision. It can be caused by infection, dry eyes, physical and chemical injury, and systemic disease. Keratitis can range from mild to severe and can be chronic. Diagnosis is usually made by an ophthalmologist using a slit lamp.

Optic Nerve Glioma

Optic nerve gliomas are present in two forms. In adults, they are malignant glioblastomas; in children, they are benign pilocytic astrocytomas. They appear in children younger than age 10 years of age and are highly associated with neurofibromatosis, a condition associated with café-au-lait lesions of the skin. In children, gliomas may appear as the rapid onset of vision loss with headache. Of the malignant optic nerve gliomas, nearly 75% present with unilateral, rapidly progressive vision loss with pain.

Craniopharyngioma

Craniopharyngiomas are tumors that arise from squamous epithelial cells of the brain. They are most common in the first 2 decades of life but also may occur in adults 50 to 70 years old. Children's presenting symptoms include headache and visual disturbance caused by increased intracranial pressure. Nystagmus and bitemporal hemianopsia are pathognomonic for this tumor. In older patients, visual deficit is common in the presence of normal optic discs.

Chemical or Thermal Trauma

A chemical burn is an ophthalmic emergency. Alkaline solutions denature eye proteins and lyse cell membranes, allowing the chemical to penetrate the eye. Acid burns can also cause severe damage, but the acid solution precipitates proteins, decreasing the amount of penetration damage.

Congenital Infection

Congenital TORCH infections can cause vision problems in infants. Postnatal screening is performed to diagnose a TORCH infection.

▶ **DIFFERENTIAL DIAGNOSIS OF** *Common Causes of Vision Loss*

CONDITION	HISTORY	PHYSICAL FINDINGS	DIAGNOSTIC STUDIES
Strabismus	Family reports child's eyes cross, family history	Extraocular movements abnormal, cover/uncover test result positive	Refer
Amblyopia	May have history of premature birth, Down syndrome, cerebral palsy, hydrocephalus	Vision decreased in one eye	Refer
Refractive errors	Sitting close to television, squinting	Loss of visual acuity	Screen with Snellen chart, tumbling E, or figures; refer
Cataracts	Blurred vision, glare, distortion and change in color perception, increased age, history of infection, trauma, or chronic disease	Whitish appearance of pupil, bilateral or unilateral	Refer
Optic neuritis	History of multiple sclerosis, viral infection, pain with eye movement, rapid vision loss	Decreased visual acuity, reduced color perception, afferent pupil defect and central scotoma	Refer
Optic nerve hypoplasia	History of vision loss, may have central vision but no peripheral vision	Optic nerve is half to one third normal size, pale to gray in color, surrounded by yellow halo	Refer
Injury, penetrating injury	History suggesting head or eye trauma (blunt or sharp)	Directed by history	Refer
Retinoblastoma	Family history, child up to 2 yr old	Partial or absent red reflex, strabismus	Refer
Nystagmus	History of eyes moving repetitively, searching	Rhythmic, repetitive oscillation of eyes	Refer
Retinopathy of prematurity	Premature birth <36 wk, weight 1500 g, oxygen administered, may be a twin	Abnormalities of retinal vessels	Refer

▶ DIFFERENTIAL DIAGNOSIS OF *Common Causes of Vision Loss—cont'd*

CONDITION	HISTORY	PHYSICAL FINDINGS	DIAGNOSTIC STUDIES
Central retinal artery occlusion	Sudden onset of painless vision loss, may come and go	Macular edema, cherry red spot; may see vessel narrowing	Refer
Glaucoma	Most often painless, gradual vision loss, blurring, and halos; more common in older adults; history of systemic disease	Decreased visual acuity; may have increased intraocular pressure on palpation of eye globe	Refer for tonometry
Retinal detachment	Sensation of flashing light accompanied by shower of floaters; history of trauma to head or face	Retina markedly elevated; appears gray with dark blood vessels; may lie in folds	Refer
Macular degeneration	Older than 60 yr, decreased central vision, blue eyes, image larger in one eye	Hyaline (drusen) deposits on retina near macula, gray-green areas of pigment under retina, decreased visual acuity	Amsler grid
Diabetic retinopathy	History of diabetes, floaters, gradual vision loss	Venous dilation, retinal hemorrhages	Refer
Uveitis	History of infection or chronic inflammation, mild to moderate pain, photophobia, tearing	Findings vary according to cause and severity	Refer
Keratitis	History of infection, trauma, mild to severe pain, blurred vision, itching with blinking	Conjunctivitis	Refer for evaluation with a slit lamp
Optic nerve glioma	Dimness of vision with loss of fields; may be unilateral rapid vision loss with pain	Visual field defects, optic atrophy	Refer
Craniopharyngioma	Unilateral vision loss, headache, child or adult	Funduscopic examination may be normal	Refer
Chemical burn	History of acid or alkaline exposure	Treat first; then examine	Immediate eye irrigation and referral
Thermal burns	History of exposure to high heat, occupational risk	Corneal opacities	Refer
Congenital infections	TORCH, maternal exposure to measles	Retinitis, optic nerve hypoplasia	Screen for TORCH; refer

TORCH, toxoplasmosis, rubella, cytomegalovirus, and herpes simplex.

Unintentional Weight Loss or Gain

Unintentional weight loss is an involuntary decrease in body weight. Weight loss in an adult is clinically significant when it exceeds 5% of usual body weight over a 6- to 12-month period. Weight loss in the newborn may occur immediately after birth, but weight should begin to increase by 2 weeks of age. Weight loss can result from a decrease in body fluid, muscle mass, or fat. It will occur with reduced energy (food) intake and increased metabolism or energy output. Individuals adjust energy balance daily to maintain a healthy weight through healthy eating and regular physical activity. Malignancy and endocrine disorders are the most common causes of unintentional weight loss followed by gastrointestinal (GI), cognitive, behavioral, and functional disorders, as well as age-related changes.

Weight gain occurs when caloric intake exceeds body requirements, causing the body to store fat. Most adults do not intentionally gain weight, but with aging, a decrease in physical abilities leads to a decrease in metabolic rate (amount of energy used in a given period), which in turn contributes to weight gain. Unexplained weight gain may be more difficult to identify, especially in the United States, where 70% of adults are overweight, and more than one third are obese, with a body mass index (BMI) greater than 40 kg/m².

The prevalence of obesity in youth is 17% and increasing. Unexplained weight gain may be endocrine related, age related, or associated with cognitive impairments.

DIAGNOSTIC REASONING: FOCUSED HISTORY

Unexplained Weight Loss

Has the patient lost weight? Is the weight loss really unexplained?

Key Questions
- How do you know that you (or the child) have lost weight?
- What is your age?
- How is your appetite?
- How would you describe your typical diet and activity patterns?
- If an infant is breastfeeding, ask the caretaker: How is breastfeeding going?
- If an infant is taking formula, ask the caretaker: What kind of formula do you use? How do you prepare it?

Measuring weight

Individuals might note that their clothes are too loose or too tight. Weight is usually measured by asking the patient to step on a balance or electric scale clothed and without shoes. Height is measured by asking the patient to stand with the back against a wall with heels touching the wall. There are several ways to classify and measure body weight, but the most commonly used method is the BMI formula, which is BMI = weight (kg)/height (m²). BMI is an indirect measure of body fat, and BMI categories are subject to errors related to age and muscle mass. To enhance the reliability of measurement of weight changes, ask the patient to weigh himself or herself at the same time each day using the same scale.

Weight and height in infants and children are measured using a scale and plotted on a National Center for Health Statistics growth chart. Infants and children should be measured in a supine position until the age of 2 years. Head circumference is also measured and plotted.

Age

Aging can be associated with both weight loss and weight gain. Normally with aging, there is less lean muscle tissue, fat is deposited more in the trunk and less in the limbs, and metabolism slows. In an older adult, it is especially important to assess what medications are being taken that could suppress appetite, cognitive status, and memory. Functional limitations that may impact nutrition include the ability to chew and swallow, prepare meals, and shop for food. Social isolation can also contribute to eating less.

Appetite

Appetite can be suppressed because of the presence of acute or chronic illness. Cachexia will result from inadequate energy intake and pathological wasting of muscle or fat tissue. The key symptom in cachexia is anorexia, or loss of appetite. Psychosocial factors, such as anxiety or depression, can contribute to a loss of appetite or lifestyle habits that include skipping meals or eating foods of poor nutritional value.

Eating habits, nutritional adequacy, and physical activity

Weight maintenance is a balance of energy expended and energy consumed. General healthy dietary guidelines can be found in the Dietary Guidelines for Americans (Box 39.1) and at http://www.choosemyplate.gov. Daily caloric needs vary by age, gender, pregnancy, and level of physical activity. Athletes in training may underestimate their caloric needs (Box 39.2).

Excess intake of fruit juices may decrease a child's appetite and cause weight loss. Conversely, excess intake of fruit juices with high caloric content may cause weight gain.

Breastfeeding

Observing and discussing issues regarding breastfeeding with the mother may reveal

---

| Box 39.1 | **Key Recommendations for Maintaining a Healthy Weight** |

- Balance calories with physical activity to manage weight.
- Consume more of certain foods and nutrients such as fruits, vegetables, whole grains, fat-free and low-fat dairy products, and seafood.
- Consume fewer foods with sodium (salt), saturated fats, trans fats, cholesterol, added sugars, and refined grains.

KEY RECOMMENDATIONS FOR SPECIFIC POPULATION GROUPS

- **Those who need to lose weight:** Aim for a slow, steady weight loss by decreasing calorie intake while maintaining an adequate nutrient intake and increasing physical activity.

- **Overweight children:** Reduce the rate of body weight gain while allowing growth and development. Consult a health care provider before placing a child on a weight-reducing diet.
- **Pregnant women:** Ensure appropriate weight gain as specified by a health care provider.
- **Breastfeeding women:** Moderate weight reduction is safe and does not compromise weight gain of the nursing infant.
- **Overweight adults and overweight children with chronic diseases or taking medication:** Consult a health care provider about weight loss strategies before starting a weight-reducing program to ensure appropriate management of other health conditions.

From US Department of Health and Human Services, US Department of Agriculture: Dietary guidelines for Americans, 2010. Available at http://www.health.gov/dietaryguidelines/2010.asp.

Box 39.2   Key Recommendations for Physical Activity

Engage in regular physical activity and reduce sedentary activities to promote health, psychological well-being, and healthy body weight.

- **To reduce the risk of chronic disease in adulthood:** Engage in at least 30 minutes of moderate-intensity physical activity, above usual activity, at work or home on most days of the week.
- For most people, greater health benefits can be obtained by engaging in physical activity of more vigorous intensity or longer duration.
- **To help manage body weight and prevent gradual, unhealthy body weight gain in adulthood:** Engage in approximately 60 minutes of moderate- to vigorous-intensity activity on most days of the week while not exceeding caloric intake requirements.
- **To sustain weight loss in adulthood:** Participate in at least 60 to 90 minutes of daily moderate-intensity physical activity while not exceeding caloric intake requirements. Some people may need to consult with a health care provider before participating in this level of activity.

Achieve physical fitness by including cardiovascular conditioning, stretching exercises for flexibility, and resistance exercises or calisthenics for muscle strength and endurance.

KEY RECOMMENDATIONS FOR SPECIFIC POPULATION GROUPS

- **Children and adolescents:** Engage in at least 60 minutes of physical activity on most, preferably all, days of the week.
- **Pregnant women:** In the absence of medical or obstetric complications, incorporate 30 minutes or more of moderate-intensity physical activity on most, if not all, days of the week. Avoid activities with a high risk of falling or abdominal trauma.
- **Breastfeeding women:** Be aware that neither acute nor regular exercise adversely affects the mother's ability to successfully breastfeed.
- **Older adults:** Participate in regular physical activity to reduce functional declines associated with aging and to achieve the other benefits of physical activity identified for all adults.

From US Department of Health and Human Services, US Department of Agriculture: Dietary guidelines for Americans, 2010. Available at http://www.health.gov/dietaryguidelines/2010.asp.

---

important information. Infants should be breastfed 8 to 12 times in a 24-hour period. Breastfeeding requires more energy expenditure from the infant, and occasionally infants fall asleep while feeding and thus do not receive an adequate amount of breast milk. Nipple soreness caused by improper positioning or poor latching or unlatching can lead to a diminished milk supply. Maternal hydration is important for adequate milk supply.

Formula-fed infant

Investigating what formula the infant is being fed and how the formula is prepared is important. Formulas come in powder and liquid forms. Powder formula requires reconstitution with water. Liquid formula comes in two forms: concentrated (requiring the addition of water) and ready-to-feed forms. Reviewing how the formula is prepared is important to determine whether incorrect preparation is causing weight loss.

What cues indicate a pathological process?

Key Questions

- Have you had a fever or any signs of illness?
- Have you ever been diagnosed with cancer?
- Have you had a change in urinary or bowel habits?
- Do you experience fatigue?
- In a room where others are comfortable, are you often too cold or too warm?
- Have you had a change in appetite or thirst?
- If a child: Has your child's appetite changed?
- If a child: Has your child's activity level changed?

Acute or chronic conditions

Fever associated fatigue and lymphadenopathy may indicate an infection. Chronic conditions, such as cough, shortness of breath, nausea, vomiting, anemia, fatigue, weakness, change in moles, pain, abnormal menstrual bleeding, breast discharge, or headaches, can contribute to unintentional weight loss. Crohn disease is an inflammatory bowel disease that can be associated with reduced appetite.

Unintentional weight loss is a red flag for cancer occurrence or recurrence. Weight loss can occur from loss of appetite and decreased caloric intake or from the body's inability to absorb nutrients because of the cancer.

Endocrine disorder

Diabetes is an endocrine disorder caused by insulin secretion deficiency and insulin resistance, resulting in elevated blood glucose levels that do not allow nutrients to enter cells. Along with weight loss, untreated diabetes is often associated with increased hunger, excessive thirst, and frequent urination.

Hyperthyroidism speeds up metabolism, thus burning more calories. It is the most common thyroid function disorder. Symptoms include trembling, insomnia, and hair loss.

In hypothyroidism, thyroid hormones are insufficient. In developing countries, it is most often because of iodine deficiency; in the United States, autoimmune processes are the major cause. Onset of symptoms is insidious and involves every organ system. A history will reveal symptoms of lethargy, dry skin, dry and brittle hair, cold intolerance, deepening of voice, and facial puffiness. Cushing syndrome is a result of prolonged exposure to excessive levels of glucocorticoid cortisol, which has a catabolic effect on most tissues. Muscle wasting and weakness are caused by generalized protein catabolism.

Appetite or activity level change

A change in an infant or child's appetite and activity level is a good indicator of illness. Appetite can decrease with an inactive lifestyle or the presence of chronic pain, irritable bowel syndrome, or other conditions that might be exacerbated by eating.

Are emotional issues contributing to weight loss?

Key Questions

- Have you recently had a stressful event in your life? How are you coping?
- Do you or anyone in your family have a problem with anxiety or depression?
- How are you doing in school or at work?
- If a child: Is the child gaining weight appropriately?

Psychosocial factors

Emotions have a big impact on appetite and eating behavior. One reaction to extreme stress or depression may be a loss of appetite. Individuals may have patterns of coping with stress by controlling food intake. Anorexia nervosa and bulimia are eating disorders most often diagnosed in young women. With these two disorders, despite the low or normal weight, the individual perceives herself or himself as overweight. Anorexia nervosa carries a high risk of complications caused by electrolyte imbalances.

Failure to thrive

Failure to thrive in infants may have a nonorganic etiology. Causes include but are not limited to caretaker's employment status, social isolation, family stress, substance abuse, postpartum depression, and poor parenting skills.

What other symptoms might help narrow the possibilities?

Key Questions

- When was your last cancer screening?
- If a child: Has your child recently switched to solid food?
- Do you have a family history of cystic fibrosis (CF)?
- Does anyone in your household have a history of tuberculosis?

Cancer screening

Cancer screening recommendations vary by gender and age and include colon cancer screening, screening mammography for breast cancer and Pap smears and human papilloma virus (HPV) tests for cervical cancer screening. Other cancer screening will depend on associated symptoms and history of risk factors and may include skin, lung, and prostate. The United States Preventive Services Task Force (USPSTF) conducts rigorous assessments of the scientific evidence for the effectiveness of a range of clinical preventive services, including screening, counseling, and preventive medications (http://www.ahrq.gov/clinic/uspstfix.htm). Lack of regular screening places patients at an increased risk for undetected cancer. Involuntary weight loss may be a symptom of cancer.

Diet change

Infants who were on formula or breast milk but switched to solid food may exhibit malabsorption conditions (e.g., lactose intolerance or celiac disease) that can cause weight loss or slowed weight gain.

Family history

The CF gene is autosomal recessive. Four percent of white people in the United States are estimated to be carriers (heterozygous) of the CF gene. CF may present as lack of weight gain between the first and sixth months.

Tuberculosis is often associated with reduced appetite and weight loss and is contracted among individuals who are exposed to an active infection, especially within a family or household.

What self-treatment was used? Did it help?

Key Questions
- Are you taking any prescribed or over-the-counter preparations to lose weight?
- How would you describe your eating habits and dietary practices?

Medication history

There are numerous weight loss drugs on the market, and many of them contain ephedrine, a stimulant that suppresses appetite. These drugs can be associated with cardiac arrhythmia and blood pressure elevation. In general, drugs to lose weight are not commonly prescribed but are readily available over the counter. Some drugs cause an altered taste sensation and decreased appetite. Maternal ingestion of drugs while nursing may affect breast milk supply. Dopamine agonists, such as cabergoline, reduce prolactin and are sometimes used therapeutically to stop lactation. Dopamine antagonists, such as metoclopramide and most antipsychotics, may increase prolactin and milk production. Other drugs that have been associated with hyperprolactinemia include selective serotonin reuptake inhibitors and opioids.

Dietary practices

Individuals may use fasting or purging as a method of rapid weight loss; fasting is also often done as a religious or spiritual practice. Healthy weight loss diets aim for gradual weight loss over weeks and months.

How serious is this situation? Is this a recent change?

Key Questions
- How long have you been concerned about your weight loss?
- Is anyone else concerned about your weight loss?
- What is your ideal or usual weight?

Validate weight change

A careful history may document changes in activity level, food intake, or a precipitating incident before weight loss was noticed as a problem.

Concern about weight loss

Patients with anorexia do not believe they have a weight loss problem and have a morbid fear of weight gain. Often family members or friends become concerned and refer the patient to be evaluated.

Ideal or usual weight

Normal or ideal weight for age and gender can be checked against actuarial tables, such as the 1999 Metropolitan Height and Weight Tables for Men and Women (http://www.bcbst.com/mpmanual/hw.htm). Unintended weight loss noted for more than 6 months should be evaluated. Weight can be verified by using a reliable weight scale. Clothing should be lightweight. Note if the person was weighed with or without shoes.

Unexplained Weight Gain

Is the weight gain explained by diet and exercise habits?

Key Questions

• Can you describe what you eat in a typical day?

• Has your eating pattern changed?
• Can you describe your level of physical activity?

Balance of energy intake and expenditure

Maintaining an ideal body weight depends on achieving a balance of energy intake and energy expenditure (Table 39.1). Calorie intake can exceed expenditure when a person consumes large quantities of food and food with high calorie content but gets little aerobic exercise. Factors that contribute to inactivity are sedentary jobs, television watching, and reliance on the automobile. Environmental and genetic factors contribute to a small percentage of cases of obesity.

Table 39.1 Estimated Calorie Needs/Day (in kilocalories) by Age, Sex, and Physical Activity Level[a]

The estimates are rounded to the nearest 200 calories. An individual's calorie needs may be higher or lower than these average estimates.

SEX	AGE (YR)	ACTIVITY LEVEL[b, c, d, e]		
		SEDENTARY	MODERATELY ACTIVE	ACTIVE
Child	2–3	1000	1000–1400[e]	1000–1400
Female	4–8	1200	1400–1600	1400–1800
	9–13	1600	1600–2000	1800–2200
	14–18	1800	2000	2400
	19–30	2000	2000–2200	2400
	31–50	1800	2000	2200
	51+	1600	1800	2000–2200
Male	4–8	1400	1400–1600	1600–2000
	9–13	1800	1800–2200	2000–2600
	14–18	2200	2400–2800	2800–3200
	19–30	2400	2600–2800	3000
	31–50	2200	2400–2800	2800–3200
	51+	2000	2200–2400	2400–2800

[a]Based on Estimated Energy Requirements from the Institute of Medicine Dietary Reference Intakes Macronutrients Report, 2002, calculated by sex, age, and activity level for reference-sized individuals. "Reference size," as determined by the Institute of Medicine, is based on median height and weight for ages up to age 18 years to give a body mass index of 21.5 for adult women and 22.5 for adult men.
[b]Sedentary means a lifestyle that includes only light physical activity associated with typical day-to-day life.
[c]Moderately active means a lifestyle that includes physical activity equivalent to walking about 1.5 to 3 miles per day at 3 to 4 miles/hr in addition to the light physical activity associated with typical day-to-day life.
[d]Active means a lifestyle that includes physical activity equivalent to walking more than 3 miles/day at 3 to 4 miles/hr in addition to the light physical activity associated with typical day-to-day life.
[e]The calorie ranges shown are to accommodate needs of different ages within the group. For children and adolescents, more calories are needed at older ages. For adults, fewer calories are needed at older ages.
From US Department of Health and Human Services, US Department of Agriculture: Dietary guidelines for Americans, 2010. Available at http://www.health.gov/dietaryguidelines/2010.asp.

Is the weight gain associated with age?

Key Questions
- What is your age?
- When was your last menstrual period?

Age

Normal aging is associated with slower metabolism and reduced energy requirements.

Menopause

Menopause is defined as the absence of a menstrual period for 1 year. About 90% of menopausal adults gain some weight between the ages of 35 and 55 years with an average age of 51 years. Hormones have a direct impact on appetite, metabolism, and fat storage. Lower levels of progesterone, androgen, and testosterone contribute to lower metabolism and weight gain.

Could weight gain be related to other behaviors?

Key Questions
- How much alcohol do you consume in a week or a day?
- Do you smoke? If so, how much do you smoke? How long have you smoked? At what age did you start smoking? Have you recently quit?
- Do you take any medications?

Alcohol and smoking

Drinking multiple glasses or bottles of alcohol daily or weekly will increase calorie intake. Many adults gain 5 to 10 lb in the first few months after quitting smoking and report an increased appetite. Adults at greatest risk for excessive weight gain with smoking cessation are those who smoke more and are less physically active.

Medications

Corticosteroids, lithium, tranquilizers, phenothiazines, and tricyclic antidepressants may lead to fluid retention.. Selective serotonin reuptake inhibitors may suppress appetite and result in weight loss.

Could this be caused by an endocrine disorder?

Key Questions
- Has the weight gain been sudden or gradual?
- How much do you weigh now compared with 1 year ago?
- Have you noticed any other symptoms or changes in your appearance?

Acuity of weight gain

An adult who is premenopausal may note gradual weight gain over a few years. Some medications, such as β-blockers, corticosteroids, and antidepressants, are associated with weight gain. Edema from congestive heart failure or renal failure can cause weight gain in a few days or weeks.

Endocrine symptoms

Hypothyroidism is associated with fatigue, constipation, and an inability to tolerate cold temperatures. Cushing syndrome is associated with truncal weight gain, moon facies, and a "buffalo hump." Both of these disorders may develop over an extended period of time. Polycystic ovary syndrome is associated with obesity and hirsutism.

DIAGNOSTIC REASONING: FOCUSED PHYSICAL EXAMINATION

A thorough health history and general physical examination, including screening for psychosocial causes (see Chapter 4), will help to identify behavioral risk factors or a pattern of associated symptoms that suggest a systemic disorder.

Note General Appearance

Observe the patient entering the room. Especially note the fit of clothing as well as general hygiene and signs of stress, anxiety, or confusion.

When examining an infant, observe interaction with the caregiver. Infants with failure to thrive may avoid eye contact, may not smile or make sounds, and have poor interaction with their environment. The infant may also prefer not to be cuddled and be difficult to comfort and may appear withdrawn even from the caregiver.

Take Vital Signs

Vital signs will provide information on cardiovascular and respiratory function. Height and weight can be compared to actuarial tables to see norms for weight by age and gender. Calculate BMI. Bradycardia may indicate hypothyroidism; tachycardia may indicate anemia, dehydration, or hyperthyroidism. Fever may indicate infection.

Weigh and Measure Newborn

A decrease in weight of more than 8% necessitates follow up within 48 hours, and a bilirubin level should be drawn to assess for hyperbilirubinemia. A loss of more than 10% of birth weight warrants careful assessment of possible causes and consideration of hospital admission.

Assess Mental Status

The major cognitive changes to detect as related to weight loss or gain are dementia and depression (see Chapter 9). The Montreal Cognitive Assessment (MoCA) test is a 30-point instrument administered in 10 minutes to assess domains of cognitive function. Whereas a score of 26 or above is considered normal, a lower score indicates mild cognitive impairment. Screen for the presence of an eating disorder.

Conduct a Comprehensive Physical Examination

Assess the skin

Examine the skin for intactness, turgor, and presence of lesions to determine hydration status and overall nutrition status. Hypothyroidism is associated with dry, flaky skin; skin darkening occurs with Addison disease.

Assess the heart

Palpate the anterior thorax for the point of maximal impulse, lifts, and heaves. Auscultate for adventitious sounds (see Chapter 8).

EVIDENCE-BASED PRACTICE *Does Screening for Obesity in Adults Have an Impact on Long-Term Health Outcomes?*

The United States Preventive Services Task Force (USPSTF) found adequate evidence that intensive, multicomponent behavioral interventions for obese adults can lead to an average weight loss of 4 to 7 kg (8.8–15.4 lb) in the first year with 12 to 26 treatment sessions compared with little or no weight loss in a control group. These interventions also improve glucose tolerance and other physiological risk factors for cardiovascular disease. The USPSTF found inadequate direct evidence about the effectiveness of these interventions on long-term health outcomes (e.g., death, cardiovascular disease, and hospitalizations). The USPSTF concluded with moderate certainty that screening for obesity in adults has a moderate net benefit. There is also benefit to offering or referring obese adults to intensive behavioral interventions to improve weight status and other risk factors for important health outcomes. The USPSTF recommends that clinicians screen adults for obesity. Clinicians should offer or refer patients with a body mass index of 30 kg/m² or greater to intensive, multicomponent behavioral interventions.

This is a B recommendation.

Reference: Moyer, U.S. Preventive Services Task Force: 2012.

Examine the head and neck

Assess the head and neck for presence of lymphadenopathy. Moon facies, also called moon face, indicates Cushing syndrome. Palpate the thyroid for masses or asymmetry.

Assess the condition of the teeth and gums. Test the patient's ability to swallow using water or test for the gag reflex. Patients with diabetes may have xanthomas associated with hyperlipidemia.

Examine the abdomen

Observe for contour. Patients with diabetes tend to have truncal obesity. Redistribution of fat in older patients may also cause them to have truncal obesity. Palpate for tenderness or lumps, auscultate for bowel sounds, and check for rebound tenderness. Patients with malabsorption may have ascites.

Examine the extremities

Conduct a musculoskeletal exam to assess strength, mobility, and balance (see Chapters 22 and 23). Assess for loss of muscle mass and subcutaneous fat associated with cachexia, malabsorption, and aging. Frailty syndrome involves a loss of muscle with aging along with muscle weakness and slowing; decreased energy; lower activity; and, when severe, unintended weight loss. Patients with hypothyroidism may have generalized edema and delayed recovery of deep tendon reflexes. Patients with hyperthyroidism may have overly brisk deep tendon reflexes. Patients with diabetes may have peripheral neuropathy.

LABORATORY AND DIAGNOSTIC STUDIES

Complete Blood Count with Indices and Differential

A complete blood count with indices will provide information about the degree and cause of anemia; microcytic hypochromic anemia reflects chronic blood loss and normocytic normochromic anemia suggests acute blood loss. An elevated white blood cell count indicates the presence of inflammation or infection.

Fasting Blood Glucose

A fasting blood glucose (FBG) is a blood specimen taken at least 8 hours after a meal. The reference value for FBG is below 100 mg/dL of glucose; an FBG level of 100 to 125 mg/dL indicates prediabetes. If a random blood glucose is obtained within 2 hours after a meal, the reference value is 140 mg/dL or less.

Glycosylated Hemoglobin

Glycosylated hemoglobin (A_{1c}) reflects the average blood glucose over a 3-month period. An A_{1c} below 5.7% is normal, between 5.7 to 6.4% indicates prediabetes, and 6.5% or above is diagnostic for diabetes. The reference value is at or below 7% for someone with diagnosed diabetes. The A_{1c} result is not dependent on when the most recent meal was consumed, but the results may be affected by the presence of anemia or sickle cell disease. The A_{1c} result may be a poor reflection of blood glucose when severe anemia or sickle cell disease is present.

Thyroid-Stimulating Hormone

Hypothyroidism is characterized by a deficient in thyroid hormone production by the thyroid gland, which can be severe or moderate. Severe deficit of thyroid hormones defines overt hypothyroidism. The moderate form, called subclinical hypothyroidism, seldom has signs and symptoms and is defined by an elevated serum thyroid-stimulating hormone (TSH) concentration and within-normal-range thyroid hormone levels. A low or undetectable level of TSH indicates hyperthyroidism.

Bilirubin

Bilirubin values are usually reported as two fractions: conjugated (direct) and unconjugated (indirect). Conjugated hyperbilirubinemia is present if more than 50% of elevated total bilirubin is the conjugated form. The reference value for total conjugated bilirubin in newborns is less than 2 mg/dL; the level peaks at 12.9 mg/dL at 3 to 4 days of life and then decreases. A tool designed to help clinicians assess the risks of the development of hyperbilirubinemia in newborns older than 35 weeks' gestational age can be found at http://www.bilitool.com. CF can lead to liver failure and hyperbilirubinemia.

Total Serum Protein

A total serum protein measures the amount of total protein and albumin (from the liver) and globulin (from the liver and immune system) in the blood. Normally, there is more albumin than globulin with a ratio of greater than 1. Albumin checks kidney function and reflects dietary protein. Elevated globulin may indicate infection.

Sweat Chloride Test

The quantitative pilocarpine iontophoresis test measures the amount of chloride and sodium in the sweat of patients with CF. Normal sweat contains less than 60 mEq/L of chloride and sodium. Two tests on different occasions are needed for accurate diagnosis of CF.

Urinalysis

The extent of diagnostic investigation of urine will depend on history and physical examination findings. Dipstick urinalysis can point out infection, proteinuria, and glycosuria (see Chapter 34).

QuantiFERON-TB Gold

QuantiFERON-TB Gold (QFT) is highly specific and sensitive: a positive result is strongly predictive of infection with *Mycobacterium tuberculosis*. However, the QFT cannot distinguish between active tuberculosis disease and latent tuberculosis infection.

Fecal Occult Blood Testing

The fecal occult blood test is an initial screening method to detect GI bleeding (see Chapter 29).

Chest Radiography

A chest x-ray study can reveal the presence of consolidation, lung lesions, and heart contour.

Tests of the Gastrointestinal Tract

A barium upper GI series is used to examine the upper GI region, but small lesions may not be detected. Any abnormality needs to be evaluated by endoscopy. The lower GI tract is evaluated using sigmoidoscopy or colonoscopy. A colonoscopy will detect the presence of polyps and lesions along the entire large intestine (see Chapter 3).

Computed Tomography

Computed tomography (CT) scanning can be done on different body regions. Abdominal CT examines the uterus, pancreas, GI tract, and other abdominal organs.

Mammography

Screening mammograms consist of two views, craniocaudal and medial lateral oblique, to detect nonpalpable breast lesions. Compare the results with previous screening mammograms (see Chapter 6).

Cervical Cancer Screening

The Pap test is designed to detect cancer cells in the cervix and vagina. HPV testing detects high-risk HPV strains (16 and 18) associated with cervical cancer.

Metabolic Rate

Estimated energy needs should be based on resting or basal metabolic rate (BMR). BMR decreases with age and loss of lean body mass. An equation using actual weight, height, gender, and age is the most accurate for estimating BMR and calculating daily caloric requirements (Box 39.3).

Box 39.3 Basal Metabolic Rate (BMR) Formula

WOMEN
BMR = 65.5 + (4.35 × Weight in pounds) + (4.7 × Height in inches) − (4.7 × Age in years)

MEN
BMR = 66 + (6.23 × Weight in pounds) + (12.7 × Height in inches) − (6.8 × Age in years)

DIFFERENTIAL DIAGNOSIS

Unintentional Weight Loss

Cancer

Cancer alters the body's appetite signals and metabolism, resulting in cachexia, a condition in which body fat stores are depleted and muscle mass decreases. The most common malignancies that cause weight loss are GI, lung, hematologic, and musculoskeletal. As many as 40% of people diagnosed with cancer reported unexplained weight loss at the time of diagnosis. Some people notice weight loss despite a good appetite. Others lose their appetite and may even become nauseated by food or have difficulty swallowing.

Nutritional status

Assess nutritional status by obtaining a history of dietary habits and physical activity patterns, as well as anthropometric measures (e.g., height and weight to calculate BMI and waist and hip circumference to determine distribution of body fat). One 24-hour or two consecutive days of 24-hour recall are reliable methods to assess dietary intake. Poor or inadequate nutrition in severe forms is most often found in developing countries and is manifested in two forms: kwashiorkor, which is a protein deficiency, and marasmus, which is caused by inadequate food intake. Weight loss not explained by dietary intake is most likely caused by systemic disease.

Frailty Syndrome

Estimates are that 7% to 16% of community-dwelling older adults have frailty syndrome. Loss of muscle mass is normal with aging. It is also a marker of a syndrome of frailty, with associated muscle weakness and slowing; decreased energy; lower activity; and, when severe, unintended weight loss. Frailty syndrome is associated declines in physiologic reserve and function across multiorgan systems, leading to increased vulnerability for adverse health outcomes.

Endocrine disorders

Diabetes Mellitus

More than 90% of all cases of diabetes are type 2. Type 1 diabetes is more often associated with weight loss despite increased appetite. Persons with type 2 diabetes may experience increased thirst and urinary frequency but often are asymptomatic. Some symptoms, such as blurred vision or peripheral neuropathy, may reflect long-term manifestations of an undiagnosed disease. Despite weight loss, patients tend to exhibit central obesity.

Hyperthyroidism

Patients with hyperthyroidism may report a variety of signs and symptoms such as palpitations, nervousness, emotional lability, fatigue, muscle weakness, weight loss despite good appetite, hyperdefecation, heat intolerance, menstrual changes (oligomenorrhea), increased appetite, insomnia, and tremors. On physical examination, exophthalmos, warm skin, onycholysis, increased sweating, and thinning hair may be evident. Patients may have localized myxedema (edematous skin thickening) of the legs (pretibial) or dorsa of the feet. The thyroid may be enlarged and a bruit may be present. Deep tendon reflexes may be brisk. High fever, congestive heart failure, and mental status changes suggest thyroid storm. TSH level will be low or undetectable.

Gastroesophageal reflux in infants

Caregivers report a child with a history of frequent regurgitation, persistent wheezing, and gagging or choking with feeding. Physical findings are normal. When symptoms persist and the lower esophageal sphincter fails to develop, the condition is known as gastroesophageal reflux disease. Upper GI or barium swallow will detect lesions of the upper GI tract.

Addison Disease

Addison disease occurs when the adrenal glands do not produce enough of their hormones. Associated symptoms may include changes in blood pressure or heart rate, darkening of the skin, weakness, salt craving, and loss of appetite.

Malabsorption

In malabsorption, the absorption and digestion of nutrients are disrupted. The disorder is caused by an insufficiency of a variety of digestive enzymes. In celiac disease, there is an immunologic response to gluten. The degree of weight loss varies and is accompanied by chronic diarrhea and growth retardation. Patients exhibit muscle wasting and loss of subcutaneous fat. In the presence of severe hypoproteinemia, ascites may be present.

Anorexia nervosa

Anorexia most often affects young women who, despite weight loss, have a self-image of being overweight and an intense fear of gaining weight. The diagnosis is based on a body weight 15% below what is expected, a distorted body image, and the absence of at least three menstrual periods. Examination demonstrates loss of body fat and dry, scaly skin.

Depression or anxiety

Mood regulation through eating is a way some individuals cope with depression or anxiety (see Chapter 4). Major depression is diagnosed by the presence of a depressed mood or loss of interest or pleasure in usual activities. Bipolar disorder involves episodes of mania or hypomania, often followed by depression. In mania, the patient experiences an elevated or irritable mood, often described as a "high" (see Chapter 4).

Cognitive impairment

Dementia or compromised cognitive function can disrupt normal self-regulation of appetite and hunger (see Chapter 9). Dementia is a nonspecific syndrome in which affected areas of cognition may include memory, attention, language, and problem solving. When it occurs early in life, it is labeled a neurocognitive disorder. In adults, dementia has a rate of memory and cognitive loss that exceeds that of normal aging (see Chapter 9).

Psychosocial factors (alcohol use, social isolation, and economic status)

Excessive alcohol intake may reduce appetite, which can lead to poor nutrition. Individuals are generally social beings, and social isolation may reduce any motivation to prepare balanced meals or to eat when alone. Older adults and young families may have financial constraints in purchasing healthy foods because fresh fruits and vegetables cost more than fast foods and snack foods (see Chapter 4).

Human immunodeficiency virus/acquired immune deficiency syndrome

Acquired immune deficiency syndrome is a disease of the immune system caused by the human immunodeficiency virus (HIV). This condition progressively reduces the effectiveness of the immune system and leaves individuals susceptible to opportunistic infections and tumors. Risk factors for infection include multiple sexual partners, unprotected sex, and intravenous drug use. HIV is transmitted through direct contact of a mucous membrane or the bloodstream with a bodily fluid containing HIV, such as blood, semen, vaginal fluid, preseminal fluid, and breast milk. Persons with HIV infection develop opportunistic infections because of their impaired immune response, and they often have systemic symptoms of infection such as fevers, sweats (particularly at night), swollen glands, chills, weakness, and weight loss.

Gastroesophageal reflux in infants

Regurgitation is commonly seen in newborns and young infants while feeding. Immature upper GI motility is thought to be the cause. Excessive reflux may cause caloric deprivation, resulting in weight loss.

Crohn disease

Crohn disease is an inflammatory bowel disease that presents with abdominal cramping, rectal bleeding, and bloody diarrhea. Weight loss is common because of malabsorption. There is a genetic link in families with a two- to fourfold increase in risk when a first-degree relative has the disease. The disease can affect any part of the tract from the mouth to the anus. Disease affecting the small bowel affects nutritional status and weight loss.

Tuberculosis

Tuberculosis is caused by *M. tuberculosis* and is spread by droplets through the respiratory tract (see Chapter 11). Weight loss is a common symptom of tuberculosis. The diagnosis of active TB infection is based on a positive sputum culture.

Nonorganic failure to thrive

Nonorganic failure to thrive is a condition in children 2 years or younger when no known pathologic condition is present to retard growth. Causes relate to the child's environment and maternal health. Physical examination reveals decreased skin fold thickness and subcutaneous fat.

Cystic fibrosis

Cystic fibrosis is an exocrine gland disorder that produces mucus blockage in major organs and is associated with an autosomal recessive trait (see Chapter 11). Growth retardation and weight loss are common symptoms of CF.

Unintentional Weight Gain

Energy balance

A 24-hour food intake history is the first approach to assessing nutritional and caloric intake. A history of physical activity or energy expenditure is done to assess the balance between calories consumed and energy expended.

Aging

In women, cessation of estrogen secretion during menopause is associated with lower levels of progesterone, androgen, and testosterone, which can lead to weight gain and greater truncal fat deposition.

Endocrine disorders

Hypothyroidism

Hypothyroidism (myxedema) is associated with weight gain and symptoms of cold intolerance, constipation, hoarseness, depression, and fatigue. Physical examination reveals bradycardia, dry skin, and delayed recovery of deep tendon reflexes. In overt hypothyroidism, the TSH is elevated and thyroid hormone level is low.

Cushing Syndrome

Cushing syndrome is associated with weight gain. The diagnosis is made through the presence of associated symptoms, glucose tolerance tests, and the dexamethasone suppression test. Cushing syndrome is associated with central truncal obesity, moon facies, supraclavicular fat pads, and thin extremities.

DIFFERENTIAL DIAGNOSIS OF *Common Causes of Unintentional Weight Loss/Gain*

CONDITION	HISTORY	PHYSICAL FINDINGS	DIAGNOSTIC STUDIES
WEIGHT LOSS			
Cancer	Loss of appetite	None or may look cachectic	Diagnostic imaging studies, CT, MRI, radiography, CBC
Undernutrition	Poor calorie or nutrient intake, error in formula preparation	Loss of body mass	Total serum protein
Frailty syndrome	Decreased energy, lower activity, weight loss	Muscle weakness, slowness of movement	CBC
Diabetes mellitus	Polyuria, polyphagia, polydipsia	Truncal obesity; xanthomas	FBG, hemoglobin A_{1c}, glucose tolerance test
Hyperthyroidism	Tachycardia, heat intolerance, sweating	Exophthalmos, warm skin, onycholysis, thinning hair, pretibial myxedema, enlarged thyroid, brisk DTRs	TSH, T_4
Gastroesophageal reflux (infants)	History of regurgitation, wheezing, difficulty feeding	None	Upper GI, barium swallow
Addison disease	Salt craving, fatigue	Darkening of the skin	Serum electrolytes, 24-hr urine for aldosterone
Malabsorption	Intolerance to gluten; chronic diarrhea, growth retardation	Muscle wasting, loss of subcutaneous fat; may have ascites	Colonoscopy, stool culture, fecal fat
Anorexia nervosa	Female-to-male ratio, 10:1; perfectionist, high achiever; amenorrhea	Cachexia, hair loss, dry skin, orthostatic hypotension	Thyroid function tests, serum electrolytes
Depression or anxiety	Loss of appetite or interest in food	None or may have poor personal hygiene	Thyroid function tests, refer for psychological evaluation
Cognitive impairment	Disorientation to person, time, or place	None or loss of body mass; poor personal hygiene	MMSE
Psychosocial factors	Alcohol consumption, social isolation, financial resources	None or poor personal hygiene with chronic alcoholism	Liver function tests
HIV/AIDS	Fever, fatigue, multiple sexual partners, unprotected sex, IV drug use	Redness or swelling of tissues or lymph nodes	Blood or tissue culture, CBC
Crohn disease	Weight loss, fever, diarrhea, family history	Perirectal fissure, anal skin tag	CBC, colonoscopy, barium enema, small bowel follow-through

Continued

> **DIFFERENTIAL DIAGNOSIS OF** *Common Causes of Unintentional Weight Loss/Gain—cont'd*

CONDITION	HISTORY	PHYSICAL FINDINGS	DIAGNOSTIC STUDIES
Tuberculosis (TB)	Contact with person who has TB, travel to endemic area, HIV	Cough, weight loss	PPD, HIV, chest radiography, QFT
Nonorganic failure to thrive	Weight loss, maternal isolation, maternal depression	Decreased skin fold thickness, decrease subcutaneous fat	Normal laboratory results
Cystic fibrosis	Weight loss, cough, chronic diarrhea, positive family history	Digital clubbing, growth retardation, weight loss	Sweat test
WEIGHT GAIN			
Intake/energy balance	Excessive calorie intake; inactivity	Generalized excess of subcutaneous fat	None
Aging	Menopause history; metabolism change	Truncal obesity; loss of peripheral subcutaneous fat; loss of muscle mass	Serum estrogen level
Hypothyroidism	Cold intolerance, weight gain, constipation; medication history	Bradycardia, dry skin, generalized edema, delayed recovery of DTRs	TSH, T_4
Cushing syndrome	Thirst, polyuria	Moon facies, truncal obesity, thin extremities	FBG, dexamethasone suppression test

CBC, complete blood count; *CT*, computed tomography; *DTR*, deep tendon reflex; *FBG*, fasting blood glucose; *GI*, gastrointestinal; *HIV*, human immunodeficiency virus; *IV*, intravenous; *MMSE*, Mini Mental State Examination; *MRI*, magnetic resonance imaging; *PPD*, purified protein derivative; *QRT*, QuantiFERON-TB Gold test; T_4, thyroxine; *TB*, tuberculosis; *TSH*, thyroid-stimulating hormone.

40 Abdominal X-ray

The abdominal x-ray is used primarily for acute conditions and has a more limited use than the chest x-ray. Often the abdominal x-ray may require additional imaging and the use of contrast radiographic substances to make structures more visible. Generally, abdominal images are taken to help in diagnosing pain, vomiting, and lack of or abnormal bowel sounds. They are also useful in finding stones in the kidneys, ureter, bladder, and gallbladder; ingested foreign objects; and air distribution. Frequently, a chest image is done at the same time. Every patient with a uterus should be asked about possible pregnancy is before an image is taken.

DIAGNOSTIC REASONING: VIEWING THE ABDOMINAL IMAGE

What are the first steps in reviewing the image?

Key Questions (to self)

- Does the image being examined belong to the correct patient?
- Do I have all views of the area being examined?
- Is the image correctly displayed on the view box or screen?
- Is the image of good quality?
- Do I know the anatomy of the abdomen?

Image and Patient Identification

As with the chest x-ray, it is important to determine that the image being viewed is from the patient being evaluated. Pertinent information about the patient should be found on the image in the upper corner and verified.

Views

Flat plate or anteroposterior view

For an anteroposterior (AP) view, the patient lies in a supine position on the x-ray table. A cassette is placed beneath the patient, with the x-ray machine above the patient. The beam passes from front to back. The patient is asked to exhale and the x-ray is taken. Because of the size of the cassette, a second image may be needed while the patient is in this position to see the entire abdomen from the diaphragm to the groin.

Left lateral decubitus view

In a left lateral decubitus image, the x-ray machine moves to a position where the beam is horizontal to the patient and the left chest is closest to the image. This view is obtained when an obstruction or perforation may have occurred, resulting in free air in the abdomen.

Erect view

For an erect view, an x-ray of the abdomen is taken as the patient is standing. A standing erect x-ray is used to assess for free air; however, this is seen only when an excessive amount of air is present.

Chest X-ray

A chest x-ray may be ordered to rule out free air collection beneath the diaphragm, a pneumonia that may be causing abdominal symptoms, a pleural effusion, or a subphrenic abscess.

Kidneys, ureter, and bladder

The term *kidneys, ureter, bladder (KUB)* is often used to indicate a flat plate of the abdomen. A KUB x-ray is done to look for stones or abnormalities.

Image Box Placement

The image, if an x-ray film, is placed on the lighted view box with the patient's left side facing the reader's right side. The image is labeled with an R or L on the bottom. Digital imaging is common where the x-ray image is viewed on a computer screen.

Image Quality

The amount of x-ray beamed through the patient affects the details seen on the image. If too few beams were delivered, the image will be underexposed and appear lighter than normal. If too many beams were delivered, the image will be overexposed and appear darker than normal. An underexposed abdominal image is not usually a problem. However, an overexposed image (darker than normal) requires a high-density spotlight looking for any free air. If the spine is visible, most other structures should be seen.

Reviewing Anatomy

Reviewing the normal anatomy of the structures of the abdomen is helpful when learning how to interpret an abdominal image. Superimposing the anatomy onto the image will help to correlate the normal structures to the shadows. The abdomen, unlike the chest image, is more difficult to read because of soft-tissue organs. The principles of radiology help explain this. Radiodense objects, such as bone and calcium, are easy to see (white). Radiolucent objects, such as air and fat, are also easy to see (dark). Structures of intermediate density are more difficult to see because they appear gray (e.g., solid organs of the abdomen), and gray densities next to each other are invisible. Organs that have varying densities next to each other (e.g., the liver border next to fat) assist in identification. Careful viewing and knowledge of anatomy are important (Fig. 40.1).

> *What approach should be used when viewing the image?*

Key Questions (to self)
- What is my initial impression?
- Am I using a systematic examination technique?

Initial Impression

When beginning to view the image, it is helpful to ask why you ordered the image, what you expect to see based on the history and physical examination, and if you see it. Initially, view the gas pattern and look for any extraluminal air, soft tissue masses, or calcifications.

Systematic Examination

Systematic examination of the image after an initial overview is mandatory. All parts of the abdominal anatomy are evaluated at 2 to 4 feet from the image, concentrating on one part of the image at a time to observe any

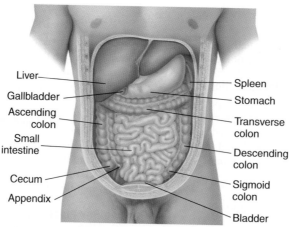

FIGURE 40.1 Normal abdominal anatomy. (From Seidel HM, Ball JW, Dains JE, et al: *Mosby's guide to physical examination*, ed. 8, St. Louis, 2015, Mosby.)

abnormalities. A suggested systematic examination follows.

DIAGNOSTIC REASONING: SYSTEMATIC EXAMINATION

How do I assess the AP view?

Bones

Identify the lower rib cage, lumbar spine, sacrum, pelvis, and hip joints. In each instance, look for fracture, cortical density, and joint and disc space.

Bladder

The inferior aspect of the bladder projects 5 to 10 mm above the symphysis pubis. If the bladder is full, it will appear as a soft-tissue density in the pelvis (Fig. 40.2).

Uterus

The uterus sits on top of the bladder, possibly indenting the bladder, and is often not seen on plain x-ray.

Liver

Observe for homogeneous density in the right upper abdominal quadrant. The lower border of the liver is found in the right flank near the right costal margin. The adjacent fat provides the contrast showing the liver edge (Fig. 40.3).

Spleen

The spleen is found in the left upper quadrant between the diaphragm and fundus of the stomach. It is the size of the adult fist and is usually not seen. Because the spleen must be very enlarged to be seen, ultrasound may be more beneficial (see Fig. 40.3).

Psoas Muscle

The psoas muscle shadows are visible as diverging lines on both sides of the spine starting from the first lumbar vertebra towards the pelvis (see Fig. 40.3).

Kidneys

The kidneys are retroperitoneal organs that are visualized on the x-ray because of the presence of perirenal fat. Visualization may be obscured by bowel loops. The left kidney is higher than the right. The shadow should appear smooth with the superior pole closest to the midline. Kidneys are located on either side of the lower thoracic and upper lumbar spine between the upper border of the eleventh thoracic vertebra and the lower border of the third lumbar vertebra (see Fig. 40.3).

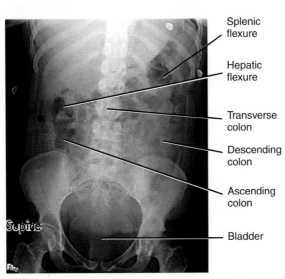

Splenic flexure

Hepatic flexure

Transverse colon

Descending colon

Ascending colon

Bladder

FIGURE 40.2 Supine abdominal radiograph showing colon, bladder, and flexures. (Modified from Johns Hopkins University, Piccini J, Nilsson K: *The Osler medical handbook,* ed. 2, Philadelphia, 2006, Saunders.)

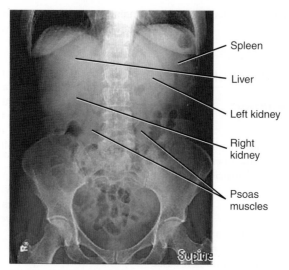

Spleen

Liver

Left kidney

Right kidney

Psoas muscles

FIGURE 40.3 Supine abdominal radiograph showing kidneys, spleen, liver, and psoas muscle. (Modified from Johns Hopkins University, Piccini J, Nilsson K: *The Osler medical handbook,* ed. 2, Philadelphia, 2006, Saunders.)

Stomach

The stomach can be identified in its location above the transverse colon by the bandlike shadows of the gastric rugae in the supine view and by the gas fluid level beneath the left hemidiaphragm in the erect view. When supine, air in the stomach will rise anteriorly and fluid will pool posteriorly (Fig. 40.4).

Colon

The colon often has a bubbly appearance representing a mixture of gas and fecal material. It lies on the periphery of the abdomen and may be filled with air or feces. The colon begins at the hepatic flexure and goes to the rectum. Fecal matter in the bowel gives a "mottled" appearance. This is seen as a mixture of grey densities representing a gas-liquid-solid mixture (Fig. 40.5). A mechanical obstruction causes the large bowel to become dilated more than 6 cm. The dilated colon is above the obstruction and no air in the colon appears below the point of obstruction (Fig. 40.6). A paralytic ileus (postsurgery) shows a bowel that is dilated but has gas throughout the small and large intestine with no delineation.

Small Bowel

The small bowel lies in the center of the abdomen within the "frame" of the large bowel; often little small bowel is seen on the image. The normal small bowel diameter should not exceed 3 cm. A small bowel obstruction presents as multiple dilated loops in the central abdomen with no air in the large bowel (Fig. 40.7).

Calcifications

Whiteness of calcifications is caused by the absorption of the x-rays. Calcifications seen in the pancreas, kidney (Fig. 40.8), gallbladder, and aorta are abnormal. Occasionally, one may see a calcification in the area of the appendix called an appendicolith. In women, fibroids may become calcified and visible.

Gas Patterns and Extraluminal Air

Air is naturally swallowed and can be seen in the stomach. When a patient is in the supine position, the gas will rise to the anterior portion of the stomach. Gas in the small bowel is located in the left midabdomen and the lower central abdomen. Gas in the colon often has a bubbly appearance representing a mixture of

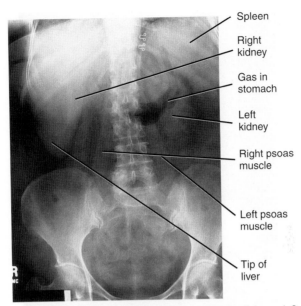

FIGURE 40.4 Normal gas in the stomach. (From Mettler F: *Essentials of radiology,* ed. 2, Philadelphia, 2005, Elsevier.)

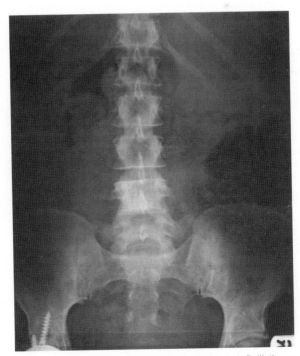

FIGURE 40.5 Constipation. (From Walsh T, Caraceni A, Fainsinger R, et al: *Palliative medicine,* Philadelphia, 2009, Elsevier.)

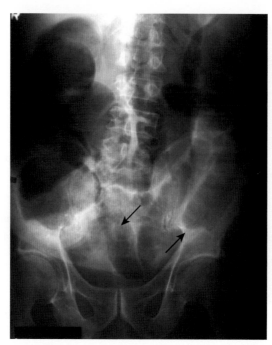

FIGURE 40.6 Mechanical large bowel obstruction *(arrows)*. (From Herring W: *Learning radiology: Recognizing the basics,* St. Louis, 2007, Elsevier.)

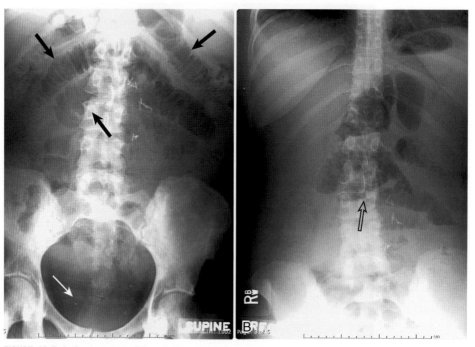

FIGURE 40.7 A, Supine view of the abdomen showing mechanical small bowel obstruction *(black arrows)* and no air in the rectum *(white arrow)*. **B,** Erect view of the abdomen showing small bowel obstruction *(arrow)*. (From Herring W: *Learning radiology: Recognizing the basics,* St. Louis, 2007, Elsevier.)

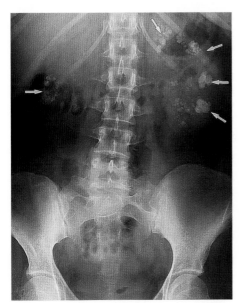

FIGURE 40.8 Nephrocalcinosis *(arrows).* (From Mettler F: *Essentials of radiology,* ed. 2, Philadelphia, 2005, Saunders.)

gas and fecal material. Gas within the peritoneal cavity outside the sealed gastrointestinal (GI) tract is abnormal and is termed pneumoperitoneum (Fig. 40.9).

Artifacts

Artifacts may be immediately obvious. Piercing of the umbilicus is very popular,

especially in young women; genital piercing is not infrequent. Metallic objects are obvious. There may be clips or materials from previous surgeries.

> *If the patient has abdominal pain, what other x-ray should I consider?*

Key Questions (to self)
- What are the indications for ordering other x-rays?

Upright Abdominal X-ray and Standing Chest X-ray

If an obstruction or ileus is suspected, an upright abdominal x-ray and a standing chest x-ray are ordered. The upright abdominal x-ray provides a view of the air/fluid levels within the bowel to differentiate between an obstruction and an ileus. Additionally, if free air in the abdomen is a concern, the standing image will demonstrate free air underneath the hemidiaphragm, which is unable to be seen on the plain abdominal x-ray. A standing chest image should be viewed using the procedure outlined in Chapter 41. When looking for free air in the abdomen, pay particular attention to the area under the right diaphragm. Extraluminal free air appears as a crescent of radiolucent gas between the diaphragm and the liver and usually indicates a perforated viscus (see Fig. 40.9).

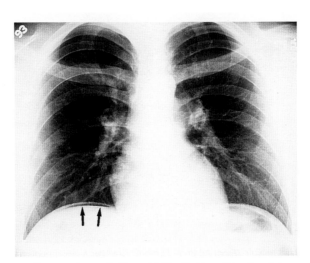

FIGURE 40.9 Pneumoperitoneum *(arrows).* (From Mettler F: *Essentials of radiology,* ed. 2, Philadelphia, 2005, Saunders.)

Left Lateral X-ray

If the patient is too ill to stand, a left lateral x-ray will be useful in finding free air in the abdomen. In the left lateral decubitus image, the patient is lying on the left side for 10 to 15 minutes and a horizontal beam is used. In this image, small amounts of free air can be seen over the lateral aspect of the right lobe of the liver. Often the free air is seen as a dark shadow between the white of the abdominal wall and the liver (Fig. 40.10).

Additional Causes of Abdominal Pain

Abdominal pain may also be caused by chest pathology mimicking abdominal pain, such as pleurisy, pneumonia, and pleural effusion. A chest x-ray should be ordered.

> ### What other imaging studies should I consider?

Key Questions (to self)
- What other common imaging studies are available for the abdomen?
- What imaging studies would give me the best information for a particular patient concern?

Upper Gastrointestinal Series

For an upper GI series, the patient drinks a barium solution that passes through the digestive tract and fills and coats the esophagus, stomach, and first part of the small intestine, making them more visible with the x-ray. A fluoroscope is held over the body part being examined and transmits continuous images to a video monitor. This test is used to diagnose hiatal hernia, reflux, narrowing of upper GI tract, and esophageal conditions.

Small Bowel Series

For a small bowel series, the barium ingested for the upper GI series is allowed to pass through the stomach into the small bowel and images are taken. This test is used to detect tumors and malabsorption syndrome.

Lower Gastrointestinal Series

In a lower GI series, barium enemas are used to examine the large intestine and the rectum. For this test, barium or an iodine-containing liquid is introduced gradually into the colon through a tube inserted into the rectum. As the barium passes through the lower intestines, it fills the colon. As in the upper GI series, a fluoroscope transmits continuous images to the video monitor. A lower GI series is used to diagnose colon polyps, tumors, diverticular disease, narrowing or obstructions, ulcerative colitis, or Crohn disease.

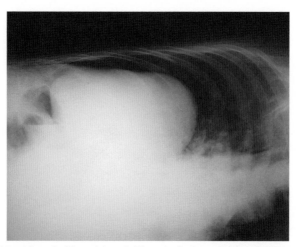

FIGURE 40.10 Left lateral free air. (From Adam A, Dixon A: *Grainger & Allison's diagnostic radiology*, ed. 5, Philadelphia, 2008, Churchill Livingstone.)

EVIDENCE-BASED PRACTICE *Should Abdominal X-Rays Be Obtained in Patients with Undifferentiated Abdominal Pain?*

Thirty-eight studies on the use of abdominal x-rays in undifferentiated abdominal pain were reviewed. The studies were evaluated for the diagnostic value and outcome of the use of the abdominal x-ray. In one study, 75% of cases had normal x-ray findings. In the 25% of cases with abnormal x-ray findings, more than half of the abnormalities were unrelated to the final diagnosis. Because the radiation exposure of an abdominal x-ray is 35 times that of a chest x-ray, the authors concluded that plain abdominal x-ray should not be used routinely in patients with undifferentiated abdominal pain unless there is clinical suspicion of bowel obstruction.

Data from Smith J. Hall E: The use of plain abdominal x-rays in the emergency department. Emerg Med J 26:160, 2009.

Colonoscopy

In a colonoscopy, a colonoscope is inserted into the rectum and advanced through the large intestine and part of the small bowel. The scope has a fibrotic light and camera projecting images onto a monitor. Polyps can be identified, biopsied, or entirely removed. Colonoscopy is used to evaluate intestinal bleeding, inflammatory bowel disease, colorectal polyps, or cancer.

Sigmoidoscopy

In a sigmoidoscopy, a flexible sigmoidoscope is passed through the rectum to view the last 2 feet of the colon. The scope transmits images of the inside of the rectum and colon. Biopsies may be taken of polyps or suspicious tissue on the intestinal wall. This test is useful for viewing inflammatory conditions in the rectum and lower colon, polyps, bleeding, and ulcerations.

Computed Tomography

Computed tomography (CT), or computed axial tomography, provides a cross-sectional slice of the area examined (see Chapter 41). CT is useful for diagnosing sigmoid diverticulitis, appendicitis, bowel obstruction, and extracolonic causes of abdominal pain.

Endoscopy

A flexible fiberoptic tube called an endoscope is equipped with a camera at the end. The camera is connected to either an eyepiece for direct viewing or a video screen that displays the images on a monitor. The endoscope is inserted into the mouth and threaded down the esophagus to the stomach and small intestine. Endoscopy is useful for diagnosing gastric bleeding, hiatal hernia, and swallowing difficulties; for removing stuck objects such as food; and for obtaining biopsy samples.

Ultrasonography

Ultrasonography is a noninvasive examination that uses high-frequency sound waves to produce images. The ultrasound images are captured in real time. They can show the size, structure, and movement of the body's internal organs, as well as blood flowing through blood vessels and pathological lesions. It is useful for evaluating the size of the spleen, gallstones, aortic aneurysm, kidney stones, and abdominal masses.

DIFFERENTIAL DIAGNOSIS OF *The Abdominal Image*

WHAT TO LOOK AT	NORMAL FINDING	ABNORMAL FINDING	SUGGESTED CAUSE
Visible spine	Image of good quality	Spine not visible	Poor-quality image
Metallic objects	History of piercing	Present without history	Foreign object ingested
Gastric air bubble	Present on the right	Not visible	Image placement error, label error

Continued

▶ **DIFFERENTIAL DIAGNOSIS OF** *The Abdominal Image—cont'd*

WHAT TO LOOK AT	NORMAL FINDING	ABNORMAL FINDING	SUGGESTED CAUSE
Liver	Right upper quadrant	Enlarged	Many causes: CHF, alcohol abuse, hepatitis
Spleen	Left upper quadrant, usually not seen	Must be very enlarged to be visualized	Many causes: infectious, anemia, trauma, cancers
Kidneys	Left higher than right, three vertebrae in size	Enlarged, calcifications	Renal calculi, hydronephrosis
Small bowel	Central portion of image, loops normally 2–3 cm, little air	Dilated >3 cm, multiple distended loops	Constipation, ileus, small bowel obstruction
Large bowel	Periphery of image, slight air in rectum	Dilated >5 cm, multiple dilated loops Mottled appearance	Large bowel obstruction Constipation
Fluid	In erect image, present in stomach, two to three levels in small bowel; never in large bowel	Fluid present in small bowel	Small bowel obstruction
Free air	Normally not seen	Free air in abdomen	Rupture of hollow viscus
Diaphragm	Right higher than left; right at level of sixth rib	Elevated	Collapsed lobe or multi-segmental collapse; pleural effusion
		Radiolucent line present that follows the curvature of the diaphragm	Free air present
		Flattened diaphragm	Emphysema, asthma, tension pneumothorax
		Elevation on left	Perforated ulcer or gas distention of stomach
		Bilateral elevation	Pregnancy, obesity, peritoneal fluid
Bladder	Usually not visible	Visible when full	Full bladder, bladder stone
Uterus	Sits on top of bladder, usually not visible	Visible with uterine fibroids	Possible fibroids
Aorta	Usually not visible	Calcifications in abdominal aorta	Abdominal aortic aneurysm
			Ultrasonography often used for diagnosis of size

CHF, congestive heart failure.

41 Chest X-ray

The chest x-ray is the most commonly performed diagnostic x-ray examination. It is performed to evaluate the lungs, heart, and chest wall. A chest image is typically the first imaging test used to help diagnose symptoms such as shortness of breath, persistent cough, trauma, chest pain, and fever. Chest images are also used to diagnose and monitor conditions such as pneumonia, lung cancer, and congestive heart failure.

DIAGNOSTIC REASONING: VIEWING THE CHEST IMAGE

What are the first steps in reviewing an image?

Key Questions (to self)

- Do the images being examined belong to the correct patient?
- Do I have two views of the area being examined?
- Is the image correctly displayed on the view box?
- Are the images of good quality?
- Do I have any old x-rays available?
- Do I know the anatomy of the chest?

Identification of the Image and Patient

Before viewing an image, it is important to verify that the image being viewed is from the patient being evaluated. Pertinent information about the patient should be found on the image in the upper corner and should be verified.

Views

Frontal and lateral views

Generally, two images are taken when a chest x-ray is requested. One is a frontal view; it is usually a posteroanterior (PA) view, in which the patient is standing 6 feet from the cassette and the image is taken from back (posterior) to front (anterior) (Fig. 41.1, *A*). A second image is the lateral view (Fig. 41.1, *B*), in which the patient is standing with the hands held above the head and the lateral thorax is against the cassette. A left lateral view (in which the left thorax is against the image cassette) is usually ordered instead of a right lateral view because it provides a better view of the area behind the heart and the bases of the lower lungs. Additional views are occasionally ordered for specific reasons.

Anteroposterior chest image

The AP view is created when the beam passes from the anterior to the posterior surface of the chest and then onto the image. These images are usually ordered for patients who are confined to bed or who cannot stand. Infants have a single supine AP image, and an erect AP is used with toddlers. When a child is old enough to cooperate, a PA image is also taken. When viewing the AP images, the heart and mediastinum appear larger because they are located in the anterior chest, and in this position the chest is farther from the image cassette.

Expiration image

An expiration image is ordered when a pneumothorax is suspected. A maximum expiration by the patient will cause the lung tissue to compress. The lung tissue is then compared with the pleural air. With a pneumothorax, the pleural air will occupy more space.

Lateral decubitus image

The lateral decubitus view is used to assess fluid and air levels in the pleural spaces. The patient is lying on his or her side with the image cassette upright against the patient's chest. The beam is sent perpendicular to the image cassette. Air rises and fluid falls to the dependent area.

Oblique image

The oblique image is used to distinguish anterior from posterior lesions by avoiding bony structures. It is also used for examining the trachea. Oblique images can be right or left obliques. In a right oblique, the patient's anterior right side is against the image cassette.

Lordotic image

The lordotic image identifies right and left middle lung fields. The x-ray machine is tilted to a 45-degree angle. This position offers a better view of lung apices that can otherwise be obscured by clavicles and upper ribs on the PA view.

Image Box Placement

The PA image is placed on the lighted view box with the patient's left side facing the reader's right side. The image is labeled with an R or L. If there is no labeling, look for the aortic arch. The arch is the first bump seen on the image and is on the patient's left or the viewing clinician's right. In the rare patient with dextrocardia, the reverse is true. The left lateral image should be placed on the view box such that the left side of the patient is facing the reader.

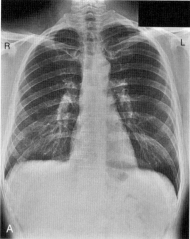
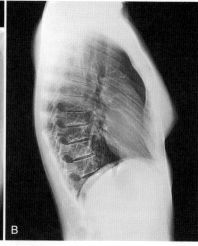

FIGURE 41.1 A, A patient positioned for a posteroanterior projection of the chest. **B,** Proper patient position for a left lateral chest view. Note the left side of the patient is placed against the image receptor. (From Ballinger PW, Frank ED: *Merrill's atlas of radiographic positions and radiographic procedures,* ed. 10, vol. 1, St. Louis, 2003, Mosby.)

Digital imaging is being increasingly used to obtain x-rays. The advantage of digital images is the ability to manipulate the images. The technique also allows for easier storage and the ability to send electronic images to consultants.

Image Quality

The number of x-rays beamed through the patient onto the image affects the details seen on the image. If not enough beams were delivered, the image will be underexposed and appear lighter than normal. If too many beams were delivered, the image will become overexposed and will be darker than normal. On the PA view, thoracic vertebral bodies should be barely visible through the heart shadow; on the lateral view, the spinal bodies should be visible.

To obtain a good chest image, the x-ray is taken with the patient in full inspiration. If the image is taken on expiration or poor inspiration, the heart appears larger, and the lungs look cloudy. The 10 posterior ribs above the diaphragm should be evident in a good-quality image.

The angle of the beam should be direct, and the patient should be positioned properly. If the patient is at an improper angle, the beam will be more scattered, and details will be lost. To determine if the patient is positioned correctly, note the clavicles. The medial heads of the clavicles should be positioned over the spine. If the heads are not centered, alignment may not be correct, causing the image to be slightly oblique. The costophrenic angle and the lateral lung fields should be visible.

Children frequently rotate when being x-rayed, which may cause the film to be misinterpreted. Note that both clavicles are equal in length and the trachea is straight.

Previous X-rays

Comparison x-rays are often important when viewing newer images side by side. View the older PA x-ray first and then the newer image.

Reviewing Anatomy

Reviewing the normal anatomy of the structures of the chest is helpful when learning how to interpret a chest image.

Superimposing the anatomy onto a chest image will help to correlate the normal structures to the shadows (Fig. 41.2). An infant's chest is more triangular shaped and deeper when seen on the AP film. As the child grows, the chest will take on a more adult appearance.

What approach should be used when viewing an image?

Key Questions (to self)
- What is your initial impression?
- Are you using a systematic examination technique?

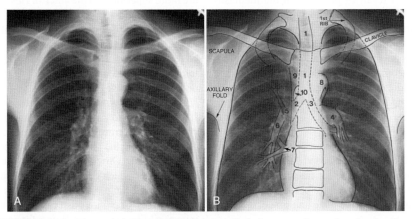

FIGURE 41.2 Normal posteroanterior image. **A,** Unlabeled. **B,** A diagrammatic overlay showing the normal anatomic structures numbered or labeled: *1,* trachea; *2,* right main bronchus; *3,* left main bronchus; *4,* left pulmonary artery; *5,* right upper lobe pulmonary artery; *6,* right interlobar artery; *7,* right lower and middle lobe vein; *8,* aortic arch; *9,* superior vena cava; and *10,* azygos vein. (From Fraser R: *Fraser and Paré's diagnosis of diseases of the chest,* ed. 4, vol. 1, Philadelphia, 1999, Saunders.)

Initial Impression

Most clinicians view images initially by standing 6 to 8 feet from the image and giving the image a once-over glance. This is to observe for any obvious abnormality as well as to obtain an overall impression of the thorax for size, shape, and symmetry.

Systematic examination of the image after an initial overview is mandatory. All parts of the chest anatomy are evaluated at 2 to 4 feet from the image, concentrating on one part of the image at a time, to observe any abnormalities. A suggested systematic examination follows.

DIAGNOSTIC REASONING: SYSTEMATIC EXAMINATION

How do I assess the PA view?

Soft Tissue

Examine the periphery of the image to evaluate the amount of soft tissue present (for obesity or cachexia), calcifications, or gas collections indicating subcutaneous emphysema. Note the presence of the breasts. Be aware that breast tissue may cover the lower lung fields.

Trachea

Located in the anterior mediastinum, the trachea should be checked for size and position. The trachea will appear deviated in a rotated patient. Abnormal pathological deviations may be a result of pressure on the mediastinum, including tumors, pneumothorax, or emphysema. A mass will push the trachea away from midline. The trachea will deviate toward a large pneumothorax and away from a tension pneumothorax. Thickening of the trachea may indicate lymph node enlargement or an upper mediastinal tumor.

Clavicles

The clavicles should be present and symmetrical and located at the second and third intercostal spaces. Scrutinize for fracture lines, which appear black on the image because of air space surrounded by white bone and tissue.

Bony Thorax

Note the size and shape of the thorax. Whereas scoliosis is visible on the frontal image, kyphosis and funnel chest are best seen on the lateral view. Examine individual shoulder girdles for shape, size, and contour. Bony structures are evaluated for deformity, mineralization, density, and cortical thickness, as well as for fractures.

Scapulae

The distance between the scapulae is increased when the shoulders are rotated forward in the PA image. This position also ensures that the scapulae will be out of the way so the lung fields can be observed. Observe for fractures and symmetry.

Thoracic Spine

Look through the mediastinum and lungs to view the spine and observe for symmetry of the rib cage. Vertebral evaluation is best done on the lateral image. Look for compression fractures, height of vertebral bodies, disc spaces, and density of bones.

Ribs and Intercostal Spaces

Count the posterior ribs; 10 should be visible. If eight or fewer ribs are visible, this is either a poor image or an expiratory image. Be careful to begin the rib count at the first thoracic vertebra. Locate the anterior end of the first rib just below the medial end of the clavicles, follow it back to its posterior end, and start counting ribs (Fig. 41.3). The posterior ribs are more superior than the anterior ribs. Check ribs side to side and completely to the lateral end. Most fractures occur on the lateral parts of the ribs. Normal ribs appear sloped at the edges; ribs that are horizontal or flattened indicate emphysema or chronic obstructive pulmonary disease (COPD).

Describe abnormalities using ribs or interspaces as location markers horizontally and chest lines as vertical markers. Interspaces are numbered using the posterior rib and according to the rib above. Observe the widths of the intercostal spaces, which should be equal bilaterally.

Decreased lung volume narrows the intercostal spaces. Conditions that cause this include interstitial fibrosis (bilateral) or a foreign body (unilateral). Increased lung volume increases the intercostal spaces in such conditions as asthma and COPD.

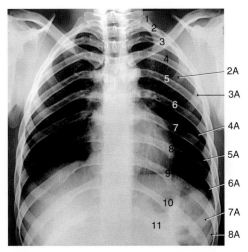

FIGURE 41.3 Respiratory lung movement. Full expiration with the ribs numbered. The anterior ribs are labeled with a suffix. (From Ballinger PW, Frank ED: *Merrill's atlas of radiographic positions and radiologic procedures,* ed. 10, St. Louis, 2003, Mosby.)

Diaphragm

The diaphragm separates the abdominal contents from the pleural cavity. Any changes in these areas can be seen radiographically to affect the diaphragm. Count down the posterior ribs near the spine; the diaphragm should be at the 10th or 11th rib. The diaphragm should have

a curve that is shaped upward. The right side is usually higher (1–2 cm) than the left because the liver is located under the right hemidiaphragm; this will be more visible on a lateral image of the diaphragm. Note if the diaphragm is elevated or flattened. In an infant the diaphragm is higher.

Suspect hepatomegaly in patients who have marked asymmetry of the right diaphragm. A unilateral elevation of the diaphragm is seen with a pneumothorax.

Patients who do not take a deep breath, who have ascites or intestinal obstruction, or who are in the third trimester of pregnancy will have elevated diaphragms. A diaphragm that is low and flat indicates enlarged structures within the thorax, as seen in COPD.

Note any free air in the peritoneum visible below the right lower diaphragm edge. The air appears as lucency (decreased opacity) under the crescent of the hemidiaphragm, typically as result of a perforated viscus.

Costophrenic Angle

The edge of the diaphragm curves downward at the costophrenic junction, meeting the ribs and forming an angle that is sometimes referred to as the letter "V" on its side. This angle should be sharp. Blunting of the angle is caused by pleural effusion, pneumonia, neoplasm, or fibrosis (Fig. 41.4). In an infant the costophrenic angles are shallower.

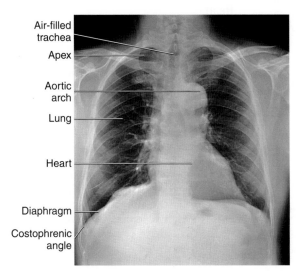

FIGURE 41.4 Normal costophrenic angle. (From Ballinger PW, Frank ED: *Merrill's atlas of radiographic positions and radiologic procedures,* ed. 10, vol. 1, St Louis, 2003, Mosby.)

Gastric Air Bubble

The gastric air bubble should always be on the examiner's right side as the image is viewed (the patient's left side). The stomach lies close beneath the left diaphragm. The liver, spleen, and kidneys are occasionally visible and should be noted for size.

Mediastinum

The mediastinum is located between the sternum anteriorly, the vertebral bodies posteriorly, and the lungs laterally. It encompasses a number of structures including the heart and its large vessels, as well as the trachea, thymus, and lymph nodes.

A prominent structure is the aortic arch (Fig. 41.5). The arch is the first prominent bulge along the left mediastinal border. Assess for size and length. As patients age, the aorta increases in thickness and length. An increase in size is also seen in an aortic aneurysm.

The ascending aorta is the small bulge on the right. The infant has a large thymus gland, which is seen as a shadow called the "sail." The shadow is caused by the margins of the thymus tissues in the intercostal space. The thymus appears less as the child ages (Fig. 41.6).

Hilar Area

The hilar area contains the roots of the lungs and is where the major bronchi and pulmonary vessels project outward.

Note the size of the hilar area. Increased fullness or size generally indicates lymphoma, metastatic carcinoma, tuberculosis, or fungal (*Histoplasma* spp.) adenopathy.

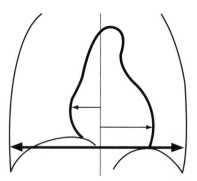

FIGURE 41.5 The normal cardiac-to-thoracic ratio is 1 to 2.

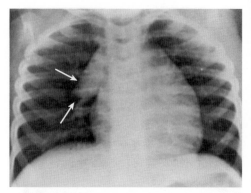

FIGURE 41.6 The classic thymic sail sign *(arrows).* (From Alves N, Sousa M: *Images in pediatrics: the thymic sail sign and thymic wave sign. Eur J Pediatr* 172:133, 2013.)

Pulmonary Vasculature

Pulmonary arteries become smaller as they progress out to the chest periphery, ending approximately 1.5 cm from the pleural surface. Normal markings extend approximately one third of the way into the lung fields.

Increased pulmonary pressure causes engorgement of the pulmonary vessels, and increased markings that resemble a branching tree are seen. When engorgement occurs, a butterfly appearance is seen. Pulmonary edema causes blurred borders and hilar clouding.

Heart

Measure the size of the heart using a ruler. The heart should be less than 50% of the transverse diameter of the thorax. The measurement should be compared with the widest thoracic diameter (found below the diaphragm and between the ribs), resulting in the cardiac/thoracic (C-T) ratio. The normal ratio is 1:2 (see Fig. 41.5). The heart size appears enlarged in supine and AP images.

Left ventricular hypertrophy extends the heart border to the left, increasing the size of the heart and increasing the C-T ratio.

Look for the silhouette sign, which occurs when two structures have the same density and are in contact with each other, resulting in a loss of borders on the x-ray. Because the right and left borders of the heart are air filled, lesions in the lung cause the differentiation of the heart border to be lost.

Pleura

Follow the pleura around the lungs and note any thickening, calcification, effusion, or pneumothorax.

Pleural thickening is seen as increased soft tissue around the periphery of the lung. An effusion will blunt the costophrenic angle. A pneumothorax will pull the visceral pleura into the lung field, away from the chest wall.

Lungs

Examine the lungs from central to peripheral. The lungs will appear whiter when looking from top to bottom because of the increasing thickness of the chest areas. The lung markings will decrease by thirds as the viewer goes from central to peripheral. The markings are also more prominent in the bases of the lungs than in the upper lung fields.

Compare the right and left lung fields, starting at the top and continuing across and down. Do this in small segments, evaluating each area carefully. Look for lesions, lung markings, and density changes such as areas of opacity (seen in white), which represent consolidation, nodules, and calcifications. Note the lung volume. Decreased volume is seen with atelectasis. Large-volume lungs with a narrow mediastinum and a flat diaphragm are typically viewed in the patient with emphysema.

Final Look

Research has shown that there are three high-risk locations where pathology is often missed: the upper lobes of the lungs, costophrenic areas, and peripheral lung margins. Take one more look at each of these areas.

How do I assess the lateral view?

Key Questions (to self)
- In what position is the patient?
- How do I know the image quality is good?
- What are the indications for a lateral image?
- Am I using a systematic approach to review the image?

The common position for the lateral view is with the patient's left chest against the image cassette. The beam passes from right to left through the patient. Remember that the right side of the patient is closer to the beam and therefore structures are magnified on the right side compared with the left. The left lateral position is preferred because the heart is less magnified and the bases of the lungs are more easily seen.

A right lateral image is ordered when the right side of the lung needs to be less magnified and sharper, such as when a tumor is suspected. In the lateral position, the ribs will seem to be superimposed on each other and the sternum will appear thin.

A good-quality lateral image shows lung markings, fissures (the septa that divide the lobes of the lung), and good visualization of the spine.

A lateral image can help localize a lesion seen on the PA view, or it may verify lobar consolidation. In addition, the lateral image allows the viewer to see behind the sternum and cardiac shadow. The lateral image is often used to detect subglottic narrowing, as seen in croup, as well as foreign body investigation.

Use a systematic approach when viewing the lateral image, similar to the PA review.

Anatomy

Review the anatomy of the lateral chest (Fig. 41.7).

Vertebral Bodies

The amount of soft tissue is greater at the lung apices than at the lung bases; therefore, the vertebral bodies appear darker as they approach the diaphragm. Kyphosis is noticeable on the lateral image. Examine each vertebra for fractures and scrutinize the intervertebral disc spaces.

Diaphragm

The right diaphragm is visible and is higher than the left because of the heart. On the left, the latter two thirds of the diaphragm should be visible. The gastric bubble is below the left diaphragm.

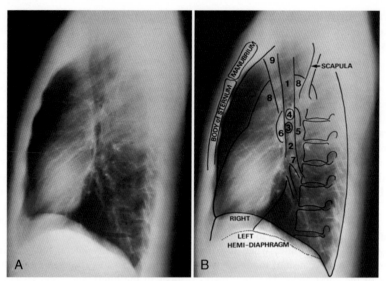

FIGURE 41.7 Lateral chest image. **A,** Unlabeled. **B,** A diagrammatic overlay showing the normal anatomic structures numbered or labeled: *1,* tracheal air column; *2,* right intermediate bronchus; *3,* left upper lobe bronchus; *4,* right upper lobe bronchus; *5,* left interlobar artery; *6,* right interlobar artery; *7,* confluence of pulmonary veins; *8,* aortic arch; and *9,* brachiocephalic vessels. (From Fraser R: *Fraser and Paré's diagnosis of diseases of the chest,* ed. 4, vol. 1, Philadelphia, 1999, Saunders.)

Costophrenic Angle

The angle is seen in the most dependent part of the lung. Both angles should be visible and sharp.

Fissures

Fissures are septa that divide the lobes of lungs. The major oblique fissure separates the left upper lobe from the left lower lobe. The right major fissure separates the right upper and middle lobes from the right lower lobe. The right minor fissure separates the right upper lobe from the right lower lobe. Fissures are generally not seen on plain images because their small surface provides no shadow or interface. However, these fissures may be seen when a pathological disorder occurs in the lung.

Pleura

Follow the pleura around the lungs from the posterior costophrenic area to the posterior sternal margin and posterior ribs.

Retrosternal Area

The retrosternal space is usually dark because of the presence of air. It is the lower one third of the sternum and appears in contact with the right ventricle. When this area is seen as opaque, air has been replaced with solid material, and anterior mediastinal disease should be considered. The area is enlarged when pulmonary overinflation occurs, as in emphysema. The retrosternal space will not be visible with an enlarged heart.

Heart and Retrocardiac Area

Identify the right ventricle, left ventricle, and left atrium. The retrocardiac area of the lateral chest image is normally dark, caused by air. If the space is opaque, then the air has been replaced with an effusion, consolidation, or mass.

Lungs

The scapulae make visualizing the upper lobe difficult in the lateral image. Lung lesions are often hidden by the heart on the PA view. Localizing a lesion in the left lung is best accomplished with the lateral image.

Final look

Take a last look at each of the areas where lesions are often missed: the upper lobes, peripheral lung margins, retrocardiac area, and costophrenic area.

What other imaging studies should I consider?

Key Questions (to self)
- What other common imaging studies are available for the chest?
- What imaging studies would give me the best information for a particular complaint?

Dual-Energy Subtraction Chest Radiography

Dual-energy subtraction chest radiography is used to detect and diagnose thoracic abnormalities. Generally, it is ordered when nodules are seen on basic chest films A major advantage of dual-energy imaging over conventional radiography is its superior sensitivity for the detection of calcification within a pulmonary nodule.

Computed Tomography

Computed tomography (CT), sometimes called computed axial tomography, provides a cross-sectional slice of the area examined. Unlike plain images, which superimpose structures onto an image, a CT scan gives only one slice. The beams of x-rays pass through the body in an axial plane as the x-ray tube moves in a continuous arc around the patient. Detectors are placed opposite the beam to catch the electrical pulses. The image is the result of the x-rays that are not absorbed by the tissues between the beam and the detectors. Detectors pick up the electrical impulses that are fed into a computer that provides the "picture." CT is used to distinguish overlapping shadows from the chest image. It is also very useful in showing fine details of the pulmonary parenchyma and hilum. Low-dose computed tomography is used to screen for lung cancer in adults older than 55 years of age who have a 30-pack year history of smoking.

Magnetic Resonance Imaging

Magnetic resonance imaging (MRI) produces a computer-based sectional image that does not use ionizing radiation. MRI uses the hydrogen molecules in the body to produce the image. A radiofrequency pulse transmitted through coils causes some of the hydrogen molecules to absorb energy and spin in a different direction from the other hydrogen ions (resonance). When the radiofrequency pulse stops, the hydrogen molecules stop spinning and release their excess stored energy. A gradient magnet located inside the main magnet, which provides the slicing capability of the image, picks up the change. The results are sent to the computer system, providing a two-dimensional image. MRI of the chest is used to view lesions of the chest wall and is less useful for examining the lungs.

Positron Emission Tomography

Positron emission tomography (PET) scans provide information on the biochemical metabolism of an organ or tissue. Positrons come from the nucleus of a proton as it decays to a neutron. When released, the positron eventually collides with an electron, resulting in the release of two high-energy gamma photons. These gamma photons are released at 180 degrees from each other. The patient is given a radiotracer that follows the destruction of the positron and the resulting gamma photons. PET scans are built with hundreds of detectors on circular rings that are located directly across from each other. The detectors allow the localization, in three-dimensional space, of the decay of the gamma photons. PET scans show the chemical function of an organ or tissue rather than its structure; very highly active metabolism is seen with cancer cells. PET scans are ordered for evaluating the effects of lung cancer therapy.

Echocardiography

In echocardiography, High-frequency sound waves are directed into the body, which are then recorded as they deflect off organs and structures. These deflections are transmitted back to a transducer that records the difference in acoustic impedance. This recording is changed into an electrical signal, which is then analyzed by a computer to produce an image. Echocardiograms are useful to evaluate heart size, valvular function, and presence of pericardial effusion.

▶ DIFFERENTIAL DIAGNOSIS OF *The Chest Image*

WHAT TO LOOK AT	NORMAL FINDING	ABNORMAL FINDING	SUGGESTED CAUSE
Clavicles	Midline, symmetrical, intact	Dark lines; clavicles not centered	Fracture; patient rotated; image taken off center
Chest wall	Chest wall has rounded contour	Sternum pushed outward (lateral image)	Pectus carinatum
		Sternum pushed inward (lateral image)	Pectus excavatum
Inspiration	Adequate inspiration	<10 ribs identified	Inadequate inspiration
Vertebral column	Straight, equal disc spaces	Curved	Kyphoscoliosis (lateral view); scoliosis (PA view)
		Collapsed disc spaces	Degenerative disc disease
Ribs	All ribs intact; able to count 10 ribs	Rib fractures present; <10 ribs identified	Trauma; inadequate inspiration
	Ribs sloped at edges	Ribs horizontal or flattened	Hyperinflated lungs, acute asthma, COPD
Trachea	Midline	Deviation from midline Widening of trachea	Atelectasis: trachea deviated toward area of atelectasis; pneumothorax: air, fluid, tumor, lymph node enlargement push trachea away from center; rotated image; chronic cough, cystic fibrosis
Hilar region	Normal size, centrally located	Area enlarged	Pulmonary artery congestion; lymph node enlargement
	Vascular markings extend <1/3 out into lung field	Vascular markings >1/3 into lung field	Bronchopneumonia or pulmonary congestion
	Bronchi invisible because air-filled bronchi have same density as air in lungs	Bronchograms present (bronchi become visible when lung tissue filled with fluid is contrasted with air-filled bronchi)	Infiltration; pulmonary edema
			Pneumonia
		Infiltrates or consolidation of lung tissue	
Gastric air bubble	Present on right	Not visible	Image placement error; image label error
Diaphragm	Right higher than left; right at level of sixth rib	Elevated	Collapsed lobe or multisegmental collapse; pleural effusion
		Radiolucent line present that follows curvature of diaphragm	Free air present
		Flattened diaphragm	Emphysema, asthma, tension pneumothorax
		Elevation on left	Perforated ulcer or gas distention of stomach
		Bilateral elevation	Pregnancy, obesity, peritoneal fluid
Costophrenic angle	Present, sharp edges	Blunted edges or absent	Pneumonia, pleural effusion

DIFFERENTIAL DIAGNOSIS OF *The Chest Image—cont'd*

WHAT TO LOOK AT	NORMAL FINDING	ABNORMAL FINDING	SUGGESTED CAUSE
Visceral pleura	Traced around chest wall	Hairline shadow, dark black with no lung markings	Pneumothorax
Heart size	Cardiac ratio <50%	Cardiac ratio >50%	Enlarged heart, patient rotated
Heart borders	Presence of heart borders	Loss of border	Infiltrates
Lungs	Translucent	Fluffy appearance	Engorged vasculature
		Honeycomb appearance	Acute respiratory distress syndrome
		Butterfly appearance	Pulmonary edema
		Density changes to consolidation	Bacterial pneumonia
		Web-shaped density	Pulmonary embolism

COPD, chronic obstructive pulmonary disease; *PA*, posteroanterior.

CHAPTER

42

Care of Transgender Patients

This chapter is intended to highlight health history questions and physical examination considerations that are specific to transgender patients in the primary care setting. The term "transgender" is used in this chapter as an umbrella term to be inclusive of transgender and gender-nonconforming patients. The chapter is not a comprehensive guideline for care of transgender patients. Not addressed in this chapter are gender dysphoria and mental health issues; transition decisions, issues, and management; criteria for hormonal and or surgical intervention; hormonal management and monitoring; surgical complications; and fertility considerations. Resources for more in-depth

care guidelines and standards are included in the chapter.

Gender identity is defined as an internal sense of self and how one fits into the world, from the perspective of gender. Sex refers to the sex assigned at birth, based on assessment of external genitalia, chromosomes, and reproductive organs. Gender identity can be congruent or incongruent with one's sex assigned at birth based on the appearance of the external genitalia. Transgender refers to gender identification and expression that is different from the sex that was assigned at birth. A transgender man (transman; female to male [FTM]) is a person with a male gender identity and female-assigned sex at

 EVIDENCE-BASED PRACTICE *Discrimination in Health Care and Poor Health Outcomes*

In a 2015 a survey of 27,715 transgender and gender-nonconforming respondents, ages 18 to 87 years from diverse backgrounds and racial and ethnic identities and from all 50 states, the District of Columbia, American Samoa, Guam, Puerto Rico, and several US military bases overseas reported high levels of mistreatment, harassment, violence and discrimination in every aspect of life, including health care, severe economic hardship and instability, and harmful effects on physical and mental health. Some specific findings:

- Nearly half (47%) have been sexually assaulted at some point in their lives, and 10% were sexually assaulted in the past year.
- More than half (54%) experienced some form of intimate partner violence. Nearly one quarter (23%) reported that they avoided seeking health care they needed in the past year because of fear of being mistreated as a transgender person.
- One-third (33%) who had seen a health care provider in the past year reported having at least one negative experience related

to being transgender, such as verbal harassment, refusal of treatment, or having to teach the health care provider about transgender people to receive appropriate care.

- Nearly one-third (31%) reported that none of their health care providers knew they were transgender.
- 15% reported that a health care provider asked them unnecessary or invasive questions about their transgender status that were not related to the reason for their visit.
- Nearly one-third (32%) limited the amount they ate or drank to avoid using the restroom in the past year. Eight percent (8%) reported having a urinary tract infection, kidney infection, or another kidney-related problem in the past year as a result of avoiding restrooms.
- 39% were currently experiencing serious psychological distress, nearly eight times the rate in the US population (5%).
- 40% have attempted suicide in their lifetime, nearly nine times the attempted suicide rate in the US population (4.6%).

Reference: James et al, 2016.

birth; a transgender woman (transwoman; male to female [MTF]) is a person with a female gender identity and male-assigned sex at birth. A nontransgender person may be referred to as cisgender (*cis* = "same side" in Latin). See Box 42.1 for a summary of terms.

Gender expression denotes the manifestation of characteristics in one's personality, appearance, and behavior that are culturally defined as masculine or feminine.

Gender role conformity is the extent to which an individual's gender expression adheres to the cultural norms prescribed for those of his or her sex. The terms *gender nonconforming* or *gender queer* denotes a person whose gender identity differs from that which was assigned at birth but may be more complex, fluid, multifaceted, or otherwise less clearly defined than a transgender person. *Nonbinary* refers to a transgender or gender-nonconforming person who identifies as neither male nor female.

Transition is the process of changing one's gender expression and/or sex characteristics to agree with one's internal sense of gender identity. Not all transgender persons choose, or are able, to have gender-affirming hormonal therapy or surgeries. The range of transition and expression in transgender persons can vary from minimal (e.g., clothing only) to complete anatomical reconstruction.

DIAGNOSTIC REASONING: FOCUSED HISTORY

How do I ascertain gender identity?

A two-step question process is recommended:

Key Questions
1. What is your gender identity?
   - Male
   - Female
   - Transgender man, transman, or FTM
   - Transgender woman, transwoman, or MTF
   - Genderqueer or gender nonconforming
   - Additional identity (fill in) _____
   - Decline to state
2. What sex were you assigned at birth?
   - Male
   - Female
   - Decline to state

The two-step method has been found to be more effective than a single question that asks gender or sex with choices of "male,"

Box 42.1	**Terms**

Gender identity: the gender with which one identifies: male, female, or elsewhere on the gender spectrum

Natal sex: the sex (male, female, or intersex) assigned at birth based on chromosomes or appearance of genitalia

Gender expression: the manifestation of appearance, behaviors, actions, and mannerisms that are culturally defined as male or female

Transgender: gender identity, gender expression, or both differs from the sex assigned at birth

Cisgender: gender identity, gender expression, or both aligns with the sex assigned at birth.

Transwoman or male to female (MTF): person assigned male sex at birth who identifies as female

Transman or female to male (FTM): person assigned female sex at birth who identifies as a male

Gender nonconforming: gender identity differs from that the sex assigned at birth but

may be more complex, fluid, multifaceted, or otherwise less clearly defined than a transgender person

Nonbinary: gender identity as neither male nor female; view of gender is on a spectrum. Similar terms include **gender neutral, genderqueer, queer, gender fluid,** and **gender free.**

Transition: an individualized process of changing one's gender expression, sex characteristics, or both to agree with one's internal sense of gender identity; may include changes to name, appearance, clothing, identity documents or undergoing medical procedures such as surgery or hormone therapy

Cross-dresser or transvestite: one who likes to dress as the opposite gender but does not identify as that gender

Sexual orientation: the direction of one's romantic and sexual attractions; an aspect of identity that is not based on gender identity or gender expression

"female," and "transgender." Querying gender identity first emphasizes to the transgender person the importance of this factor relative to that of the sex assigned at birth.

Gender identity data have been added to the requirements for the interoperability of electronic health records.

How do I provide culturally sensitive care?

Both personal behaviors and structural elements such as policies and bathrooms contribute to an environment that is sensitive to the transgender community and particular needs. Barriers to disclosure in the health care setting include embarrassment, fear of discrimination or bias, or worry that family members will be informed. Maintaining privacy and confidentiality is paramount.

Although many patients may feel vulnerable and anxious when seeking health care, these feelings are intensified in transgender patients. The fear of or experience with disrespect, discrimination, inflexible or noninclusive policies, or refusal of care make seeking health care stressful and uncomfortable. As a health care provider, it is essential to examine your own attitudes and possible internal biases that may contribute to your own stereotypes and assumptions about transgender patients.

Ask transgender patients how they prefer to be addressed. Ask about their legal names and preferred names. Some have not changed their names legally but go by another name. Address the patient by the chosen name and pronoun that coincides with the patient's gender identity. Use of the preferred name and pronoun during the entire visit and in documentation contributes to an environment that is sensitive and respectful. Failure to do so can compromise the provider–patient relationship, patient satisfaction, and quality of care and influence the patient's decision to seek follow-up care.

The preferred name and pronoun should be clearly recorded in the medical record. Specific details regarding gender-affirming interventions and an inventory of organs can be recorded in the medical and surgical history sections of the record.

Become aware of the basic terminology used by the transgender community (see Box 42.1). Terminology may change over time and vary by geographic location or language. Be mindful of terms that gender label and use phrases such as "patients with a uterus" rather than "females" or "women." Some patients prefer general terms for body parts, for example, "top" and "bottom" as opposed to specific anatomic terms; others prefer anatomical terms. Ask the patient about the preferred terms.

Culturally sensitive care extends beyond the individual provider. All personnel in a health care system, including direct care providers, administrative, clerical, lab, and x-ray personnel, should receive training on transgender health issues. Training should be integrated into the hiring and orientation process for all employees.

Specifically state that patients may choose either the women's or men's rooms based on personal preference. Having at least one gender-neutral bathroom provides a safe space for nonbinary patients as well as for those in transition who feel uncomfortable in a gender-specific space. Intake forms and policies should have language that is inclusive and gender neutral. The waiting area should reflect a commitment to the provision of transgender care.

What are the past medical and surgical history questions that I need to ask?

Key Questions
- Have you had any surgeries to alter your body or appearance?
- Do you take hormones or use other substances that may have feminizing or masculinizing effects?
- Do you have any other providers that are assisting you with these procedures or transition?

Gender-Affirming Surgeries

A wide range of gender-affirming surgeries exist. These include surgeries specific to transgender persons, as well as procedures commonly performed in nontransgender populations. Any complications that have occurred as a result of surgery should be noted.

| Box 42.2 | **Gender-Affirming Surgeries** |

FEMINIZING SURGERIES
- Feminizing vaginoplasty
- Breast augmentation
- Orchiectomy
- Facial feminization procedures
- Reduction thyrochondroplasty (tracheal cartilage shave)
- Vocal cord surgery
- Lipo suction
- Lipo filling

MASCULINIZING SURGERIES
- Metaoidioplasty (clitoral release/enlargement, may include urethral lengthening)
- Masculinizing chest surgery ("top surgery"): mastectomy and chest contouring
- Hysterectomy or oophorectomy
- Vaginectomy
- Masculinizing phalloplasty or scrotoplasty

Providers should maintain an inventory of organs to guide the assessment and management of certain specific health concerns and cancer screening. The inventory includes what gender-related organs (breasts, vagina, clitoris, ovaries, penis, prostate and testes) are present and whether they are natal or surgically constructed. The inventory also includes the organs that have been surgically removed (breasts, uterus, ovaries, penis, prostate, testes). Box 42.2 summarizes gender-affirming surgeries.

Hormone Therapy

Gender-affirming hormone therapy is a medical intervention used to allow the acquisition of secondary sex characteristics that are aligned with the gender identity. Inquiry about hormone therapy is part of medication assessment, as with any patient. Ask about past and current doses. Knowledge of hormone therapy use assists with risk assessment related to side effects or adverse consequences of the therapy. It also helps set expectations for physical examination findings. Box 42.3 summarizes information related to gender-affirming hormone therapies. Most physical changes, whether feminizing or masculinizing, occur over the course of about 2 years. The degree of physical change and the specific timeline of effects are highly variable and depend on the dose, route of administration, medications used, and patient's medical profile.

In adolescents who are at Tanner stage 2, the use of gonadotropin-releasing hormone (GnRH) agonists to suppress puberty may be appropriate. GnRH agonists allow a constant level of stimulation to the GnRH receptor. This in turn inhibits the pulsatile secretion of luteinizing hormone and follicle-stimulating hormone from the anterior pituitary, halting the progression of puberty. The progression is slow, allowing the patient time to adjust to the change, and is also reversible. Box 42.4 describes monitoring during suppression of puberty.

The use of cross-sex hormones for eligible adolescent patients beginning at or after age 16 years or Tanner stage 3 or 4 can also be used. By preventing secondary sex characteristics, patients require fewer physical interventions to make the transition if they choose to do so later.

Other Substances

Some transgender women use silicone or other soft-tissue fillers to enhance the breast contour ("silicone injections"). Medically appropriate use of soft-tissue fillers involves multiple small-volume injections by a trained practitioner. However, the cosmetic use of silicone injections is not supported in the United States, and typically the injections in transgender women are performed by an unlicensed provider. The actual composition of the filler substance is often unknown and may not be of medical grade. Additionally, the volume of the injection may exceed that used by a licensed medical provider. Silicone injections can cause breast deformity and pain and lead to serious side effects.

Other Providers

Be aware that some patients may use medically unsupervised hormonal therapy. A health care network of providers that includes primary care, and as appropriate, endocrinology, mental health, and surgery, can best provide comprehensive care.

Box 42.3	**Gender-Affirming Hormone Therapies**

FEMINIZING THERAPIES: ESTROGEN, SPIRONOLACTONE, PROGESTERONE EFFECTS

Irreversible
- Breast tissue growth
- Decreased testicular volume
- Infertility

Reversible
- Redistribution of body fat
- Decreased muscle mass
- Softening of skin
- Decreased libido
- Decreased spontaneous erections
- Decreased terminal hair growth

Possible Risks
- Venous thromboembolic diseases
- Gallstones
- Elevated liver enzymes
- Weight gain
- Hypertriglyceridemia
- Cardiovascular disease
- Hypertension
- Hyperprolactinemia or prolactinoma
- Type 2 diabetes

MASCULINIZING THERAPIES: TESTOSTERONE EFFECTS

Irreversible
- Facial hair growth
- Voice deepening
- Clitoral enlargement
- Balding

Reversible
- Increased muscle mass
- Fat redistribution
- Acne and oily skin
- Increased libido
- Decreased fertility (but does not eliminate the possibility of pregnancy)

Possible Risks
- Polycythemia
- Weight gain
- Acne
- Androgenic alopecia (balding)
- Sleep apnea
- Elevated liver enzymes
- Hyperlipidemia
- Destabilization of certain psychiatric disorders
- Cardiovascular disease
- Hypertension
- Type 2 diabetes

Box 42.4	**Follow-up Protocol During Puberty Suppression Therapy**

EVERY 3 MONTHS
- Anthropometry: height, weight, sitting height, Tanner stage
- Laboratory: luteinizing hormone, follicle-stimulating hormone, estradiol/testosterone

EVERY YEAR
- Laboratory: renal and liver function, lipids, glucose, insulin, glycosylated hemoglobin
- Bone density using dual-energy x-ray absorptiometry
- Bone age on x-ray of the left hand

What are the social history questions that I need to ask?

Key Questions

- Is your gender identity creating challenges, concerns, or difficulties for your relationships (e.g., family, friends, work)?

- Do you have concerns related to employment?
- Do you have adequate resources for your daily needs?
- Have you experienced any discrimination, bodily harm, or threats of bodily harm?
- Do you think about suicide or harming yourself?
- Do you smoke? How much?
- Do you drink alcohol or use other substances? How much?

The psychosocial history should include the patient's family, economic status, and larger social environments that may be stressful or supportive. Transgender patients experience higher rates of unemployment, employment discrimination, and income disparities. The incidence of physical and sexual abuse from intimate partners is high. The use of alcohol, drugs, and tobacco products is higher in this population compared with the national average. A substantial number of transgender patients report using drugs and alcohol specifically to cope with discrimination and mistreatment (Grant et al, 2011). Risk factors for severe psychological stress include physical violence or sexual assault. Having a supportive family mitigates some of the negative experiences related to economic stability and health (James et al, 2016).

> *What other history questions might be relevant?*

Key Questions

- Do you use any nonsurgical or nonhormonal methods to affirm your gender identity (binding, packing, tucking, voice modulation)?
- What cancer screenings have you had?

Gender-Affirming Practices

Some gender-affirming practices create special health concerns for transgender patients. These practices may or may not be relevant to the presenting health concern and should be asked only if relevant.

Binding: used by some transgender men, the practice involves the use of tight-fitting sports bras, shirts, ace bandages, or a specially made binder to flatten the breasts and provide a flat chest contour. Prolonged binding may result in breast pain, local skin breakdown, or fungal infection.

Packing: used by some transgender men, the patient places a penile prosthesis in the underwear, creating an outward appearance of the presence of a penis.

Tucking: used by some transgender women, the practice creates a visibly smooth crotch contour. The patient tucks the testicles (if present) into the inguinal canal and positions the penis and scrotum posteriorly in the perineal region. Tight-fitting underwear or a special undergarment known as a *gaffe* may be worn to maintain this alignment. Sometimes patients use adhesive or duct tape. This practice can result in urinary retention, hernias, or skin breakdown.

Voice modulation: used by some transgender persons to alter pitch, resonance, intonation, and intensity as a means to make the voice congruent with the identified gender. Patients may experience vocal fatigue. Specialty trained speech language pathologists are best equipped to facilitate overall vocal health and efficiency.

Cancer Screening

Transgender patients are less likely to have undergone routine cancer screening. There are no established guidelines for transgender patients. Routine screening should continue based on the patient's assigned sex at birth and the organs present. Therefore, for example, a transgender man with an intact uterus still needs cervical cancer screening and mammograms, and clinical breast examination should be done on patients with breasts. Prostate cancer screening should be considered in transgender patients with a prostate using the same guidelines as for nontransgender men. Box 42.5 summarizes cancer screening recommendations for transgender patients.

Box 42.5	**Cancer Screening Recommendations for Transgender Patients**

TRANSGENDER WOMEN
- Prostate cancer screening if prostate intact
  - Prostate-specific antigen not reliable if testosterone levels are low
  - Digital rectal examination
- Breast cancer screening:
  - Mammograms after age 50 yr if on estrogen for more than 5 yr
  - Clinical breast examination
- Colon cancer screening: the same age-appropriate screening recommendations and schedule as nontransgender patients

TRANSGENDER MEN
- Breast cancer screening
  - Mammogram: Follow guidelines until after breast surgery.
  - Clinical breast examination: Follow guidelines until after breast surgery.
- Cervical cancer screening (Pap smear and human papillomavirus testing)
  - Follow guidelines if the cervix is intact.
  - Clarify specimen is cervical.
  - Alert the pathologist to the use of testosterone.
  - No screening after hysterectomy unless there is a history of high-grade cervical lesions
- Colon cancer screening: the same age-appropriate screening recommendations and schedule as nontransgender patients

DIAGNOSTIC REASONING: FOCUSED PHYSICAL EXAMINATION

The physical examination should be relevant to the anatomy that is present in the patient regardless of gender identity or expression and should be specific to the presenting health concern. For example, examination of the genitalia is not appropriate for a visit for headache or cough. A prostate examination in a transgender woman and pelvic examination in a transgender man would be appropriate for a relevant presenting symptom or for cancer screening.

The physical examination should also be performed without assumptions as to anatomy or gender identity. Maintaining an organ inventory will help guide the appropriate examination. It is important to respect the patient's wishes regarding potentially sensitive examinations such as pelvic examination. It may take more than a single encounter to establish a relationship that will support the performance of such examinations.

Secondary Sex Characteristics and Physical Changes

Patients using hormone therapy may present with secondary sex characteristics that fall along a continuum of development. The degree of secondary sex characteristics are somewhat dependent on the age hormones were started, the duration of the therapy, or if the patient went through puberty suppression therapy as an adolescent. Transgender men may have facial and body hair, clitoromegaly, increased muscle mass, masculine fat redistribution, androgenic alopecia, and acne. Transgender women may have some breast development and feminine fat redistribution. The breast tissue that develops as a result of hormone therapy should not be referred to as gynecomastia. Transgender women who have had silicone injections may have disfigured breasts or hard, lumpy masses. Transgender women who have used hormone therapy may have reduced muscle mass; thinned or absent body hair; thinned or absent facial hair; softened, thinner skin; and testicles that have decreased in size or have completely retracted (see Box 42.3).

Electrolysis is commonly used by transgender women.

Patients who have undergone gender-affirming surgeries may have varying physical examination findings depending on what procedures were performed, the surgical approaches used, and sequelae from complications.

Pelvic Examination with Transgender Patients

Pelvic examination in transgender women who have had vaginoplasty—the creation of a neovagina—may be appropriate to screen for lesions, granulation tissue, stenosis, or to test for sexually transmitted infections (STIs). The differences between a natal vagina and a neovagina alter both the examination and the findings. The neovagina ends in a blind cuff, does not have a cervix or fornices, and may have a more posterior orientation. The neovagina does not self-lubricate and requires the use of a lubricant.

Pelvic examination in transgender men who have an intact vagina and cervix may be appropriate for cancer screening or to test for STIs. Transgender men are less likely to be up to date on cervical cancer screenings. When sending a specimen for Pap smear, it is essential to make clear to the laboratory that the specimen is cervical, especially if the listed gender is "male." Otherwise, the specimen may be discarded or incorrectly run as an anal Pap. The use of testosterone or presence of amenorrhea should be indicated.

Pelvic examination in a transgender patient requires special consideration and care because the examination may be anxiety producing and perceived as traumatic. Many transgender patients have experienced violence, including sexual violence, and providing patients with information, choices, decision-making ability, and a sense of control is important. In testing for STIs, some transgender patients may prefer to collect their own specimens. If a patient refuses a speculum examination, consider offering an external or bimanual examination as a beginning step. A positive experience can establish trust and comfort and may facilitate further examination in the future.

Prostate Examination in Transgender Women

In transgender women with a prostate, prostate examination may be appropriate for cancer screening or for evaluation of prostate specific symptoms or concerns (see Chapter 18). Both rectal and neovaginal approaches may be considered. In transgender women who have undergone vaginoplasty, the prostate is anterior to the vaginal wall, and a digital neovaginal examination may be more effective.

LABORATORY AND DIAGNOSTIC STUDIES

Laboratory testing and diagnostic studies will be determined by the specific presenting concerns and as indicated for hormone therapy monitoring. See the guidelines and standards for care. Box 42.4 summarizes monitoring during puberty suppression therapy.

SPECIAL HEALTH CONCERNS

Breast Pain in Transgender Men

Prolonged breast binding may result in breast pain, local skin breakdown, bruising, or fungal infection. Patients may be reluctant to remove the binder for physical examination. In some patients with larger breasts, multiple garments may be used, and breathing may be restricted. Binding can also cause back pain. The workup for breast pain for transgender women is the same as that for nontransgender patients (see Chapter 7).

Pelvic Pain in Transgender Men

The workup of pelvic pain in transgender men will be the same as that for nontransgender patients (see Chapters 35 and 36). The use of testosterone creates a hypoestrogenic state that that promotes tissue atrophy, increases vaginal pH, and increases the risk of vaginitis and cervicitis. As with cisgender women, the atrophic tissue is susceptible to traumatic irritation from sexual contact and can result in in dyspareunia or vaginitis.

Transgender men may have decreased access to or use of screening for and treatment of STIs. Genital or pelvic surgery may cause adhesions, scarring, bladder dysfunction, or nerve injury, which cause or contribute to pain.

Vaginal Bleeding in Transgender Men

For transgender men using testosterone, cessation of menses is expected, typically within 6 months of initiation of therapy. Cessation of menses driven by endometrial atrophy and testosterone-induced ovulation suppression may be incomplete. The time to cessation of menses may vary depending on dose and frequency of testosterone, presence and functioning of ovaries, and body habitus.

Patients with intact organs not taking testosterone will continue to have menses, and the workup for abnormal bleeding will be the same as that for nontransgender patients (see Chapter 36). The workup includes ruling out pregnancy in transgender men who have sex with partners who produce sperm.

Breast Pain in Transgender Women

Early potential adverse effects from soft-tissue fillers include localized skin papules and inflammatory nodules that may be infected. Noninflammatory nodules may also develop. Causing pain, itching, and abnormal pigmentation.

Potential long-term adverse effects include migration of silicone with associated pain or deformity. Silicone granulomas may develop, which can produce pain, swelling, ulcerations, and lymphadenopathy.

Scrotal Pain in Transgender Women

A common cause of scrotal contents pain in transgender women is the practice of "tucking," described previously. Many transgender women find this practice to be gender affirming and may maintain positioning throughout the night while asleep. The scrotal pain may be of traumatic, mechanical, or neuropathic origin. Prolonged tucking may also result in urinary reflux and symptoms of epididymitis, orchitis, prostatitis, or cystitis. Prolonged positioning of the urethral meatus near the anus may serve as a portal of infection.

Acute scrotal contents pain requires a workup to rule out conditions requiring emergency treatment (see Chapter 18).

Voice Issues and Vocal Health

Lowering of voice pitch may occur as a desired effect of hormone therapy in transgender men. Transgender women may use strategies to increase the tension in the vocal folds to elevate pitch. This requires continuous muscular effort, and patients may report a sensation of vocal effort or fatigue. Vocal cord surgeries have been designed to elevate pitch by altering vocal fold tension, mass, or both. Voice surgery undertaken by transgender persons to alter the pitch of their voice can injure the delicate tissue of the vocal folds and negatively alter normal vocal quality.

Patients may have voice-related issues not related to transition (see Chapter 21).

GUIDELINES AND STANDARDS FOR CARE

The following sources provide guidelines and standards for care of transgender patients.

- Deutsch M (ed): Guidelines for the Primary and Gender-Affirming Care of Transgender and Gender Nonbinary People (ed 2). Center of Excellence for Transgender Health (CoE) at the University of California, Davis – San Francisco, 2016 http://transhealth.ucsf.edu/trans?page= guidelines-home

- Eckstrand K, Ehrenfeld JM: (eds) Lesbian, Gay, Bisexual, and Transgender Healthcare: A Clinical Guide to Preventive, Primary, and Specialist Care 1st ed. Springer: Switzerland, 2016.
- GLMA (Gay and Lesbian Medical Association): Guidelines for Care of Lesbian, Gay, Bisexual and Transgender Patients, 2006 http://glma.org/_data/n_0001/resources/ live/GLMA%20guidelines%202006% 20FINAL.pdf
- Hembree WC, Cohen-Kettenis P, Delemarre-van de Waal HA, Gooren LJ, Meyer, WJ III, Spack NP, Tangpricha V, Montori VM: Endocrine Treatment of Transsexual Persons: An Endocrine Society Clinical Practice Guideline. *The Journal of Clinical Endocrinology & Metabolism,* Volume 94, Issue 9, 1 September 2009, Pages 3132–3154, https:// doi.org/10.1210/jc.2009-0345.
- Makadon HJ, Mayer KH, Potter J, Goldhammer H, (eds): Fenway Guide to Lesbian, Gay, Bisexual, and Transgender Health, ed 2, American College of Physicians: Philadelphia; 2015
- WPATH (World Professional Association for Transgender Health) http://www.wpath.org/ site_home.cfm Standards of care: http://www. wpath.org/site_page.cfm?pk_association_ webpage_menu=1351

> **DIFFERENTIAL DIAGNOSIS** *Special Concerns in Transgender Patients*

TRANSGENDER MEN (FEMALE TO MALE)			
CONDITION	HISTORY	PHYSICAL FINDINGS	DIAGNOSTIC STUDIES
Breast pain	Use of binding Also see Chapter 7	Prolonged binding may result local skin breakdown, or fungal infection	See Chapter 7
Pelvic pain	Possible use of testosterone Genital or pelvic surgery Untreated sexually transmitted infection Also see Chapter 36	Atrophic vaginal tissue if taking testosterone Also see Chapter 36	See Chapter 36
Vaginal bleeding	Use of testosterone with incomplete cessation of menses Also see Chapters 35 and 36	Atrophic vaginal tissue if taking testosterone Also see Chapters 35 and 36	See Chapters 35 and 36
Vocal issues	Possible use of testosterone Vocal cord surgery Also see Chapter 21		

> **DIFFERENTIAL DIAGNOSIS** *Special Concerns in Transgender Patients—cont'd*

TRANSGENDER WOMEN (MALE TO FEMALE)

CONDITION	HISTORY	PHYSICAL FINDINGS	DIAGNOSTIC STUDIES
Breast pain	Use of silicone injections or other soft tissue fillers See also Chapter 7	Possible skin papules, inflammatory nodules; or noninflammatory nodules; migration of silicone; silicone granulomas and possible swelling, ulcerations, and lymphadenopathy	Breast ultrasonography See Chapter 7
Scrotal pain	Use of tucking Also see Chapter 18	Some patients use tight-fitting underwear, or a *gaffe* Some patients use adhesive or duct tape Possible hernias of skin breakdown Also see Chapter 18	See Chapter 18
Vocal issues	Possible use of vocal fold tension Vocal cord surgery Also see Chapter 21	See Chapter 21	See Chapter 21

References

Abbott AV. Diagnostic approach to palpitations. *Am Fam Physician.* 2005;71:743.

Aberle DR, Adams AM, National Lung Screening Trial Research Team, et al. Reduced lung-cancer mortality with low-dose computed tomographic screening. *N Engl J Med.* 2011;365:395.

Abrams P, Andersson KE, Birder L, et al. Fourth international consultation on incontinence recommendations of the international scientific committee: evaluation and treatment of urinary incontinence, pelvic organ prolapse, and fecal incontinence. *Neurourol Urodyn.* 2010;29:213.

Abrams P, Chapple C, Khoury S, Roehrborn C, de la Rosette J. Evaluation and treatment of lower urinary tract symptoms in older men. *J Urol.* 2013; 189(1):S93-S101.

Adam A, Dixon A, (eds.). *Grainger & Allison's Diagnostic Radiology.* 5th ed. Philadelphia: Churchill Livingstone, Elsevier; 2014.

Adam HM. Fever: measuring and managing. *Pediatr Rev.* 2013;34:368.

AGA Institute on "Management of Acute Pancreatitis" Clinical Practice and Economics Committee, AGA Institute Governing Board. AGA Institute medical position statement on acute pancreatitis. *Gastroenterology.* 2007;132:2019.

Aguilera ZP, Chen PL. Eye pain in children. *Pediatr Rev.* 2016;37.

Aiyer A, Hennrikus W. Foot pain in the child and adolescent. *Pediatr Clin North Am.* 2014;61:1185.

Akdemir B, Yarmohammadi H, Alraies MC, Adkisson WO. Premature ventricular contractions: reassure or refer? *Cleve Clin J Med.* 2016;83(7):524-530.

Alamiri J, Lowery AJ, Rajendran S, Hill AD. Breast clinic referrals – should mastalgia be managed in primary care? *BMC Proc.* 2013;7(suppl 1):SO7.

Albers JR, Hull SK, Wesley RM. Abnormal uterine bleeding. *Am Fam Physician.* 2004;69:1915.

Alegria CA. Transgender identity and health care: implications for psychosocial and physical evaluation. *J Am Acad Nurse Pract.* 2011;23(4):175-182.

Aletaha D, Neogi T, Silman AJ, et al. 2010 Rheumatoid arthritis classification criteria: An American College of Rheumatology/European League Against Rheumatism collaborative initiative. *Arthritis Rheum.* 2010;62:2569.

Alizadeh F, Zargham M, Nouri-Mahdavi K, Khorrami MH, Izadpanahi MH, Sichani MM. Bladder involvement in thyroid dysfunction. *J Res Med Sci.* 2013;18:167.

Alper BS, Curry SH. Urinary tract infection in children. *Am Fam Physician.* 2005;72:2483.

Altaf F, Heran MK, Wilson LF. Back pain in children and adolescents. *Bone Joint J.* 2014;96:717.

Alvarado A. A practical score for the early diagnosis of acute appendicitis. *Ann Emerg Med.* 1986;15: 557-564.

American Academy of Pediatrics Committee on Practice and Ambulatory Medicine and Section on Ophthalmology. *Procedures for the Evaluation of the Visual System by Pediatricians.* 2016. Available at: http://pediatrics.aappublications.org/content/137/1/e20153597.full. Accessed September 19, 2018.

American Academy of Pediatrics. 2017 Recommendations for preventive pediatric health care. *Pediatrics.* 2017;139(4):e20170254.

American Academy of Pediatrics. Fruit juice in infants, children and adolescents: current recommendations. *Pediatrics.* 2017;140:967.

American College of Cardiology Foundation, American Heart Association, Inc., Heart Rhythm Society. Guideline for the evaluation and management of patients with syncope: executive summary. *Heart Rhythm.* 2017;14:e218.

American Diabetes Association (ADA). Standards of medical care in diabetes 2017 abridged for primary care providers. *Clin Diabetes.* 2017;35:5.

American Gastroenterological Association, Spechler SJ, Sharma P, Souza RF, Inadomi JM, Shaheen NJ. American Gastroenterological Association Medical Position Statement on the Management of Barrett's Esophagus. *Gastroenterology.* 2011;140(3): 1084-1091.

American Gastroenterological Association. American Gastroenterological Association Medical Position Statement: guidelines on constipation. *Gastroenterology.* 2013;144:211.

American Geriatrics Society 2015 Beers Criteria Update Expert Panel. American Geriatrics Society 2015 updated Beers criteria for potentially inappropriate medication use in older adults. *J Am Geriatr Soc.* 2015;63:2227-2246.

American Psychiatric Association. *Diagnostic and Statistical Manual of Mental Disorders.* 5th ed. Arlington, VA: American Psychiatric Association: 2013.

American Urological Association. *American Urological Association Guideline: Management of Benign Prostatic Hyperplasia (BPH).* 2010, validated and confirmed 2014. Available at: http://www.auanet.org/guidelines/benign-prostatic-hyperplasia-(2010-reviewed-and-validity-confirmed-2014). Accessed October 6, 2017.

American Urological Association. *Diagnosis, Evaluation and Follow-up of Asymptomatic Microhematuria (AMH) in Adults: AUA guideline.* 2012, validated and confirmed 2016. Available at: http://www.auanet.org/guidelines/asymptomatic-microhematuria-(2012-reviewed-and-validity-confirmed-2016). Accessed October 9, 2017.

American Urological Association. *Early Detection of Prostate Cancer: AUA guideline.* 2013, validated and confirmed 2015. Available at http://www.auanet.org/guidelines/early-detection-of-prostate-cancer-(2013-reviewed-and-validity-confirmed-2015). Accessed October 9, 2017.

Amir B, Farrell SA, Sub-Committee on Urogynaecology. SOGC Committee opinion on urodynamics testing. *J Obstet Gynaecol Can.* 2008;30:717.

Amsel R, Totten PA, Spiegel CA, Chen KC, Eschenbach D, Holmes KK. Nonspecific vaginitis: diagnostic criteria and microbial and epidemiologic associations. *Am J Med.* 1983;74:14.

Andermann A, Blancquaert I, Beauchamp S, Déry V. Revisiting Wilson and Jungner in the genomic age: a review of screening criteria over the past 40 years. *Bull World Health Organ.* 2008; 86(4):317-319. Available at: www.who.int/bulletin/volumes/86/4/07-050112/en/.

Andersen JC. Is immediate imaging important in managing low back pain? *J Athl Train.* 2011;46:99.

Anderson MR, Klink K, Cohrssen A. Evaluation of vaginal complaints. *JAMA.* 2004;291:1368.

Andriole GL, Crawford ED, Grubb RL, et al. Mortality results from a randomized prostate-cancer screening trial. *N Engl J Med.* 2009;360:1310.

Antoon JW, Knudson-Johnson M, Lister WM. Diagnostic approach to fever of unknown origin. *Clin Pediatr (Phila).* 2012;51:1091.

Antoon JW, Potisek NM, Lohr JA. Pediatric fever of unknown origin. *Pediatr Rev.* 2015;36:380.

Argenziano G, Puig S, Zalaudek I, et al. Dermoscopy improves accuracy of primary care physicians to triage lesions suggestive of skin cancer. *J Clin Oncol.* 2006;24:1877.

Arnold JJ, Hehn LE, Klein DA. Common questions about recurrent urinary tract infections in women. *Am Fam Physician.* 2016;93:560.

Asplund C, Barkdull T, Weiss BD. Genitourinary problems in bicyclists. *Curr Sports Med Rep.* 2007; 6:333.

Austin J, Marks D. Hormonal regulators of appetite. *Int J Pediatr Endocrinol.* 2009;2009:141753.

Aziz Q, Fass R, Gyawali P, Miwa H, Pandolfino JE, Zerbib F. Section II: FGIDs: diagnostic groups: esophageal disorders. *Gastroenterology.* 2016;150(6): 1368-1379.

Babcock DA. Evaluating sleep and sleep disorders in the pediatric primary care setting. *Pediatr Clin North Am.* 2011;58:543.

Bagheri N, Mehta S. Acute Vision Loss. *Prim Care.* 2015;42:347.

Baird DC, Seehusen DA, Bode DV. Enuresis in children: a case based approach. *Am Fam Physician.* 2014;90:560.

Baird G, Charman T, Cox A, et al. Current topic: Screening and surveillance for autism and pervasive and developmental disorders. *Arch Dis Child.* 2001;84:468-475.

Baker ME, Nelson RC, Rosen MP, et al. *ACR Appropriateness Criteria® Acute Pancreatitis.* Reston, VA: American College of Radiology; 2013. Available at: https://guideline.gov/summaries/summary/47649/acr-appropriateness-criteria–acute-pancreatitis. Accessed August 2, 2017.

Bal SK, Hollingworth GR. Red eye. *BMJ.* 2005; 331:438.

Balagué F, Mannion AF, Pellisé F, Cedraschi C. Nonspecific low back pain. *Lancet.* 2012;379:482.

Ballesio L, Maggi C, Savelli S, et al. Role of breast magnetic resonance imaging (MRI) in patients with unilateral nipple discharge: preliminary study. *Radiol Med.* 2008;113:249.

Banfield G, Tandon P, Solomons N. Hoarse voice: an early symptom of many conditions. *Practitioner.* 2000;244:267.

Barash JH, Buchanan EM, Hillson C. Diagnosis and management of ectopic pregnancy. *Am Fam Physician.* 2014;90:34.

Barnhart DC. Gastroesophageal reflux disease in children. *Semin Pediatr Surg.* 2016;25:212.

Baron EJ, Miller JM, Weinstein MP, et al. A guide to utilization of the microbiology laboratory for diagnosis of infectious diseases: 2013 recommendations by the Infectious Diseases Society of America (IDSA) and the American Society for Microbiology (ASM). *Clin Infect Dis.* 2013;57:e22.

Barr W, Smith A. Acute diarrhea. *Am Fam Physician.* 2014;89(3):180-189.

Barry MJ, Fowler Jr FJ, O'Leary MP, et al. The American Urological Association symptom index for benign prostatic hyperplasia: the Measurement Committee of the American Urological Association. *J Urol.* 1992;148:1549.

Barton MB, Harris R, Fletcher SW. The rational clinical examination. Does this patient have breast cancer? The screening clinical breast examination: Should it be done? How? *JAMA*. 1999;282:1270.

Basson MD. *Constipation*. 2013. Available at: http://emedicine.medscape.com/article/184704-overview. Accessed November 4, 2017.

Bastian LA, Smith CM, Nanda K. Is this woman perimenopausal? *JAMA*. 2003;289:895.902.

Batra AS, Hohn AR. Consultation with the Specialist: palpitations, syncope and sudden cardiac death in children: who's at risk? *Pediatr Rev.* 2003;24:269.

Baumann LJ, Leventhal H. I can tell when my blood pressure is up, can't I? *Health Psychol.* 1985;4:203.

Bayard M, Avonda T, Wadzinski J. Restless legs syndrome. *Am Fam Physician.* 2008;78:235.

Bayne AP, Skoog SJ. Nocturnal enuresis: an approach to assessment and treatment. *Pediatr Rev.* 2014;35:327.

Beal C, Giordano B. Clinical evaluation of red eyes in pediatric patients. *J Pediatr Health Care.* 2016;30:506.

Bell AL, Rodes ME, Collier Kellar L. Childhood eye examination. *Am Fam Physician.* 2013;88:241.

Benich JJ, Carek PJ. Evaluation of the patient with chronic cough. *Am Fam Physician.* 2011;84:887.

Benjamins LJ. Practice guideline: evaluation and management of abnormal vaginal bleeding in adolescents. *J Pediatr Health Care.* 2009;23:189.

Benner P, Hughes RG, Sutphen M. Clinical reasoning, decision-making, and action: thinking critically and clinically. In: Hughes RG, ed. *Patient Safety and Quality: An Evidence-Based Handbook for Nurses.* Rockville, MD: Agency for Healthcare Research and Quality, U.S. Dept. of Health and Human Services; 2008.

Bennett AR, Gray SH. What to do when she's bleeding through: the recognition, evaluation and management of abnormal uterine bleeding in adolescents. *Curr Opin Pediatr.* 2014;26:413.

Benseler JS. *The Radiology Handbook: A Pocket Guide to Medical Imaging.* Ohio University Press. 2014.

Bent S, Nallamothu BK, Simel DL, Fihn SD, Saint S. Does this woman have an acute uncomplicated urinary tract infection? *JAMA.* 2002;287:2701.

Benun J. Balance and vertigo in children. *Pediatr Rev.* 2011;32:84.

Berliner D, Schneider N, Welte T, Bauersachs J. The differential diagnosis of dyspnea. *Dtsch Arztebl Int.* 2016;113:834-845.

Bhagavatula M, Powell C. Common superficial skin infections. *Paediatr Child Health.* 2011;21(3):132-136.

Bhargava S. Diagnosis and management of common sleep problems in children. *Pediatr Rev.* 2011;32:91.

Bickle I, Kelly B. Abdominal x-rays made easy: normal radiographs. *Student BMJ.* 2002;10:103.

Bielak KS, Harris S. *Amenorrhea, e-Medicine.* 2010. Available at: http://emedicinemedscape.com/article/953850-overview. Accessed November 4, 2017.

Biondi E. Cardiac arrhythmias in children. *Peds Rev.* 2010;31:9.

Blackmer AB, Farrington EA. Constipation in the pediatric patient: an overview and pharmacologic considerations. *J Pediatr Health Care.* 2010;24(6):385-399.

Blagaa TS, Dumitrascuc D, Galmiche JP, et al. Functional heartburn: clinical characteristics and outcome. *Eur J Gastroenterol Hepatol.* 2013;25:282.

Blume HK. Pediatric headache a review. *Pediatr Rev.* 2012;33:562.

Bochner RE, Gangar M, Belamarich PF. A clinical approach to tonsillitis, tonsillar hypertrophy, and peritonsillar and retropharyngeal abscesses. *Pediatr Rev.* 2017;38:81.

Bonomi M, Rochira V, Pasquali D, et al., Klinefelter Italian Group. Klinefelter syndrome (KS): genetics, clinical phenotype and hypogonadism. *J Endocrinol Invest.* 2017;40(2):123-134.

Bonow RO, Mann DL, Zipes DP, Libby P. *Braunwald's Heart Disease: A Textbook of Cardiovascular Medicine.* 9th ed. St. Louis: Elsevier; 2011.

Borson S, Scanlan JM, Chen P, Ganguli M. The Mini-Cog as a screen for dementia: validation in a population-based sample. *J Am Geriatr Soc.* 2003;51:1451-1454.

Bösner S, Haasenritter J, Becker A, et al. Heartburn or angina? Differentiating gastrointestinal disease in primary care patients presenting with chest pain: a cross sectional diagnostic study. *Int Arch Med.* 2009;2:40.

Boyle JT. Gastrointestinal bleeding in infants and children. *Pediatr Rev.* 2008;29:39.

Braithwaite RS. A piece of my mind. EBM's six dangerous words. *JAMA.* 2013;310:2149.

Brambilla DJ, McKinlay SM, Johannes CB. Defining the perimenopause for application in epidemiologic investigations. *Am J Epidemiol.* 1994;140:1091-1095.

Brand PL, Hoving MF, de Groot EP. Evaluating the child with recurrent lower respiratory tract infections. *Paediatr Respir Rev.* 2012;13(3):135.

Brandt LJ, Chey WD, Foxx-Orenstein AE, et al. An evidence-based position statement on the management of irritable bowel syndrome. *Am J Gastroenterol.* 2009;104:S1-35.

Braun MM, Overbeek-Wager EA, Grumbo RJ. Diagnosis and management of endometrial cancer. *Am Fam Physician.* 2016;93:468.

Brill J. Diagnosis and treatment of urethritis in men. *Am Fam Physician.* 2010;81:873.

Brodlie M, Graham C, McKean MC. Childhood cough. *BMJ*. 2012;344:e1177.

Brook I. Acute sinusitis in children. *Pediatr Clin North Am*. 2013;60:409.

Brown DL. Congenital bleeding disorders. *Curr Probl Pediatr Adolesc Health Care*. 2005;35:38.

Brown EL, Brown DF, Nadel ES. Pediatric abdominal pain. *J Emerg Med*. 2009;36(1):72-75.

Brown N, White J, Brasher A, Scurr J. The experience of breast pain (mastalgia) in female runners of the 2012 London Marathon and its effect on exercise behaviour. *Br J Sports Med*. 2014;48:320.

Browner EA. Corneal abrasions. *Pediatr Rev*. 2012; 33(6):285-286.

Buchanan MA, Muen W, Heinz P. Management of periorbital and orbital cellulitis. *Paediatr Child Health*. 2012;22:72.

Burbank KM, Stevenson JH, Czarnecki GR, Dorfman J. Chronic shoulder pain: part I. evaluation and diagnosis. *Am Fam Physician*. 2008;77:453.

Burd EM, Kehl KS. A critical appraisal of the role of the clinical microbiology laboratory in the diagnosis of urinary tract infections. *J Clin Microbiol*. 2011;49:S34.

Burns A, Iliffe S. Dementia. *BMJ*. 2009;338:b75.

Burrus M, Werner BC, Starman JS, et al. Chronic leg pain in athletes. *Am J Sports Med*. 2015;43:1538.

Buysse DJ. Insomnia. *JAMA*. 2013;309:706.

Canadian Cardiovascular Society, American Academy of Family Physicians, American College of Cardiology, American Heart Association, Antman EM, Hand M, Armstrong PW, et al. 2007 focused update of the ACC/AHA 2004 guidelines for the management of patients with ST-elevation myocardial infarction: A report of the American College of Cardiology/American Heart Association Task Force on Practice Guidelines. *J Am Coll Cardiol*. 2008;51: 210.

Canavan A, Arant Jr BS. Diagnosis and management of dehydration in children. *Am Fam Physician*. 2009;80:692.

Canning BJ. Afferent nerves regulating the cough reflex: Mechanisms and mediators of cough in disease. *Otolaryngol Clin North Am*. 2010; 43:15.

Cannon B, Wackel P. Syncope. *Pediatr Rev*. 2016;37: 159-167.

Carlat DJ. The psychiatric review of symptoms: a screening tool for family physicians. *Am Fam Physician*. 1998;58(7):1617.

Carroll CL, Sala KA. Pediatric status asthmaticus. *Crit Care Clin*. 2013;29(2):153-166.

Carson L, Lewis D, Tsou M, et al. Abdominal migraine: an under-diagnosed cause of recurrent abdominal pain in children. *Headache*. 2011;51(5): 707-712.

Carter JC, Wrede JE. Overview of sleep and sleep disorders in infancy and childhood. *Pediatr Ann*. 2017;46:e133.

Carter KA, Hathaway NE, Lettieri CF. Common sleep disorders in children. *Am Fam Physician*. 2014; 89:368.

Cartwright SL, Knudson MP. Diagnostic imaging of acute abdominal pain in adults. *Am Fam Physician*. 2015;91(7):452.

Cartwright SL, Knudson MP. Evaluation of acute abdominal pain in adults. *Am Fam Physician*. 2008;77:971.

Casablanca Y. Management of dysfunctional uterine bleeding. *Obstet Gynecol Clin North Am*. 2008; 35:219.

Casey R Gomex-Loba. Common pediatric vulvar complaints. *Contemp OB GYN*. 2014;59:40.

Casselbrant ML, Mandel EM. Balance disorders in children. *Neurol Clin*. 2005;23:807.

Cavanaugh Jr RM. Evaluating adolescents with fatigue: ever get tired of it? *Pediatr Rev*. 2002;23:337.

Centers for Disease Control and Prevention. *2015 Sexually Transmitted Diseases Treatment Guidelines*. 2015. Available at: https://www.cdc.gov/std/tg2015/default.htm. Accessed November 24, 2017.

Centers for Disease Control and Prevention. CDC Yellow Book 2018: Health Information for International Travel. New York: Oxford University Press; 2017. Available at: https://wwwnc.cdc.gov/travel/page/yellowbook-home. Accessed December 6, 2017.

Centers for Disease Control and Prevention. *Chronic Fatigue Syndrome*. 2017. Available at: http://www.cdc.gov/cfs/. Accessed September 6, 2018.

Centers for Disease Control and Prevention. *Diagnosing and Treating Foodborne Illness*, 2014. Available at: https://www.cdc.gov/foodsafety/foodborne-germs.html. Accessed October 3, 2017.

Centers for Disease Control and Prevention. *Lesbian, Gay, Bisexual, and Transgender Health*, May 2018. Available at: https://www.cdc.gov/lgbthealth/transgender.htm. Accessed December 12, 2017.

Centers for Disease Control and Prevention. Locally acquired dengue—Key West Florida, 2009-2010. *MMWR*. 2010;59:577.

Centers for Disease Control and Prevention. Seasonal influenza. 2018. Available at: http://www.cdc.gov/flu/index.htm. Accessed September 6, 2018.

Centor RM. When should patients seek care for sore throat? *Ann Intern Med*. 2013;159:636.

Chen HH, Meyers AD. *Chronic Cough, Medscape Drugs, Diseases and Procedures Reference*. 2016. Available at: http://emedicine.medscape.com/article/1048560-overview. Accessed September 6, 2018.

Chen X, Mao G, Leng SX. Frailty syndrome: an overview. *Clin Interv Aging*. 2014;9:433.

Chosidow O. Clinical practices. Scabies. *N Engl J Med*. 2006;354:1718.

Chou R, Qaseem A, Snow V, et al. Diagnosis and treatment of low back pain: a joint clinical practice guideline from the American College of Physicians and the American Pain Society. *Ann Intern Med*. 2007;147:478.

Chung KF, Widdicombe JG. Cough. In: Mason RJ, Broaddus VC, eds. *Murray and Nadel's Textbook of Respiratory Medicine*. 6th ed. St. Louis: Saunders; 2016.

Chusid MJ. Fever of unknown origin in childhood. *Pediatr Clin North Am*. 2017;64:205.

Cirilli AR, Cipot SJ. Emergency evaluation and management of vaginal bleeding in the nonpregnant patient. *Emerg Med Clin North Am*. 2012;30:991.

Clayton KM. Pediatric abdominal imaging. *Pediatr Rev*. 2010;31(12):506-510.

Clegg A, Young J, Lliffe S, Rikkert MO, Rockwood K. Frailty in elderly people. *The Lancet*. 2013;381:752-62.

Clement KD, Lapitan MCM, Omar MI, Glazener CMA. Urodynamic studies for management of urinary incontinence in children and adults. *Cochrane Database Syst Rev*. 2013;(10):CD003195.

Cohen SM, Dinan MA, Roy N, et al. Diagnosis change in voice-disordered patients evaluated by primary care and/or otolaryngology: a longitudinal study. *Otolaryngol Head Neck Surg*. 2014;150:95.

Coker TJ, Dierfeldt DM. Acute bacterial prostatitis: diagnosis and management. *Am Fam Physician*. 2016;93(2):114-120.

Coleman JS, Charlotte A. Gaydos CA, Witter F. Trichomonas vaginalis vaginitis in obstetrics and gynecology practice: new concepts and controversies. *Obstet Gynecol Surv*. 2013;68:43.

Colgan R, Williams M, Johnson JR. Diagnosis and treatment of acute pyelonephritis in women. *Am Fam Physician*. 2011;84:519.

Colombo JM, Wassom MC, Rosen JM. Constipation and encopresis in childhood. *Ped rev*. 2015;36:392.

Comkornruecha M. Gonococcal infections. *Pediatr Rev*. 2013;34:228.

Cordell CB, Borson S, Boustani M, et al. Alzheimer's Association recommendations for operationalizing the detection of cognitive impairment during the Medicare Annual Wellness Visit in a primary care setting. *Alzheimers Dement*. 2013;9:141.

Cordova J, Chugh A, Rivera Rivera ED, Young S. Recurrent pediatric perianal swelling. *Pediatr Ann*. 2016;45:e59-62.

Corrigan Jr JJ, Boineau FG. Hemolytic-uremic syndrome. *Pediatr Rev*. 2001;22:365.

Crawford P, Crop JA. Evaluation of scrotal masses. *Am Fam Physician*. 2014;89(9):723-727.

Crochet JR, Bastian LA, Chireau MV. Does this woman have an ectopic pregnancy?: the rational

clinical examination systematic review. *JAMA*. 2013;309:1722.

Cronau H, Kankanala RR, Mauger T. Diagnosis and management of red eye in primary care. *Am Fam Physician*. 2010;81:137.

Crosby NE, Greenberg JA. Ulnar-sided wrist pain in the athlete. *Clin Sports Med*. 2015;34:127.

Crownover BK, Bepko JL. Appropriate and safe use of diagnostic imaging. *Am Fam Physician*. 2013;87:494.

Cunill-De Sautu B, Gereije RS. Knee conditions. *Pediatr Rev*. 2014;35:359.

Darrow DH, Siemens C. Indications for tonsillectomy and adenoidectomy. *Laryngoscope*. 2002;112:6.

Davenport R. Headache. *Pract Neurol*. 2008;8:335.

Davidson BR, Dipiero CM, Govoni KD, Littleton SS, Neal JL. Abnormal uterine bleeding during the reproductive years. *J Midwifery Womens Health*. 2012;57:248.

Davies D, Bailey J. Diagnosis and management of anorectal disorders in the primary care setting. *Prim Care*. 2017;44:709.

Davis DH, Creavin ST, Yip JL, Noel-Storr AH, Brayne C, Cullum S. Montreal cognitive assessment for the diagnosis of Alzheimer's disease and other dementias. *Cochrane Database Syst Rev*. 2015;(10): CD010775.

Davis KF, Parker KP, Montgomery GL. Sleep in infants and young children: part two. Common sleep problems. *J Pediatr Health Care*. 2004;18:130.

Davis R, Jones JS, Barocas DA, et al. American Urological Association. Diagnosis, evaluation and follow-up of asymptomatic micro-hematuria (AMH) in adults: AUA guideline. *J Urol*. 2012;188: 2473.

De La Cruz MS, Buchanan EM. Uterine fibroids: diagnosis and treatment. *Am Fam Physician*. 2017;95:100.

Deibel JP, Cowling K. Ocular inflammation and infection. *Emerg Med Clin North Am*. 2013;31:387.

Deligeoroglou E, Athanasopoulos N, Tsimaris P, Dimopoulos KD, Vrachnis N, Creatsas G. Evaluation and management of adolescent amenorrhea. *Ann NY Acad Sci*. 2010;1205:23-32.

Deligeoroglou E, Karountzos V, Creatsas G. Abnormal uterine bleeding and dysfunctional uterine bleeding in pediatric and adolescent gynecology. *Gynecol Endocrinol*. 2013;29:74.

Deligeoroglou E, Tsimaris P. Menstrual disturbances in puberty. *Best Pract Res Clin Obstet Gynaecol*. 2010;24:157.

Deng DY. Urinary incontinence in females. *Med Clin North Am*. 2011;95:101.

Dennehy PH. Acute diarrheal disease in children: epidemiology, prevention, and treatment. *Infect Dis Clin North Am*. 2005;19:585.

DeSantis D. Amblyopia. *Pediatr Clin North Am.* 2014;61:505.

Deshpande AV, Craig JC, Smith GH, Caldwell PH. Management of daytime urinary incontinence and lower urinary tract diagnosis in children. *J Pediatr Child Health.* 2012;48:E44.

Deutsch MB, ed. *Guidelines for the Primary and Gender-Affirming Care of Transgender and Gender Nonbinary People.* 2nd ed. *Center of Excellence for Transgender Health (CoE) at the University of California, Davis – San Francisco; 2016.* Available at: http://transhealth.ucsf.edu/trans?page=guidelines-home.

Deutsch MB, Green J, Keatley J, Mayer G, Hastings J, Hall AM. Electronic medical records and the transgender patient: recommendations from the World Professional Association for Transgender Health EMR Working Group. *J Am Med Inform Assoc.* 2013;20(4):700-703.

DeVon HA, Ryan CJ. Chest pain and associated symptoms of acute coronary syndromes. *J Cardiovasc Nurs.* 2005;20:232.

Deyo RA, Rainville J, Kent DL. What can the history and physical examination tell us about low back pain? *JAMA.* 1992;268:760.

Deyo RA, Weinstein JN. Low back pain. *N Engl J Med.* 2001;344:363.

Diaz-Parker C, Bratslavsky G. Male genitourinary disease: urethritis, epididymitis, and prostatitis. *Clin Rev.* 2005;15:40.

Dickson G. Gynecomastia. *Am Fam Physician.* 2012;85(7):716-722.

Dickson G. Gynecomastia. *Am Fam Physician.* 2012;85(7):716-722.

Dillon BE, Zimmern PE. When are urodynamics indicated in patients with stress urinary incontinence? *Curr Urol Rep.* 2012;13:379.

DiNenno EA, Prejean J, Irwin K, et al. Recommendations for HIV screening in gay, bisexual, and other men who have sex with men—United States 2017. *MMWR Morb Mortal Wkly Rep.* 2017;66;830.

Divo M, Pinto-Plata V. Role of exercise in testing and in therapy of COPD. *Med Clin North Am.* 2012;96:753-766.

Dobbie AM, White DR. Laryngomalacia. *Ped Clin of North Am.* 2013;60:893-902.

Dodick DW. Pearls: headache. *Semin Neurol.* 2010; 30:74.

Downing LJ, Caprio TV, Lyness JM. Geriatric psychiatry review: differential diagnosis and treatment of the 3 D's—delirium, dementia, and depression. *Curr Psychiatry Rep.* 2013;15:365.

Drossman DA, Hasler WL. Rome IV-functional GI disorders: disorders of gut-brain interaction. *Gastroenterology.* 2016;150(6):1257-1261.

Drossman DA. Functional gastrointestinal disorders: history, pathophysiology, clinical features, and Rome IV. *Gastroenterology.* 2016;150(6):1262-1279.

Dubois RW, Goodnough LT, Ershler WB, Van Winkle L, Nissenson AR. Identification, diagnosis, and management of anemia in adult ambulatory patients treated by primary care physicians: evidence-based and consensus recommendations. *Curr Med Res Opin.* 2006;22:385.

Duke University Medical Center Library & Archives. *Introduction to Evidence-Based Practice.* n.d. Available at: http://guides.mclibrary.duke.edu/ebm. Accessed September 6, 2018.

Dupre AA, Wightman JM. Red and painful eye. In: Walls RM, Hockberger RS, Gausche M, et al. (eds.). *Rosen's Emergency Medicine: Concepts and Clinical Practice.* 9th ed. St. Louis, MO: Elsevier Inc; 2018:169-183.e2 .

Ebell MH, Hansen JG. Proposed clinical decision rules to diagnose acute rhinosinusitis among adults in primary care. *Ann Fam Med.* 2017;15:347.

Ebell MH, Lundgren J, Youngpairoj S. How long does a cough last? Comparing patients' expectations with data from a systematic review of the literature. *Ann Fam Med.* 2013;11:5-13.

Ebell MH, Smith MA, Barry HC, Ives K, Carey M. The rational clinical examination: Does this patient have strep throat? *JAMA.* 2000;284:2912.

Eddy DM. Evidence-based medicine: a unified approach. *Health Aff.* 2005;24:9.

Edlow JA, Panagos PD, Godwin SA, Thomas TL, Decker WW, American College of Emergency Physicians. Clinical policy: critical issues in the evaluation and management of adult patients presenting to the emergency department with acute headache. *Ann Emerg Med.* 2008;52:407.

Ely JW, Kennedy CM, Clark EC, Bowdler NC. Abnormal uterine bleeding: a management algorithm. *J Am Board Fam Med.* 2006;19:590.

Ely JW, Seabury Stone M. The generalized rash: part II. Diagnostic approach. *Am Fam Physician.* 2010; 81:735.

Epstein LJ, Kristo D, Strollo Jr PJ, et al. Clinical guideline for the evaluation, management and long-term care of obstructive sleep apnea in adults. *J Clin Sleep Med.* 2009;5:263.

Eslick GD, Coulshed DS, Talley NJ. Diagnosis and treatment of noncardiac chest pain. *Nat Clin Pract Gastroenterol Hepatol.* 2005;2:10.

Etoom Y, Ratnapalan S. Evaluation of children with heart murmurs. *Clin Pediatr (Phila).* 2014;53:111.

Ewing JA. Screening for alcoholism using CAGE. Cut down, annoyed, guilty, eye opener. *JAMA.* 1984; 280:1904.

Expert Panel on Detection, Evaluation, and Treatment of High Blood Cholesterol in Adults. Executive summary of the third report of the National Cholesterol Education Program (NCEP): Expert Panel on detection, evaluation, and treatment of high blood cholesterol in adults (Adult Treatment Panel III). *JAMA.* 2001;285:2486.

Fagan HB. Approach to the patient with acute swollen/painful joint. *Clin Fam Pract.* 2005;7:305.

Fairhall N, Langron C, Sherrington C, et al. Treating frailty—a practical guide. *BMC Med.* 2011;9:83.

Fallat ME, Ignacio Jr RC. Breast disorders in children and adolescents. *J Pediatr Adolesc Gynecol.* 2008;21:311.

Falloon K, Arroll B, Elley CR, Fernando A. The assessment and management of insomnia in primary care. *BMJ.* 2011;342:d2899.

Fargo MV, Latimer KM. Evaluation and management of common anorectal conditions. *Am Fam Physician.* 2012;85:624.

Fasano A, Catassi C. Clinical practice. Celiac disease. *N Engl J Med.* 2012;367:2419.

Fashner J, Bell AL. Herpes zoster and postherpetic neuralgia: prevention and management. *Am Fam Physician.* 2011;83(12):1432-1437.

Fashner J, Gitu AC. Diagnosis and treatment of peptic ulcer disease and *H. pylori* infection. *Am Fam Physician.* 2015;91(4):236-242.

Fedullo PF, Tapson VF. Clinical practice. The evaluation of suspected pulmonary embolism. *N Engl J Med.* 2003;349:1247.

Feld LG, Mattoo TK. Urinary tract infections and vesicoureteral reflux in infants and children. *Pediatr Rev.* 2010;31:451.

Feldhaus KM, Koziol-McLain J, Amsbury HL, Norton IM, Lowenstein SR, Abbott JT. Accuracy of 3 brief screening questions for detecting partner violence in the emergency department. *JAMA.* 1997;277:1357.

Fenway Health in Boston, Fenway Health Transgender Program. Available at: http://fenwayhealth.org/care/medical/transgender-health/. Accessed December 2, 2017.

Fenway Institute. The National LGBT Health Education Center. https://www.lgbthealtheducation.org/. Accessed December 2, 2017.

Ferrara LR, Saccomano SJ. Constipation in Children: diagnosis, treatment and prevention. *Nurse Pract.* 2017;42:30.

Ferreira A, Young T, Mathews C, Zunza M, Low N. Strategies for partner notification for sexually transmitted infections, including HIV. *Cochrane Database Syst Rev.* 2013;(10):CD002843. Available at: http://www.cochrane.org/CD002843/STI_strategies-for-partner-notification-for-sexually-transmitted-infections-including-hiv. Accessed November 24, 2017.

Ferzoco RM, Ruddy KJ. The epidemiology of male breast cancer. *Curr Oncol Rep.* 2016;18(1):1.

Fetter M. Assessing vestibular function: which tests, when? *J Neurol.* 2000;247:335.

Flegal KM, Carroll MD, Ogden CL, Curtin LR. Prevalence and trends in obesity among US adults, 1999-2008. *JAMA.* 2010;303:235.

Fleming A, Cutrer W, Reimschisel T, Gigante J. You too can teach clinical reasoning! *Pediatrics.* 2012;130(5):795-797.

Forbes BA, Patel R, Rosenblatt JE, et al. A guide to utilization of the microbiology laboratory for diagnosis of infectious diseases: 2013 recommendations by the Infectious Diseases Society of America (IDSA) and the American Society for Microbiology (ASM)(a). *Clin Infect Dis.* 2013;57:e22.

Ford AC, Moayyedi P, Lacy BE, et al. American College of Gastroenterology monograph on the management of irritable bowel syndrome and chronic idiopathic constipation. *Am J Gastroenterol.* 2014;109(suppl 1):S2-S26.

Ford AC, Talley NJ, Veldhuyzen van Zanten SJ, Vakil NB, Simel DL, Moayyedi P. Will the history and physical examination help establish that irritable bowel syndrome is causing this patient's lower gastrointestinal tract symptoms? *JAMA.* 2008;300:1793-1805.

Fornari ED, Suszter M, Roocroft J, Bastrom T, Edmonds EW, Schlechter J. Childhood obesity as a risk factor for lateral condyle fractures over supracondyle humerus fractures. *Clin Orthop Relat Res.* 2013;417:1193.

Fox TG, Manaloor JJ, Christenson JC. Travel-related infections in children. *Pediatr Clin North Am.* 2013;60:507.

Foxx-Orenstein AE, Umar SB, Crowell MD. Common anorectal disorders. *Gastroenterol Hepatol (N Y).* 2014;10:294.

Fraser RS, Müller NL, Colman N, Pare PD. (eds.). *Fraser and Paré's Diagnosis of Diseases of the Chest.* 4th ed. vol. 1. Philadelphia: Saunders; 1999.

Frassetto L, Kohlstadt I. Treatment and prevention of kidney stones: an update. *Am Fam Physician.* 2011;84:1234.

Friedman B, English JC, Ferris LK. Indoor tanning, skin cancer and the young female patient: a review of the literature. *J Pediatr Adolesc Gynecol.* 2015;28:275.

Friedman K, Alexander M. Chest pain and syncope in children: a practical approach to the diagnosis of cardiac disease. *J Pediatr.* 2013;163:896.

Friedman KG, Alexander ME. Chest pain and syncope in children: A practical approach to the diagnosis of cardiac disease. *J Pediatr.* 2013;163:896.

Furness S, Roberts H, Marjoribanks J, Lethaby A. Hormone therapy in postmenopausal women and risk of endometrial hyperplasia. *Cochrane Database Syst Rev.* 2012;(8):CD000402.

Gaber KA, McGavin CR, Wells IP. Lateral chest x-ray for physicians. *J R Soc Med.* 2005;98:310.

Gaddey HL, Holder K. Unintentional weight loss in older adults. *Am Fam Physician.* 2014;89:718.

Garbez R, Puntillo K. Acute musculoskeletal pain in the emergency department: A review of the literature and implications for the advanced practice nurse. *AACN Clin Issues.* 2005;16:310.

Garbez R, Puntillo K. Acute musculoskeletal pain in the emergency department: A review of the literature and implications for the advanced practice nurse. *AACN Clin Issues.* 2005;16:310.

Gargiulo KA, Spector ND. Stuffy nose. *Pediatr Rev.* 2010;31:320.

Garrett CG, Ossoff RH. Hoarseness. *Med Clin North Am.* 1999;83:115.

Gauer RL. Evaluation of syncope. *Am Fam Physician.* 2011;84:640.

Gendo K, Larson EB. Evidence-based diagnostic strategies for evaluating suspected allergic rhinitis. *Ann Intern Med.* 2004;140:278.

George BD. Anal and perianal disorders. *Medicine.* 2011;39:84.

Gereige R, Cunill-De Sautu B. Throat infections. *Pediatr Rev.* 2011;32:459.

Gereige RS, Laufer PM. Pneumonia. *Pediatr Rev.* 2013;34(10):438-56.

Ghassemi KA, Jensen DM. Lower GI bleeding: epidemiology and management. *Curr Gastroenterol Rep.* 2013;15:333.

Giesen LG, Cousins G, Dimitrov BD, van de Laar FA, Fahey T. Predicting acute uncomplicated urinary tract infection in women: a systematic review of the diagnostic accuracy of symptoms and signs. *BMC Fam Pract.* 2010;11:78.

Gilani CJ, Yang A, Yonkers M, Boysen-Osborn, M. Differentiating urgent and emergent causes of acute red eye for the emergency physician. *West J Emerg Med.* 2017;18:509.

Giordano BD. Assessment and treatment of hip pain in the adolescent athlete. *Pediatr Clin North Am.* 2014;61:1137.

Gluckman SJ. Chronic fatigue syndrome. In: Kellerman RD, Bope ET, eds. *Conn's Current Therapy, 2018.* St. Louis, MO: Saunders, an imprint of Elsevier Inc; 2018:512-514.

Godbole P. Testicular problems in children. *Paediatr Child Health.* 2012;22:6.

Goolsby MJ. Evaluating acute musculoskeletal complaints. *J Am Acad Nurse Pract.* 2001;13:195.

Goroll AH, Mulley AG. *Primary Care Medicine.* 7th ed. Philadelphia: Lippincott Williams & Wilkins; 2014.

Goswami D, Conway GS. Premature ovarian failure. *Hum Reprod Update.* 2005;11:391.

Goyal A. Breast pain. *Am Fam Physician.* 2016; 93(10):872-873.

Gradison M. Pelvic inflammatory disease. *Am Fam Physician.* 2012;85:791.

Graham KM, Levy JB. Enuresis. *Pediatr Rev.* 2009; 30:165.

Granado-Villar D, Cunill-De Sautu B, Granados A. Acute gastroenteritis. *Pediatr Rev.* 2012;33: 487.

Grant JM, Mottet LA, Tanis J, Harrison J, Herman JL, Keisling M. *Injustice at Every Turn: A Report of the National Transgender Discrimination Survey.* Washington: National Center for Transgender Equality and National Gay and Lesbian Task Force; 2011.

Gray SH. Menstrual disorders. *Pediatr Rev.* 2013; 34(1):6-17.

Grundy SM, Cleeman JI, Merz CN, et al. Implications of recent clinical trials for the National Cholesterol Education Program Adult Treatment Panel III Guidelines. *Circulation.* 2004;110:227.

Guidozzi F. Sleep and sleep disorders in menopausal women. *Climacteric.* 2013;16:214.

Guluma K, Lee JE. Opthalmology. In: *Rosen's Emergency Medicine: Concepts & Clinical Practice.* 9th ed. St. Louis: Elsevier; 2017:790-819.

Gurnari M, Birken C, Hamilton J. Childhood obesity: causes, consequences and management. *Pediatr Clin North Am.* 2015;62:821.

Haamid F, Sass AE, Dietrich JE. Heavy menstrual bleeding in adolescent. *J Pediatr Adolesc Gynecol.* 2017;30:335.

Habif TP. *Clinical Dermatology.* 6th ed. St. Louis, MO: Mosby; 2016.

Haefner J. Primary care management of depression in children and adolescents. *Nurse Pract.* 2016; 41:38.

Hainer BL, Gibson MV. Vaginitis. *Am Fam Physician.* 2011;83:807.

Halpern JA, Shoag JE, Mittal S, et al. Prognostic significance of digital rectal examination and prostate specific antigen in the Prostate, Lung, Colorectal and Ovarian (PLCO) cancer screening arm. *J Urol.* 2017;197(2):363-368.

Hamilton JL, John SP. Evaluation of fever in infants and young children. *Am Fam Physician.* 2013; 87:254.

Hampson NB, Piantadosi CA, Thom SR, Weaver LK. Practice recommendations in the diagnosis, management, and prevention of carbon monoxide poisoning. *Am J Respir Crit Care Med.* 2012;186:1095.

Harmes KM, Blackwood RA, Burrows HL, et al. Otitis media: diagnosis and treatment. *Am Fam Physician.* 2013;88(7):435-440.

Hartman-Adams H, Banvard C, Juckett G. Impetigo: diagnosis and treatment. *Am Fam Physician.* 2014; 90(4):229.

Hartnick CJ, Cotton RT. Congenital laryngeal anomalies: laryngeal atresia, stenosis, webs, and clefts. *Otolaryngol Clin North Am.* 2000;33:1293.

Harvey PT. Common eye diseases of elderly people: identifying and treating causes of vision loss. *Gerontology*. 2003;49:1.

Hauer AJ, Luiten EL, van Erp NF, et al. No evidence for distinguishing bacterial from viral acute rhinosinusitis using fever and facial/dental pain: a systematic review of the evidence base. *Otolaryngol Head Neck Surg*. 2014;150:28.

Haus BM, Micheli LJ. Back pain in the pediatric and adolescent athlete. *Clin Sports Med*. 2012;31(3): 423.

Hawryluk EB, Liang MG. Pediatric melanoma, moles, and sun safety. *Pediatr Clin North Am*. 2014;61: 279.

Hazell P. Depression in children and adolescents. *Am Fam Phys*. 2012;86:1138.

Heffner V, Gorelick M. Pediatric urinary tract infection. *Clin Ped Emerg Med*. 2008;9:233.

Heidelbaugh JJ, Gill AS, Van Harrison R, Nostrant TT. Atypical presentations of gastroesophageal reflux disease. *Am Fam Physician*. 2008;78:483.

Heiman DL. Amenorrhea. *Prim Care*. 2009;36(1): 1-17.

Herman MJ, Martinek M. The limping child. *Pediatr Rev*. 2015;36:184.

Herring W. *Learning Radiology: Recognizing the Basics*. St. Louis: Mosby; 2015.

Hersey AD. Pediatric headache, continuum: lifelong learning. *Neurology*. 2015;21:1131.

Herzig DO, Lu KC. Anal fissure. *Surg Clin North Am*. 2010;90:33.

Hess EP, Thiruganasambandamoorthy V, Wells GA, et al. Diagnostic accuracy of clinical prediction rules to exclude acute coronary syndrome in the emergency department setting: a systematic review. *CJEM*. 2008;10:373-382.

High KP, Bradley SF, Gravenstein S, et al. Clinical practice guideline for the evaluation of fever and infection in older adult residents of long-term care facilities: 2008 update by the Infectious Diseases Society of America. *Clin Infect Dis*. 2009;48:149.

Hillard J. Menstruation in adolescents: what do we know? and what do we do with the information. *Journ of Ped and Adol Gyn*. 2014;27:309.

Hing W, White S, Reid D, Marshall R. Validity of the McMurray's test and modified version of the test: a systematic literature review. *J Man Manip Ther*. 2009;17:22.

Hoebeke P, Bower W, Combs A, De Jong T, Yang S. Diagnostic evaluation of children with daytime incontinence. *J Urol*. 2010;183:699.

Hoefman E, Boer KR, van Weert HC, Reitsma JB, Koster RW, Bindels PJ. Predictive value of history taking and physical examination in diagnosing arrhythmias in general practice. *Fam Pract*. 2007; 24:636.

Hoffman RM, Sanchez R. Lung cancer screening. *Med Clin North Am*. 2017;101:769.

Hollands H, Johnson D, Hollands S, Simel DL, Jinapriya D, Sharma S. Do findings on routine examination identify patients at risk for primary open-angle glaucoma? The rational clinical examination systematic review. *JAMA*. 2013;309:2035.

Holroyd-Leduc JM, Tannenbaum C, Thorpe KE, Straus SE. What type of urinary incontinence does this woman have? *JAMA*. 2008;299:1446.

Holt JD, Garrett WA, McCurry TK, Teichman JM. Common questions about chronic prostatitis. *Am Fam Physician*. 2016;15;93(4):290-296.

Homan GJ. Failure to thrive: a practical guide. *Am Fam Physician*. 2016;94:295.

Huancahuari N. Emergencies in early pregnancy. *Emerg Med Clin North Am*. 2012;30:837.

Huang W, Molitch ME. Evaluation and management of galactorrhea. *Am Fam Physician*. 2012;85(11): 1073-1080.

Huntzinger A. Guidelines for the diagnosis and management of hoarseness. *Am Fam Physician*. 2010; 81:1292-1296.

Huppert JS, Hesse E, Kim G, et al. Adolescent women can perform a point-of-care test for trichomoniasis as accurately as clinicians. *Sex Transm Infect*. 2010;86:514.

Hyderi A, Angel J, Madison M, Perry LA, Hagshenas L. Transgender patients: providing sensitive care. *J Fam Pract*. 2016;65(7):450-461.

Hyman P. Chronic and recurrent abdominal pain. *Pediatr Rev*. 2016;37:377.

Inouye SK, van Dyck CH, Alessi CA, Balkin S, Siegal AP, Horwitz RI. Clarifying confusion: the confusion assessment method. A new method for detecting delirium. *Ann Intern Med*. 1990;113:941.

Inouye SK. Delirium in older persons. *N Engl J Med*. 2006;354:1157.

Institute of Medicine. *Clinical Practice Guidelines We Can Trust*. Washington, DC: National Academies Press; 2011.

Institute of Medicine. *The Health of Lesbian, Gay, Bisexual, and Transgender People: Building a Foundation for Better Understanding*. Washington DC: The National Academies Press; 2011. Available at: http://nap.edu/13128.

Ishiyama A. Why does air travel cause earache? *West J Med*. 1999;171:106.

Ittyachen A, Vijayan A, Isac M. The forgotten view: chest x-ray – lateral view. *Resp Med Case Rep*. 2017;22:257.

Jacobs CK, Coffey J. Clinical inquiries. Sleep apnea in adults: how accurate is clinical prediction? *J Fam Pract*. 2009;58:327.

Jacobson GP, McCaslin DL, Piker EG, Gruenwald J, Grantham S, Tegel L. Insensitivity of the "Romberg test of standing balance on firm and compliant support surfaces" to the results of caloric and VEMP tests. *Ear Hear.* 2011;32:e1-e5.

James SE, Herman JL, Rankin S, Keisling M, Mottet L, Anafi M. *The Report of the 2015 U.S. Transgender Survey.* Washington, DC: National Center for Transgender Equality; 2016.

Jamison MA. Disorders of menstruation in adolescent girls. *Ped Clin North Am.* 2015;62:943.

Jamshed N, Dubin J, Eldadah Z. Emergency management of palpitations in the elderly: epidemiology, diagnostic approaches, and therapeutic options. *Clin Geriatr Med.* 2013;29(1):205-230.

Jamshed N, Lee ZE, Olden KW. Diagnostic approach to chronic constipation in adults. *Am Fam Physician.* 2011;84:299.

Jasper J. Vulvovaginitis in the prepubertal child. *Clin Pediatr Emerg Med.* 2009;10:10.

Javed A, Tebben PJ, Fischer PR, Lteif AN. Female athlete triad and its components: toward improved screening and management. *Mayo Clin Proc.* 2013;88:996-1009. Available at: www.sciencedirect.com/science/article/pii/S0025619613005545. Accessed September 6, 2018.

Jefferis J, Perera R, Everitt H, et al. Acute infective conjunctivitis in primary care: who needs antibiotics? An individual patient data meta-analysis. *Br J Gen Pract.* 2011;61:e542.

Jensen H. Epstein-Barr virus. *Peds Rev.* 2011;32:375.

Johnson CP. Recognition of autism before age 2 years. *Pediatr Rev.* 2008;29:86.

Jones LL, Hassanien A, Cook DG, Britton J, Leonardi-Bee J. Parental smoking and the risk of middle ear disease in children: A systematic review and meta-analysis. *Arch Pediatr Adolesc Med.* 2012;166:18.

Juckett G, Trivedi R. Evaluation of chronic diarrhea. *Am Fam Physician.* 2011;84:1119.

Jung I, Kim JS. Approach to dizziness in the emergency room. *Clin Exp Emerg Med.* 2015;2:75.

Kabbouche MA, Cleves C. Evaluation and management of children and adolescents presenting in an acute setting. *Semin Pediatr Neurol.* 2010;17:105.

Kahrilas PJ, Shaheen NJ, Vaezi MF, et al. American Gastroenterological Association. American Gastroenterological Association medical position statement on the management of gastroesophageal reflux disease. *Gastroenterology.* 2008;135:1383.

Kallvik E, Putus T, Simberg S. Indoor air problems and hoarseness in children. *J Voice.* 2016;30:109.

Kalra MG, Higgins KE, Perez ED. Common questions about streptococcal pharyngitis. *Am Fam Physician.* 2016;94:24-31.

Kapoor WN. Syncope. *N Engl J Med.* 2000;343:1856.

Karnani NG, Reisfield GM, Wilson GR. Evaluation of chronic dyspnea. *Am Fam Phys.* 2005;71(8):1529-1537.

Karnes JB, Usatine RP. Management of external genital warts. *Am Fam Physician.* 2014;90:312.

Kaslovsky R, Sadof M. Chronic cough in children a primary care and subspecialty collaborative approach. *Pediatr Rev.* 2013;34(11):498-508.

Katz PO, Gerson LB, Vela MF. Guidelines for the diagnosis and management of gastroesophageal reflux disease. *Am J Gastroenterol.* 2013;108:308.

Kellerman R, Kintanar T. Gastroesophageal reflux disease. *Prim Care.* 2017;44(4):561-573.

Kelvin R. Depression in children and young people. *Ped and Child Health.* 2016;26:540.

Kenny RA. Syncope in the elderly: diagnosis, evaluation, and treatment. *J Cardiovasc Electrophysiol.* 2003;14:S74.

Kersten LD. *Comprehensive Respiratory Nursing.* Philadelphia: Saunders; 1989.

Khan FU, Ihsan AU, Khan HU, et al. Comprehensive overview of prostatitis. *Biomed Pharmacother.* 2017; 94:1064-1076.

Khandelwal C, Kistler C. Diagnosis of urinary incontinence. *Am Fam Physician.* 2013;87:543.

Kirsch DB. PRO: sliding into home: portable sleep testing is effective for diagnosis of obstructive sleep apnea. *J Clin Sleep Med.* 2013;9:5.

Klein DA, Poth MA. Amenorrhea: An approach to diagnosis and management. *Am Fam Physician.* 2013;87:781.

Klein S. Evaluation of palpable breast masses. *Am Fam Physician.* 2005;71:1731.

Kleinman A, Benson P. Anthropology in the clinic: the problem of cultural competency and how to fix it. *PLoS Med.* 2006;3:e294.

Kleyman I, Weimer LH. Syncope: case studies. *Neurol Clin.* 2016;34:525.

Kmetova A, Kralikova E, Stepankova L, et al. Factors associated with weight changes in successful quitters participating in a smoking cessation program. *Addict Behav.* 2014;39:239.

Knight JR, Shrier LA, Bravender TD, Farrell M, Vander Bilt J, Shaffer HJ. A new brief screen for adolescent substance abuse. *Arch Pediatr Adolesc Med.* 1999;153:591.

Kochhar GS, Singh T, Gill A, Kirby DF. Celiac disease: managing a multisystem disorder. *Cleve Clin J Med.* 2016;83(3):217-227.

Kodner CM, Thomas Gupton EK. Recurrent urinary tract infections in women: Diagnosis and management. *Am Fam Physician.* 2010;82:638.

Koes BW, van Tulder MW, Ostelo R, Kim Burton A, Waddell G. Clinical guidelines for the management of low back pain in primary care: an international comparison. *Spine (Phila Pa 1976).* 2001;26:2504.

Kraft M. Approach to the patient with respiratory disease. In: Goldman L, Schafer AI, eds. *Goldman's Cecil Medicine.* 25th ed. St. Louis: Elsevier; 2016.

Kramer BS, Croswell JM. Cancer screening: the clash of science and intuition. *Annu Rev Med.* 2009;60:125-137.

Kravets I. Hyperthyroidism: diagnosis and treatment. *Am Fam Physician.* 2016;93(5):363-370.

Krieger JN, Nyberg Jr L, Nickel JC. NIH consensus definition and classification of prostatitis. *JAMA.* 1999;282:236.

Kundu RV, Patterson S. Dermatologic conditions in skin of color: part II. Disorders occurring predominately in skin of color. *Am Fam Physician.* 2013;87:859.

Lachs MS, Pillemer KA. Elder abuse. *N Engl J Med.* 2015;373:1947.

Lacy BE, Mearin F, Chang L, et al. Section II: FGIDs: diagnostic groups: bowel disorders. Gastroenterology. 2016;150(6):1393-1407.

Lacy BE, Weiser K, Chertoff J, et al. The diagnosis of gastroesophageal reflux disease. *Am J Med.* 2010; 123(7):583-592.

Lacy BE, Weiser K. Common anorectal disorders: diagnosis and treatment. *Curr Gastroenterol Rep.* 2009; 11:413.

Landay MJ. *Interpretation of the Chest Roentgenogram.* Boston: Little Brown; 1987.

Lane JR, Ben-Shachar G. Myocardial infarction in healthy adolescents. *Pediatrics.* 2007;120:e938-943.

Lane VA, Sugarman ID. Investigation of rectal bleeding in children. *Paediatr Child Health.* 2010;20:465.

Lange RA, Hills LD. Clinical practice. Acute pericarditis. *N Engl J Med.* 2004;351:2195.

Last AR, Hulbert K. Chronic low back pain: evaluation and management. *Am Fam Physician.* 2009; 79:1067.

LeBlanc KE, LeBlanc LL, LeBlanc KA. Inguinal hernias: diagnosis and management. *Am Fam Physician.* 2013;87(12):844-848.

Leddy R, Irshad A, Zerwas E, et al. Role of breast ultrasound and mammography in evaluating patients presenting with focal breast pain in the absence of a palpable lump. *Breast J.* 2013;19:582.

Lee R, Elder A. Dizziness in older adults. *Medicine.* 2017;45(1):19-22.

Lee TH, Goldman L. Evaluation of the patient with acute chest pain. *N Engl J Med.* 2000;342:1187.

Leech S. Recurrent urticaria. *Paediatr Child Health.* 2011;22(7):281-286.

Lehman PJ, Carl RL. Growing pains. *Sports Health.* 2017;9:132.

Leibowitz HM. The red eye. *N Engl J Med.* 2000;343:345.

Levin B, Lieberman DA, McFarland B, et al. Screening and surveillance for the early detection of colorectal cancer and adenomatous polyps: a joint guideline from the American Cancer Society, the U.S. Multi-Society Task Force on Colorectal Cancer, and the American College of Radiology. *Gastroenterology.* 2008;134:1570.

Lewandowski AS, Ward TM, Palermo TM. Sleep problems in children and adolescents with common medical conditions. *Pediatr Clin North Am.* 2011; 58:699.

Lewis SJ, Heaton KW. Stool form scale as a useful guide to intestinal transit time. *Scand J Gastroenterol.* 1997;32(9):920-924.

Li JC. *Otalgia.* Available at https://emedicine.medscape.com/article/845173-overview. Accessed September 6, 2018.

Lieberman JA III. BATHE: an approach to the interview process in the primary care setting. *J Clin Psychiatry.* 1997;58:3.

Lieberthal AS, Carroll AE, Chonmaitree T, et al. American Academy of Pediatrics Clinical Practice Guideline: The diagnosis and management of acute otitis media. *Pediatrics.* 2013;131:e964.

Lightdale JR, Gremse DA. Gastroesophageal reflux: management guidance for the pediatrician. *Pediatrics.* 2013;131:e1684.

Linder JA. Sore throat: avoid overcomplicating the uncomplicated. *Ann Intern Med.* 2015;162:311-12.

Linzer M, Yang EH, Estes NA III, Wang P, Vorperian VR, Kapoor WN. Diagnosing syncope. Part 1: Value of history, physical examination, and electrocardiography. Clinical Efficacy Assessment Project of the American College of Physicians. *Ann Intern Med.* 1997;126:989.

Lipton RB, Bigal ME, Steiner TJ, Silberstein SD, Olesen J. Classification of primary headaches. *Neurology.* 2004;63:427.

Long SS. Distinguishing among prolonged, recurrent, and periodic fever syndromes: Approach of a pediatric infectious diseases subspecialist. *Pediatr Clin North Am.* 2005;52:811.

Loo JT, Duddalwar V, Chen FK, Tejura T, Lekht I, Gulati M. Abdominal radiograph pearls and pitfalls for the emergency department radiologist: a pictorial review. *Abdom Radiol (NY).* 2017;42:987.

Lowe RM, Hashkes PJ. Growing pains: a noninflammatory pain syndrome in early childhood. *Nat Clin Pract Rheumatol.* 2008;4:542.

Loyd RA, McClellan DA. Update on the evaluation and management of functional dyspepsia. *Am Fam Physician.* 2011;83:547.

Lu SH, Leasure AR, Dai YT. A systematic review of body temperature variations in older people. *J Clin Nurs.* 2009;19:4-16.

Lukacz ES, Santiago-Lastra Y, Albo ME, Brubaker L. Urinary Incontinence in Women: a review. *JAMA.* 2017;318:1592.

Lunny C, Taylor D, Hoang L, et al. Self-collected versus clinician-collected sampling for chlamydia and gonorrhea screening: a systemic review and meta-analysis. *PLoS One.* 2015;10:e0132776. doi:10.1371/journal.pone.0132776.

Luthy KE, Larimer SG, Freeborn DS. Differentiating between lactose intolerance, celiac disease and irritable bowel syndrome diarrhea. *The Jour of Nurs Practitioner*. 2017;13:348.

Ma JF, Shortliffe LM. Urinary tract infection in children: etiology and epidemiology. *Urol Clin North Am*. 2004;31:517.

Maarsingh OR, Dros J, Schellevis FG, et al. Causes of persistent dizziness in elderly patients in primary care. *Ann Fam Med*. 2010;8:196.

Macbeth AE, Grindlay DJ, Williams HC. What's new in skin cancer? An analysis of guidelines and systematic reviews published in 2008–2009. *Clin Exp Dermatol*. 2011;36:453.

Maciosek MV, Coffield AB, Edwards NM, Flottemesch TJ, Goodman MJ, Solberg LI. Priorities among effective clinical preventive services: results of a systematic review and analysis. *Am J Prev Med*. 2006;31:52.

MacNeill EC, Vashist S. Approach to syncope and altered mental status. *Pediatr Clin North Am*. 2013;60:1083.

Madani S, Tsang L, Kamat D. Constipation in children a practical review. *Pediatr Ann*. 2016;45:189.

Majumdar S, Wu K, Bateman ND, Ray J. Diagnosis and management of otalgia in children. *Arch Dis Child Educ Pract Ed*. 2009;94:33.

Manchikanti L, Singh V, Datta S, Cohen SP, Hirsch JA, American Society of Interventional Pain Physicians. Comprehensive review of epidemiology, scope, and impact of spinal pain. *Pain Physician*. 2009;12:E35.

Manzoni GC, Torelli P. Headache screening and diagnosis. *Neurol Sci*. 2004;25:S255.

Marcus C, Schechter M. Updated guidelines for childhood sleep apnea. *Contemp Pediatr*. 2013;11:36.

Marin JR, Alpern ER. Abdominal pain in children. *Emerg Med Clin North Am*. 2011;29(2):401-428.

Markle W, Conti T, Kad M. Sexuality transmitted diseases. *Prim Care*. 2013;40:557.

Marple BF, Stankiewicz JA, Baroody FM, et al. Diagnosis and management of chronic rhinosinusitis in adults. *Postgrad Med*. 2009;121:121.

Marsh CA, Grimstad FW. Primary amenorrhea: diagnosis and management. *Obstet Gynecol Surv*. 2014;69:603.

Marshall GS. Prolonged and recurrent fevers in children. *J Infec*. 2014;68:S83.

Martin JL, Williams KS, Abrams KR, et al. Systematic review and evaluation of methods of assessing urinary incontinence. *Health Technol Assess*. 2006;10:1.

Maslow GR, Dunlap K Chung RJ. Depression and suicide in children and adolescents. *Pediatr Rev*. 2015;36:299.

Matta NS, Silbert D. Pediatric vision screening. *Int Ophthalmol Clin*. 2014;54:41.

Matthews PJ, Aziz Q. Functional abdominal pain. *Postgrad Med J*. 2005;81:448.

Matthews SJ, Lancaster JW. Urinary tract infections in the elderly population. *Am J Geriatr Pharmacother*. 2011;9:286.

Maurer DM. Screening for depression. *Am Fam Physician*. 2012;85(2):139.

McCabe M, Branowicki P. Fatigue in acute care and ambulatory settings. *Journ Ped Nurs*. 2014;29:344.

McCallum IJ, Ong S, Mercer-Jones MM. Chronic constipation in adults. *BMJ*. 2009;338:b831.

McConaghy JR, Oza RS. Outpatient diagnosis of acute chest pain in adults. *Am Fam Physician*. 2013;87:177.

McConaghy JR, Panchal B. Epididymitis: an overview. *Am Fam Physician*. 2016;94(9):723-726.

McGrath NA, Howell JM, Davis JE. Pediatric genitourinary emergencies. *Emerg Med Clin North Am*. 2011;29(3):655-666.

McKertich K. Urinary incontinence assessment in women: stress, urge or both? *Aust Fam Physician*. 2008;37:112.

McKinnon Jr HD, Howard T. Evaluating the febrile patient with a rash. *Am Fam Physician*. 2000;62:804.

McMurray JS. Disorders of phonation in children. *Pediatr Clin North Am*. 2003;50:363.

McPhee SJ, Papadakis MA. *Current medical diagnosis and treatment*. 57th ed. New York: McGraw-Hill; 2018.

Medina-Bombardó D, Jover-Palmer A. Does clinical examination aid in the diagnosis of urinary tract infections in women? A systematic review and meta-analysis. *BMC Fam Pract*. 2011;12:111.

Meister L, Morley EJ, Scheer D, Sinert R. History and physical examination plus laboratory testing for the diagnosis of adult female urinary tract infection. *Acad Emerg Med*. 2013;20:631.

Meites E, Gaydos CA, Hobbs MM, et al. A review of evidence-based care of symptomatic trichomoniasis and asymptomatic trichomonas vaginalis infections. *Clin Infect Dis*. 2015;15(suppl 8):S837.

Metalidis C, Knockaert DC, Bobbaers H, Vanderschueren S. Involuntary weight loss. Does a negative baseline evaluation provide adequate reassurance? *Eur J Intern Med*. 2008;19:345.

Mettler F. *Essentials of Radiology*. 3rd ed. Philadelphia: Saunders; 2014.

Michaudet C, Malaty J. Chronic cough: evaluation and management. *Am Fam Physician*. 2017;96:575.

Michels TC, Sands JE. Dysuria: evaluation and differential diagnosis in adults. *Am Fam Physician*. 2015;92:778.

Michels TC, Sands JE. Dysuria: evaluation and differential diagnosis in adults. *Am Fam Physician*. 2015;92(9):778-786.

Milisen K, Braes T, Fick DM, Foreman MD. Cognitive assessment and differentiating the 3 Ds (dementia, depression, delirium). *Nurs Clin North Am.* 2006;41:1.

Mills BB. Vaginitis: beyond the basics. *Obstet Gynecol Clin North Am.* 2017;44:159.

Mills R, Nnadi C, Wilkinson N. Evaluation of back pain. *Paediatr Child Health.* 2011;21:534.

Misiri J, Candler S, Kusumoto FM. Evaluation of syncope and palpitations in women. *J Womens Health.* 2011;20(10):1505-1515.

Mitchell H. ABC of sexually transmitted infections: Vaginal discharge—causes, diagnosis, and treatment. *BMJ.* 2004;328:1306.

Mmbaga BT, Houpt ER. Cryptosporidium and giardia infection in children: a review. *Pediatr Clin North Am.* 2017;64:837.

Moayyedi P, Talley NJ, Fennerty MB, Vakil N. Can the clinical history distinguish between organic and functional dyspepsia? *JAMA.* 2006;295:1566.

Moi H, Blee K, Horner PJ. Management of non-gonococcal urethritis. *BMC Infect Dis.* 2015;15:294.

Moodley M. Clinical approach to syncope in children. *Semin Pediatr Neurol.* 2013;20:12.

Moragas-Garrido M, Davenport R. Acute headache. *Medicine.* 2013;41:164.

Morel JC, Iqbal A, Peacock C, et al. A comparison of the accuracy of digital breast tomosynthesis with supplementary views in the diagnostic workup of mammographic lesions. *Breast Cancer Res.* 2011; 13(suppl 1):O6.

Morris AM, Regenbogen SE, Hardiman KM, Hendren S. Sigmoid diverticulitis: a systematic review. *JAMA.* 2014;311:287-297.

Morris-Jones R, Morris-Jones S. Travel-associated skin disease. *Infect Dis Clin North Am.* 2012;26:675.

Morton RL, Sheikh S, Corbett ML, Eid NS. Evaluation of the wheezy infant. *Ann Allergy Asthma Immunol.* 2001;86:251.

Mostbeck G, Adam EJ, Nielsen MB, et al. How to diagnose acute appendicitis: ultrasound first. *Insights Imaging.* 2016;7(2):255-263.

Mounsey AL, Halladay J, Sadiq TS. Hemorrhoids. *Am Fam Physician.* 2011;84:204.

Moy L, Heller SL, Bailey L, et al. ACR appropriateness criteria® palpable breast masses. *J Am Rad.* 2014;14:(5):S203-S224.

Moyer JE, Brey JM. Shoulder injuries in the pediatric athlete. *Orthop Clin North Am.* 2016;47:749.

Moyer VA, U.S. Preventive Services Task Force. Screening for and management of obesity in adults: US Preventive Services Task Force recommendation statement. *Ann Intern Med.* 2012;157:373.

Mulle BA. Prostatitis: What NPs need to know about diagnosis and treatment. *Am J Nurse Pract.* 2005;9:33.

Muncie HL, Sirmans SM, James E. Dizziness: approach to evaluation and management. *Am Fam Physician.* 2017;95:154.

Murdin L, Seemungal BM, Bronstein AM. Dizziness. *Medicine.* 2012;40:431.

Murphy N, Alderman P, Voege Harvey K, Harris N. Women and heart disease: an evidence-based update. *J Nurse Pract.* 2017;13(9):610-616.

Musson RE, Bickle I, Vijay RK. Gas patterns on plain abdominal radiographs: a pictorial review. *Postgrad Med J.* 2011;87:274.

Nasseri YY, Osborne MC. Pruritus ani: diagnosis and treatment. *Gastroenterol Clin North Am.* 2013;42:801.

National Asthma Education and Prevention Program. Expert panel report 3: guidelines for the diagnosis and management of asthma-summary report 2007. *J Allergy Clin Immunol.* 2007;120:S94.

National Collaborating Centre for Nursing and Supportive Care. *Irritable Bowel Syndrome in Adults: Diagnosis and Management of Irritable Bowel Syndrome in Primary Care.* London, UK: National Institute for Health and Care Excellence; 2015.

National Institute for Health and Care Excellence, Clinical Guideline. *Chest Pain of Recent Onset.* 2016. Available at: http://guidance.nice.org.uk/CG95. Accessed September 6, 2018.

National Lung Screening Trial Research Team, Aberle DR, Adams AM, et al. Reduced lung-cancer mortality with low-dose computed tomographic screening. *N Engl J Med.* 2011;365:395.

Neikrug AB, Ancoli-Israel S. Sleep disorders in the older adult—a mini-review. Gerontology. 2010;56: 181.

Nelson KA, Zorc JJ. Asthma update. *Pediatr Clin North Am.* 2013;60(5):1035-1048.

Nelson RL, Thomas K, Morgan J, Jones A. Non surgical therapy for anal fissure. *Cochrane Database Syst Rev.* 2012;(2):CD003431.

Newman-Toker DE, Edlow JA. TiTrATE: a novel, evidence-based approach to diagnosing acute dizziness and vertigo. *Neurol Clin.* 2015;33(3):577-599.

Nickel JC, Shoskes D, Wang Y, et al. How does the pre-massage and post-massage 2-glass test compare to the Meares-Stamey 4-glass test in men with chronic prostatitis/chronic pelvic pain syndrome? *J Urol.* 2006;176:119.

Nierengarten MB. Diagnosis and management of croup in children. *Contemp Pediatr.* 2015;32:31.

Norton I. Practical ophthalmology—a survival guide for doctors and optometrists. *Emerg Med Australas.* 2005;17:524.

Novelline RA. *Squire's Fundamentals of Radiology.* 5th ed. Cambridge: Harvard University Press; 1997.

Novelline RA. *Squire's Fundamentals of Radiology.* 6th ed. Cambridge, MA: Harvard University Press; 2004.

Numans ME, Lau J, de Wit NJ, Bonis PA. Short-term treatment with proton-pump inhibitors as a test for gastroesophageal reflux disease: a meta-analysis of diagnostic test characteristics. *Ann Intern Med.* 2004;140:518.

Nye C. A child's vision. *Ped Clin North Am.* 2014; 61:495.

O'Donnell LJ, Virjee J, Heaton KW. Detection of pseudodiarrhoea by simple clinical assessment of intestinal transit rate. *BMJ.* 1990;300(6722): 439-440.

Onstad M, Stuckey A. Benign breast disorders. *Obstet Gynecol Clin North Am.* 2013;40:459-473.

Pääkkönen M, Peltola H. Bone and joint infections. *Pediatr Clin North Am.* 2013;60:425.

Page C, Mounsey A, Rowland K. PURLs: is self-swabbing for STIs a good idea? *J Fam Pract.* 2013; 62:651.

Palmer LS. Hernias and hydroceles. *Pediatr Rev.* 2013;34:457.

Papadakis MA, McPhee SJ, Rabow MW. *Current Medical Diagnosis and Treatment.* 56th ed. New York: McGraw Hill; 2017.

Papadakis MA, McPhee SJ, Rabow MW. *Current Medical Diagnosis and Treatment.* 57th ed. New York: Lange Series, McGraw-Hill; 2018.

Park CJ, Kim EK, Moon HJ, Yoon JH, Kim MJ. Reliability of breast ultrasound BI-RADS final assessment in mammographically negative patients with nipple discharge and radiologic predictors of malignancy. *J Breast Cancer.* 2016;19(3):308-315.

Park JK. Palpitations and arrhythmias and sudden cardiac arrest/sudden cardiac death in children and adolescents. *Pediatr Ann.* 2015;44:e279.

Paruthi S, Brooks LJ, D'Ambrosio C, et al. Recommended amount of sleep for pediatric populations: a consensus statement of the American Academy of Sleep Medicine. *J Clin Sleep Med.* 2016;212(6):785-786. Available at: http://www.aasmnet.org/Resources/pdf/Pediatricsleepdurationconsensus.pdf.

Paudel B, Paudel K. The diagnostic significance of the holter monitoring in the evaluation of palpitation. *J Clin Diagn Res.* 2013;7(3):480-483.

Pearson R, Williams PM. Common questions about the diagnosis and management of benign prostatic hyperplasia. *Am Fam Physician.* 2014;90(11):769-774.

Pelletier AL, Rojas-Roldan L, Coffin J. Vision loss in older adults. *Am Fam Physician.* 2016;94:219.

Pelton SI. Otitis media: Re-evaluation of diagnosis and treatment in the era of antimicrobial resistance, pneumococcal conjugate vaccine, and evolving morbidity. *Pediatr Clin North Am.* 2005;52:711.

Pepper VK, Stanfill AB, Pearl RH. Diagnosis and management of pediatric appendicitis, intussusception, and Meckel diverticulum. *Surg Clin North Am.* 2012;92(3):505-526.

Petersen EE, Staples JE, Meaney-Delman D, et al. Interim guidelines for pregnant women during zika virus outbreak—United States. *MMWR Morb Mortal Wkly Rep.* 2016;65:30.

Phillips J, Fein-Zachary VJ, Mehta TS, Littlehale N, Venkataraman S, Slanet PJ. Breast imaging in the transgender patient. *AJR Am J Roentgenology.* 2014;202:1149-1156.

Pilcher TA, Saarel EV. A teenager fainter (dizziness, syncope, postural orthostatic tachycardia syndrome). *Pediatr Clin North Am.* 2014;61:29.

Pinching A. Chronic fatigue syndrome: believing in ME. *Nurse Prescribing.* 2009;7:358.

Pinsky PF, Prorok PC, Yu K, et al. Extended mortality results for prostate cancer screening in the PLCO trial with median follow-up of 15 years. *Cancer.* 2017;123(4):592-599.

Piscitelli JT, Simel DL. Update: Vaginitis. In: Simel DL, Drummond R, eds. *The Rational Clinical Examination: Evidence-Based Clinical Diagnosis.* New York: McGraw Hill; 2009.

Polackwich AS, Shoskes DA. Chronic prostatitis/chronic pelvic pain syndrome: a review of evaluation and therapy. *Prostate Cancer Prostatic Dis.* 2016;19(2):132-138.

Polites SF, Mohamed MI, Habermann EB, et al. A simple algorithm reduces computed tomography use in the diagnosis of appendicitis in children. *Surgery.* 2014;156(2):448.

Powell J, Wilson JA. An evidence-based review of peritonsillar abscess. *Clin Otolaryngol.* 2012;37:136.

Powers KS. Dehydration: isonatremic, hyponatremic and hypernatremic recognition and management. *Pediatr Crit Care.* 2015;36:274.

Practice Committee of American Society for Reproductive Medicine. Current evaluation of amenorrhea. *Fertil Steril.* 2008;90:S219-225.

Preti M, Scurry J, Marchitelli CE, Micheletti L. Vulvar intraepithelial neoplasia. *Best Pract Res Clin Obstet Gynaecol.* 2014;28:1051.

Pruthi S, Jones KN, Boughey JC, Simmons PS. Breast masses in adolescents: clinical pearls in the diagnostic evaluation. *Am Fam Physician.* 2012;86:325.

Purdy RA. Clinical evaluation of a patient presenting with headache. *Med Clin North Am.* 2001;85:847.

Putz K, Hayani K, Zar FA. Meningitis. *Prim Care.* 2013;40(3):707-726.

Quan M. Vaginitis: diagnosis and management. *Postgrad Med.* 2010;122:117.

Rajkomar A, Dhaliwal G. Improving diagnostic reasoning to improve patient safety. *Perm J.* 2011;15(3): 68-73.

Ramaswamy K, Jacobson K. Infectious diarrhea in children. *Gastroenterol Clin North Am.* 2001;30: 611.

Rao SS, Ozturk R, Laine L. Clinical utility of diagnostic tests for constipation in adults: A systematic review. *Am J Gastroenterol.* 2005;100:1605.

Raoof S, Feigin D, Sung A, Raoof S, Irugulpati L, Rosenow EC. Interpretation of plain chest roentgenogram. *Chest.* 2012;141:545.

Ratner RE; Diabetes Prevention Program Research. An update on the diabetes prevention program. *Endocr Pract.* 2006;12:20-24.

Ravi C, Rodrigues G. Accuracy of clinical examination of breast lumps in detecting malignancy: a retrospective study. *Indian J Surg Oncol.* 2012;3(2):154-157.

Rayala BZ, Morrell DS. Common skin conditions in children: skin infections. *FP Essent.* 2017;453:26.

Reddy SR, Singh HR. Chest pain in children and adolescents. *Pediatr Rev.* 2010;31:e1-9.

Rees J, Abrahams M, Doble A, Cooper A. The Prostatitis Expert Reference Group. Diagnosis and treatment of chronic bacterial prostatitis and chronic prostatitis/chronic pelvic pain syndrome: a consensus guideline. *BJU Int.* 2015;116(4):509-525.

Reeves AG, Swenson RS. *Disorders of the Nervous System: A Primer.* Dartmouth Medical School; 2008. Available at: https://www.dartmouth.edu/~dons/. Accessed November 2017.

Reife CM. Involuntary weight loss. *Med Clin North Am.* 1995;79:299.

Reifsnider E. Common adult infectious skin conditions. *Nurse Pract.* 1997;22:17.

Reust CE, Williams A. Acute abdominal pain in children. *Am Fam Physician.* 2016;93:830.

Richens J. Main presentations of sexually transmitted infections in men. *BMJ.* 2004;328:1251.

Rietveld RP, ter Riet G, Bindels PJE, Sloos JH, van Weert HC. Predicting bacterial cause in infectious conjunctivitis: cohort study on informativeness of combinations of signs and symptoms. *BMJ.* 2004;329:206.

Rivera RF, Chambers P, Ceresnak SR. Evaluation of children with palpitations. *Clin Pediatr Emerg Med.* 2011;12(4):278-288.

Roberts DM, Stallard TC. Emergency department evaluation and treatment of knee and leg injuries. *Emerg Med Clin North Am.* 2000;18:67.

Roberts KB. Urinary tract infection: clinical practice guideline for the diagnosis and management of the initial UTI in febrile infants and children 2 to 24 months. *Pediatrics.* 2011;128:595.

Robins DL, Casagrande K, Barton M, Chen CM, Dumont-Mathieu T, Fein D. Validation of the modified checklist for autism in toddlers, revised with follow-up (M-CHAT-R/F). *Pediatrics.* 2014;133:37.

Rodrignez-Galindo C, Orbach D, VanderVeen D. Retinoblastoma. *Pediatr Clin North Am.* 2015;62:201.

Roepke SK, Ancoli-Israel S. Sleep disorders in the elderly. *Indian J Med Res.* 2010;131:302.

Rogers RG. Urinary stress incontinence in women. *N Engl J Med.* 2008;358:1029.

Rogers SJ, Talbott MR. Chapter eight—early identification and early treatment of autism spectrum disorder. *Int Rev Res Dev Disabil.* 2016;50:233.

Rosa-Olivares J, Porro A, Rodriguez-Varela M, Riefkohl G, Niroomand-Rad I. Otitis media: to treat, to refer, to do nothing: a review for the practitioner. *Pediatr Rev.* 2015;36:480.

Rose AS, Thorp BD, Zanation AM, Ebert Jr CS. Chronic rhinosinusitis in children. *Pediatr Clin North Am.* 2013;60:979.

Rosenfeld RM, Andes D, Bhattacharyya N, et al. Clinical practice guideline: adult sinusitis. *Otolaryngol Head Neck Surg.* 2007;137:S1.

Rosenfeld RM, Shin JJ, Schwartz SR, et al. Clinical practice guideline otitis media with effusion executive summary (update). *Otolaryngol Head Neck Surg.* 2016;154:201.

Rosenthal TC, Majeroni BA, Pretorius R, Malik K. Fatigue: an overview. *Am Fam Physician.* 2008;78:1173.

Roser T, Bonfert M, Ebinger F, Blankenburg M, Ertl-Wagner B, Heinen F. Primary versus secondary headache in children: a frequent diagnostic challenge in clinical routine. *Neuropediatrics.* 2013;44:34.

Ross A, LeLeiko NS. Acute abdominal pain. *Pediatr Rev.* 2010;31:135.

Rothman KJ. BMI-related errors in the measurement of obesity. *Int J Obes (Lond).* 2008;32(suppl 3):S56-9. doi:10.1038/ijo.2008.87.

Runcie I. Interpreting the chest radiograph. *Anaesth Intensive Care.* 2011;12:513.

Ryan MW. Evaluation and management of the patient with "sinus." *Med Clin North Am.* 2010;94:881.

Sahn B, Bitton S. Lower gastrointestinal bleeding in children. *Gastrointest Endosc Clin N Am.* 2016;26:75.

Sahnan K, Adegbola SO, Tozer PJ, Watfah J, Phillips RK. Perianal abscess. *BMJ.* 2017;356:j475.

Salzman B, Fleegle S, Tully AS. Common breast problems. *Am Fam Physician.* 2012;86:343-349.

Salzman B, Fleegle S, Tully AS. Common breast problems. *Am Fam Physician.* 2012;6:343-349.

Sanfilippo AM, Barrio V, Kulp-Shorten C, Callen JP. Common pediatric and adolescent skin conditions. *J Pediatr Adolesc Gynecol.* 2003;16(5):269-283.

Sayuk GS, Gyawali CP. Irritable bowel syndrome: modern concepts and management options. *Am J Med.* 2015;128(8):817-827.

Scarpero H. Urodynamics in the evaluation of female LUTS: when are they helpful and how do we use them? *Urol Clin North Am.* 2014;41:429.

Schiller LR. Chronic diarrhea. *Gastroenterology.* 2004;127:287.

Schmidt B, Copp HL. Work-up of pediatric urinary infection. *Urol Clin North Am.* 2015;42:519.

Schmiemann G, Kniehl E, Gebhardt K, Matejczyk MM, Hummers-Pradier E. The diagnosis of urinary tract infection: a systematic review. *Dtsch Arztebl Int.* 2010;107:361.

Schmulson MJ, Drossman DA. What is new in Rome IV. *J Neurogastroenterol Motil.* 2017;23(2):151-163.

Schnipper JL, Kapoor WN. Diagnostic evaluation and management of patients with syncope. *Med Clin North Am.* 2002;85:423.

Scholler I, Nittur S. Understanding failure to thrive. *Paediatr Child Health.* 2012;22:438.

Schröder FH, Hugosson J, Roobol MJ, et al. Screening and prostate-cancer mortality in a randomized European study. *N Engl J Med.* 2009;360:1320.

Schürks M, Rist PM, Bigal ME, Buring JE, Lipton RB, Kurth T. Migraine and cardiovascular disease: systematic review and meta-analysis. *BMJ.* 2009;339:b3914.

Schutte-Rodin S, Broch L, Buysse D, Dorsey C, Sateia M. Clinical guideline for the evaluation and management of chronic insomnia in adults. *J Clin Sleep Med.* 2008;4:487.

Searcy JAR. Geriatric urinary incontinence. *Nurs Clin North Am.* 2017;52:447-455.

Sedaghat-Yazdi F, Koenig PR. The teenager with palpitations. *Pediatr Clin North Am.* 2014;16(1):63-79.

Seemungal BM, Bronstein AM. A practical approach to acute vertigo. *Pract Neurol.* 2008;8:211.

Selbst S. Approach to the child with chest pain. *Pediatr Clin North Am.* 2010;57(6):1221-1234.

Selius BA, Subedi R. Urinary retention in adults: diagnosis and initial management. *Am Fam Physician.* 2008;77(5):643-650.

Semelka M, Wilson J, Floyd R. Diagnosis and treatment of obstructive sleep apnea in adults. *Am Fam Physician.* 2016;94:355.

Shaheen NJ, Falk GW, Iyer PG, Gerson LB. ACG clinical guideline: diagnosis and management of Barrett's esophagus. *Am J Gastroenterol.* 2016;111:30-50.

Shaikh N, Morone NE, Lopez J, et al. Does this child have a urinary tract infection? *JAMA.* 2007;298:2895.

Sharp VJ, Barnes KT. Assessment of asymptomatic microscopic hematuria in adults. 2013;88:747.

Sharp VJ, Barnes KT. Assessment of asymptomatic microscopic hematuria in adults. *Am Fam Physician.* 2013;88(11):747-754.

Sharp VJ, Kieran K, Arlen AM. Testicular torsion: diagnosis, evaluation, and management. *Am Fam Physician.* 2013;88(12):835-840.

Sharp VJ, Takacs EB, Powell CR. Prostatitis: diagnosis and treatment. *Am Fam Physician.* 2010;82:397.

Sheerin NS. Urinary tract infection. *Medicine.* 2011;39:384.

Shekelle P, Aronson MD, Melin JA. *Overview of Clinical Practice Guidelines. UpToDate*; 2017. Available at: https://www.uptodate.com/contents/overview-of-clinical-practice-guidelines#!. Accessed September 6, 2018.

Sheperd C. The debate: myalgic encephalomyelitis and chronic fatigue syndrome. *Br J Nurs.* 2006;15:662.

Shulman ST, Bisno AL, Clegg HW, et al. Clinical practice guideline for the diagnosis and management of group A streptococcal pharyngitis: 2012 update by the Infectious Diseases Society of America. *Clin Infect Dis.* 2012;55:1279.

Shumer DE, Nokoff NJ, Spack NP. Advances in the care of transgender children and adolescents. *Adv Pediatr.* 2016;63:79.

Silverstein MJ, Recht A, Lagios MD, et al. Special report: consensus conference III. Image-detected breast cancer: state-of-the-art diagnosis and treatment. *J Am Coll Surg.* 2009;209(4):504-520.

Silvis ML. Common musculoskeletal problems in the ambulatory setting. *Med Clin North Am.* 2014;98:xvii. doi:10.1016/j.mcna.2014.04.005.

Simmons BB, Hartmann B, DeJoseph D. Evaluation of suspected dementia. *Am Fam Physician.* 2011;84(8):895.

Simon JW, Kaw P. Commonly missed diagnoses in the childhood eye examination. *Am Fam Physician.* 2001;64:623.

Simren M, Palsson, OS, Whitehead WE. Update on Rome IV criteria for colorectal disorders: implications for clinical practice. *Curr Gastroenterol Rep.* 2017;19(4):15.

Siu AL, US Preventive Services Task Force (USPSTF), Bibbins-Domingo K, et al. Screening for Depression in Adults: US Preventive Services Task Force Recommendation Statement. *JAMA.* 2016;315(4):380.

Skoner DP. Allergic rhinitis: definition, epidemiology, pathophysiology, detection, and diagnosis. *J Allergy Clin Immunol.* 2001;108:S2.

Smith GD, Fry MM, Taylor D, Morgans A, Cantwell K. Effectiveness of the Valsalva manoeuvre for reversion of supraventricular tachycardia. *Cochrane Database Syst Rev.* 2015;(2):CD009502. doi:10.1002/14651858.CD009502.pub3.

Smith JE, Hall EJ. The use of plain abdominal x-rays in the emergency department. *Emerg Med J.* 2009;26:160.

Smith RL, Pruthi S, Fitzpatrick LA. Evaluation and management of breast pain. *Mayo Clin Proc.* 2004;79:353.

Sneider EB, Maykel JA. Anal abscess and fistula. *Gastroenterol Clin North Am.* 2013;42:773.

Sneider EB, Maykel JA. Diagnosis and management of symptomatic hemorrhoids. *Surg Clin North Am.* 2010;90:17.

Snow V, Lascher S, Mottur-Pilson C. Evidence base for management of acute exacerbations of chronic obstructive pulmonary disease. *Ann Intern Med.* 2001;134:595.

Snyder J, Fisher D. Pertussis in childhood. *Pediatr Rev.* 2012;33(9):412-420.

Snyder MJ, Bepko J, White M. Acute pericarditis: diagnosis and management. *Am Fam Physician.* 2014;89:553.

Snyderman D, Rovner B. Mental status exam in primary care: a review. *Am Fam Physician.* 2009;80:809.

Sobol SE, Zapata S. Epiglottitis and croup. *Otolaryngol Clin North Am.* 2008;41:551.

Söderström HF. Carlsson A. Börjesson A, Elfving M. Vaginal bleeding in prepubertal girls: etiology and clinical management. *J Pediatr Adolesc Gynecol.* 2013;29:280.

Sokkary N, Dietrich JE. Management of heavy menstrual bleeding in adolescents. *Curr Opin Obstet Gynecol.* 2013;24:275.

Sokol RJ, Martier SS, Ager JW. The T-ACE questions: practical prenatal detection of risk-drinking. *Am J Obstet Gynecol.* 1989;160:863.

Solebo AL, Rahi J. Epidemiology aetiology, and management of visual impaired children. *Arch Dis Child.* 2014;99:375.

Soloman ML, Weiss-Kelly AK. Approach to the underperforming athlete. *Peds Annals.* 2016;45: e91.

Solomon DH, Simel DL, Bates DW, Katz JN, Schaffer JL. The rational clinical examination. Does this patient have a torn meniscus or ligament of the knee? Value of the physical examination. *JAMA.* 2001;286:1610.

Solomon L, Reeves WC. Factors influencing the diagnosis of chronic fatigue syndrome. *Arch Intern Med.* 2004;164:2241.

Srikrishna S, Robinson D, Cardozo L, Vella M. Management of overactive bladder syndrome. *Postgrad Med J.* 2007;83:481.

Stafstrom CE, Rostasy K, Minster A. The usefulness of children's drawings in the diagnosis of headache. *Pediatrics.* 2002;109:460.

Stanghellini V, Chan FKL, Hasler WL, et al. Section II: FGIDs: diagnostic groups: gastroduodenal disorders. *Gastroenterology.* 2016;150(6):1380-1392.

Stein L, Chellman-Jeffers M. The radiologic workup of a palpable breast mass. *Cleve Clin J Med.* 2009; 76:175-180.

Stevens D. A sore throat or something else? *Pract Nurs.* 2008;19:83.

Stewart JM. Common syndromes of orthostatic intolerance. *Pediatrics.* 2013;131:968.

Stollman N, Smalley W, Hirano I, AGA Institute Clinical Guidelines Committee. American Gastroenterological Association Institute guideline on the management of acute diverticulitis. *Gastroenterology.* 2015;149:1944-1949.

Straus SE, Richardson WS, Glasziou P, Haynes RB. *Evidence-based Medicine: How to Practice and Teach It.* 4th ed. London, UK: Churchill Livingstone: 2010.

Strickberger SA, Benson DW, Biaggioni I, et al. AHA/ACCF scientific statement on the evaluation of syncope. *J Am Coll Cardiol.* 2006;47:473.

Strickland J, Gibson EJ, Levine SB. Dysfunctional uterine bleeding in adolescents. *J Pediatr Adolesc Gynecol.* 2006;19:49.

Sullivan JS, Sundaram SS. Gastroesophageal reflux. *Pediatr Rev.* 2012;33:243.

Sund-Levander M, Grodzinsky E. Time for a change to assess and evaluate body temperature in clinical practice. *Int J Nurs Pract.* 2009;15:241.

Suzuki K, Miyamoto M, Hirata K. Sleep disorders in the elderly: diagnosis and management. *J Gen Fam Med.* 2017;18(2):61-71.

Sveum R, Bergstrom J, Brottman G, et al. *Diagnosis and Management of Asthma,* Bloomington, Minn: Institute for Clinical Systems Improvement; 2012.

Sweet MG, Schmidt-Dalton TA, Weiss PM, Madsen KP. Evaluation and management of abnormal uterine bleeding in premenopausal women. *Am Fam Physician.* 2012;85:35.

Syed I, Daniels E, Blach NR. Hoarse voice in adults: an evidenced-based approach to 12 minute consultation. *Clin Otolarnygol.* 2009;34:54.

Takhellambam YS, Lourembam SS, Sapam, OS, Kshetrimayum RS, Ningthoujam BS, Khan T. Comparison of ultrasonography and fine needle aspiration cytology in the diagnosis of malignant breast lesions. *J Clin Diagn Res.* 2013;7(12):2847-2850.

Talley NJ, American Gastroenterological Association. American Gastroenterological Association medical position statement: evaluation of dyspepsia. *Gastroenterology.* 2005;129:1753.

Talley NJ. American Gastroenterological Association medical position statement: evaluation of dyspepsia. *Gastroenterology.* 2005;129:1753.

Tang MH, Pinsky EG. Mood and affective disorders. *Peds in Rev.* 2015;36:52.

Tarrac SE. A systematic approach to chest x-ray interpretation in the perianesthesia unit. *J Perianesth Nurs.* 2009;24:41.

Task Force on Sudden Infant Death Syndrome, Moon RY. SIDS and other sleep-related infant deaths: expansion of recommendations for a safe infant sleeping environment. *Pediatrics.* 2011;128:1030.

Ternent CA, Bastawrous AL, Morin NA, et al. Standards Practice Task Force of the American Society of Colon and Rectal Surgeons. Practice parameters for the evaluation and management of constipation. *Dis Colon Rectum.* 2007;50:2013.

Thanavaro JL. Evaluation and management of syncope. *Clin Schol Rev.* 2009;2:65.

Thavendiranathan P, Bagai A, Khoo C, Dorian P, Choudhry NK. Does this patient with palpitations have a cardiac arrhythmia? *JAMA.* 2009;302:2135.

Thielman NM, Guerrant RL. Clinical practice. Acute infectious diarrhea. *N Engl J Med.* 2004;350:38.

Thiene G, Carturan E, Corrado D, Basso C. Prevention of sudden cardiac death in the young and in athletes: dream or reality? *Cardiovasc Pathol.* 2010; 19:207.

Thomas JL, Christensen JC, Kravitz SR, et al. The diagnosis and treatment of heel pain: a clinical practice guideline-revision. *J Foot Ankle Surg.* 2010;49(3 suppl):S1-S19.

Thompson L, Kaufman LM. The visually impaired child. *Pediatr Clin North Am.* 2003;50:225.

Tice JA, O'Meara ES, Weaver DL, Vachon C, Ballard-Barbash R, Kerlikowske K. Benign breast disease, mammographic breast density, and the risk of breast cancer. *J Natl Cancer Inst.* 2013;105(14):1043-1049.

Tingley DH. Vision screening essentials: screening today for eye disorders in the pediatric patient. *Pediatr Rev.* 2007;28:54.

Tobias N, Mason D, Lutkenhoff M, Stoops M, Ferguson D. Management principles of organic causes of childhood constipation. *J Pediatr Health Care.* 2008;22:12.

Todd PS, Orlowski T, Schumacher-Kim W. A review of annular eruptions in children. *Pediatr Ann.* 2015; 44:e199.

Trent M. Pelvic inflammatory disease. *Pediatr Rev.* 2013;34:163.

Trinite T, Loveland-Cherry C, Marion L. The U.S. Preventive Services Task Force: an evidence-based prevention resource for nurse practitioners. *J Am Acad Nurse Pract.* 2009;21:301.

Trojian TH, Lishnak TS, Heiman D. Epididymitis and orchitis: an overview. *Am Fam Physician.* 2009;79:583.

Trowbridge RL, Rutkowski NK, Shojania KG. Does this patient have acute cholecystitis? In: Simel DL, Rennie D, eds. *The Rational Clinical Examination: Evidence-Based Clinical Diagnosis.* New York, NY: McGraw-Hill; 2009.

Tsang MY, Calvin AD, Reeder GS, Ammash NM, Hammack JE, Melduni RM. New-onset chest pain and palpitation. Coronary embolism. *Heart.* 2014;100(22):1769, 1814-1815.

Tsipouras S. Nonabdominal causes of abdominal pain—finding your heart in your stomach! *Aust Fam Physician.* 2008;37:620.

Tsirlin A, Oo Y, Sharma R, Kansara A, Gliwa A, Banerji MA. Pheochromocytoma: a review. *Maturitas.* 2014;77:229.

Tuck J. *Evaluation and Treatment of Common Upper Extremity Problems and Injuries.* Available at: https://lecom.edu/content/uploads/2017/03/J-Tuck-Hand-and-upper-ext-2017-Compatibility-Mode.pdf. Accessed December 2017.

Tumyan L, Hoyt AC, Bassett LW. Negative predictive value of sonography and mammography in patients with focal breast pain. *Breast J.* 2005;11:333.

Tuong W, Cheng LS, Armstrong AW. Melanoma: epidemiology, diagnosis, treatment, and outcomes. *Dermatol Clin.* 2012;30(1):113-124.

Türk C, Petřík A, Sarica K, et al. EAU Guidelines on conservative management of urolithiasis. *Eur Urol.* 2016;69:468.

U.S. Department of Agriculture. *The Dietary Guidelines for Americans 2015-2020.* Washington, DC: Author; 2017. Available at: https://health.gov/dietaryguidelines/2015. Accessed September 6, 2018.

U.S. Department of Health and Human Services, National Center for Health Statistics. *Health. United States, 2016.* Pub # 2017-1232. April 2018. Available at: http://www.cdc.gov/nchs/hus/index.htm. Accessed September 6, 2018.

U.S. Department of Health and Human Services, US Department of Agriculture. *2015-2020 Dietary guidelines for Americans.* December, 2017. Available at: http://www.health.gov/dietaryguidelines/2015/. Accessed September 6, 2018.

U.S. Preventive Services Task Force, Bibbins-Domingo K, Grossman DC, Curry SJ, et al. Screening for colorectal cancer, US Preventive Services Task Force Recommendation statement. *JAMA.* 2016;315(23):2564-2575.

U.S. Preventive Services Task Force, Moyer VA. Screening for hearing loss in older adults: U.S. Preventive Services Task Force Recommendation Statement. *Ann Intern Med.* 2012;157:655.

U.S. Preventive Services Task Force. Intimate Partner Violence and Abuse of Elderly and Vulnerable Adults: Screening. 2013. Available at: www.uspreventiveservicestaskforce.org/Page/Document/RecommendationStatementFinal/intimate-partner-violence-and-abuse-of-elderly-and-vulnerable-adults-screening. Accessed September 19, 2018.

U.S. Preventive Services Task Force. Recommendation statement screening for prostate cancer. *Ann Intern Med.* 2012;157:120. Available at: http://www.uspreventiveservicestaskforce.org/prostate-cancerscreening/prostatefinalrs2.htm#copyright. Accessed October 10, 2017.

U.S. Preventive Services Task Force. *Recommendations.* November 2017. Available at: https://www.uspreventiveservicestaskforce.org/.

U.S. Preventive Services Task Force. *Screening for Colorectal Cancer Recommendation Statement.* 2016. Available at: https://www.uspreventiveservices

taskforce.org/Page/Document/Recommendation-StatementFinal/colorectal-cancer-screening2. Accessed September 19, 2018.

Ungar A, Mussi C, Del Rosso A, et al. Diagnosis and characteristics of syncope in older patients referred to geriatric departments. *J Am Geriatr Soc*. 2006; 54:1531.

University of Iowa Health Care, Carver College of Medicine. *Clinical and Diagnostic Reasoning*. Available at: https://medicine.uiowa.edu/internal-medicine/education/master-clinician-program/information-students/clinical-and-diagnostic-reasoning. Accessed October 31, 2017.

Usmani ZA, Chai-Coetzer CL, Antic NA, McEvoy RD. Obstructive sleep apnoea in adults. *Postgrad Med J*. 2013;89:148.

Uy J, Forciea MA. In the clinic. Hearing loss. *Ann Intern Med*. 2013;158:ITC4-1.

Valensi P, Lorgis L, Cottin Y. Prevalence, incidence, predictive factors and prognosis of silent myocardial infarction: a review of the literature. *Arch Cardiovasc Dis*. 2011;104:178.

Valente M, McCaslin DL. Vestibular disorders and evaluation of the pediatric patient. *ASHA Lead*. 2011;16(3)12-15.

Van den Bruel A, Haj-Hassan T, Thompson M, et al. Diagnostic value of clinical features at presentation to identify serious infection in children in developed countries: a systematic review. *Lancet*. 2010; 375:834.

Vennemann MM, Hense HW, Bajanowski T, et al. Bed sharing and the risk of sudden infant death syndrome: can we resolve the debate? *J Pediatr*. 2012;160:44.

Vincent MT, Celstin N, Hussain AN. Pharyngitis. *Am Fam Physician*. 2004;69:1465.

Wackel P, Cannon B. Heart rate and rhythm disorders. *Pediatr Rev*. 2017;38:243.

Wagg A, Gibson W, Ostaszkiewicz J, Johnson T III, et al. Urinary incontinence in frail elderly persons: Report from the 5th International Consultation on Incontinence. *Neurourol Urodyn*. 2015;34:398.

Wagner J, Shojania K. Update: does this adult patient have appendicitis? In: Simel DL, Rennie D, eds. *The Rational Clinical Examination: Evidence-Based Clinical Diagnosis*. New York, NY: McGraw-Hill; 2009.

Wagner RS, Aquino M. Pediatric ocular inflammation. *Immunol Allergy Clin North Am*. 2008;28: 169.

Wald ER, Applegate KE, Bordley C, et al., American Academy of Pediatrics. Clinical practice guideline for the diagnosis and management of acute bacterial sinusitis in children aged 1 to 18 years. *Pediatrics*. 2013;132:e262.

Walia R, Mahajan L, Steffen R. Recent advances in chronic constipation. *Curr Opin Pediatr*. 2009;21: 661.

Walker NA, Challacombe B. Managing epididymoorchitis in general practice. *Practitioner*. 2013; 257:21.

Walker S, Harris Z. Detecting the serious visual disorders of childhood. *Pediatr Child Health*. 2011; 22:25.

Wallace DV, Dykewicz MS, Bernstein DI, et al. The diagnosis and management of rhinitis: an updated practice parameter. *J Allergy Clin Immunol*. 2008;122:S1.

Walsh T, Caraceni A, Fainsinger R, et al. *Palliative Medicine*. Philadelphia: Saunders; 2009.

Wang W, Bourgeois T, Klima J, Berlan ED, Fischer AN, O'Brien SH. Iron deficiency and fatigue in adolescent females with heavy menstrual bleeding. *Hemophilia*. 2013;19:225.

Watford KE. 5-minute diagnosis of dizziness. *J Nurse Pract*. 2013;9(10):712-713.

Watts NB. The Fracture Risk Assessment Tool (FRAX^R): applications in clinical practice. *J Womens Health (Larchmt)*. 2011;20:525.

Watts P. Preseptal and orbital cellulitis in children: a review. *Paediatr Child Health*. 2012;22:1.

Webster LR. Opioid-induced constipation. *Pain Med*. 2015;16(suppl 1):S16-S21.

Wei LA, Fearing MA, Sternberg EJ, Inouye SK. The Confusion Assessment Method: a systematic review of current usage. *J Am Geriatr Soc*. 2008;56:823.

Weidinger S, Novak N. Atopic dermatitis. *Lancet*. 2016;387:1109.

Weinberger M, Abu-Hasan M. Perceptions and pathophysiology of dyspnea and exercise intolerance. *Pediatr Clin North Am*. 2009;56:33.

Weinberger M, Fischer A. Differential diagnosis of chronic cough in children. *Allergy Asthma Proc*. 2014;35:95.

Welt CK, Carmina E. Clinical review: lifecycle of polycystic ovary syndrome (PCOS): from in utero to menopause. *J Clin Endocrinol Metab*. 2013; 98:4629.

Wernli KJ, Henrikson NB, Morrison CC, Nguyen M, Pocobelli G, Blasi PR. Screening for skin cancer in adults. Updated evidence report and systematic review for the US Preventive Services Task Force. *JAMA*. 2016;316:436-447. doi:10.1001/jama.2016.5415.

Wessels MR. Clinical practice: streptococcal pharyngitis. *N Engl J Med*. 2011;364:648.

Wexler RK, Pleister A, Raman S. Outpatient approach to palpitations. *Am Fam Physician*. 2011;84:63.

Whooley MA, Avins AL, Miranda J, Browner WS. Case-finding instruments for depression. Two questions are as good as many. *J Gen Intern Med.* 1997;12:439.

Wiatrak BJ. Congenital anomalies of the larynx and trachea. *Otolaryngol Clin North Am.* 2000;33:91.

Wichinski KA. Providing culturally proficient care for transgender patients. *Nursing.* 2015;45(2):58-63.

Wiener-Vacher SR. Vestibular disorders in children. *Int J Audiol.* 2008;47:578.

Wiers SG, Keilman LJ. Improving care for women with urinary incontinence in primary care. *J Nurs Pract.* 2017;13(10):675.

Wiglesworth A, Austin R, Corona M, et al. Bruising as a marker of physical elder abuse. *J Am Geriatr Soc.* 2009;57:1191.

Wilbur J, Shian B. Diagnosis of deep venous thrombosis and pulmonary embolism. *Am Fam Physician.* 2012;86:913.

Wilkins T, Baird C, Pearson AN, Schade RR. Diverticular bleeding. *Am Fam Physician.* 2009;80:977.

Wilkins T, Embry K, George R. Diagnosis and management of acute diverticulitis. *Am Fam Physician.* 2013;87(9):612-620.

Williams Jr JW, Steffens D. Update: depression. In: Simel DL, Drummond R, eds. *The Rational Clinical Examination: Evidence-Based Clinical Diagnosis.* New York: McGraw Hill; 2009.

Williams T, Mortada R, Porter S. Diagnosis and treatment of polycystic ovary syndrome. *Am Fam Physician.* 2016;94:106.

Wilson GR, Haddad JE, Haddad CJ. Amenorrhea: common causes and evaluation. *Compr Ther.* 2005;31:270.

Wilson JJ, Furukawa M. Evaluation of the patient with hip pain. *Am Fam Physician.* 2014;89:27.

Wilson S, Thompson J. *Respiratory Disorders.* St. Louis: Mosby; 1990.

Wing R, Dor MR, McQuilkin PA. Fever in the pediatric patient. *Emerg Med Clin North Am.* 2013; 31:1073.

Wöber-Bingöl C. Epidemiology of migraine and headache in children and adolescents. *Curr Pain Headache Rep.* 2013;17:341.

Wolkove N, Elkholy O, Baltzan M, Palayew M. Sleep and aging: 1. Sleep disorders commonly found in older people. *CMAJ.* 2007;176:1299.

Wong CL, Holroyd-Leduc J, Simel DL, Straus SE. Does this patient have delirium? Value of bedside instruments. *JAMA.* 2010;304:779.

Wong CL, Holroyd-Leduc J, Straus SE. Does this patient have a pleural effusion? *JAMA.* 2009; 301:309.

Wong MM, Anninger W. The pediatric red eye. *Pediatr Clin North Am.* 2014;61:591.

Woods CR. Rocky Mountain spotted fever in children. *Pediatr Clin North Am.* 2013;60(2):455-470.

Woodworth BA, Gillespie MB, Lambert PR. The canalith repositioning procedure for benign positional vertigo: a meta-analysis. *Laryngoscope.* 2004;114:1143-6.

World Gastroenterology Organisation Global Guidelines. *Acute Diarrhea in Adults and Children: A Global Perspective,* 2012. Available at: http://www.worldgastroenterology.org/assets/export/userfiles/Acute%20Diarrhea_long_FINAL_120604.pdf. Accessed October 30, 2017.

World Gastroenterology Organisation Global Guidelines. *Constipation, a Global Perspective.* Available at: http://www.worldgastroenterology.org/guidelines/global-guidelines/constipation/constipation-english. Accessed October 30, 2017.

World Gastroenterology Organisation Global Guidelines. *Irritable Bowel Syndrome: a Global Perspective, Update September 2015.* Available at: http://www.worldgastroenterology.org/guidelines/global-guidelines/irritable-bowel-syndrome-ibs/irritable-bowel-syndrome-ibs-english. Accessed October 30, 2017.

World Health Organization. *Visual impairment and blindness.* Fact Sheet 282, 2017. Available at: http://www.who.int/mediacentre/factsheets/fs282/en/.

Xue, QL. The frailty syndrome: definition and natural history. *Clin Geriatr Med.* 2011;27:1-15.

Yang S, Werner BC, Singla A, Abel MF. Low back pain in adolescents: a 1 year analysis and eventual diagnosis. *J Pediatr Orthop.* 2017;37:344.

Yang WC, Lee J, Chen CY, Chang YJ, Wu HP. Westley score and clinical factors in predicting the outcome of croup in the pediatric emergency department. *Pediatr Pulmonol.* 2017;52:1329.

Yang YX, Brill J, Krishnan P, Leontiadis G, The Clinical Guidelines Committee. American Gastroenterological Association Institute guideline on the role of upper gastrointestinal biopsy to evaluate dyspepsia in the adult patient in the absence of visible mucosal lesions. *Gastroenterology.* 2015;140:1082-1087.

Yao CK, Tuck CJ. The clinical value of breath hydrogen testing. *J Gastroenterol Hepatol.* 2017;32(suppl 1): 20-22.

Yarbrough ML, Burnham CA. The ABCs of STIs: an update on sexually transmitted infections. *Clin Chem.* 2016;62:811.

Yeh J. Syncope in children and adolescents. *Pediatr Ann.* 2015;44:e287.

Yeh TK, Yeh J. Chest pain in pediatrics. *Pediatr Ann.* 2015;44:e274.

Young J, Inouye SK. Delirium in older people. *BMJ.* 2007;334:842.

Youssef NN, Sanders L, Di Lorenzo C. Adolescent constipation: evaluation and management. *Adolesc Med Clin.* 2004;15:37.

Zeevenhooven J, Koppen IJ, Benninga MA. The New Rome IV criteria for functional gastrointestinal disorders in infants and toddlers. *Pediatr Gastrol Hepatol Nutr.* 2017;20:1.

Zeiter D. Abdominal pain in children. *Pediatr Clin North Am.* 2017;64:525.

Zella GC, Israel EJ. Chronic diarrhea in children. *Pediatr Rev.* 2012;33:207.

Zerbib F, Bruley des Varannes S, Simon M, Galmiche JP. Functional heartburn: definition and management strategies. *Curr Gastroenterol Rep.* 2012;14: 181.

Zoorob R, Sidani M, Murray J. Croup: an overview. *Am Fam Physician.* 2011;83(9):1067-1073.

Zuckerman A, Romano M. Clinical Recommendation: vulvovaginitis. *J Pediatr Adolesc Gynecol.* 2016; 29:673.

Index